The Periodontal Ligament
in Health and Disease

The Periodontal Ligament in Health and Disease

Editors

B. K. B. Berkovitz
Department of Anatomy (Oral Biology),
University of Bristol

B. J. Moxham
Department of Anatomy (Oral Biology),
University of Bristol

H. N. Newman
Department of Periodontology,
Institute of Dental Surgery,
Eastman Dental Hospital, London

PERGAMON PRESS

OXFORD · NEW YORK · TORONTO · SYDNEY · PARIS · FRANKFURT

U.K.	Pergamon Press Ltd., Headington Hill Hall, Oxford OX3 0BW, England
U.S.A.	Pergamon Press Inc., Maxwell House, Fairview Park, Elmsford, New York 10523, U.S.A.
CANADA	Pergamon Press Canada Ltd., Suite 104, 150 Consumers Rd., Willowdale, Ontario M2J 1P9, Canada
AUSTRALIA	Pergamon Press (Aust). Pty. Ltd., P.O. Box 544, Potts Point, N.S.W. 2011, Australia
FRANCE	Pergamon Press SARL, 24 rue des Ecoles, 75240 Paris, Cedex 05, France
FEDERAL REPUBLIC OF GERMANY	Pergamon Press GmbH, 6242 Kronberg-Taunus, Hammerweg 6, Federal Republic of Germany

First edition 1982

Library of Congress Catalog Card No. 81–83022
British Library Cataloguing in Publication Data
The Periodontal ligament in health and
  disease.
  1. Periodontium
  I. Berkovitz, B. K. B.
  II. Moxham, B. J.
  III. Newman, H. N.
  612′,31   RK305
  ISBN 0–08–024412–2 Hard cover
  ISBN 0–08–024411–4 Flexicover

Printed in Great Britain by
A. Wheaton & Co. Ltd., Exeter

To Our Families

PREFACE

This book is built upon the belief that the periodontal ligament is a tissue worthy of study because of its biological interest as a connective tissue adapted to specialized functions and because clinically it is involved in one of the most common causes of tooth loss in man – chronic inflammatory periodontal disease. Our purpose in writing this book was to gather together knowledge of the periodontal ligament which, having been obtained from diverse disciplines, has been scattered in the literature. As work proceeded, however, we became aware that the book's value lies not only in what information it can supply but also in revealing the many things which remain to be discovered. It is our fervent hope that this will encourage researchers to greater efforts.

There are two things which this book is not. First, it is not a text dealing with all the tooth-supporting tissues. Although for some topics it has been necessary to widen the field to include tissues other than the periodontal ligament (particularly in those chapters dealing with the periodontal ligament in disease), we have restricted discussion as many texts already cover the periodontium as a whole. However, the periodontium is a complex field of study with an enormous literature and in our opinion such texts have not given the periodontal ligament the importance it deserves. Second, we have not concerned ourselves with therapy.

It is clear to us that if we are to gain a proper understanding of the periodontal ligament its study must be multi-disciplinary. Furthermore, it is necessary to be aware of how advances in connective tissue biology in general have a bearing upon our study, even if we can only claim a fugitive up-to-dateness.

In choosing authors, we have not only picked colleagues from the various fields of dental sciences and dental surgery who wanted to write specifically about the periodontal ligament but have included some who, because of the lack of information, could only write about the ligament as a connective tissue. We have found both approaches instructive and perhaps even those interested primarily in soft connective tissues can also learn from study of the periodontal ligament. We are particularly glad to have been able to bring together colleagues in the fields of periodontal biology and pathology and would be pleased if this resulted in more integrated research.

It is fashionable nowadays for scientists to decry the scholarship involved in writing books, contending that books lend themselves to desultory speculation. Whilst speculation based upon tendentious argument has been discouraged, we believe that reasoned discursiveness is advantageous, furnishing debate and encouraging the development of hypotheses for future research. It is obvious that in any newly emerging area of research there exist uncertainty and extensive gaps of ignorance. Consequently, it is not surprising that, despite our initial intention to present a consistent story, in places different authors maintain different views about some aspects of the biology or pathology of the periodontal ligament. We trust that where controversy exists, this will not be found burdensome to the reader but will fire his imagination. It is to persons such as this that this book is dedicated.

B. K. B. BERKOVITZ
B. J. MOXHAM
H. N. NEWMAN

ACKNOWLEDGEMENTS

We express our warmest appreciation to the authors who contributed to this book. Although we did not think it desirable to wield our editorial power too heavily, they were magnanimous enough to take note of our suggestions. We also acknowledge the invaluable support of the publishers, Pergamon Press, and especially Mr. J. Lavender and his colleagues. It is with much gratitude that we acknowledge those colleagues and publishers who graciously gave us permission to reproduce their photographs and diagrams:

Chapter 3

Fig. 1b.	B. K. B. Berkovitz and P. Sloan. *Journal of Zoology (Lond.)*.
Fig. 6.	P. Sloan, R. P. Shellis and B. K. B. Berkovitz. *Archives of Oral Biology*.
Fig. 11.	P. Sloan. *Archives of Oral Biology*.
Fig. 17.	A. D. G. Beynon.
Fig. 18.	E. H. Jennings.

Chapter 4

Fig. 5.	E. D. Harris and E. C. Cartwright. Research Monographs in Cell and Tissue Physiology.

Chapter 5

Fig. 3.	D. A. Hulmes and A. Miller. *Nature*.
Fig. 5.	L. G. Gathercole and A. Keller. *Structure of Fibrous Biopolymers*. Butterworths.
Figs. 6 & 7.	P. Sloan.

Chapter 6

Fig. 1.	Modified after M. Fukuda and S. Hakomori. *Journal of Biological Chemistry*.
Fig. 5.	J. M. Plecash.

Chapter 7

Fig. 1.	W. A. Castelli. *Journal of Dental Research*.
Fig. 2.	M. Kindlová. *Archives of Oral Biology*.
Figs. 3 & 4.	B. Orban. *Journal of the American Dental Association*.
Fig. 5.	L. E. A. Folke and R. E. Stallard. *Journal of Periodontal Research*.
Figs. 6–8.	P. Gängler and K. Merte. *Zahn-, Mund- und Kieferheilkunde mit Zentralblatt*.
Figs. 9 & 10.	K. Körber. *Journal of Periodontology*.
Fig. 11.	L. Myhre, H. R. Preuss and H. Aars. *Acta Odontologica Scandinavica*.
Fig. 12.	K. G. Palcanis. *Journal of Dental Research*.
Fig. 13.	L. Edwall and M. Kindlová. *Acta Odontologica Scandinavica*.
Figs. 14 & 15.	M. P. Ruben, J. R. Prieto-Hernandez, F. K. Gott, G. M. Kramer and A. A. Bloom. *Journal of Periodontology*.

Chapter 8

Figs. 1–4.	K. H. Andres and M. Düring. *Handbook of Sensory Physiology*. Springer-Verlag.
Fig. 5.	M. R. Chambers, K. H. Andres, M. Düring and A. Iggo. *Quarterly Journal of Experimental Physiology*.
Fig. 6.	K. H. Andres and M. Düring. *Handbook of Sensory Physiology*. Springer-Verlag.
Fig. 7.	M. R. Byers and G. R. Holland. *Anatomical Record*.
Fig. 8.	R. Martinez and J. M. Pekorthy. *American Journal of Anatomy*.
Fig. 9.	V. Everts, W. Beertsen and A. van den Hooff. *Anatomical Record*.
Fig. 10.	B. K. B. Berkovitz and P. Sloan. *Journal of Zoology (Lond.)*.
Fig. 11.	R. Rapp, W. D. Kirstine and J. K. Avery. *Journal of the Canadian Dental Association*.
Fig. 12.	B. K. B. Berkovitz and R. C. Shore. *Archives of Oral Biology*.
Fig. 14.	A. G. Hannam. *Archives of Oral Biology*.
Fig. 15.	A. G. Hannam and T. J. Farnsworth. *Archives of Oral Biology*.
Fig. 16.	A. G. Hannam. *Archives of Oral Biology*.
Fig. 17.	R. S. Johansson and K. A. Olsson. *Brain Research*.
Fig. 18.	A. G. Hannam. *Archives of Oral Biology*.

Chapter 9

Figs. 1–16.	D. A. Grant and S. Bernick. *Journal of Periodontology*.

Acknowledgements

Figs. 17–19.   D. A. Grant, S. Bernick, B. M. Levy and S. Dreizen. *Journal of Periodontology.*

Chapter 10

Figs. 1 & 2.   A. I. Darling and B. G. H. Levers. *The Eruption and Occlusion of Teeth.* Butterworths.

Fig. 3.   G. G. T. Fletcher. *Transactions of the British Society for the Study of Orthodontics.*

Fig. 4.   S. Siersbaek-Nielson. *Tandlaegebladet.*

Figs. 5–7.   B. J. Moxham. *Archives of Oral Biology.*

Fig. 9.   R. C. Shore and B. K. B. Berkovitz. *Archives of Oral Biology.*

Fig. 10.   H. J. Van Hassel and R. G. McMinn. *Archives of Oral Biology.*

Figs. 11–17.   B. J. Moxham. *Archives of Oral Biology.*

Chapter 11

Figs. 1 & 2.   G. J. Parfitt. *Journal of Dental Research.*

Fig. 3a.   D. C. A. Picton. *Dental Practitioner.*

Fig. 3b.   D. C. A. Picton. *Archives of Oral Biology.*

Fig. 4.   D. J. Wills, D. C. A. Picton and W. I. R. Davies. *Journal of Biomechanics.*

Fig. 5.   S. M. Bien. New York Academy of Sciences.

Fig. 6.   D. C. A. Picton, R. B. Johns, D. J. Wills and W. I. R. Davies. *Oral Sciences Review.*

Fig. 7.   D. C. A. Picton and D. J. Wills. *Journal of Prosthetic Dentistry.*

Figs. 8–11.   B. J. Moxham and B. K. B. Berkovitz. *Archives of Oral Biology.*

Chapter 12

Fig. 1.   H. R. Mühlemann. *Journal of Periodontology.*

Fig. 2.   G. G. Ross, C. S. Lear and R. DeCou. *Journal of Biomechanics.*

Fig. 3.   C. J. Burstone, R. J. Pryputniewicz and W. W. Bowley. *Journal of Periodontal Research.*

Figs. 4 & 5.   K. Reitan. *Current Orthodontic Concepts and Techniques.* Saunders.

Fig. 6.   K. Reitan. *American Journal of Orthodontics.*

Fig. 17.   K. Reitan.

Fig. 18.   P. Rygh and K. Reitan. *Transactions of the European Orthodontic Society.*

Fig. 19.   P. Rygh and K. A. Selvig. *Scandinavian Journal of Dental Research.*

Fig. 20.   P. Rygh. *Angle Orthodontics.*

Chapter 14

Fig. 1.   P. Dowell.

Fig. 2.   R. B. Johns.

Fig. 3.   S. Seltzer. *Oral Surgery, Oral Medicine, Oral Pathology.*

Fig. 4.   J. O. Andreasen. *International Journal of Oral Surgery.*

Fig. 5.   A. H. R. Rowe.

Fig. 6.   S. Seltzer. *Journal of Endodontics.*

Fig. 7.   K. Langeland. *Dental Clinics of North America.*

Chapter 15

Figs. 1–3.   K. A. Selvig. *Journal of Periodontal Research.*

Fig. 4.   H. M. Fullmer.

Fig. 5.   R. C. Page. *Journal of Periodontal Research.*

Fig. 6.   C. Michel and R. M. Frank. *Parodontologie.*

Figs. 7 & 8.   B. M. Eley and J. D. Harrison. *Journal of Periodontal Research.*

Fig. 9.   M. Bouyssou.

Figs. 10–14.   T. H. Morton. *Journal of Endodontics.*

Figs. 15 & 16.   S. O. Krols. *Journal of Oral Medicine.*

Fig. 17.   P. Reichart. *Journal of Periodontology.*

Chapter 17

Fig. 1.   H. D. Glenwright.

Fig. 2.   W. A. S. Alldritt.

Fig. 5.   J. G. Burland.

Chapter 19

Fig. 4.   H. M. Fullmer. *Archives of Pathology.*

Fig. 5.   A. F. Gardner. *Journal of Dental Research.*

Chapter 20

Fig. 1.   S. Shapiro. *Journal of Periodontology.*

Fig. 2.   A. C. G. Pinto. *Journal of Periodontology.*

Fig. 3.   I. Glickman. *Oral Surgery, Oral Medicine, Oral Pathology.*

Fig. 4.   S. Dreizen. *Journal of Periodontology.*

Fig. 5.   A. W. Sallum. *Journal of Periodontology.*

Fig. 6.   G. Sklar. *Journal of Periodontology.*

Fig. 7.   I. Glickman. *Journal of Periodontology.*

Fig. 8.   G. Sklar. *Journal of Periodontology.*

Fig. 9.   T. N. Chawla. *Oral Surgery, Oral Medicine, Oral Pathology.*

Fig. 10.   S. Dreizen. *Journal of Periodontal Research.*

Figs. 11 & 12.   W. M. Oliver. *Journal of Periodontal Research.*

Fig. 13.   B. S. Moskow. *Archives of Oral Biology.*

Fig. 14.   H. Fahmy. *Journal of Dental Research.*

CONTENTS

LIST OF AUTHORS

A. K. ADATIA
Department of Dental Medicine, University of Bristol Dental School, Lower Maudlin Street, Bristol, BS1 2LY, United Kingdom.

B. K. B. BERKOVITZ
Department of Anatomy (Oral Biology), The Medical School, University of Bristol, University Walk, Bristol, BS8 1TD, United Kingdom.

S. BERNICK
Department of Anatomy, University of Southern California, School of Medicine, Los Angeles, California 90033, U.S.A.

A. H. BROOK
Department of Children's Dentistry, University of Hong Kong Dental School, Hong Kong.

R. M. BROWNE
Department of Oral Pathology, The Dental School, University of Birmingham, Birmingham, B46 6NN, United Kingdom.

D. J. CARMICHAEL
Faculty of Dentistry, The University of Alberta, Edmonton, Alberta, T6G 2N8, Canada.

D. M. CHISHOLM
Department of Dental Surgery, The Dental School, University of Dundee, Park Place, Dundee, DD1 4HN, United Kingdom.

L. G. A. EDWALL
Faculty of Dentistry, Karolinska Institute, Box 3207, S103 64 Stockholm, Sweden.

M. M. FERGUSON
Department of Oral Medicine and Pathology, Glasgow Dental Hospital and School, 378 Sauchiehall Street, Glasgow, G2 3J2, United Kingdom.

L. J. GATHERCOLE
H. H. Wills Physics Laboratory, University of Bristol, Tyndall Avenue, Bristol, BS8 1TL, United Kingdom.

D. A. GRANT
Department of Anatomy, University of Southern California, School of Medicine, Los Angeles, California 90033, U.S.A.

A. G. HANNAM
Department of Oral Biology, University of British Columbia, 2199 Westbrook Mall, Vancouver 8, British Columbia, V6T 1W5, Canada.

A. KELLER
H. H. Wills Physics Laboratory, University of Bristol, Tyndall Avenue, Bristol, BS8 1TL, United Kingdom.

K. W. LEE
Department of Oral Pathology, Institute of Dental Surgery, Eastman Dental Hospital, 256 Gray's Inn Road, London, WC1X 8LD, United Kingdom.

B. J. MOXHAM
   Department of Anatomy (Oral Biology), The Medical School, University of Bristol, University Walk, Bristol, BS8 1TD, United Kingdom.

H. N. NEWMAN
   Department of Periodontology, Institute of Dental Surgery, Eastman Dental Hospital, 256 Gray's Inn Road, London, WC1X 8LD, United Kingdom.

C. H. PEARSON
   Department of Oral Biology, Faculty of Dentistry, University of Alberta, Edmonton, Alberta, T6G 2N8, Canada.

P. RYGH
   Department of Orthodontics, School of Dentistry, University of Bergen, Årstadveien 17, N-5000, Bergen, Norway.

R. P. SHELLIS
   MRC Dental Unit, University of Bristol Dental School, Lower Maudlin Street, Bristol, BS1 2LY, United Kingdom.

R. C. SHORE
   Department of Anatomy (Oral Biology), The Medical School, University of Bristol, University Walk, Bristol, BS8 1TD, United Kingdom.

P. SLOAN
   Department of Dental Surgery, University of Newcastle upon Tyne, The Dental School, Framlington Place, Newcastle upon Tyne, NE2 4BW, United Kingdom.

J. D. STRAHAN
   Department of Periodontology, Institute of Dental Surgery, Eastman Dental Hospital, 256 Gray's Inn Road, London WC1X 8LD, United Kingdom.

INTRODUCTORY REMARKS

This book has been written primarily for the graduate dentist and dental research worker. Nevertheless, it also contains information which should be of relevance to those engaged in the study of connective tissues in general. For example, even though the periodontal ligament is often considered to be specialized, such specializations, being essentially modifications of systems already existing in other connective tissues, provide important insights into how connective tissues are adapted to function. Again, knowledge concerning the biomechanical properties of connective tissue *in vivo* is difficult to obtain without the use of invasive techniques. Because of the nature of the attachment of the tooth, tooth-borne loading allows an examination of such properties. We think it appropriate, therefore, to provide some general and elementary information about the periodontal ligament for those without a background in dental science.

The periodontal ligament is the fibrous connective tissue which occupies the periodontal space between the root of a tooth and its bony socket (Fig. 1). At the cervical region of the tooth, above the alveolar crest, the periodontal ligament merges with the gingival connective tissue. At the root apex, it merges with the dental pulp. Together with cementum, alveolar bone and the lamina propria of the gingiva it forms the tissues which support the tooth in the jaw. These tissues often are referred to collectively as the periodontium. This type of attachment is not common to all dentitions, being restricted to mammals and a few groups of reptiles.

Although the term 'periodontal ligament' appears to be used most frequently, many other names have been given (e.g. periodontal membrane, alveolo-dental ligament, desmodont, pericementum, dental periosteum and gomphosis). According to many dictionaries (e.g. the *Concise Oxford Dictionary, Gould's Medical Dictionary, Black's Medical Dictionary,* the *Faber Medical Dictionary*), a ligament is defined as a band of fibrous tissue binding together skeletal elements. To us, this definition does not seem inappropriate for the periodontal ligament.

The average width of the periodontal ligament usually is quoted as 0.2 mm. However, the dimensions of the periodontal space vary around the tooth. Kronfeld (1931) and Coolidge (1937) have reported that the periodontal space is often hour-glass shaped, being narrowest in the mid-root region near the fulcrum about which the tooth moves. The periodontal ligament usually is widest cervically. Its width also varies according to the functional state of the tissue. Coolidge (1937) has published data showing

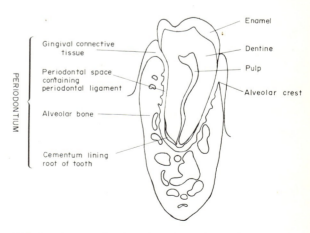

FIG. 1. Diagram showing the relationships of the tissues comprising the periodontium to the tooth.

that teeth in heavy function tend to have wider ligaments than non-functioning teeth. Furthermore, the periodontal space narrows with age.

As other fibrous connective tissues, the periodontal ligament consists of a fibrous stroma (mainly collagen) in a gel of ground substance containing cells, blood vessels and nerves. In many respects the periodontal ligament appears to be a specialized fibrous connective tissue. For example, it appears to be comparatively well vascularized and innervated and it has a relatively high rate of turnover (that of its collagen being about 15 times faster than in skin (Sodek, 1977)). It would be wrong, however, to over-emphasize its specializations to the extent of losing sight of the many features it has in common with other fibrous connective tissues. It can be argued that the periodontal ligament has features more in common with foetal than with adult connective tissues. The presence of intercellular contacts between the fibroblasts (e.g. Ross and Greenlee, 1966; Shore, Berkovitz and Moxham, in press), the high rate of turnover (Sodek, 1977) and the pattern of its collagen fibril diameter distribution (Parry, Barnes and Craig, 1978; Berkovitz *et al.,* in press) are suggestive of it being foetal-like.

Functionally, the periodontal ligament is considered primarily to be the tissue responsible for resisting displacing forces impinging upon the tooth. This is usually referred to as the tooth support mechanism. In this capacity the ligament serves to protect the tissues, especially those in the periapical region, against damage. The periodontal ligament also is responsible for the processes whereby a tooth attains, and then maintains, its functional position. These processes include the mechanism which generates the forces effecting tooth eruption and the mechanism responsible for drifting of teeth. We should also include the tooth support mechanism, particularly that part which allows recovery following tooth displacement. The cells of the periodontal ligament form, maintain and repair not only the ligament itself but also the adjacent alveolar bone and cementum. Sensory nerves and receptors within the periodontal ligament appear to have an important proprioceptive function and they may play a part in

the control of masticatory movements. In addition, sensations of pain from the periodontal ligament may have a protective role.

Study of the periodontal ligament has attracted the biologist more than the pathologist. Indeed, the term 'periodontal disease' is synonymous to most clinicians with chronic inflammatory periodontal disease, because of its association with widespread tooth loss. Curiously, in this condition the ligament ahead of the main lesion remains uninvolved. However, a survey of the literature shows that the periodontal ligament is subject to a large number of less frequent disorders. Even if a number of these spread from the surrounding tissues (particularly the overlying gingiva), others originate within the periodontal ligament itself (e.g. periodontal cysts). Altogether, it is now clear that the periodontal ligament is liable to as wide a range of disease as other tissues.

REFERENCES

BERKOVITZ, B. K. B., WEAVER, M. E., SHORE, R. C. & MOXHAM, B. J. Fibril diameters in the extracellular matrix of the periodontal connective tissues of the rat. *Conn. Tissue Res.* (in press).

COOLIDGE, E. D. (1937) The thickness of the human periodontal membrane. *J. Am. dent. Assoc.* **24,** 1260–1270.

KRONFELD, R. (1931) Histologic study of the influence of function on the human periodontal membrane. *J. Am. dent. Assoc.* 18, 1242–1274.

PARRY, D. A. D., BARNES, G. R. G. & CRAIG, A. S. (1978) A comparison of the size distribution of collagen fibrils in connective tissues as a function of age and a possible relation between fibril size distribution and mechanical properties. *Proc. R. Soc. Lond.* B203, 305–321.

ROSS, R. & GREENLEE, T. K. Jr. (1966) Electron microscopic attachment sites between connective tissue cells. *Science* 153, 997–999.

SHORE, R. C., BERKOVITZ, B. K. B. & MOXHAM, B. J. Intercellular contacts between fibroblasts in the periodontal connective tissues of the rat. *J. Anat.* (in press).

SODEK, J. (1977) A comparison of the rates of synthesis and turnover of collagen and non-collagenous protein in adult rat periodontal tissues and skin using a microassay. *Archs. oral Biol.* 23, 977–982.

Chapter 1

COMPARATIVE ANATOMY OF TOOTH ATTACHMENT

R. P. Shellis

INTRODUCTION

Among the vertebrates there have evolved dentitions adapted to dealing with every kind of diet. Adaptation of tooth form has been accompanied by adaptation of the means by which the teeth are linked to the jaws, the source of power for tooth function. The teeth may be supported rigidly or the attachment tissues may provide a support with some degree of deformability, ranging from a slight resilience to the most elaborate hinge mechanism. The resulting diversity of structure and arrangement of the tissues involved often obscures the relationships between the different kinds of attachment, in particular between the socketed attachment in mammals and some reptiles and the forms of attachment in other vertebrates.

The main objective of this review is to present the information available in the literature on development and structure of the attachment, together with some original observations, mainly on fishes. From this information, it is hoped to present a coherent picture of tooth attachment with emphasis on two main aspects. Firstly, the study of development of the attachment in a number of vertebrates should throw some light on the relationships between the various tissues involved. Secondly, the form of attachment will be related where possible to tooth function. Consideration also will be given to the relationship between attachment and the processes of growth, eruption and tooth succession.

TYPES OF TOOTH ATTACHMENT: NOMENCLATURE

Although there exist many forms of tooth attachment, a feature common to all is that the linkage between tooth and jaw is mediated by collagenous tissues (which may be partly or wholly mineralized). The different forms of attachment can be classified in terms of the extent of mineralization and of the distribution of the mineralized and unmineralized components. Since these factors determine the mechanical and other properties of the attachment, the types listed below represent broadly adaptations to different functional requirements. However, it will become obvious that absolute divisions do not exist.

A. *Ankylosis*. Here completely mineralized union exists between tooth and bone, giving rigid support. It is found in many bony fishes and in nearly all living reptiles. For the latter, it is customary to distinguish between *acrodont* ankylosis (when the teeth rest on the crest of the jaw) and *pleurodont* ankylosis (when the teeth are attached to the lingual wall of a labial flange of the jaw). In some extinct reptiles, labial and lingual flanges of bone formed a groove in the jaw and the teeth were ankylosed to the inner walls of this groove. This is referred to as the *protothecodont* condition. The tissue connecting ankylosed teeth to bone will be referred to as the bone of attachment (Tomes, 1904). This has a spongy structure and differs from the more compact bone of the jaw proper. It is formed in association with each new tooth and is resorbed when the tooth is shed. It may form a thin cementing layer, as in pleurodont or acrodont reptiles, but may also form a substantial mass, especially in some fishes.

B. *Fibrous attachment*. Here the collagen fibres providing attachment are partly unmineralized, so that some degree of tooth movement relative to the jaw is possible. In a *direct fibrous attachment* (elasmobranchs, some teleosts), collagen fibres arising from the base of the tooth run into the bone of the jaw or, in the case of the elasmobranchs, into connective tissue covering the jaw cartilage. In an *indirect* or *pedicellate fibrous attachment* (perhaps most teleosts, all living amphibians), fibres from the tooth base run into a discrete mineralized structure, the *pedicel*, which is in turn ankylosed to the jaw bone.

C. *Socketed (thecodont) attachment*. The term thecodonty is a collective term for all forms of attachment in which the teeth have roots which are implanted into sockets or grooves in the jaw bone and which are attached to the surrounding bone by means of a fibrous periodontal ligament. Among living vertebrates it is found only in mammals and a single group of reptiles, the crocodilians, but a number of extinct reptilian groups had some form of thecodont attachment. The mammalian attachment has a number of distinctive features, such as subdivision of the roots in molars, constricted root apices and the formation *de novo* of sockets for replacement teeth. This is termed *gomphosis* to distinguish it from other forms of thecodonty.

TEETH IN EARLY FISHES. DERMAL DENTICLES

True teeth were absent in the earliest vertebrates, the agnathans, but these animals had homologous structures, the dermal denticles, at the surface of their bony armour (Ørvig, 1967). These denticles were generally attached by ankylosis (Fig. 1A), as were those of the later acanthodians and crossopterygians (Bystrow, 1939; Gross, 1957). However, in the thelodonts the bony armour was lost and the denticles were attached by fibres (Fig. 1B), like those of elasmobranchs. The rostral teeth of sawfishes (*Pristis*) are presumably derivatives of dermal denticles and deserve special mention. These teeth are continuously growing structures and are not replaced (Slaughter and Springer, 1968). Unusually for elasmobranchs, they are seated in sockets in the cartilage of the rostrum; they are anchored in the connective tissue filling the socket by fibres embedded in an outer layer of mineralized tissue (Engel, 1909; Schmidt and Keil, 1971; Berkovitz and Shellis, unpublished) but it is not known how this attachment adjusts itself in relation to growth and eruption of the tooth.

In the acanthodian placoderms, some teeth were attached to jaw bones by ankylosis (Fig. 1C) but other teeth resembled those of sharks and were probably attached to cartilaginous parts of the jaws by fibres (Fig. 1D). In addition, some teeth formed rows which, unlike the tooth families in elasmobranchs, were attached to a common basal plate (Fig. 1E; Gross, 1957). The tissue forming the undersurface of the plate contained cell spaces (Fig. 1D,E) and the presence of Sharpey fibres in the plate indicates that it was anchored on the jaw by a fibrous attachment. These whorls were shed and replaced *in toto* (Gross, 1957; Peyer, 1968).

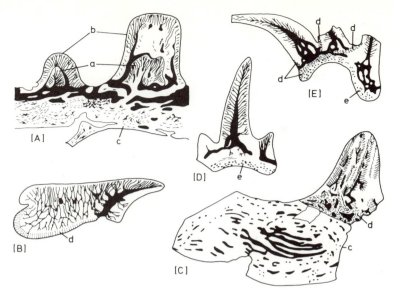

FIG. 1. Diagrams of the structure of dermal denticles and teeth in early fishes. A, Vertical section through dermal armour of *Cephalaspis* (agnathan). B, Vertical section of thelodont scale. C–E, *Gomphodus* (acanthodian placoderm). C, Section of jaw bone fragment with ankylosed tooth. D, Isolated tooth which would in life have had a fibrous attachment. E, Section of tooth whorl (two teeth broken). (a) First generation denticles; (b) second generation denticles; (c) bone; (d) Sharpey fibres; (e) cell spaces. After Ørvig (1961) and Gross (1957).

ELASMOBRANCHS

All sharks and rays share the same type of attachment. At the base of the tooth is a specialized structure, the basal plate (Hertwig, 1874), which is composed of mineralized collagenous tissue and is anchored to the jaw by unmineralized fibres (Fig. 2). In the teeth of larger sharks and some rays (e.g. *Myliobatis*), the plate is filled with spongy, hard tissue permeated by vascular canals (Jacobshagen, 1923), which is osteodentine *sensu* Ørvig (1967). In dogfishes and most rays, however, the plate has an undivided pulp and the nature of the hard tissue surrounding it is disputed. Hertwig (1874) likened it to cementum, while Jacobshagen (1923) and Peyer (1968) regarded it as dentine. Moss (1970), Grady (1970a) and Reif (1978) regarded the plate as a two-layered structure, the outer layer being composed of acellular bone or cementum (formed by connective tissue cells) while the inner layer was composed of dentine. The controversy arises because the tissue forming the plate in

small teeth tends to have an ill-defined structure, with tubules and cell spaces being rare or absent.

In the thornback ray (*Raia clavata*), basal plate formation begins with the deposition of tracts of coarse fibres which run out of the base of the papilla and lie immediately next to the rim of the dental epithelium (Fig. 3). These fibres are laid down by connective tissue cells but, as dentine formation in the body of the tooth advances, odontoblasts differentiate near the base of the papilla and form dentine which incorporates the fibres in this region. Subsequently, the fibre tracts are consolidated by deposition of collagenous matrix. During this process, the fibrous tissue, which represents the rudimentary lateral wall of the plate, is covered on the outer aspect by connective tissue cells and on the inner by odontoblasts (Fig. 4). The plate is completed by formation of the horizontal 'floor', again in conjunction with distinct outer and inner cell layers (Figs. 4 and 5). Autoradiographs prepared from animals injected with tritiated proline confirm that the odontoblast layer secretes protein into the matrix

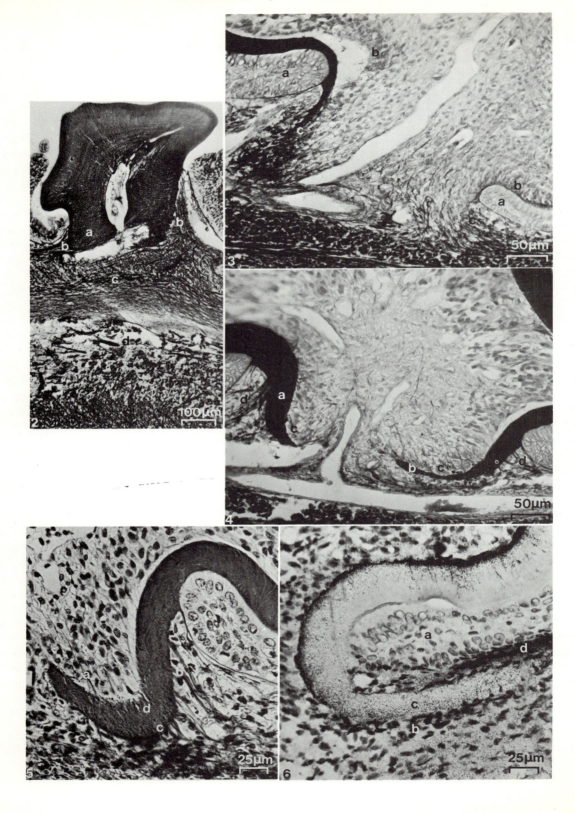

of the plate (Fig. 6). The coarse fibres which make up the first rudiment of the plate ultimately connect the plate with the jaw. They are incorporated into the plate as mineralized Sharpey fibres and their presence gives the atubular, acellular, outer layer a coarse texture (Fig. 5). Dentinal tubules are visible, although in small numbers, in the inner layer of the plate (Fig. 5) and their presence is confirmed by their becoming labelled in the autoradiographs (Fig. 6).

In the larger teeth of the blue shark (*Prionace glauca*), the formation of the basal plate follows essentially the same pattern. In addition, however, spongy osteodentine is formed within the pulp, on a network of coarse fibres laid down by pre-odontoblasts which seem to migrate inwards from the walls of the plate (Fig. 7). In a basal plate of this type, dentinal tubules are clearly visible in the osteodentine but are absent from the outer layer of the plate (Fig. 8); this was also observed by Jacobshagen (1923).

The conclusion to be drawn from these results is that the basal plate is not a structure of a single developmental origin. Some regions, formed early in development, are probably a joint product of odontoblasts and connective tissue cells. Later-formed tissue would be formed by only one cell type; the inner dentine layer by odontoblasts and the outer, atubular layer by connective tissue cells. This substantiates the view of Moss (1970), Grady (1970a) and Reif (1978), although it is debatable whether the outer layer should be referred to as bone. Although in the two species discussed the outer layer is smoothly continuous with the dentine, this may not always be so. Figure 9 shows the basal plate of an unidentified shark (probably *Galeorhinus*) in which the outer layer forms a perforated shell around the dentine

component of the plate. In developing teeth this outer layer seems to form independently, in advance of the basal dentine.

The basal plate is linked to a dense fibrous band which underlies the whole tooth field (Fig. 2). The band forms in parallel with development of the teeth, moves forward with the teeth as they erupt and may have a role in tooth eruption (Poole and Shellis, 1976; Reif, McGill and Motta, 1978). Between the fibrous band and the perichondrium is an intermediate layer of less dense fibre texture. In the region of the functional teeth this layer is much thickened (Fig. 2) and is rich in elastic fibres. It may therefore provide a resilient pad cushioning the teeth during function.

The fibrous attachment confers mobility on elasmobranch teeth but the degree of mobility is extremely variable. It is governed by the spacing of the teeth, by the lengths of the attachment fibres, by the mobility of the fibrous band and by the morphology of the basal plate. The rectangular, closely packed teeth of eagle rays (e.g. *Myliobatis*) are the least mobile. The most mobile teeth are found in sharks. This may be related to the fact that large tensile stresses are exerted on the teeth during function by the struggles of the prey and by the sawing action of the dentition. In predatory elasmobranchs, the fibrous attachment performs a further function. The grasping or cutting teeth must be erect during function but can be depressed when the mouth is shut (Fig. 10). As the mouth opens the teeth are brought forward by tension in the fibrous band. Although the teeth are displaced for only a short distance, they become erect by being brought over the crest of the jaw, which has a small radius of curvature.

The basal plate in sharks is commonly fusiform or elongated in the mesiodistal direction, parallel with the blade of the tooth. In dogfishes and other forms,

---

PLATE 1 (*opposite*)

FIG. 2. Section of functional tooth of thornback ray *Raia clavata in situ*. (a) Basal plate; (b) attachment fibres; (c) fibrous band; (d) zone of loose connective tissue between fibrous band and perichondrium. Gomori's reticulin method.

FIG. 3. Developing attachment in *Raia*. (a) Dental epithelium; (b) odontoblasts; (c) fibrous rudiment of basal plate. Heidenhain's azan.

FIG. 4. *Raia*; more advanced attachment formation. (a) Wall of basal plate; (b) rudiment of plate floor; (c) odontoblasts; (d) attachment fibres. Heidenhain's azan.

FIG. 5. *Raia*; basal plate of mature but unerupted tooth. (a) Odontoblasts; (b) connective tissue cells among attachment fibres; (c) outer, coarse-fibred layer of plate; (d) dentinal tubules in inner layer of plate. Masson's trichrome.

FIG. 6. Developing wall of basal plate in *Raia*. Autoradiograph, 4 hours after injection of ^{3}H-proline, (a) dental epithelium; (b) odontoblasts; (c) labelled wall of plate, with highest grain density near odontoblasts; (d) artefactual fold. Harris's haematoxylin.

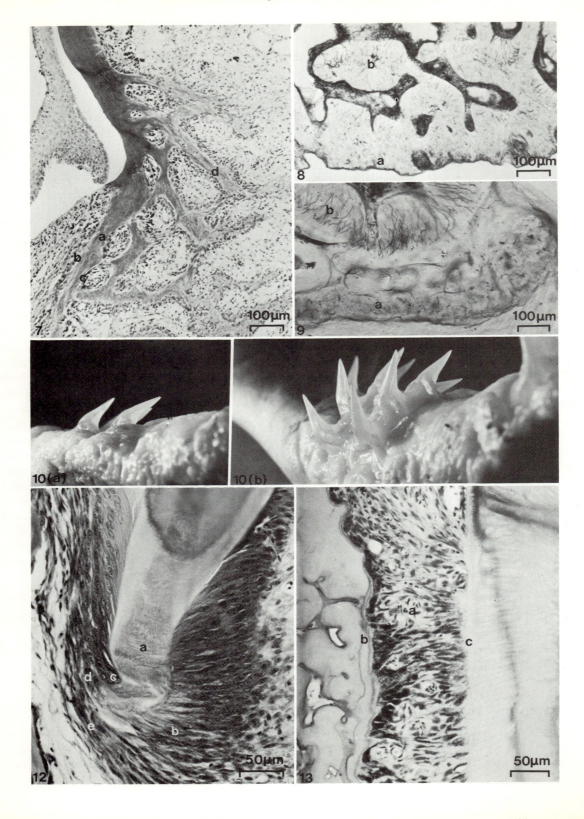

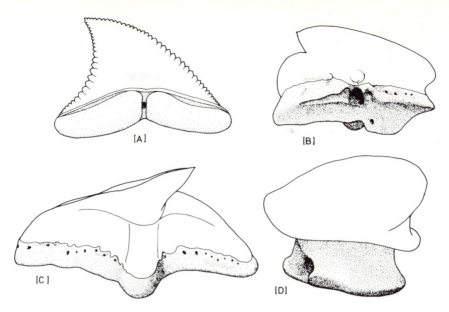

FIG. 11. Morphology of basal plate in elasmobranchs. A, Blue shark. B, Spiny dogfish, *Squalus acanthias.* C, Monkfish (cf. Fig. 10). D, Thornback ray. From SEM specimens. Basal plate regions shaded. A, B and C side views; D viewed from above.

the plate bears lateral processes which presumably stabilize the tooth. In rays, stability is achieved by the plate having a round, flattened shape (Fig. 11).

ACTINOPTERYGIANS

In the living palaeoniscoid fish *Polypterus,* the teeth are attached by ankylosis (Moy-Thomas, 1934; Kerr, 1960). In both living holosteans, *Amia* and *Lepisos-*

teus, the teeth are also ankylosed (Moy-Thomas, 1934; Peyer, 1968). The attachment in the extinct members of these groups has not been studied.

Among teleosts there are three basic forms of attachment: ankylosis, direct fibrous attachment and pedicellate fibrous attachment. A great variety of hinged attachments have evolved in this group. Although hinged attachments will be dealt with separately, they are always a form of fibrous attachment. Soule (1969) described a periodontal ligament in the trigger fish *Balistes.* However, Soule's figures

---

PLATE 2 (*opposite*)

FIG. 7. Developing basal plate in blue shark, *Prionace glauca.* (a) Rudiment of plate wall; (b) connective tissue cells forming outer layer of plate wall and attachment fibres; (c) odontoblasts; (d) osteodentine trabeculae forming inside plate. Van Gieson.

FIG. 8. Ground section of basal plate of tiger shark, *Galeocerdo cuvieri.* (a) Outer, atubular layer; (b) central osteodentine with tubules.

FIG. 9. Ground section of basal plate of unidentified shark (?*Galeorhinus*). (a) Spongy atubular outer layer of plate; (b) inner layer of orthodentine.

FIG. 10. Erection of mandibular teeth during mouth opening in unfixed, recently killed specimen of the monkfish, *Squatina squatina,* which is carnivorous. (a) Mandible elevated; (b) mandible depressed.

(FIG. 11. See above.)

FIG. 12. Formation of basal part of erupting tooth in the ballan wrasse, *Labrus bergylta.* (a) Dentine; (b) odontoblasts; (c) basal limit of Hertwig's sheath; (d) connective tissue cells; (e) follicle. Haematoxylin and eosin.

FIG. 13. *Labrus.* Follicle (a) immediately before bone formation. Note horizontal or oblique orientation of cells and fibres (cf. Fig. 12) and attachment of fibres to bone (b) and tooth surface (c). Autoradiograph, 1 hour after injection of ³H-proline. Cells of follicle are heavily labelled and some labelled matrix has been secreted, notably at the bone surface. Harris's haematoxylin.

show that the teeth are actually attached to the bone by a direct fibrous attachment at the base and that the fibrous 'ligament' is located only between the teeth. Nevertheless, this finding deserves further investigation.

Ankylosis

This rigid form of attachment is commonly found in dentitions adapted to crushing, where lateral displacement of the teeth under compressive loads would reduce efficiency. Examples are found among the parrot fishes (Pflugfelder, 1930) and the wrasses. However, ankylosis is not restricted to durophagous dentitions. The marginal teeth of many predatory fishes (e.g. the mackerel (Tomes, 1904) and the barracuda (Beust, 1938)) are ankylosed. In the pike and hake, ankylosed teeth co-exist with hinged teeth (Levi, 1939b, 1940).

The basal portion of an ankylosed tooth is embedded to some extent within the jaw bone. The base develops within a cavity formed by exfoliation of the previous tooth. The space between tooth and bone is then filled in by new bone of attachment. This process is illustrated by material from the ballan wrasse (*Labrus bergylta*).

In this species, the teeth form in crypts beneath the bone supporting the functional teeth. The developing tooth is enclosed by a follicle of connective tissue, the fibres of which are continuous with those of the dental papilla. As the body of the tooth nears completion, the tooth begins to erupt through a channel formed by osteoclastic removal of the overlying tooth and bone (Poole and Shellis, 1976, Fig. 17). Simultaneously, Hertwig's epithelial root sheath ceases to grow but coarse-fibred dentine continues to form beyond it. On the outer surface of this tissue additional matrix is laid down by cells of connective tissue origin (Fig. 12). This matrix appears to incorporate fibres of the follicle, which meanwhile has become more prominent. As the tooth emerges into the mouth spongy bone begins to form. At first this bone is laid down within the region around the tooth base occupied by the follicle, then up the sides of the tooth and finally beneath the tooth. It is interesting that just before bone forms lateral to the tooth there is a change in orientation of the follicular fibres. Previously more or less parallel with the tooth surface, they are now aligned obliquely and are inserted into the bone and the outer layer of the teeth (Fig. 13). This appearance is reminiscent of a thecodont attachment.

At the base of the tooth, the fibres of the dentine mingle with the matrix of the bone. The latter tissue is formed by small osteoblasts continuous with the odontoblast layer (Fig. 14).

PLATE 3 (*opposite*)

FIG. 14. *Labrus.* Bone formation around newly erupted tooth. Autoradiograph, 2 hours after injection of ^{3}H-proline. Bone deposition is almost completed at the sides of the tooth, except in the more superficial regions (a). Here, and in the region beneath the pulp (b), there is active osteogenesis, shown by the heavy labelling of the bone surfaces. Harris's haematoxylin.

FIG. 15. Formation of the rudiments of the fibrous attachment (a) and pedicel (b) in the eel, *Anguilla anguilla.* The forming tissues are covered at this stage by Hertwig's sheath (c). (d) Bone. Haematoxylin and eosin.

FIG. 16. *Anguilla.* Later stage of formation of the attachment. The pedicel (a) is now mineralized, so that the fibrous attachment (b) is distinct. Hertwig's sheath has retracted to (c) and its place on the pedicel surface is taken by connective tissue cells, (d). Note the odontoblast layer, (e), on the inner surface of the attachment tissues. Haematoxylin and eosin.

FIG. 17. *Anguilla.* Same stage of development as in Fig. 15. Autoradiograph, 2 hours after injection with ^{3}H-proline. In mixed incident and transmitted light, so that the silver grains appear white. Osteogenesis, shown by deposition of labelled matrix, is beginning around the point of contact of the pedicel (a) with the bone (b). Harris's haematoxylin.

FIG. 18. *Anguilla.* Same stage of development as in Fig. 16. Autoradiograph under same illumination as in Fig. 17. Note labelling on both inner and outer surfaces of the pedicel (a) and the active osteogenesis over the whole surface of the bone (b) underlying the tooth. Harris's haematoxylin.

FIG. 19. Scanning electron micrograph of part of jaw bone of the sea bream, *Sparus auratus*, from which the organic material has been removed by treatment with sodium hypochlorite. The teeth have been lost by dissolution of the fibrous attachment. This reveals the pedicels (a), which are partly submerged in the jaw. Each is surrounded by a ring of bone of attachment (b), which is clearest around the newest pedicel (c).

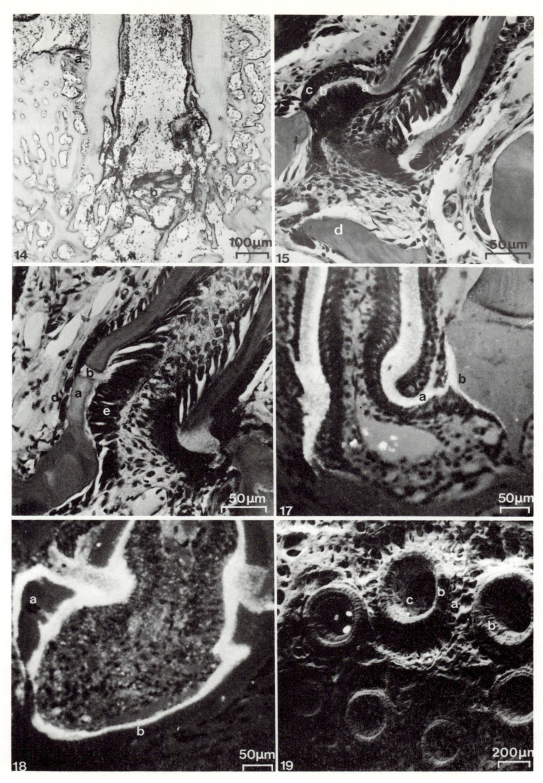

Direct fibrous attachment

This was described in the piranha (*Serrasalmus rhombeus*) by Shellis and Berkovitz (1976) and may also be the mode of attachment in the wolf fish (*Anarrhichas*; Lühmann, 1954). Fibres arising from the base of the tooth traverse a narrow gap to form a fibrous attachment and enter the spongy bone of attachment at the jaw crest. The fibres embedded in the jaw appear to be formed jointly by odontoblasts and by connective tissue cells. This form of attachment differs from ankylosis only by the presence of an unmineralized zone between tooth and jaw. In piranhas this zone is so narrow and the attachment fibres so short, that the teeth are not perceptibly mobile (Shellis and Berkovitz, 1976).

Indirect (pedicellate) fibrous attachment

Probably the most common form of attachment in teleosts is by way of a pedicel, a calcified structure, usually in the form of a squat cylinder ankylosed to the jaw at the basal end. Usually, the pedicel rests within a shallow depression in the bone surface but can also be embedded partially or wholly within the bone.

It has long been accepted that both the fibrous attachment and the pedicel form as extensions of the tooth (Bhatti, 1938; Levi, 1939 a, b, 1940; Lühmann, 1955; Kerr, 1960). They are laid down in continuity with the tooth before fixation to the jaw occurs, in association with a layer of odontoblasts continuous with those of the tooth pulp. Collagen fibres extend from the dentine through the fibrous attachment into the pedicel. Usually, however, the pedicel is atubular but may contain a few cell spaces. It does not therefore resemble dentine. An exception is the vasodentine pedicel of *Lutianus* (Ribeiro and Monteiro, 1971).

Probably most pedicellate teeth form in the corium superficial to the jaw bone, as in the eel (see below), but in some species (e.g. the sea breams) they form in crypts below the bone supporting the functional teeth.

Formation of the pedicellate attachment will be illustrated in the common eel (*Anguilla anguilla*).

Following completion of the tooth tip, the rest of the tooth is formed by a rapid downgrowth of Hertwig's sheath accompanied by differentiation of odontoblasts and formation of dentine. Hertwig's sheath continues to extend until it is close to the bone, odontoblasts differentiate on its inner aspect and the first thin rudiment of the attachment tissues appears between the two layers of cells (Fig. 15). Soon thereafter the sheath retracts so that it extends only to the site of the fibrous attachment. Simultaneously, cells derived from the connective tissue become applied to the outer surface of the pedicel. Subsequent growth of the pedicel involves secretion by both odontoblasts and the connective tissue cells (Figs. 16—18).

During growth of the tooth, there is no sign in autoradiographs of osteogenesis on the surface of the underlying bone. However, as the base of the forming pedicel contacts the jaw bone labelled matrix appears at the bone surface, at first near the point of contact (Fig. 17) and later over a wider area (Fig. 18). Most of this matrix deposition takes place on the bone forming the base of the pulp (Fig. 18). Osteogenesis becomes less active after the teeth have been in function for some time.

In other species, where the teeth erupt from a crypt, the pedicel is ankylosed laterally instead of basally (Fig. 19). In such teeth, a follicle is present and bone is formed within it. Beust (1938) observed in *Sargus* the same re-orientation of the follicular fibres prior to ankylosis as was described above in the wrasse.

Hinged teeth

In a hinged attachment the freedom of the tooth to move during function is restricted more or less completely to the labiolingual plane. In addition, there is usually a mechanism preventing or restricting movement in the labial direction. The most well-known hinged teeth are found in carnivorous fishes, such as the pike, the hake and the angler fish. In such fishes the teeth are easily depressed in a lingual direction, so that entry of prey into the mouth is facilitated, but become fixed in the erect position when pushed labially, so that escape of the prey is prevented. Hinged teeth are, however, also found in some herbivorous fishes.

Modifications of the pedicellate form of attachment providing a hinge effect are known in several species and might prove to be more widespread if a systematic study were made. In the haddock and gurnard the base of the tooth rests partially inside the rim of the pedicel to form a ball-and-socket joint (Mummery, 1924; Levi, 1939a). In the herbivorous cichlid *Tilapia* (Fig. 20A,B), both the morphology of the tooth and pedicel and the disposition of the fibres of attachment are modified so as to form a fulcrum on one aspect about which the tooth swings (Körber and Weismann, 1973). The teeth on the upper and lower pharyngeal plates of *Tilapia* are curved and also hinged in opposite directions; this facilitates trituration of vegetable matter in the pharynx (Fig. 20C). The most specialized hinged pedicellate attachment known is found in the herbivorous fish *Girella,* where a labiolingual flange on the pedicel articulates in a groove in the tooth base (Fig. 20D; Norris and Prescott, 1959). Movement in the labial direction is limited by a fibrous band on the lingual aspect of the joint. The hinged attachment in this species allows close adaptation of the hoe-shaped teeth to rough surfaces and thus promotes an efficient grazing action.

The well-known hinged teeth in the hake and the pike have what seems to be a modified direct fibrous attachment. In the pike (Fig. 20E), the teeth are attached by fibres to the bone only at the lingual aspect of the basal margin to form a hinge (Tomes, 1904). However, they are also attached centrally by unmineralized longitudinal trabeculae running down through the pulp chamber. When the teeth are depressed these trabeculae are strained. Their elastic recoil restores the tooth to the erect position when the applied force is removed. In the hake (Fig. 20F), the tooth rotates about an anterior fibrous attachment arising from the inner surface of the labial wall of the tooth. The restoring force is generated by the storage of strain energy in a thick, dense, fibrous layer on the lingual aspect of the joint, which seems to be a partly mineralized layer of dentine (Mummery, 1924; Levi, 1939b). Depression of the tooth causes buckling of this tissue and as the

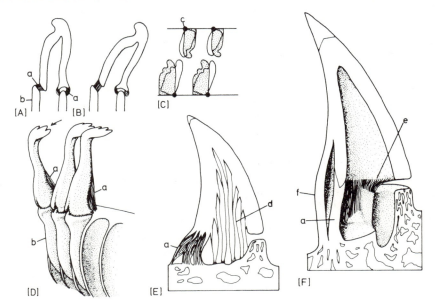

FIG. 20. Diagrams of various forms of hinged attachment in teleosts. A, B, *Tilapia* pharyngeal tooth. C, Tooth form and function on the pharyngeal plates of *Tilapia.* D, Jaw teeth of *Girella,* from the labial aspect. E, Pike, *Esox lucius.* F. Hake, *Merluccius.* After Körber and Weismann (1973), Norris and Prescott (1959), Tomes (1904), Mummery (1924). (a) Fibrous attachment; (b) pedicel; (c) fulcrum; (d) unmineralized trabeculae; (e) anterior fibrous hinge; (f) outer, partly mineralized layer of dentine.

load on the tooth is removed the layer straightens out and erects the tooth. In both the pike and the hake, movement in the labial direction is prevented by the base of the tooth abutting against a raised labial shelf of bone.

CROSSOPTERYGIANS

Only four forms (the coelacanth *Latimeria* and three species of lungfish) survive today but the Devonian representatives of this group are important because of their close relation to the tetrapod stock. In the early rhipidistians, the teeth were characteristically formed of elaborately folded plicidentine and were ankylosed into shallow pits in the bone (Bystrow, 1939). Dentine and bone seemed to merge imperceptibly into each other at the base but bone of attachment tissue also extended some way up the tooth and formed a distinct surface layer.

In the living coelacanth (a distant relative of the early rhipidistians), the conical teeth are ankylosed in small groups to plates of spongy bone. These plates are in turn linked with the jaw bones proper by a fibrous layer (Isokawa *et al.,* 1968; Castanet *et al.,* 1975). As in rhipidistians, the bases of the teeth rest in shallow pits and are attached laterally by bone of attachment which also extends as a diminishing layer for some way up the tooth (Miller and Hobdell, 1968; Hobdell and Miller, 1969; Grady, 1970b; Smith, 1978; Shellis and Poole, 1978). Polarized light reveals the penetration of longitudinal fibres from the dentine into the bone of attachment, and the latter tissue appears to grow outwards from the dentine (Shellis and Poole, 1978). These facts indicate a mode of development similar to that seen in the piranha.

The dentition of early dipnoans consisted of separate denticles or tooth ridges ankylosed to the jaw bones (Smith, 1977). In later dipnoans, including those alive today, the jaws bear ridged tooth plates which have a complex, trabecular arrangement of dentinal tissues (Smith, 1977, 1979; Kemp, 1979). Each plate is attached at its margin to an underlying mass of trabecular bone. Growth of the tooth plate, and compensation for wear, involve resorption of

bone of attachment at the base of the pulp chamber and its replacement by dentine (Smith, 1979).

AMPHIBIANS

The earliest amphibians, the labyrinthodonts, evolved from Devonian crossopterygians. As implied by their name, these animals had folded plicidentine teeth which were ankylosed into the jaw bone, the gap between tooth and bone being filled with trabecular bone of attachment (Bystrow, 1938). Genuine plicidentine was not present in a later group, the lepospondylids, although small ribs of bone were formed at the tooth base (Peyer, 1968).

The very small teeth of extant amphibians are not composed of plicidentine and are attached not by ankylosis but by way of a pedicel. This seems to be universal among all three orders; Parsons and Williams (1962) found that an externally visible division into 'crown' and pedicel was lacking in only one species, *Siren lacertina,* out of a very large number examined.

In general, the length of the pedicel is equal to or greater than that of the tooth proper (Oltmanns, 1952), the reverse of the pattern in teleosts where the pedicel is relatively short. This may be related to the fact that the pedicel in amphibians is usually ankylosed in a pleurodont fashion to the lingual wall of the jaw bone. The pedicel is composed of atubular, acellular hard tissue. The pulp chamber is usually undivided but in some species (e.g. *Proteus, Ceratophrys*) may be invaded by trabeculae arising from the pedicel wall (Oltmanns, 1952). Teeth with such a structure tend to be attached in a more acrodont fashion near the crest of the jaw bone. The junction between the base of the tooth and pedicel is often poorly defined in histological sections. It is probably always hypomineralized. Oltmanns (1952) believed that the junctional region was unmineralized in newly erupted teeth but later mineralized. On the other hand, in the frog (Gillette, 1955), a number of urodeles (Kerr, 1960) and gymnophionans (Parsons and Williams, 1962; Lawson, 1965) there has been observed a distinct ring of fibrous tissue which may act as a rudimentary hinge.

There is no doubt that the pedicel develops as an

extension of the tooth. Not only does it form in association with odontoblasts, like the teleost pedicel, but it is covered during development by Hertwig's sheath (Oltmanns, 1952; Gillette, 1955; Kerr, 1960; Parsons and Williams, 1962; Howes, 1977, 1978 a,b). Autoradiographic evidence suggests, in fact, that the epithelium contributes to the matrix of the pedicel (Smith and Miles, 1969; Chibon, 1972). The pedicel forms rapidly during eruption and the movement of the tooth brings the base of the pedicel close to the bone of the jaw (Gillette, 1955; Kerr, 1960). Development is completed by deposition of bone of attachment between the pedicel and jaw bone and also between the pedicel and those of adjacent teeth.

REPTILES

Ankylosis is the predominant mode of attachment among the reptiles. The relationship of the teeth to the jaws can be acrodont, pleurodont or protothecodont. The bone of attachment, which is often referred to as cementum (Cooper, 1963; Edmund, 1969), contains cells and coarse fibres. It forms as the tooth comes into function and is resorbed during tooth replacement (Edmund, 1969). It forms a thin layer between the tooth and the bone, fills the spaces between the teeth in pleurodont forms and is also laid down on the surface of acrodont teeth. The bone of attachment can form a substantial mass in protothecodont forms.

Even in the oldest fossil reptiles (the cotylosaurs) there was diversification of the attachment. In the captorhinomorphs, attachment was acrodont but in *Diadectes* and its relatives the teeth were protothecodont and the alveoli were well developed (Edmund, 1969). In later reptiles, there has been even greater variety of form of the attachment. The following account is drawn mainly from the reviews of Edmund (1960, 1969) and Peyer (1968).

Pleurodont ankylosis is the predominant mode of attachment among the extant lizards and snakes and their ancestors. In most lizards, ankylosis involves a considerable length of the labial wall of the tooth, the free 'coronal' region being relatively short (Fig. 21A). Even among lizards the degree of pleurodonty can be reduced and in some species (e.g. the horned

lizard *Phrynosoma*) attachment can be almost acrodont. In the armoured teyou (*Dracaena*), which has rounded crushing teeth, there is a low lingual wall which with the labial wall forms a groove in the jaw. This is roofed over by a substantial thickness of bone of attachment supporting the teeth (Jacobshagen, 1955). Thus, in this species the attachment approaches the protothecodont condition (Fig. 21B). In snakes, the teeth are attached in a near-acrodont fashion in shallow craters in the bone (Fig. 21C); the bone of attachment is well developed (Tomes, 1904).

Among living reptiles, acrodont ankylosis occurs in the tuatara *Sphenodon* and in the agamid and chamalaeonid lizards (Fig. 21D). It was also the mode of attachment in some extinct reptiles such as the cotylosaur *Captorhinus* and the synapsid *Edaphosaurus*, animals in which the teeth were arranged in multiple rows. In all these forms, tooth replacement is reduced. It is confined to juvenile stages in the chamaeleonids (Edmund, 1969) and to a small anterior group of pleurodont teeth in agamids (Cooper, Poole and Lawson, 1970). In the agamid *Uromastix,* and also in *Sphenodon* and the extinct *Captorhinus*, tooth replacement does not occur at all (Edmund, 1969; Cooper, Poole and Lawson, 1970). In *Uromastix,* the non-replaced teeth eventually wear away and their place is taken by cutting edges of bone (Cooper and Poole, 1973).

Protothecodont teeth, attached by ankylosis to the walls of alveoli or grooves, were present in a number of groups which appeared early in reptile evolution and subsequently became extinct: some cotylosaurs such as *Diadectes,* the protorosaurians, and the pelycosaurs. The latter two groups were succeeded by forms with thecodont attachment.

Thecodonty evolved in several major groups of reptiles. Some of the mosasaurs (an extinct group of lizards) had teeth with barrel-shaped roots seated in separate alveoli (Fig. 21E). Very similar teeth, although lying in a common dental groove (Schmidt and Keil, 1971), were present in the primitive birds *Archaeopteryx* and *Hesperornis*. In plesiosaurs and the earlier (Triassic) ichthyosaurs, the teeth were seated in separate alveoli. In the later Jurassic and Cretaceous ichthyosaurs, however, the interdental alveolar walls were lost and the teeth were held in a common dental groove. This was accompanied by infolding of the tooth bases and increased cementum

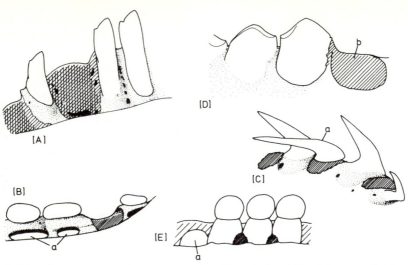

FIG. 21. Diagrams of tooth attachment in reptiles. A, Green lizard, *Lacerta*: pleurodont. B, *Dracaena* and C, *Python*: modified pleurodont. D, *Agama* sp. (acrodont).
Posterior end of tooth row; the tooth that will occupy the space (b) will not be
replaced. E, Extinct mosasaur, *Globidens,* with thecodont attachment. Bone of
attachment stippled, resorption cavities for new teeth hatched. (a) Successional teeth.
After Jacobshagen (1955), Edmund (1960, 1969) and from SEM specimens.

deposition. Most archosaurs (including the dinosaurs
and the pterosaurs) had separate alveoli, as do the
surviving representatives of this group, the crocodilians. In the ceratopsids and hadrosaurs, however,
a dental groove was present instead. This was related
to the possession of a 'dental battery' — cutting
plates composed of a number of generations of teeth
cemented together by bone or cementum. Implantation of teeth in a common dental groove, rather
than in sockets (as found in some fossil forms),
may be a retention of a neotenous character. In
crocodilians, interdental walls are added progressively
during life and a groove may persist posteriorly for
a considerable period (Miller, 1968). Implantation
in a groove presumably increased tooth mobility and
may have given the attachment more resilience
(Schmidt and Keil, 1971).

The only example of thecodonty in living reptiles
is found in the crocodilians; its structure has by now
been studied in some detail by Kvam (1960), Miller
(1968), Soule (1967) and Berkovitz and Sloan
(1979). It differs macroscopically from the mammalian
gomphosis in several respects. Firstly, the sockets
are persistent. Thus, the replacement tooth grows
within the base of the socket and as it enlarges and
erupts the root of its predecessor is progressively

resorbed. Secondly, the root is almost cylindrical,
with a wide apical opening. Microscopically, attachment tissues are essentially similar to those of
mammals but with some notable differences. Both
acellular and cellular cementum are formed but the
greatest thickness of cementum is at the level of the
alveolar crest. The fibres of the periodontal ligament
are arranged in bundles which run horizontally at the
alveolar crest but obliquely at the sides of the tooth.
At the ultrastructural level, collagen fibrils of normal
diameter (55 nm) and oxytalan fibres are present but
larger collagen fibrils with diameters up to 250 nm
have been observed (Berkovitz and Sloan, 1979).
The presence of these large fibrils (together with the
cytology of the fibroblasts) has prompted the suggestion that collagen turnover in the crocodilian ligament
may be slower than in the mammalian ligament. The
fibres are embedded less deeply in the alveolar bone
than in mammals.

It appears that in crocodilians the alveolar portion
of the ligament of a tooth that is being replaced may
be retained and become incorporated into that of
the successional tooth. This contrasts with mammals,
where the ligament of a deciduous tooth is resorbed
completely (Berkovitz and Sloan, 1979).

Berkovitz and Sloan (1979) observed in the

ligament of *Caiman* a number of ovoid bodies made up of lamellae of flattened cells surrounding a central cell resembling an axon. If they are pressure receptors, their presence indicates that the crocodilian ligament has an important sensory as well as a supportive function.

MAMMALS

The conical teeth of the earlier mammal-like reptiles (the pelycosaurs) had a protothecodont attachment (Edmund, 1969). In the later mammal-like reptiles (the therapsids) attachment was thecodont (Edmund, 1969, Noble, 1969). At first the roots were single and barrel-shaped, with open apices, but in therapsids the features of the mammalian gomphosis emerged. Tapered roots with constricted apices became the rule and multiple roots in cheek teeth appeared. These changes occurred in parallel with the extensive modifications to the skull, jaws, teeth and associated soft tissues which contributed to the evolution of mastication, a uniquely mammalian activity. The modification of tooth support was an integral part of this evolutionary process. Several features of gomphosis contribute to its being the most appropriate form of tooth support in the masticatory dentitions of mammals, in which the teeth are morphologically differentiated and in which there exist precise occlusal relationships.

One such feature, probably the most important, is that gomphosis permits movement of the teeth relative to the bone without any accompanying weakening of the support provided. Growth of the dentition in non-mammalian vertebrates is achieved by the continuous replacement of teeth, each successive generation being a little larger than the last. Any change in tooth morphology during life, and any repositioning of teeth necessitated by jaw growth, are achieved by the same mechanism. However, continuous tooth replacement would markedly reduce the efficiency of a masticatory dentition, not only because of the periodic loss of tooth surface but, because to become fully effective, most mammalian teeth have to be 'worn in'. The edges of cutting teeth are sharpened by wear while the cusps of molars are removed by attrition so that the tooth surface acquires a pattern of enamel ridges which increases the efficiency of the grinding surface. Mammalian tooth replacement is therefore limited. The resulting prolongation of the functional life of the tooth introduces the problem of maintaining occlusal relationships as the jaw grows and as tooth substance is lost by attrition. This was solved by the ability of the periodontal ligament and alveolar bone to remodel without the tooth support being weakened. The process of eruption maintains the occlusal surfaces of teeth in contact despite wear at the surface, while the teeth are also able to drift laterally to compensate for wear at the approximal surfaces.

This property has been most important in the dentitions of herbivores, where attrition is potentially a severe problem. The hypsodont molars of ungulates allow for compensation for occlusal wear by continuing eruption over a long period despite being teeth of limited growth. The mechanism is developed to the extreme when the teeth continue to grow indefinitely, most notably in the dentitions of rodents and lagomorphs.

The multiplicity of roots in molar teeth of mammals improves support. Since molars are subjected to complex stress patterns during mastication, improved support is obtained by increasing the surface area of attachment and by re-orientating and distributing the stresses on the tooth. True masticatory movements require much closer neuromuscular control than the simpler hinge movements involved in the seizing or crushing of food by non-mammalian vertebrates and the sensory functions of the mammalian periodontal ligament play a large part in this control.

The long functional life of a mammalian tooth creates a problem at the potentially weak point where the tooth protrudes through the body surface. In non-mammalian vertebrates, the mucosa surrounding the teeth shows no structural differentiation from that in the rest of the mouth. Bacteria and toxins are hindered from entering the body at this junction between tooth and epithelium mainly by the mucus secreted by the oral epithelium. When the teeth are replaced fairly frequently, this may be of little long-term significance. In the crocodiles, however, which replace their teeth relatively infrequently (Edmund, 1962), there is evidence that the circumdental epithelium becomes progressively infiltrated with white cells as the tooth ages and that bleeding may occur through the damaged epithelium around a tooth near the end of its functional life (Miller, 1968). In the mammals, specializations of the gingivae and of the epithelial attachment have evolved and provide a more efficient barrier to micro-organisms and their products.

Periodontal ligament

Whilst the full extent of variation in the mammals is unknown, the structure of the periodontal ligament has been studied intensively in certain mammals, notably the rodents (e.g. Hunt, 1959; Bernick, 1960; Zwarych and Quigley, 1965) and primates (e.g. Arnim and Hagerman, 1953; Hall, Grupe and Claycomb, 1967; Smukler and Dreyer, 1969; Avery and Simpson, 1973; Levy, Dreizen and Bernick, 1972; Grant, Chase and Bernick, 1973; Sloan, 1979), largely because of the interest in them as potential models in experimental periodontal research. In these animals, and also in insectivores and related mammals (Shellis, unpubl.), the fibres are orientated horizontally near the alveolar crest and obliquely down the sides of the roots of the teeth, as in man. It seems, however, that there are marked differences in fibre organization between teeth of continuous and limited growth (Sloan, 1978, 1979; Chapter 3).

Cementum

The two-layered arrangement of cementum well described in man is by no means typical of all mammals. A primary layer of acellular cementum is a constant feature of the roots but great variation exists in the thickness and distribution of cellular cementum. In non-human primates, for example, there are differences between the Old World monkeys and apes on the one hand, and the New World monkeys, marmosets and prosimians on the other. In the first group, the distribution of cementum is similar to that in man, although even here there are wide variations in the abundance of cementocytes. In the latter group, the cementum is thin and acellular over most of the root surfaces and cellular cementum is found only around the apices, where it may form bulbous masses or may form an extension of the root (Lavelle, Shellis and Poole, 1977).

Although comparative information on cementum is fragmentary, enough is available to suggest that both of these patterns of radicular cementum distribution are widespread among mammals.

Concentrations of cellular cementum around the apices are found on the molars of a number of relatively small mammals, including insectivores (Fig. 22) and tree shrews (Shellis, unpubl.), carnivores (Kronfeld, 1938) and some rodents such as the rat, where the roots of these teeth tend to be slender and pointed. In contrast, cellular cementum is very thick on the stout roots of the large molars of ungulates and the teeth of odontocete whales (Kronfeld, 1938; Schmidt and Keil, 1971). In pigs, the distribution of cementum is similar to that in man (Kronfeld, 1938).

Kronfeld (1938) pointed out that in general the roots of herbivore teeth have more cementum than those of carnivores. However, the amount seems to vary with tooth size rather than with the diet of the animal. Thus, the functionally distinct molars of carnivores, small primates and insectivores share the same pattern of cementum distribution. Moreover, in the cat the cementum is thicker on the stout root of the canine than on the molar roots (Schmidt and Keil, 1971). Factors which possibly control this relationship directly are the time available during root formation for cementum deposition, and also the functional life of the tooth, as cementum continues to form after eruption. It seems likely that such a tooth size/cementum thickness relationship would have functional significance but without more comparative information, on both adult and growing animals, and without a clearer concept of the role of cementum in tooth support, hypotheses on this matter cannot be evaluated.

Cementum is as variable in continuously growing teeth as it is in teeth of limited growth. On the incisors of rodents, lagomorphs, hyraxes and the aye-aye, only a thin layer of acellular cementum is present (Schmidt and Keil, 1971; Lavelle et al., 1977). The much larger canines or incisors (tusks) of the hippopotamus, elephant and narwhal have a substantial covering of cellular cementum (Schmidt and Keil, 1971). The continuously growing molars of lagomorphs and some rodents are invested with a thin layer of acellular cementum like the incisors. In the molars of the guinea pig, however, the cementum is present as small islands scattered over the tooth surface and forming attachment points for the attachment fibres (Schmidt and Keil, 1971; Listgarten and Shapiro, 1974). The cementum covering the teeth of sloths is thicker and contains cementocytes (Schmidt and Keil, 1971). In these animals enamel is lacking on the molars so that cementum is laid down on dentine as on teeth of limited growth, but in the continuously growing molars of lagomorphs and rodents cementum is deposited on enamel.

Alveolar bone

The sockets of mammalian teeth are lined by a layer of coarsely fibrous bundle bone into which periodontal ligament fibres are inserted. In the smaller insectivores (e.g. shrews) the mandible may consist only of bundle bone lining the sockets and an outer plate of cortical bone, with no intervening layer (Shellis, unpubl.). Usually, however, the two are separated by a mass of 'supporting bone' which varies considerably in structure among the mammals. In small forms, this bone tends to be compact throughout, whereas in larger forms it is usually trabecular in

the central regions and compact towards the cortical plate and the bundle bone of the sockets. The vascular canals usually have a reticular arrangement but in insectivores and primates they are longitudinally orientated. In artiodactyls, a plexiform structure is prevalent (Enlow and Brown, 1958). The extent of secondary remodelling varies considerably and is partly, though not entirely, correlated with body size (Enlow and Brown, 1958). Thus, in insectivores and rodents the primary structure may persist throughout life (Fig. 22) or be only partially reconstructed, while in large mammals most of the bone undergoes secondary remodelling.

In many mammals, including man, the posterior molars develop within an alveolar bulb which lies within the mandibular ramus or at the back of the maxilla. In many large herbivores, particularly elephants and sirenians, the bulb forms a very prominent structure (Mummery, 1924; Wegner, 1951). The posterior molars form at a stage before the jaws have grown large enough to accommodate them and the alveolar bulb appears to provide support for the teeth during their development. Later, the teeth within the bulb emerge into occlusion and the bulb itself becomes incorporated into the alveolar process

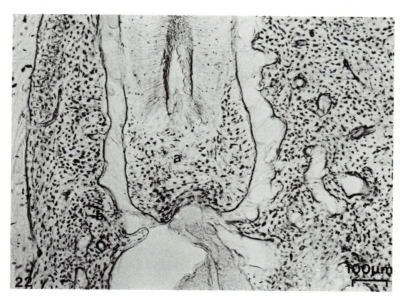

FIG. 22. Ground section of mandible of a shrew, *Crocidura occidentalis*. Note the concentration of cellular cementum around the apex (a). The bone has a primary structure throughout, with no Haversian osteones. Sharpey fibres can be seen in the bundle bone lining the socket at (b).

proper. The bulb may be most important, and is most highly developed, in elephants and sirenians. Here there is complete horizontal replacement of the dentition (Mummery, 1924; Wegner, 1951). Wegner (1951) suggested that in these animals the anterior wall of the bulb prevents premature forward movement of the teeth.

DISCUSSION

Although the dermal denticles of the earliest known vertebrates were attached to bone by ankylosis, this was not necessarily the primitive form of attachment of true teeth. The teeth of placoderms were ankylosed where bone was present but, where the jaws were cartilaginous, the mineralized tissue which would otherwise connect tooth and bone served to link unmineralized attachment fibres to the tooth. This fibrous attachment was retained in the elasmobranchs and has become adapted to various functional demands. On the other hand, the early actinopterygians, the crossopterygians and, through the latter, the early tetrapods all inherited ankylosis. This mode of attachment is widespread among bony fishes of all kinds but the rigid support it provides was probably especially important for the evolution of crushing dentitions among the holosteans and teleosts. However, fibrous attachments have secondarily and independently evolved among both teleosts and amphibians. Such attachments provide a resilience which, without preventing the teeth of carnivores from gripping prey, reduces the likelihood of the teeth being broken. The various modifications resulting in hinged attachments among teleosts led to increased efficiency of carnivorous dentitions on the one hand, and on the other must have contributed significantly to the emergence of dentitions adapted to scraping and triturating vegetable matter.

Among reptiles, the attachment also became modified; either by changes in the positioning of the teeth relative to the bone or, as in teleosts and amphibians, by the development of a fibrous attachment. In the reptiles, the fibrous attachment was a thecodont type which in one line evolved into the gomphosis of mammals. An important factor in the evolution of the attachment in tetrapods may have

been the problem of increasing mechanical strength while allowing for continuous replacement of teeth. It is likely that crossopterygian teeth developed superficially in the corium between the functional teeth, as in *Latimeria* and many teleosts. This leads to each functional tooth being shed at a relatively early stage of formation of its successor to create space for the latter to complete its development. The result would be that the dentition would always have several unfilled tooth positions and that these gaps would be filled relatively slowly; both features are seen in the trout (Berkovitz and Moore, 1974).

The problem has been solved in some teleosts, like the wrasse and the piranha, by intra-osseous development of the successional teeth. In the piranha the tooth positions are empty for only a few days during tooth replacement (Berkovitz and Shellis, 1978). In pleurodont reptilian and amphibian teeth, the surface area of attachment is increased by fixation to a labial wall of bone. The successional tooth begins to develop near the base of the functional tooth and can grow to a large size before the latter has to be shed (Smith, 1958; Cooper, 1963). The added lingual support in protothecodonty and thecodonty results in a further delay in tooth shedding. Thecodonty may have evolved because a fibrous attachment can be resorbed more easily than a mineralized one. However, if the claim (Berkovitz and Sloan, 1979) that a successional crocodilian tooth can in part adopt the ligament of its predecessor proves correct, remodelling rather than wholesale resorption would suffice.

Attachment of the teeth in sockets is not a feature unique to mammals and reptiles. Many, if not most, ankylosed teeth among bony fishes are embedded deeply into the bone and sockets exist even among elasmobranchs (in the rostral teeth of the sawfishes). The transient organization of the follicular fibres in the wrasse and *Sargus* and the more persistent fibre arrangement in *Balistes* and *Pristis* suggest that the potential to form a periodontal ligament is present even in fishes. In *Balistes* and *Pristis*, however, the fibres do not connect the tooth to bone. In the wrasse and *Sargus*, the fibres merely form a basis for bone deposition. Quite probably the same was true in the protothecodont attachment. The characteristic feature of thecodonty is that hard tissue is formed only on the outer surface of the ligament as bone, and on the inner as cementum. This implies the evolution among the reptiles of a mechanism for localizing formation of hard tissue to these surfaces and inhibiting it elsewhere.

Despite the great variation that exists in tooth attachment among the vertebrates, the development of the tooth and the complex of tissues that mediates attachment is always closely co-ordinated. This is obviously essential for the orderly eruption and prompt fixation of the tooth and it may be that comparative studies can shed some light on how it is achieved.

In mammals, the tooth and its attachment tissues (comprising cementum, periodontal ligament and at least part of the alveolar bone) appear to form a developmental unit. This was expressed by Mummery (1924) and Baume (1956) on morphological and histological grounds. Wegner (1951) remarked that the alveolar bulb in elephants and sirenians seemed superfluous for protection of the tooth it enclosed as this function was already served by the sphenoid or the mandibular ramus. This is supported by the fact that the bulb begins to form only after mineralization of the crown, i.e. after the stage when the tooth is most vulnerable. It thus seems best to regard formation of the bulb as part of the programme of development of a tooth/attachment complex.

The morphological evidence is supported by experimental embryology. In work with rodents, it has been established that bone and periodontal ligament are formed as well as teeth when tooth primordia (Lumsden, 1979) or more advanced tooth germs, either with or without their follicles (Hoffman, 1960; Ten Cate, 1976), are transplanted to sites where bone does not normally form (see Chapter 9).

Mesenchymal cells from outside the tooth germ are involved at some stage in the formation of the attachment in all vertebrates. The experimental work noted above does not distinguish between two possibilities for the origin of these cells in mammals. They could arise from undifferentiated mesenchymal cells in the connective tissue under the influence of some stimulus from the tooth germ. Alternatively, they could originate from the dental papilla itself by migration. For present purposes, it is not important to know the answer to this problem; both alternatives seem equally likely. There are no *a priori* grounds for supposing either that the mesenchymal cells should

have any special derivation, such as from the neural crest, or that they should have the same origin in all vertebrates. The point is that these cells form a developmental unit with the tooth germ. It is the timing of the onset of the activity of the mesenchymal cells, and the pattern of their subsequent activity, which determine the form of the attachment and co-ordinate its formation with the processes of tooth development and eruption.

Histological evidence suggests that both the dental epithelium and the dental papilla are involved in morphogenesis of the attachment tissues. The role of the epithelium seems to be regulatory rather than initiative, in that attachment tissues form only where it is absent. In mammals and crocodilians, cementogenesis is dependent on disintegration of Hertwig's sheath. In other vertebrates, structures such as bone of attachment and the basal plate form only beyond the limits of the dental epithelium. Hard tissue forms ectopically on the roots of transplanted tooth germs where Hertwig's sheath is accidentally damaged (Hoffman, 1960; Howes, 1977). These observations suggest two hypotheses, which are not mutually exclusive. Firstly, the dentine may always be a potential substrate for deposition of hard tissue and a prime role of the dental epithelium may be to regulate the distribution of such tissues in the formation of the attachment by acting as a physical barrier at the dentine surface (Howes, 1978a). Secondly, the epithelium might regulate the activity of the papilla in inducing mesenchymal cells to form hard tissue. It seems to be a prerequisite for the initiation of hard tissue production by the mesenchymal cells that they should come into contact with partly or fully differentiated odontoblasts. In most vertebrates this can occur only beyond the limit of the dental epithelium. In mammals, the contact may be with the terminal ends of odontoblast processes. These have been shown by recent work to extend to the outer surface of the forming roots in the dog (Owens, 1975, 1978). The presence of an intact Hertwig's sheath might suppress any inductive activity by the odontoblasts. Alternatively, the odontoblasts might be inductively potent at all stages and the sheath might simply prevent access to inducible mesenchymal cells. Indeed, the sheath itself shows activity which might represent a response to such a continuously present stimulation by the odontoblasts. In the teleosts and amphibians the sheath cells secrete protein into the outer layer of dentine (Smith and Miles, 1969, 1971; Chibon, 1972; Shellis and Miles, 1974) and it has been suggested that in mammals the cells of the sheath contribute to a thin layer of matrix at the root surface (Slavkin and Boyde, 1974; Owens, 1978).

Some structures related to attachment, notably the teleost pedicel and the elasmobranch basal plate, form outside the limits of the dental epithelium. This epithelium thus cannot play any part in their morphogenesis. Odontoblasts differentiate within the rudiments of these structures and it seems reasonable to suggest that the shape of the structure might represent the contour of a mass of cells which migrate out of the papilla, stimulate the differentiation of adjacent mesenchyme and also form hard tissue. It is difficult, however, to suggest factors which would set limits to this migration or control the shape which, in the case of the basal plate, can be very elaborate.

The hypothesis that the tooth germ together with an adjacent population of mesenchymal cells are a developmental unit responsible for forming in concert both the tooth and its attachment leads to the view that the diversity of attachments among the vertebrates represents a range of modulations of this unit. In the foregoing discussion, an attempt has been made to identify, from comparative studies, some of the factors which might contribute to the great developmental plasticity of the unit. Although much is known of the comparative anatomy of tooth attachment, a great deal of the information available is rather superficial. It is to be hoped that more detailed comparative studies of structure and development will be carried out. Such studies, with the aim of elucidating patterns of cell behaviour and interaction during development of the attachment, would make a valuable contribution to knowledge of the biology of the mammalian and human periodontium as well as to increased understanding of the evolution of tooth attachment.

ACKNOWLEDGEMENTS

I am indebted to Mr. J. E. Linder and Mr. A. Churchland, of the London Hospital Medical College, for much assistance in preparation of histological material. I thank Mr. M. S. Gillett for assistance with scanning electron microscopy and for photographing the specimen in Fig. 10, Mrs. M. Coomber for preparing the plates and Mrs. D. Jelfs for typing the manuscript. Dr. J. S. Cooper kindly donated several specimens of reptilian jaws for study. I am grateful to Dr. D. F. G. Poole for many interesting discussions.

REFERENCES

ARNIM, S. S. & HAGERMAN, D. A. (1953) The connective tissues of the marginal gingiva. *J. Amer. dent. Assoc.* **47**, 271–281.

AVERY, B. E. & SIMPSON, D. M. (1973) The baboon as a model system for the study of periodontal disease: clinical and light microscopic observations. *J. Periodontol.* **44**, 675–686.

BAUME, L. J. (1956) Tooth and investing bone: a developmental entity. *Oral Surg.* **9**, 736–741.

BERKOVITZ, B. K. B. & MOORE, M. H. (1974) A longitudinal study of replacement patterns of teeth in the lower jaw and tongue in the rainbow trout *Salmo gairdneri*. *Archs. oral Biol.* **19**, 1111–1119.

BERKOVITZ, B. K. B. & SHELLIS, R. P. (1978) A longitudinal study of tooth succession in piranhas (Pisces: Characidae), with an analysis of the tooth replacement cycle. *J. Zool. Lond.* **184**. 545–561.

BERKOVITZ, B. K. B. & SLOAN, P. (1979) Attachment tissues of the teeth in *Caiman sclerops* (Crocodilia). *J. Zool. Lond.* **187**, 179–194.

BERNICK, S. (1960) The organization of the periodontal membrane fibres of the developing molars of rats. *Archs. oral Biol.* **2**, 57–63.

BEUST, T. B. (1938) Genesis of the periodontium. *J. Amer. dent. Assoc.* **25**, 114–118.

BHATTI, H. K. (1938) The integument and dermal skeleton of Siluroidea. *Trans. Zool. Soc. Lond.* **24**, 1–79.

BYSTROW, A. P. (1938) Zahnstruktur der Labyrinthodonten. *Acta zool.* **19**, 387–425.

BYSTROW, A. P. (1939) Zahnstruktur der Crossopterygier. *Acta zool.* **20**, 283–338.

CASTANET, J., MEUNIER, F., BERGOT, C. & FRANÇOIS, Y. (1975) Données préliminaires sur les structures du squelette de *Latimeria chalumnae* I. Dents, écailles, rayons et nageoires. In: *Problèmes actuels de paléontologie — évolution des vertébrés*, pp. 161–167. (Colloques int. C.N.R.S. No 218.) Paris, Centre National de la Recherche Scientifique.

CHIBON, P. (1972) Etude ultrastructurale et autoradiographique des dents chez les amphibiens. Rélations entre la morphogénèse dentaire et l'activité thyroïdienne. *Bull. Soc. Zool. Fr.* **97**, 437–448.

COOPER, J. S. (1963) *The dental anatomy of the genus* Lacerta. Ph.D. Thesis, University of Bristol.

COOPER, J. S. & POOLE, D. F. G. (1973) The dentition and dental tissues of the agamid lizard *Uromastyx*. *J. Zool. Lond.* **169**, 85–100.

COOPER, J. S., POOLE, D. F. G. & LAWSON, R. (1970)

The dentition of agamid lizards with special reference to tooth replacement. *J. Zool. Lond.* **162**, 85–98.

EDMUND, A. G. (1960) Tooth replacement phenomena in lower vertebrates. *Contr. Life Sci. Div. R. Ont. Mus.* **52**, 1–190.

EDMUND, A. G. (1962) Sequence and rate of tooth replacement in the Crocodilia. *Contr. Life Sci. Div. R. Ont. Mus.* **56**, 1–42.

EDMUND, A. G. (1969) Dentition. In: *Biology of the reptilia*, vol. 1, *Morphology A*, C. GANS, A. d'A. BELLAIRS & T. S. PARSONS (eds.), pp. 117–200. London, Academic Press.

ENGEL, H. (1909) Die Zähne am Rostrum der Pristiden. *Zool. Jahrb.* **29** (Abt. Anat. Ontog.), 51–100.

ENLOW, D. H. & BROWN, S. O. (1958) A comparative histological study of fossil and recent bone tissues, Part III. *Tex. J. Sci.* **10**, 187–230.

GILLETTE, R. (1955) The dynamics of continuous succession of teeth in the frog (*Rana pipiens*). *Amer. J. Anat.* **96**, 1–36.

GRADY, J. E. (1970a) Tooth development in sharks. *Archs. oral Biol.* **15**, 613–619.

GRADY, J. E. (1970b) Tooth development in *Latimeria chalumnae*. *J. Morph.* **132**, 377–388.

GRANT, D. A., CHASE, J. & BERNICK, S. (1973) Biology of the periodontium in primates of the *Galago* species. *J. Periodontol.* **44**, 540–550.

GROSS, W. (1957) Mundzähne und Hautzähne der Acanthodier und Arthrodiren. *Palaeontographica* **109A**, 1–40.

HALL, W. B., GRUPE, H. E. & CLÁYCOMB, C. K. (1967) The periodontium and periodontal pathology in the howler monkey. *Archs. oral Biol.* **12**, 359–365.

HERTWIG, O. (1874) Ueber Bau und Entwickelung der Placoidschuppen und der Zähne der Selachier. *Jena. Z. Naturw.* **8**, 331–405.

HOBDELL, M. H. & MILLER, W. A. (1969) Radiographic study of the teeth and tooth supporting tissues of *Latimeria chalumnae*. *Archs. oral Biol.* **14**, 855–858.

HOFFMAN, R. L. (1960) Formation of periodontal tissues around subcutaneously transplanted hamster molars. *J. dent. Res.* **39**, 781–798.

HOWES, R. I. (1977) Root formation in ectopically transplanted teeth of the frog, *Rana pipiens* I. Tooth morphogenesis. *Acta anat.* **97**, 151–165.

HOWES, R. I. (1978a) Root formation in ectopically transplanted teeth of the frog, *Rana pipiens* II. Comparative aspects of the root tissues. *Acta anat.* **100**, 461–470.

HOWES, R. I. (1978b) Regeneration of ankylosed teeth in the adult frog premaxilla. *Acta anat.* **101**, 179–186.

HUNT, A. M. (1959) A description of the molar teeth and investing tissues of normal guinea pigs. *J. dent. Res.* **38**, 216–243.

ISOKAWA, S., TODA, Y. & KUBOTA, K. (1968) A histological observation of a coelacanth (*Latimeria chalumnae*). *J. Nihon Univ. Sch. Dent.* **10**, 102–114.

JACOBSHAGEN, E. (1923) Placoidorgane und Selachierzähne. Kritik der morphologischen Herleitung von Zement und Knochen nach O. Hertwig. *Anat. Anz.* **57** (Ergänz. Heft), 174–179.

JACOBSHAGEN, E. (1955) Wie kam es zum Wurzelbau und der Befestigung der Menschen- und der Säugetierzähne? *Anat. Anz.* **102**, 249–270.

KEMP, A. (1979) The histology of tooth formation in the

Australian lungfish *Neoceratodus forsteri* Kneff. *Zool. J. Linn. Soc. Lond.* **66**, 251–288.

KERR, T. (1960) Development and structure of some actinopterygian and urodele teeth. *Proc. zool. Soc. Lond.* **133**, 401–422.

KÖRBER, E. & WEISMANN, K. (1973) Die Zahnhalteapparat bei Buntbarschen (*Tilapia*). *Dtsch. zahnärztl. Z.* **28**, 329–332.

KRONFELD, R. (1938) The biology of cementum. *J. Amer. dent. Assoc.* **25**, 1451–1461.

KVAM, T. (1960) The teeth of *Alligator mississipiensis* Daud. VI. Periodontium. *Acta odont. Scand.* **18**, 67–82.

LAVELLE, C. L. B., SHELLIS, R. P. & POOLE, D. F. G. (1977) *Evolutionary changes to the primate skull and dentition.* Springfield, Illinois, Charles C. Thomas.

LAWSON, R. (1965) The teeth of *Hypogeophis rostrata* (Amphibia, Apoda) and tooth structure in the Amphibia. *Proc. zool. Soc. Lond.* **145**, 321–325.

LEVI, G. (1939a) Etudes sur le développement des dents chez les téléostéens I. Les dents de substitution chez les genres *Ophidium, Trigla, Rhombus, Belone. Arch. Anat. micr.* **35**, 101–146.

LEVI, G. (1939b) Etudes sur le développement des dents chez les téléostéens II. Développement des dents pourvues de dentine trabéculaire (*Esox, Sphyraena*). *Arch. Anat. micr.* **35**, 201–221.

LEVI, G. (1940) Etudes sur le développement des dents chez les téléostéens III. Développement des dents de substitution de *Merluccius, Chrysophrys. Cepola, Lophius. Arch. Anat. micr.* **35**, 415–455.

LEVY, B. M., DREIZEN, S. & BERNICK, S. (1972) *The marmoset periodontium in health and disease.* Basel, S. Karger.

LISTGARTEN, M. A. & SHAPIRO, B. L. (1974) Fine structure and composition of coronal cementum in guinea pig molars. *Archs. oral Biol.* **19**, 679–696.

LÜHMANN, M. (1954) Die histogenetischen Grundlagen des periodischen Zahnwechsels der Katfische und Wasserkatzen (Fam. Anarrhichidae, Teleostei). *Z. Zellforsch. mikr. Anat.* **40**, 470–509.

LÜHMANN, M. (1955) Die histogenetische Grundlagen des Zahnwechsels der nordeuropäischen *Pleuronectes*-Arten (Heterosomata, Teleostei). *Z. Zellforsch. mikr. Anat.* **42**, 443–480.

LUMSDEN, A. G. S. (1979) Pattern formation in the molar dentition of the mouse. *J. Biol. bucc.* **7**, 77–103.

MILLER, W. A. (1968) Periodontal attachment apparatus in the young *Caiman sclerops*. *Archs. oral Biol.* **13**, 735–743.

MILLER, W. A. & HOBDELL, M. H. (1968) Preliminary report on the histology of the dental and paradental tissues of *Latimeria chalumnae* (Smith) with a note on tooth replacement. *Archs. oral Biol.* **13**, 1289–1291.

MOSS, M. L. (1970) Enamel and bone in shark teeth: with a note on fibrous enamel. *Acta anat.* **77**, 161–187.

MOY-THOMAS, J. A. (1934) On the teeth of the larval *Belone vulgaris* and the attachment of teeth in fishes. *Q. J. micr. Sci.* **76** NS, 481–498.

MUMMERY, J. H. (1924) *The microscopic and general anatomy of the teeth, human and comparative.* Oxford University Press.

NOBLE, H. W. (1969) The evolution of the mammalian periodontium. In: *Biology of the periodontium,*

A. H. MELCHER & W. H. BOWEN (eds.), Chap. 1. London, Academic Press.

NORRIS, K. S. & PRESCOTT, J. H. (1959) Jaw structure and tooth replacement in the opaleye, *Girella nigricans* (Ayres), with notes on other species. *Copeia* 1959, 275–283.

OLTMANNS, E. (1952) Zur Morphologie der Zähne rezenter Amphibien. *Anat. Anz.* 98, 369–389.

ØRVIG, T. (1961) Notes on some early representatives of the Drepanaspida (Pteraspidomorphi, Heterostraci). *Ark. Zool.* 12, 515–535.

ØRVIG, T. (1967) Phylogeny of tooth tissues: evolution of some calcified tissues in early vertebrates. In: *Structural and chemical organization of teeth*, Vol. I, A. E. W. MILES (ed.), Chap. 2. London, Academic Press.

OWENS, P. D. A. (1975) The fine structure of the coronal root region of premolar teeth in dogs. *Archs. oral Biol.* 20, 705–708.

OWENS, P. D. A. (1978) Ultrastructure of Hertwig's epithelial root sheath during early root development in premolar teeth in dogs. *Archs. oral biol.* 23, 91–104.

PARSONS, T. W. & WILLIAMS, E. E. (1962) The teeth of Amphibia and their relation to amphibian phylogeny. *J. Morph.* 110, 375–389.

PEYER, B. (1968) *Comparative odontology*. Chicago University Press.

PFLUGFELDER, O. (1930) Das Gebiss der Gymnodonten. Ein Beitrag zur Histogenese des Dentins. *Z. Anat. Entw.* 93, 543–556.

POOLE, D. F. G. & SHELLIS, R. P. (1976) Eruptive tooth movements in non-mammalian vertebrates. In: *The eruption and occlusion of teeth*, D. F. G. POOLE & M. V. STACK (eds.) (Colston Papers no. 27), pp. 65–79. London, Butterworth.

REIF, W-E. (1978) A note on the distinction between acellular bone and atubular dentine in fossil shark teeth. *N. Jb. Geol. Paläont. Mh.* 7, 447–448.

REIF, W-E., McGILL, D. & MOTTA, P. (1978) Tooth replacement rates of the sharks *Triakis semifasciata* and *Ginglymostoma cirratum*. *Zoll. Jb. Anat.* 99, 151–156.

RIBEIRO, M. C. L. & MONTEIRO, M. P. (1971) Structure histologique des dents du *Lutianus* sp. (Caranha). *Arch. Biol. Liège* 82, 529–541.

SCHMIDT, W. J. & KEIL, A. (1971) *Polarizing microscopy of dental tissues*. (Translated and edited by D. F. G. POOLE.) Oxford, Pergamon Press.

SHELLIS, R. P. & BERKOVITZ, B. K. B. (1976) Observations on the dental anatomy of piranhas (Characidae) with special reference to tooth structure. *J. Zool. Lond.* 180, 69–84.

SHELLIS, R. P. & MILES, A. E. W. (1974) Autoradiographic study of the formation of enameloid and dentine matrices in teleost fishes using tritiated amino acids. *Proc. R. Soc. Lond.* B185, 51–72.

SHELLIS, R. P. & POOLE, D. F. G. (1978) The structure of the dental hard tissues of the coelacanthid fish *Latimeria chalumnae* Smith. *Archs. oral Biol.* 23, 1105–1113.

SLAUGHTER, B. H. & SPRINGER, S. (1968) Replacement of rostral teeth in sawfishes and sawsharks. *Copeia* 1968, 499–506.

SLAVKIN, H. C. & BOYDE, A. (1974) Cementum: an epithelial secretory product? *J. dent. Res.* 53 Spec. Iss. (Proc. 52nd Session Int. Assoc. Dent. Res.), 157 (Abstr.)

SLOAN, P. (1978) Scanning electron microscopy of the collagen fibre architecture of the rabbit incisor periodontium. *Archs. oral Biol.* 23, 567–572.

SLOAN, P. (1979) Collagen fibre architecture in the periodontal ligament. *J. R. Soc. Med.* 72, 188–191.

SMITH, H. M. (1958) Evolutionary lines in tooth attachment and replacement in reptiles: their possible significance in mammalian dentition. *Kans. Acad. Sci.* 61, 216–225.

SMITH, M. M. (1977) The microstructure of the dentition and dermal ornament of three dipnoans from the Devonian of Western Australia. *Phil. Trans. R. Soc. Lond.* 281, 29–72.

SMITH, M. M. (1978) Enamel in the oral teeth of *Latimeria chalumnae* (Pisces, Actinistia). A scanning electron microscope study. *J. Zool. Lond.* 185, 355–369.

SMITH, M. M. (1979) Structure and histogenesis of tooth plates in *Sagenodus inaequalis* Owen considered in relation to the phylogeny of post-Devonian dipnoans. *Proc. R. Soc. Lond.* B204, 15–39.

SMITH, M. M. & MILES, A. E. W. (1969) An autoradiographic investigation with the light microscope of proline-H^3 incorporation during tooth development in the crested newt (*Triturus cristatus*). *Archs. oral Biol.* 14, 479–490.

SMITH, M. M. & MILES, A. E. W. (1971) The ultrastructure of odontogenesis in larval and adult urodeles: differentiation of the dental epithelial cells. *Z. Zellforsch. mikr. Anat.* 121, 470–498.

SMUKLER, H. & DREYER, C. J. (1969) Principal fibres of the periodontium. *J. periodont. Res.* 4, 19–25.

SOULE, J. D. (1967) Oxytalan fibres in the periodontal ligament of the Caiman and the Alligator (Crocodilia, Reptilia). *J. Morph.* 122, 169–174.

SOULE, J. D. (1969) Tooth attachment by means of a periodontium in the trigger-fish (Balistidae). *J. Morph.* 127, 1–6.

TEN CATE, A. R. (1976) Development of the periodontal membrane and collagen turnover. In: *The eruption and occlusion of teeth*, D. F. G. POOLE & M. V. STACK (eds.) (Colston Papers No. 27). London, Butterworths.

TOMES, C. S. (1904) *A manual of dental anatomy, human and comparative*, 6th edn. London, Churchill.

WEGNER, R. N. (1951) Der Tütenfortsatz (Processus cucullaris mandibulae) beim Elefanten, den Sirenen, Rhinozerotiden und Suiden. *Anat. Anz.* 98, 66–82.

ZWARYCH, P. D. & QUIGLEY, M. B. (1965) The intermediate plexus of the periodontal ligament: History and further observations. *J. dent. Res.* 44, 383–391.

Chapter 2

CELLS OF THE PERIODONTAL LIGAMENT
B. K. B. Berkovitz and R. C. Shore

INTRODUCTION

The cells of the periodontal ligament may be classified into four groups: connective tissue cells, epithelial cells, defence cells and those associated with the neurovascular elements. The connective tissue cells include fibroblasts, osteoblasts, cementoblasts, osteoclasts, cementoclasts and undifferentiated mesenchymal cells. The most numerous are the fibroblasts which occupy approximately 50% by volume of the periodontal ligament excluding the blood vessels (Beertsen and Everts, 1977; Shore and Berkovitz, 1979). Aggregations of epithelial cells (rests of Malassez) are a normal feature of the ligament and represent the remains of the developmental epithelial root sheath. Several types of defence cell (e.g. macrophages, eosinophils and mast cells) may be observed in apparently undiseased periodontal tissue. Cells associated with the neurovascular elements are considered elsewhere (Chapters 7 and 8). One general point concerning this topic which must be borne in mind is the fact that most studies have relied upon animal tissue (particularly the rodent molar) and not human periodontal ligament.

FIBROBLASTS

These cells are found between the collagen fibres and consequently their general orientation will be related to that of the fibres. In teeth sectioned longitudinally, therefore, fibroblasts appear obliquely orientated to the tooth surface in the middle portion of the ligament, perpendicular to the tooth surface in the alveolar crest, root apex and interradicular regions and have a more variable orientation in transitional regions (Fig. 1). The fibroblasts in the loose connective tissue associated with the neurovascular bundles appear to have a more random orientation.

Determination of cell shape is difficult in routine histological sections because the fibroblast cytoplasm takes up little stain. The shape is deduced mainly from the position and orientation of the nucleus which stains more intensely. In the human, the fibroblasts have been described as 'ovoid' or 'flattened' in appearance (Fullmer, 1967). Examination of the ligament suggests that fibroblasts are often fusiform. This appearance, however, may simply be the product of viewing a disc-shaped structure in one plane only. From a scanning electron microscopic

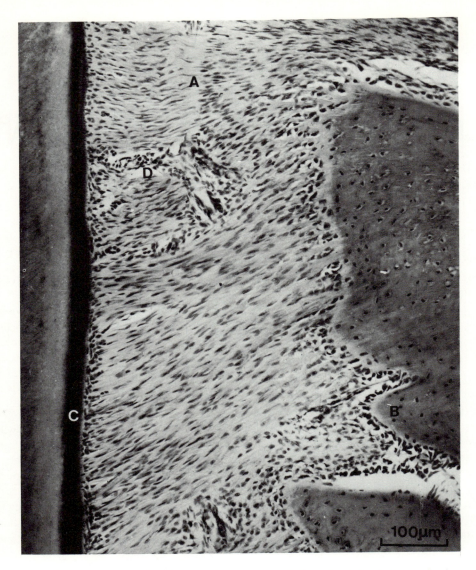

FIG. 1. Longitudinal section of periodontal ligament showing general distribution and orientation of cells. Note the orientation of fibroblasts perpendicular to the root surface in the alveolar crest region (A), whilst apically the cells are aligned more obliquely. Osteoblasts are seen adjacent to the alveolar bone (B) and cementoblasts adjacent to cementum (C). D = blood vessels.

study of rat molar periodontal ligament, Roberts and Chamberlain (1978) concluded that the cells were pleomorphic (varying in size, shape and surface morphology) but identified four general cell types. However, care must be taken before accepting this classification since it is conceivable that artefacts resulting from specimen preparation could have been produced. In tissue culture, the fibroblasts of the periodontal ligament show morphologies varying from spindle-shaped to trapezoid (Brunette, Melcher and Moe, 1976). However, this does not necessarily reflect the *in vivo* situation. Indeed, Ross (1968) has noted that the environment in which fibroblasts are situated has an important influence on cell shape.

The morphology of periodontal fibroblasts can be determined by ultrathin sectioning of the periodontal ligament in different planes, though interpretation is still difficult when cells are randomly orientated. The outline of any individual cell can only ultimately be determined by serial reconstruction and this has yet to be undertaken. However, information exists concerning fibroblast morphology in the rat incisor (Shore and Berkovitz, 1979). In the cemental aspect of the ligament, the cells have an ordered orientation. From measurements taken in longitudinal and transverse section of this tissue, it seems that the fibroblast is a flattened disc having an average diameter of about 30 μm. The outline of the cell is irregular due to cytoplasmic processes.

Since fibroblasts are responsible for secreting the extracellular proteins of connective tissue, they contain all the intracellular organelles necessary for their synthesis. These organelles are particularly abundant in the periodontal ligament where there is a rapid turnover of extracellular protein (e.g. Rippin, 1976; Sodek, 1977).

The periodontal fibroblast, like other actively secreting cells, has a prominent nucleus (Fig. 2) which generally shows at least one nucleolus. In the rat incisor at least, the nucleus conforms to the general shape of the cell, being a flattened disc (Shore and Berkovitz, 1979) and occupying approximately 25% of the cell by volume (Beertsen and Everts, 1977).

The cytoplasmic organelles abundant in periodontal fibroblasts are rough endoplasmic reticulum, mitochondria, Golgi complex and vesicles (Fig. 3). The rough endoplasmic reticulum consists of a series of inter-connected tubular structures dispersed throughout the whole of the cytoplasm except for the finest processes of the cell and occupies approximately 7% of the cytoplasm by volume (Beertsen and Everts, 1977); the tubes are studded with chains of ribosomes of between 15—20 nm diameter and the cisternae are filled with a material which has a more electron-dense appearance than that of the surrounding cytoplasm. The rough endoplasmic reticulum may be arranged in relatively ordered, parallel arrays or have a more random configuration. Areas may be evident where the cisternae are markedly dilated, a

situation which may be related to increased protein synthesis. Numerous free ribosomes are also present. The Golgi complex consists of a series of smooth-membraned, flattened lamellae with vesicles of varying size. The complex is usually situated close to the nucleus (Fig. 3a). Mitochondria are randomly distributed throughout the cytoplasm. Their profile varies from elongated to round. This variation may reflect differences in plane of section and/or form. Vesicles of varying size and density are seen throughout the cytoplasm. Since vesicles are also associated with the cell membrane (Fig. 3b), this is taken as evidence that some, at least, are involved in either endocytosis or exocytosis of substances such as procollagen, enzymes related to collagen maturation and breakdown, and ground substance and its associated enzymes. Large, membrane-bound, dense vesicles occur within the cytoplasm and are probably lysosomes (Fig. 3b).

Microfilaments with a diameter of approximately 5 nm may be seen as a network throughout the cytoplasm or gathered together into recognizable bundles beneath the cell membrane (Fig. 3b). In other cell types, filaments have been seen to bind with heavy meromyosin (Schroeder, 1973). It is deduced, therefore, that they are comprised of actin. Myosin is not positively identifiable by electron microscopy in non-muscle cells but its presence can be confirmed by specific histochemical methods (Allison, 1973). Microfilaments are present within many diverse types of cell and are involved in endocytosis, exocytosis and cell locomotion and motility (Allison, 1973). Indeed, active migration of periodontal fibroblasts has been implicated in generating the force responsible for tooth eruption (see Chapter 10). However, in the periodontal ligament of the continuously growing rat incisor where eruption rates are high, microfilament bundles within fibroblasts appear to be less numerous and to lack the preferential orientation that might be expected of cells undergoing rapid unidirectional locomotion (Shore and Berkovitz, 1979).

Microtubules are present as a system of randomly orientated, non-branching cylinders with an approximate diameter of 22 nm (Fig. 3). They play a part in intracellular transport and in the formation and/or maintenance of cell shape (Allison, 1973). Drugs which affect microtubular structure (e.g. colchicine)

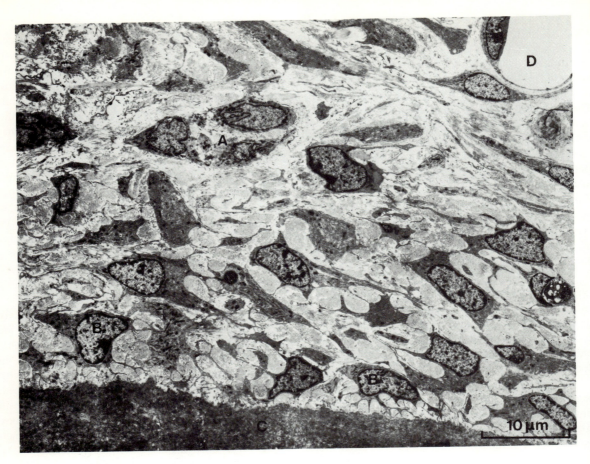

FIG. 2. Electron micrograph of periodontal ligament showing general appearance of fibroblasts. Note also epithelial cell rest (A) and cementoblasts (B) adjacent to the cementum (C). D = lumen of blood vessel.

can inhibit the export of secretory products. In fibroblasts this can result in an intracellular accumulation of procollagen (Ehrlich and Bornstein, 1972) or polymerized collagen fibrils (Cho and Garant, 1978). Microtubules are also associated with centrioles and cilia. The centriole consists of a small cylinder of microtubules up to 2 μm in diameter. Solitary cilia (Fig. 4) have been described as lying within cell invaginations in approximately 70% of mouse incisor periodontal fibroblasts (Beertsen, Everts and Houtkooper, 1975), where they are described as containing no more than nine tubule doublets as opposed to the normal 9 + 2 configuration. The significance of cilia in fibroblasts is not known.

Three types of cell contacts between periodontal fibroblasts have been described, namely simplified desmosomes, tight junctions (zonula occludentes) and gap junctions (nexus) (Beertsen, Everts and van den Hooff, 1974; Azuma et al., 1975; Frank, Fellinger and Steuer, 1976) (Fig. 5). However, little information exists concerning their distribution and functions. In a recent quantitative study of cell contacts in the various periodontal tissues within the rat mandible, no significant differences were observed in the distribution of desmosomes and gap junctions between the periodontal ligaments of the continuously growing incisor and of the molar (Shore, Berkovitz and Moxham, in press). However, desmosomes (which were overall the most common type of contact) were found in significantly greater numbers in the connective tissue adjacent to the enamel organ of the continuously growing incisor.

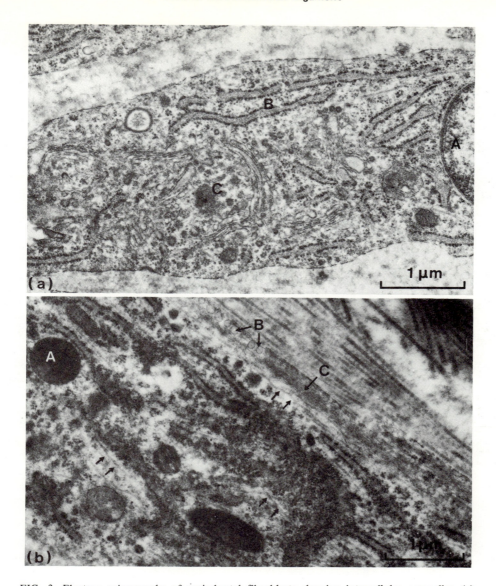

FIG. 3. Electron micrographs of periodontal fibroblasts showing intracellular organelles. (a) A = nucleus. B = rough endoplasmic reticulum. C = Golgi complex. Note the vesicles, mitochondria, free ribosomes and microtubules. (b) A = lysosome. B = vesicles associated with cell membrane. C = microfilament bundle lying beneath cell membrane. Microtubules (arrowed) are present throughout the cytoplasm.

Much attention has been paid in recent years to the presence of intracellular collagen profiles within periodontal fibroblasts and these have been linked with collagen degradation (Ten Cate, 1972; Listgarten, 1973; Beertsen *et al.*, 1974; Eley and Harrison, 1975; Frank *et al.*, 1976; Beertsen and Everts, 1977; Melcher, Chan and Svoboda, 1978; Shore and Berkovitz; 1979). Previously, collagen degradation had been regarded as an extracellular process. However, intracellular collagen profiles also have been observed in other sites of rapid collagen breakdown such as cranial sutures, wound repair (Ten Cate and Freeman,

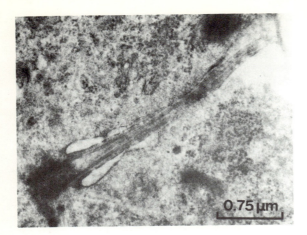

FIG. 4. Electron micrograph of a solitary cilium lying within an invagination of the fibroblast cell membrane.

1974) and the involuting uterus (Parakkal, 1969). Indeed, Ten Cate and Deporter (1975) have suggested that in healthy tissue all collagen degradation is intracellular; where degradation is occurring slowly the scarcity and the small sampling area imposed by electron microscopy make detection of intracellular profiles unlikely. In the periodontal ligament profiles are of three main types: (1) where a banded fibril is surrounded by an electron-lucent zone (Fig. 6a), (2) where a banded fibril is surrounded by an electron-dense zone, with or without swellings along its length (Fig. 6b), and (3) where a fibril is unbanded

(Fig. 6c). Ten Cate, Deporter and Freeman (1976) suggest that these represent a temporal sequence in the intracellular digestion of collagen. In the first stage, a well-defined collagen fibril is phagocytosed by the fibroblast to form a phagosome consisting of the fibril in a clear matrix surrounded by a unit membrane. Primary lysosomes fuse with the phagosome to form a phagolysosome in which there is a gradual increase in electron density of the matrix. Further enzymatic degeneration of the fibril results in a progressive loss of its characteristic structure.

In mouse incisor periodontal ligament, Beertsen and Everts (1977) reported a preponderance of intracellular collagen profiles in the central part of the ligament, a part they consider to correspond to a zone of shear. However, such a localized concentration was not reported for the rat incisor (Shore and Berkovitz, 1979).

It might be argued that the intracellular appearance of collagen profiles results from oblique sectioning across surface invaginations. Alternatively, the profiles could be internally polymerized fibrils which have never been secreted into the extracellular space. Indeed, biochemical studies have demonstrated that fibroblasts in vitro can degrade considerable amounts of newly synthesized collagen within the cell before secretion (Bienkowski, Baum and Crystal, 1978).

Attempts have been made to clarify these questions by the injection of the electron-dense marker thorium

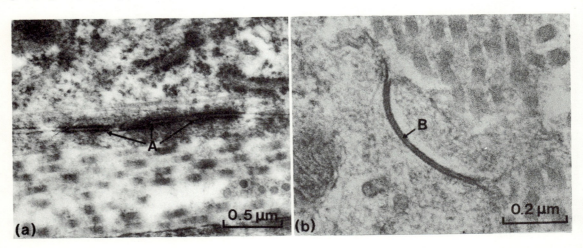

FIG. 5. Electron micrographs of intercellular contacts between fibroblasts. A = intermediate or simplified desmosome type. B = gap junction.

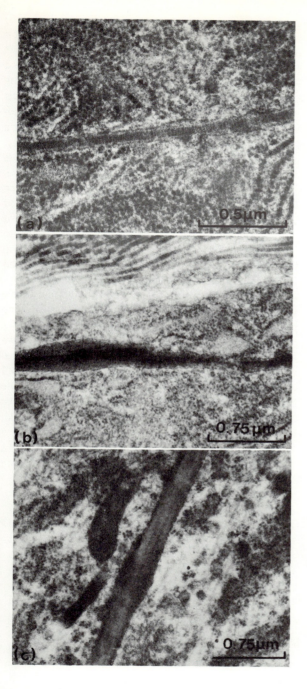

FIG. 6. Electron micrographs of intracellular collagen profiles.
(a) Banded fibril surrounded by an electron-lucent zone.
(b) Banded fibrils surrounded by an electron-dense zone.
(c) Fibrils with indistinct banding surrounded by an electron-dense zone.

dioxide (Ten Cate *et al.*, 1976), and by histochemical techniques for the localization of alkaline and acid phosphatases (Deporter and Ten Cate, 1973; Ten Cate and Syrbu, 1974). The identification of these substances within the profiles was regarded by the authors as evidence that profiles were intracellular and that the collagen had once been in the extracellular environment. Ultimately, however, it would seem that this problem can only be resolved by serial sectioning and an initial study using this method has been undertaken by Svoboda, Brunette and Melcher (1979). These authors examined periodontal fibroblasts cultured on tendon collagen. The fibroblasts appeared to phagocytose the collagen and serial sectioning revealed many of the collagen profiles to be intracellular. It is notable that the cells in culture seem to have a larger number of more randomly orientated intracellular collagen fibrils than cells *in vivo*. Further evidence that intracellular collagen fibrils had once been in the extracellular compartment has been deduced from examination of the periodontal ligaments of scorbutic guinea-pigs where the synthetic phase is inhibited. The continuing presence of intracellular collagen under these conditions (Ten Cate *et al.*, 1976) has been explained on the basis of phagocytosis by the fibroblast. However, under experimental conditions where the microtubular structure (and therefore protein export) is disrupted by colchicine, there is a build-up of intracellular collagen profiles resulting from polymerization of unsecreted collagen (Cho and Garant, 1978).

Even if the collagen profiles are intracellular and are the result of phagocytosis, the question remains as to whether there are sufficient profiles to account for collagen turnover or whether extracellular digestion is also involved. If it is assumed that collagen within rat molar periodontal ligament constitutes a homogeneous pool and turns over in about 2 days (Sodek, 1978), then calculations based upon the volume of electron-dense profiles indicate that intracellular degradation within any profile must take place within approximately 25 minutes to account for the complete turnover of all the collagen (Shore and Berkovitz, 1979). If electron-lucent profiles are also taken into account (since these may also be intracellular (Svoboda *et al.*, 1979)), the time for intracellular degradation could be increased to approximately 50 minutes (Berkovitz and Shore, unpublished data). This latter rate is similar to the time derived for rat incisor ligament (Shore and Berkovitz, 1979), assuming a turnover time of about 12 days (Beertsen and Everts, 1977; Orlowski, 1978). In rat incisor fibroblasts nearly all the profiles appear electron-dense (Berkovitz and Shore, unpublished data). However, if Sodek's (1978) calculation of 3 days for the half life of incisor ligament collagen is correct, then the degradation time must be correspondingly shortened.

When collagen turnover rates are increased by making rat incisors unimpeded, any subsequent increase in the rate of intracellular collagen degradation must involve either an increase in the total number of collagen profiles and/or a decrease in the time required for intracellular digestion within each profile. As Beertsen and Everts (1977) found a slight reduction in the number of profiles, the latter alternative seems more probable. Unfortunately, no information is yet available concerning the time that is required for intracellular degradation of collagen.

Finally, the question should be asked: what advantages would intracellular collagen degradation have over extracellular degradation? In view of the high rate of turnover of collagen in the ligament, intracellular degradation may represent the most efficient method in terms of energy expenditure and material conservation. Furthermore, it may allow the cell to isolate more specifically the aggregative and degradative processes. Much still needs to be learned concerning how these two processes can occur simultaneously and in such close proximity. (Further consideration is given to this topic in Chapter 4.)

MYOFIBROBLASTS

In addition to the typical fibroblast, a cell type having characteristics of both fibroblasts and smooth muscle cells has been observed. These myofibroblasts possess a crenulated nucleus and prominent bundles of microfilaments throughout the cell (Fig. 7). They are seen in wounds where they are thought to be responsible for generating the force associated with wound

contraction (Gabbiani, 1979). Myofibroblasts have also been described within the periodontal ligament of rat molars by Azuma et al. (1975). They implicated them in the generation of the force of tooth eruption. However, we do not believe that the cells described within the ligament as myofibroblasts have features significantly different from typical periodontal fibroblasts. Furthermore, myofibroblasts have not been described by any other worker studying the periodontal ligament.

OSTEOBLASTS

Osteoblasts within the periodontal ligament are found adjacent to the surface of alveolar bone. When most active, they form a layer of columnar cells which exhibit a strongly basophilic cytoplasm. The prominent round nucleus tends to lie towards the basal end of the cell. A pale juxtanuclear area indicates the site of the Golgi complex (Fig. 8). Like fibroblasts of the ligament, active osteoblasts contain an extensive rough endoplasmic reticulum and numerous mitochondria and vesicles. However, their Golgi appears more localized and extensive than that found in fibroblasts (Fig. 8). Microtubules and microfilaments are also seen, their presence presumably being associated with morphogenesis and secretion. Microfilaments are prominent beneath the cell membrane distally at the secreting surface (Fig. 8). The cells contact one another by means of desmosomes and tight junctions. The cell surface adjacent to bone has many fine cytoplasmic processes some of which contact underlying osteocytes by tight junctions to form part of a transport system throughout the bone tissue (Holtrop and Weinger, 1972). As bone deposition proceeds, osteoblasts become incorporated into the bone as osteocytes (in which the quantity of cytoplasmic organelles becomes reduced).

Cells which may be osteoblast precursors are often seen immediately beneath the osteoblast layer (Fig. 8). These cells have a reduced cytoplasm and few organelles.

When osteogenesis is not occurring, a distinct layer of osteoblasts is not usually evident at the bone surface. Indeed, in other sites in mature animals,

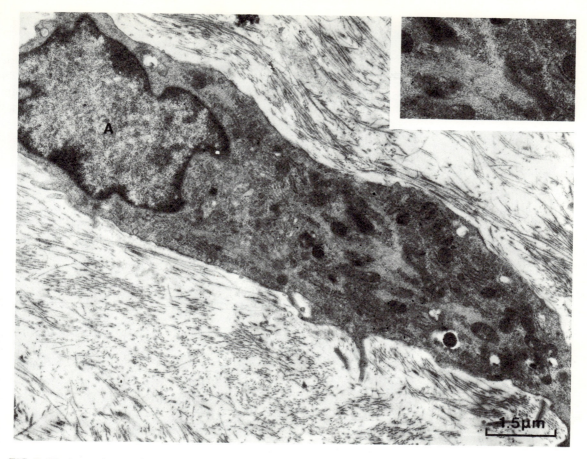

FIG. 7. Electron micrograph of a myofibroblast from the pubic symphysis of a pregnant mouse. Note the crenulated nucleus (A) and the prominent bundles of microfilaments throughout the cytoplasm. Inset shows details of microfilaments.

osteoblasts and osteoclasts are present only over about 10–15% of bone surfaces (Jowsey *et al.,* 1965), the remaining 85–90% of the bone surface being covered by flattened cells with scanty cytoplasm.

The pathway for synthesis and release of extracellular proteins would seem to be similar to that for the fibroblast, namely from rough endoplasmic reticulum to Golgi complex and then via vesicles to the cell membrane (Weinstock and Leblond, 1974). The subsequent process of mineralization may be initiated within matrix vesicles that are budded off from the osteoblast (Anderson, 1976), though once mineralization has begun it then proceeds extracellularly.

CEMENTOBLASTS

Cementoblasts resemble osteoblasts and their appearance depends upon their functional state. When active, they form a recognizable layer of cells adjacent to the cementum (especially during root formation). Their shape is not as regular as that of osteoblasts (Fig. 2) and their intracytoplasmic organelles associated with protein synthesis are less prominent and well ordered (Fig. 9). Cells depositing acellular cementum lack prominent cytoplasmic processes unlike those associated with the formation of cellular cementum. Apart from their location immediately adjacent to cementum, it may be difficult to dis-

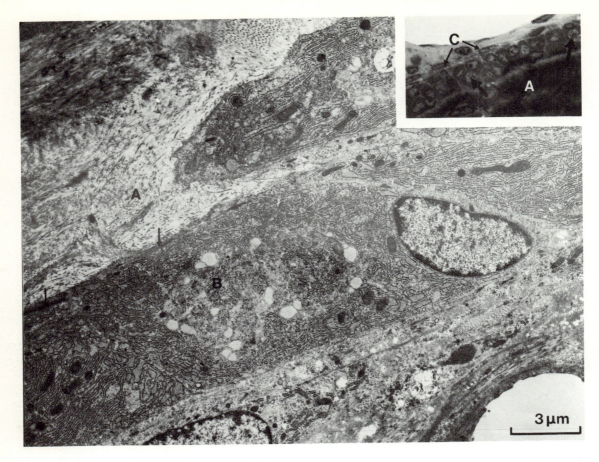

FIG. 8. Electron micrograph of osteoblasts lying adjacent to a forming bone surface (A). The cells exhibit extensive arrays of rough endoplasmic reticulum and a prominent Golgi complex (B). Note bundles of microfilaments (arrowed) beneath the cell membrane adjacent to the bone. Inset shows longitudinal section of periodontal ligament with a layer of osteoblasts adjacent to a forming bone surface (A). Note extensive areas of Golgi complex (arrowed) appearing as a pale zone within the cytoplasm. Note also the flattened cells (C) immediately adjacent to the osteoblasts, which may represent osteoblast precursors.

tinguish cementoblasts from periodontal fibroblasts. Indeed, since some of the processes of cementoblasts do not approach the cementum and their cytoplasmic contents are not polarized, the cells may contribute some protein to the ligament. The synthetic pathway of cementoblasts is presumably similar to that of the osteoblast and fibroblast.

OSTEOCLASTS

Surface resorption of bone is carried out by osteo-clasts though it has been claimed that osteolysis within bone can occur under the influence of osteo-cytes (Bélanger, 1971). Typically, osteoclasts are large multinucleated cells lying within resorption lacunae at the surface of bone (Fig. 10). They do not appear to cover the entire resorbing bone surface at any one time (Owen and Shetlar, 1968) and tissue culture studies have shown them to be mobile (Hancox, 1972). The bone surface between osteoclasts is covered by uninucleated cells whose function is uncertain but which may be osteoclast precursors (Owen, 1971). Though most osteoclasts have between ten

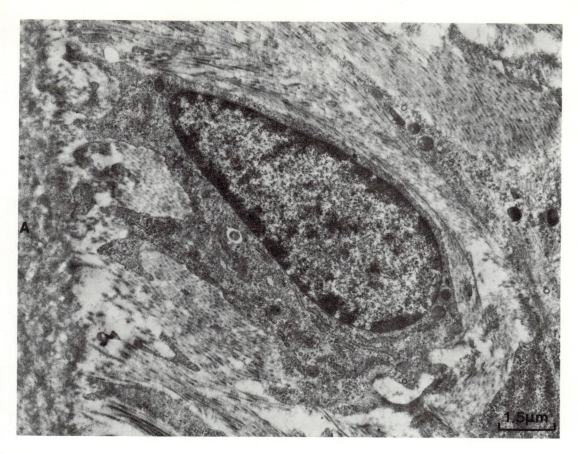

FIG. 9. Electron micrograph of a cell (presumably a cementoblast) lying adjacent to the surface of the cementum (A). The cytoplasm contains the organelles associated with protein synthesis, but not in significant quantities.

and twenty nuclei, there may be several hundred or only one or two (Hancox, 1972). Using tritiated thymidine, Kember (1960), Tonna and Cronkite (1961) and Young (1963) have demonstrated that osteoclast nuclei do not synthesize DNA and therefore do not divide. Evidence is available to show that the nuclear population may be continually changing during the life of the cell, with new nuclei entering and others leaving. It has been suggested that the nuclei leaving an osteoclast may return to the osteoprogenitor pool (Young, 1962). At the light-microscope level, the cell surface in contact with the bone forms a 'brush border'. Beneath this border, the cytoplasm has a characteristic 'foamy' appearance. Ultrastructurally, the brush border is comprised of many tightly packed microvilli which may be coated

with fine bristle-like structures (Kallio, Garant and Minkin, 1971). At the circumference of the brush border, the plasma membrane tends to become smooth (Fig. 10) and the cytoplasm beneath it more dense. It has been suggested that this modified 'annular' zone may serve to limit the diffusion of hydrolytic enzymes, thereby creating a microenvironment in which resorption can take place (Malkani, Luxembourger and Rebel, 1973). This arrangement might be the most efficient in terms of energy expenditure and material conservation. The osteoclast contains numerous mitochondria distributed throughout the cytoplasm, except for the region immediately beneath the brush border (Fig. 10). The rough endoplasmic reticulum is less conspicuous than in osteoblasts, but Golgi complexes are prominent (especially in

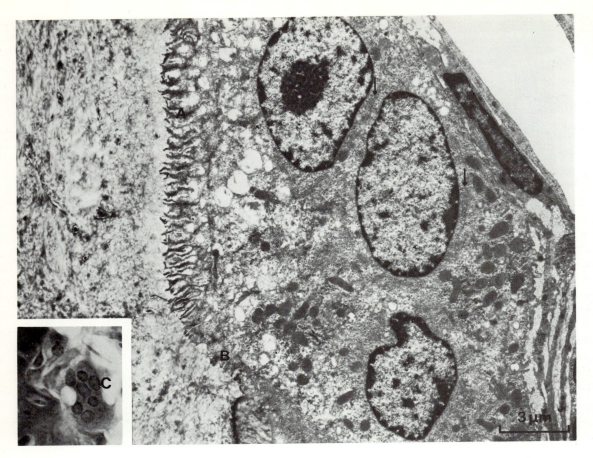

FIG. 10. Electron micrograph of a multinucleated osteoclast showing general distribution of organelles. There is an abundance of vesicles and a lack of mitochondria beneath the brush border (A). Note the lack of microvilli in the 'annular zone' (B). The Golgi complex lies in a juxtanuclear position (arrow) and there is little endoplasmic reticulum. Inset shows longitudinal section of periodontal ligament with a multinucleated osteoclast (C) lying within a lacuna at the alveolar bone surface.

juxtanuclear areas). Most of the remaining cytoplasm contains large numbers of vesicles of different sizes and types. Some have been identified on morphological and histochemical grounds as lysosomes containing acid phosphatase (Doty, Schofield and Robinson, 1967), while others are presumably related to endocytosis or exocytosis. Though in tissue culture the osteoclast is seen to be mobile (Hancox, 1972), microfilament bundles and also microtubules are sparsely distributed.

Unlike periodontal fibroblasts, intracellular collagen profiles have not been observed within osteoclasts, suggesting extracellular digestion of bone collagen. This may be related either to the presence of a localized extracellular microenvironment (delineated by the annular zone of the osteoclast) or to differences in the physical or chemical properties of bone and periodontal ligament collagen. Another explanation may be that the osteoclast is only involved in the initial stages of resorption and that the final degradation of collagen is undertaken by adjacent fibroblasts (Heersche and Deporter, 1979). That osteoclasts are not responsible for the complete degradation of bone has also been suggested by Dorey and Bick (1977), adjacent perivascular macrophages also being implicated. For a review of bone resorption the reader is referred to Melcher (1978).

Though the multinucleated cells associated with resorption of cementum and dentine have sometimes been termed 'cementoclasts' and 'odontoclasts', evidence suggests that all resorptive cells associated with vertebrate mineralized tissues are morphologically similar (Yaeger and Kraucunas, 1969; Freilich, 1971; Addison, 1979).

In spite of considerable research, the mechanisms ultimately responsible for switching on and off osteogenesis and osteoclasis are unknown. Among the important factors which play a role in skeletal homeostasis are: (1) biochemical substances (such as hormones) and dietary factors and (2) mechanical stresses (as illustrated by changes following orthodontic tooth movement, exercise or disuse, and weightlessness during space flight). However, the response of the individual bone cells will presumably be governed by factors in their immediate microenvironment such as pH and oxygen tension (for review see Melcher, 1978). In reviewing control mechanisms associated with bone remodelling, Bassett (1971) highlighted the possible role of piezoelectricity and streaming potentials.

EPITHELIAL CELLS

These are distinguishable from adjacent fibroblasts by the close packing of their cuboidal cells and their tendency to stain more deeply (Fig. 11). They often appear as separate clusters of cells, the shape of which may be related to tension in the surrounding collagen fibres (Grant and Bernick, 1969). However, when cut tangentially the clusters are seen to be part of a continuous network, though this may not be the case for all species (e.g. monkey (Valderhaug, 1974)).

From light-microscopical examination, Reeve and Wentz (1962) described three cell types: resting, degenerated and proliferated. Wentz, Weinmann and Schour (1950) suggested that these represent successive stages in the life history of epithelial cell rests. However, since these studies were based only on haematoxylin and eosin preparations, the validity of such a classification awaits further investigation.

The cell rests are located close to the cementum surface. Valderhaug and Zander (1967) found that the average distance from the cementum to the epithelial cells in humans was 27 μm in the apical region, increasing gradually to 41 μm cervically. Though these authors did not observe epithelial cell rests in direct contact with cementum, Lester (1969) and Grant and Bernick (1969) found that some cells were incorporated into cementum in experimental animals during mineralization.

Differences have been noted in the distribution of epithelial cells in humans according to age and site. They appear to be more numerous in children than in adults (Reitan, 1961). Reeve and Wentz (1962) noted that during the first and second decades of life the epithelial cells were found most commonly in the apical region of the periodontal ligament, whereas between the third and seventh decades the majority of cells were located cervically in the gingiva above the alveolar crest. The authors related this change in distribution to the presence of chronic inflammation in the area of the gingival sulcus. It has been suggested that some of the epithelial cells in the cervical region may originate from the epithelium of the gingiva or from the junctional epithelium (Wentz *et al.,* 1950). In studying the development and fate of epithelial rests in miniature swine, Grant and Bernick (1969) described a possible continuity between the epithelial cells and the reduced enamel epithelium before eruption and the junctional epithelium after eruption. The authors suggested that this continuity may be of significance in periodontal disease.

Reitan (1961) has studied the behaviour of epithelial cell rests in teeth subjected to orthodontic loads. He observed that on the 'compression' side hyalinization of the periodontal ligament occurred and, whilst there was subsequent regeneration of the connective tissue, there was no regeneration of the epithelial cells.

At the ultrastructural level, the epithelial cells are seen to be separated from surrounding connective tissue by a basal lamina. Listgarten (1975) has shown that this lamina may be fragmented (Fig. 11). The nucleus of each cell is prominent and often shows invaginations (Fig. 11). The scanty cytoplasm is characterized by the presence of tonofibrils some of which insert into the frequent desmosomes between

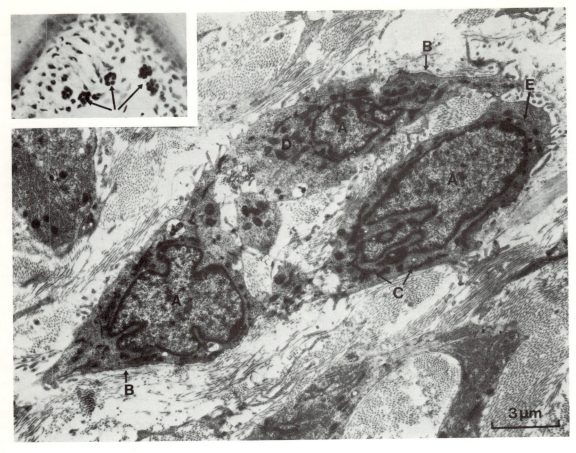

FIG. 11. Electron micrograph of an epithelial cell rest. Note the indented nuclei (A), fragmented basal lamina (B), tono-filaments (C), mitochondria (D) and a small amount of rough endoplasmic reticulum (E). Inset shows longitudinal section of periodontal ligament in the interradicular region with a collection of epithelial cell rests (arrowed).

adjacent cells and into hemidesmosomes between the cells and the basal lamina; tight junctions also occur between the cells (Fig. 12). Mitochondria are distributed throughout the cytoplasm, whilst the rough endoplasmic reticulum and the Golgi complex are poorly developed. Other cell inclusions such as vesicles and granules are present in varying amounts (Valderhaug and Nylen, 1966). Though these cells have been considered to be metabolically inactive, histochemical studies by Ten Cate (1965, 1967) have shown that they possess enzymes associated with glycolysis and the pentose-shunt.

The functional significance of epithelial cells within the periodontal ligament is unknown (for review see Grant and Bernick, 1969). However,

they have considerable clinical significance since they may be stimulated to proliferate and become involved in certain types of periodontal disease.

DEFENCE CELLS

The macrophages, eosinophils and mast cells within the periodontal ligament are similar to those in other connective tissues, though studies of their distribution are lacking.

Macrophages are responsible primarily for phago-cytosing particulate debris and are derived from blood monocytes (e.g. Sutton and Weiss, 1966) which in turn are thought to originate in the bone marrow from

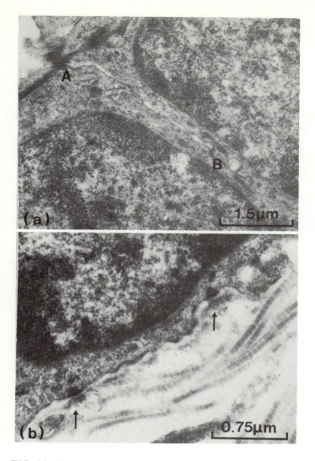

FIG. 12. Electron micrographs showing types of cell contacts associated with epithelial cell rests. (a) Junction between two epithelial cells showing a desmosome with associated tonofilaments (A) and a tight junction (B). (b) An epithelial cell showing hemidesmosomes (arrow) between the cell membrane and the basal lamina.

teristic presence of many lysosomes and other membrane-bound vesicles of varying density. Like fibroblasts, however, they contain Golgi complex and mitochondria (Fig. 13). When active, macrophages have many mitochondria and vesicles and may possess large branching processes. In addition to their phagocytic activity there is evidence that they secrete such substances as the enzymes lysosyme, elastase and collagenase, interferons and certain proteins of the complement system (Goldberg and Rabinovitch, 1977). Recently, a macrophage-dependent factor has been demonstrated that stimulates the proliferation of fibroblasts *in vitro* (Leibovich and Ross, 1976). Further evidence that there may be interactions between macrophages and other cell types is indicated by the observations of Birkdal-Hansen *et al.* (1976). They found that in rabbit alveolar macrophages cultured *in vitro,* there was a 5—10-fold increase in the production of latent collagenase when exposed to a soluble bovine lymphocyte extract.

Eosinophils are seen occasionally within the periodontal ligament. The shape of the cell is generally round or ovoid and the nucleus is polymorphic. Microvilli may project from the cell surface. The characteristic feature of the eosinophil is the presence of many peroxisomes which possess one or more crystalloid structures (Fig. 14). The cells are capable of phagocytosis and increase in number in certain pathological conditions (see Chapter 17).

Mast cells are often associated with blood vessels. In histological sections, the nucleus of the cell is comparatively pale and undefined, unlike that of surrounding fibroblasts where the nucleus is the most prominent feature. Mast cells can be readily distinguished because of their intense staining reaction with basic aniline dyes such as toluidine blue (Fig. 15). The staining property is due primarily to the presence of large numbers of intracytoplasmic granules. The granules are seen as dense membrane-bound vesicles of varying sizes (Fig. 15). Other cytoplasmic organelles are relatively sparse although more abundant in younger cells (Combs, 1966). It has been suggested that the dense granular state represents a resting phase and that when the cell is stimulated it degranulates (Barnett, 1973). Numerous functions have been ascribed to mast cells (for review see Selye, 1965), the most important relating to the production of histamine, heparin and factors associated with ana-

a pluripotential stem cell (van Furth, 1975). The morphology and internal organization of the macrophage depends upon its state of activity and the tissue within which it is found. When resting, they assume a round or ovoid shape and may not be readily distinguishable histologically from fibroblasts (though it has been stated that their nuclei are small and indented and stain more intensely (Leeson and Leeson, 1970)). Ultrastructurally, features which help distinguish the resting macrophage from active fibroblasts are: (1) the paucity of rough endoplasmic reticulum, (2) the presence of thin finger-like projections from the cell surface and (3) the charac-

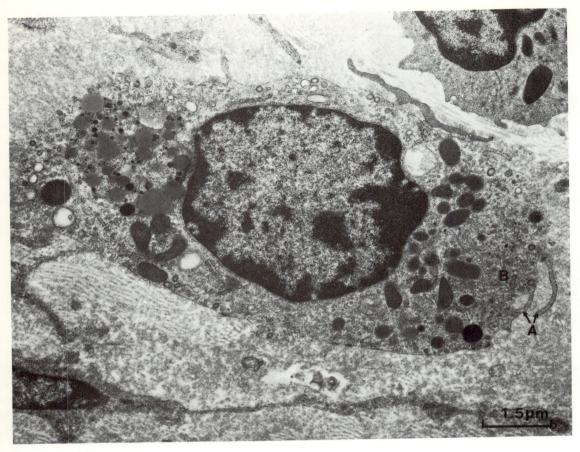

FIG. 13. Electron micrograph of a macrophage. There are a larger number of lysosomes and mitochondria. Note the paucity of rough endoplasmic reticulum. A = microvilli. B = Golgi complex.

phylaxis (Austen, 1974). They may also produce prostaglandins which appear to be important in the regulation of histamine release (Whittle, 1977).

CELLULAR AGE CHANGES

A decrease in cellularity of the periodontal ligament with age has been reported in the molars of the rat (Klingsberg and Butcher, 1960; Jensen and Toto, 1968; Toto, Rubenstein and Gargiulo, 1975), hamster (Klingsberg and Butcher, 1960), mouse (Toto and Borg, 1968) and monkey (Klingsberg and Butcher, 1960). Toto *et al.* (1975) calculated the average cell density associated with the mesial root of rat first molars to be 93 ± 9 cells/110 μm^2 at 1 month and 69 ± 7 cells/110 μm^2 at 15 months of age. Grant and Bernick (1972) found a decrease in cellularity of the ligament following examination of post-mortem material from four humans aged 55, 72, 76 and 92 years. They also noted that epithelial cells were distributed more randomly across the width of the ligament in this group than the normal aggregations close to the cementum in younger age groups. The possible significance of this observation is not known.

In addition to the reduction in cell density with age, it has also been shown by autoradiographic studies using tritiated thymidine that there is a reduction in the number of mitotic cells within the periodontal ligament in the molars of the rat (Jensen

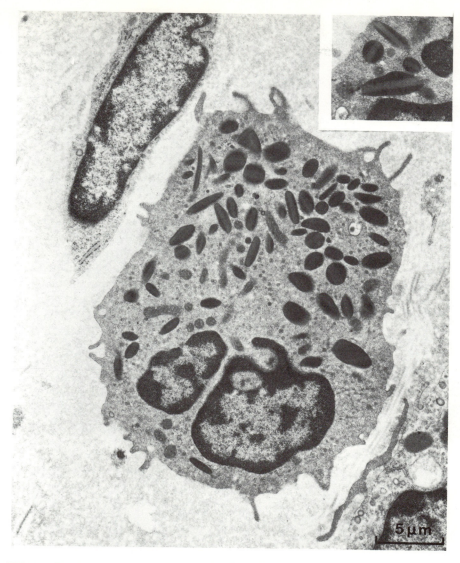

FIG. 14. Electron micrograph of an eosinophil with characteristic granules (peroxisomes). Inset shows the crystalloid inclusions of the granules.

and Toto, 1968; Toto *et al.,* 1975) and mouse (Toto and Borg, 1968). For example, the labelling index of fibroblasts decreases from 104 ± 3 cells/1000 at 1 month to 44 ± 1.5 cells/1000 at 15 months for rat molars (Toto *et al.,* 1975). These authors also suggested that the fibroblasts of ageing tissue had longer 'lives' than those of younger tissue.

Tonna and Stahl (1974) demonstrated that, following gingivectomy in mice, cells in the perio-

dontal ligament some distance from the site of trauma show a cell proliferative response which decreases with age. The reasons for such a response are un-known. For a general review of factors controlling the rate of mitosis the reader is referred to Melcher (1978).

Toto and Borg (1968) have suggested that cellular age changes may be associated with increasing insolu-bility of collagen and with a comparative reduction

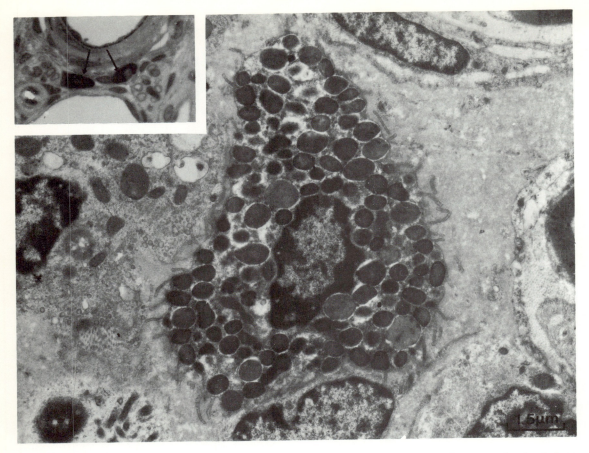

FIG. 15. Electron micrograph of a mast cell showing the cytoplasm filled with numerous dense granules. Inset shows section of the periodontal ligament with two intensely stained mast cells (arrowed) between blood vessels. Stained with toluidine blue.

in the amount of acid mucopolysaccharides. This is thought to result in a decrease in movement and availability of DNA precursors. In addition, degenerative age changes have been reported within the vascular system (e.g. Grant and Bernick, 1972; Levy, Dreizen and Bernick, 1972) and these may also have an effect on cellular ageing. However, little information exists concerning these hypotheses. Furthermore, since atrophic changes within the periodontal ligament have been reported in association with loss of function (e.g. Cohn, 1965, 1966), and cell density and kinetics may be responsive to inflammatory changes (e.g. Tonna and Stahl, 1974), it is important that the functional state of a tooth

be carefully assessed before attributing any cellular changes directly to ageing.

CELL KINETICS WITHIN THE PERIODONTAL LIGAMENT

As osteoblasts and cementoblasts of the periodontal ligament become incorporated into alveolar bone and cellular cementum, replacing cells must be formed to permit osteogenesis and cementogenesis to continue. Periodontal fibroblasts are also formed throughout life. Though progenitor cells may be identified by their ability to incorporate substances such as tritiated thymidine, little is known about their origin and nature within the periodontal ligament.

During the main eruptive phase in mouse molars, Ten Cate (1972) observed that the majority of new fibroblasts originated from precursor cells located around blood vessels at the root apex. In the molars of the mouse (Toto and Borg, 1968) and rat (Toto and Kwan, 1970), it was noted that the majority of cells labelled soon after injection of tritiated thymidine were located near the root apex though there was also a smaller peak near the alveolar crest. However, McHugh and Zander (1965) observed little uptake of label around the developing root apex in erupting monkey molars, though there was significantly more label in the bifurcation region between the roots. Weiss, Stahl and Tonna (1968) similarly noted a high uptake of tritiated thymidine at the interradicular crest region. This they related to functional activity, the region being said to be subjected to considerable occlusal loads. However, no evidence is available to show that such a distribution of force exists. Toto and Kwan (1970) found that approximately 1% of cells in rat molar periodontal ligament were initially labelled with tritiated thymidine. The doubling time of such cells was 16–18 hours.

Assuming that labelled cells (1) adjacent to bone are osteoblast precursors, (2) adjacent to cementum are cementoblast precursors, (3) in the remainder of the periodontal ligament are fibroblast precursors, Weiss *et al.* (1968) concluded that fibroblasts had the highest cellular proliferative activity, followed by osteoblasts and then cementoblasts. The low rate of cementoblast proliferation has also been noted by Tonna and Stahl (1974) and Gould, Melcher and Brunette (1977). The latter authors speculated that the precursor population of osteoblasts is located perivascularly in the vicinity of the alveolar bone, that the precursor population of fibroblasts is located perivascularly in the body of the ligament but that the progenitor population of cementoblasts is located near cementum away from blood vessels.

Though the longevity of periodontal fibroblasts is not known, it may be surmised from the data above that this is probably to be measured in terms of days or weeks rather than months. The eventual fate of ligament fibroblasts is not known. Certainly there is no record of large-scale degeneration of cells

within the ligament. It may be that fibroblasts 'migrate' out of the periodontal ligament.

Though cell kinetics of osteoblasts within the periodontal ligament has received little attention, a considerable literature exists concerning that of osteoblasts from other sites (particularly from growing long bones; for review see Owen, 1971).

In summary, though information exists concerning the distribution of progenitor cells within the ligament, the fundamental question which still remains to be answered is whether periodontal osteoblasts, fibroblasts and cementoblasts all arise from a common (and therefore pluripotent) precursor or whether each cell type has its own specific precursor. In addition, it is not known whether the progenitor cell population is intrinsic to the ligament or whether it is supplemented by migration of cells from an external source.

The origin of the osteoclast has been the subject of considerable research and much controversy. The topic has been reviewed by Owen (1970), Hall (1975) and Gothlin and Ericsson (1976). The main experimental systems used to determine the origin of osteoclasts are growing long bones and fracture callus. Two fundamental problems relate to whether there is a common precursor for both osteoblasts and osteoclasts and whether the precursors of osteoclasts lie within the immediate vicinity of bone or migrate from outside. Using tritiated thymidine to study cell proliferation, Kember (1960) and Young (1962, 1963, 1964) were of the opinion that osteoprogenitor cells could become either osteoblasts or osteoclasts, depending on the cellular environment. In this context, Wong and Cohn (1974) have identified a sub-population of cells separated from mouse calvaria which respond *in vitro* to both parathyroid hormone and to calcitonin. If the cell population is homogeneous, the authors claim that such a response provides evidence that the same population of cells (but not necessarily the same cell) is a precursor to both osteoclasts and osteoblasts. However, further work is necessary to assess the validity of the separation technique employed. Tonna (1960) postulated that osteoclasts may arise from the fusion of osteoblasts, whilst Rasmussen and Bordier (1974) suggested that osteoclasts may give rise to osteoblasts. However, there is growing evidence that osteoblasts and osteoclasts are derived from different stem-cell populations and that the progenitor cells of osteoclasts originate from fusion of non-skeletal cells.

Scott (1967) and Luk, Nopagaroonsri and Simon (1974) claim that they can distinguish precursors of osteoblasts from those of osteoclasts by their ultrastructure. A distinction has also been made histochemically on the basis that 'preosteoblasts' are rich in alkaline phosphatase and 'preosteoclasts' are rich in succinic dehydrogenase (Walker, 1961). Furthermore, Bingham, Brazell and Owen (1969) reported that parathyroid extract had opposite effects on the precursors of osteoblasts and osteo-clasts. However, it could be argued that in these studies a pluripotent type of precursor cell had already undergone some differentiation into two cell lines.

That osteoclasts can originate from fusion of non-skeletal cells has been demonstrated by Jee and Nolan (1963), Gothlin and Ericsson (1973 a and b) and Jotereau and Le Douarin (1978). Jee and Nolan (1963) injected a suspension of bone charcoal into the nutrient artery of rabbit femurs. Subsequently, the marker was first seen within the cytoplasm of macrophages and later within osteoclasts on resorb-ing bone surfaces. Gothlin and Ericsson (1973a) described an experiment where thorium dioxide solution was initially injected into the peritoneum of rats. The particles were phagocytosed by monocyte-like cells and macrophages and these cells were isolated by centrifugation. The cells were then injected into other rats which had their right femurs fractured. Subsequently, osteoclasts containing thorium label were identified in the fracture callus. Gothlin and Ericsson (1973b) irradiated parabiotic rats to destroy the haemopoietic tissues. However, the hindlimb of one was shielded. The right femur of each rat was fractured 1 day after irradiation and tritiated thymidine administered to the pro-tected rat at intervals of 4 days. Osteoclasts were seen to be labelled in the regenerating blastemas of the femurs in both rats. Jotereau and Le Douarin (1978) carried out interspecific grafts of limb buds and femurs between quail and chick embryos. Due to their different nuclear features, the cells of the two species can be identified in the chimeric bones. It was possible to show that the osteoblasts and osteoclasts were derived from different cell lines; the osteoblasts were derived from the limb bud

mesenchyme, the osteoclasts from haemopoietic cells brought into the bone marrow via the circula-tion.

The only work on the periodontal ligament which relates to the origin of osteoclasts is that of Roberts (1975). He studied cell kinetics in the rat maxillary first molar following the injection of parathyroid extract to stimulate osteoclast formation and found that an increased cellularity resulted which could be accounted for only partially by local cell proliferation. He concluded that there must have been an influx of migrating cells into the periodontal ligament.

TISSUE CULTURE OF THE PERIODONTAL LIGAMENT

Tissue culture studies of the periodontal ligament have utilized three different experimental systems: (1) culture of a whole tooth (or teeth) and its sur-rounding periodontal tissues (e.g. Melcher and Turnbull, 1976), (2) culture of portions of perio-dontal ligament attached to tooth and/or bone fragments (e.g. Grupe, Ten Cate and Zander, 1967), (3) culture of isolated periodontal ligament or suspen-sions of periodontal cells (e.g. Brunette et al., 1976).

Melcher and Turnbull (1976) cultured mouse mandibular first molars and surrounding alveolar bone for up to 7 days. During this time there was continued protein synthesis as evidenced by uptake of tritiated proline. However, some areas of the periodontal ligament (especially in the bifurcation region of the roots) became devoid of cells and extracellular protein and there was resorption of alveolar bone. In a further study on the bone resorp-tion seen in such explants, Melcher et al. (1978) observed an increase in both number and size of osteoclasts compared with the appearance in vivo, though the numbers of nuclei per osteoclast were similar in the two groups. The origin of these osteo-clasts in vitro has not been determined, though non-skeletal cells from the marrow spaces of transplanted bone are an obvious source.

Yen and Melcher (1978) studied the effects of oxygen tension on organ culture of mouse jaw fragments containing either one or all three mandibular molars. They observed a considerable improvement in the histological appearance and in the uptake of tritiated proline with a high oxygen tension. This was especially noticeable at the periphery of the explant, the effect being reduced towards the centre.

Grupe *et al.* (1967) developed a method for preparing cell suspensions from portions of periodontal ligament. Culture of the suspension resulted in the growth of two morphologically distinct cell types, one epithelial-like (presumably derived from the epithelial cell rests), the other fibroblast-like. Techniques have also been reported for separating these two cell populations (Kanoza *et al.*, 1978; Rao, Moe and Heersche, 1978). Brunette *et al.* (1976) reported that few cells of the explanted porcine periodontal ligament survived initially; most cells died and underwent autolysis. Indeed, many of the surviving connective tissue-like cells which constituted the progenitor pool of the culture (as evidenced by uptake of tritiated thymidine) appeared to be located in the vicinity of blood vessels. The death of many ligament cells during the early stage after explantation may partly explain the observations of Rossman, Rosenbloom and Robinson (1975). These authors reported that when excised periodontal ligament from humans and hamsters was incubated *in vitro* for periods of 30 minutes to 6 hours, only a small percentage of the protein synthesized was collagen.

A fundamental question to be answered is whether the periodontal ligament cells grown *in vitro* retain the specialized properties of cells seen in this site *in vivo*. Gabbiani (1979) has stated that cultured fibroblasts are cytologically very different from fibroblasts *in vivo,* especially with regard to the content and organization of filaments and contractile proteins. Thus, immunofluorescent staining of human or animal tissues with anti-actin, anti-myosin or anti-tubulin antibodies does not show selective fixation to tissue fibroblasts. However, immunofluorescent staining of cultured fibroblasts with antibodies against cytoskeletal proteins results in a typical pattern of fixation which indicates a highly organized arrangement of such proteins. Though such immunofluorescent studies have not been undertaken on cultured periodontal fibroblasts, ultrastructural studies on such cells (Brunette *et al.*,

1977; Svoboda *et al.*, 1979) have not led to accounts of features uncharacteristic of periodontal fibroblasts. Rose, Yajima and Mahan (1978) reported that the ultrastructural characteristics of cultured human gingival fibroblasts were similar to those *in vivo*.

Epithelial-like cells in culture show characteristic bundles of tonofilaments and desmosomes (Brunette *et al.*, 1977). However, they differ from those *in vivo* in their abundance of cytoplasm with an increased number of lateral processes and by the marked alterations in number, arrangement and morphology of organelles and inclusions (Nylen and Grupe, 1969). The presence of lipid within epithelial cells *in vitro* (Grupe *et al.*, 1967; Nylen and Grupe, 1969) can be correlated with a histochemical study demonstrating pentose-shunt activity in these cells (Grupe *et al.*, 1967).

Marmary, Brunette and Heersche (1976) cultured monkey periodontal and skin fibroblasts under identical conditions. The differences they noted were: (1) cells from the periodontal ligament required an inoculum of 0.6×10^4 cells/cm^2 in order to reach confluency within 6 days, whereas skin cells required an inoculum of 0.3×10^4 cells/cm^2; (2) in the stationary phase of the growth curve, there were 2.7 times more periodontal ligament cells per unit area of culture dish than skin cells; (3) cells from the periodontal ligament contained less than half the concentration of $3'5'$c-AMP than skin cells; (4) significantly more periodontal cells were attached to the plastic substratum 10 and 20 minutes after inoculation (though the numbers were equal after 90 minutes of culture); (5) prostaglandin E_1 (2.5 μg/ml) increased c-AMP levels in periodontal cells after 3 minutes about 30-fold and those of skin cells about 10-fold. However, the significance of such differences in terms of deciding whether periodontal fibroblasts in culture functionally resemble those *in vivo* remains obscure. Limeback, Sodek and Brunette (1978) investigated the nature of collagens synthesized by monkey periodontal ligament fibroblasts *in vitro* and compared them with those synthesized by skin fibroblasts cultured under identical conditions. Though Type-I and Type-III collagens were synthesized by periodontal fibroblasts, the pattern of collagen synthesis was not markedly different from that obtained with skin fibroblasts. Neither was there any indication of lower metabolism of collagen in skin fibroblast cultures compared with periodontal ligament as might be expected from studies *in vivo* (e.g. Sodek, 1976, 1977). Limeback *et al.* (1978) have suggested that this similarity in collagen synthesis may reflect the fact that both sources of fibroblast-like cells in culture may have a similar origin, being derived from progenitor cells lying in the vicinity of blood vessels.

To observe whether periodontal fibroblasts from monkeys would phagocytose collagen *in vitro* (as these cells appear to do *in vivo*), Svoboda *et al.* (1979) prepared confluent cells which were then cultured together with rat-tail tendon collagen (the fibrils of which have a larger diameter than those produced normally by the fibroblasts *in vitro*). Ultrastructural serial sectioning showed that the fibroblasts phagocytosed the extracellular rat tail collagen. However, little further digestion occurred, the cells accumulating excessive amount of collagen compared with cells *in vivo*. Whether this relates to the 'foreign' nature of the extracellular collagen used is not known. Similar results for human gingival fibroblasts *in vitro* have been described (Yajima and Rose, 1977).

In summary, care should be taken before extrapolating from the *in vitro* to the *in vivo* state since the evidence suggests that the cells in the two situations are not identical. In view of the loss of normal architecture and function which occurs in the periodontal ligament *in vitro,* this may not seem surprising.

A clinical situation where tissue culture of the periodontal ligament has assumed some importance is that of tooth reimplantation. Following reimplantation of human teeth, Andreasen and Hjorting-Hansen (1966 a and b) reported that ankylosis resulted and there was always some evidence of tooth resorption. However, small areas with normal periodontal ligament were present. In order to encourage the formation of a viable periodontal ligament on human teeth to be reimplanted, Litwin, Lundquist and Söder (1971) described techniques for maintaining extracted teeth *in vitro* so that the remaining cells were kept viable and were able to multiply. Such techniques involved placing the extracted teeth in Eagle's culture medium and incubating them at 37°C. Söder and Lundquist (1972) developed this technique for the autotransplantation of fully developed roots. Following culture for up to 22

weeks, roots (endodontically treated and root filled) were autotransplanted into surgically prepared sockets. Following healing, crowns or bridges were placed on the implanted roots. Radiographic examination showed evidence of the formation of new bone around the transplants and an apparently normal radiolucent periodontal space after 3 years. Reinholdt *et al.* (1977) studied the cultivation of periodontal fibroblasts on extracted monkey incisors. After 2 days, most of the periodontal ligament showed signs of extensive cell necrosis. By 3 days, the first signs of cell proliferation were observed (either around blood vessels or as a surface layer). After 7 days, an almost complete cover of multi-layered connective tissue had formed on the root surface. No further significant changes took place with extended periods of culture.

In an histological study involving reimplantation of incisors of monkeys, Andreasen *et al.* (1978) found that, though some ankylosis occurred in all teeth, those cases where extracted incisors were kept in tissue culture medium for 5 to 14 days before reimplantation showed improved periodontal healing and significantly less inflammatory resorption than control teeth which had been reimplanted immediately. The reasons for this difference are obscure.

ACKNOWLEDGEMENTS

The authors are grateful to the British Medical Research Council for financing their work described in this review.

REFERENCES

ADDISON, W. C. (1979) The distribution of nuclei in human odontoclasts in whole cell preparations. *Archs. oral Biol.* **23,** 1167–1171.

ALLISON, A. C. (1973) The rôle of microfilaments and microtubules in cell movement, endocytosis and exocytosis. In: *Locomotion of tissue cells: Ciba Symposium 14,* pp. 110–143. Amsterdam, Elsevier.

ANDERSON, H. C. (1976) Matrix vesicles of cartilage and bone. In: *The biochemistry and physiology of bone,* Vol. IV (2nd ed.), G. H. BOURNE (ed.), pp. 135–158. London, Academic Press.

ANDREASEN, J. O. & HJORTING-HANSEN, E. (1966a) Replantation of teeth. I. Radiographic and clinical study of 110 human teeth replanted after accidental loss. *Acta odont. Scand.* **24**, 263–286.

ANDREASEN, J. O. & HJORTING-HANSEN, E. (1966b) Replantation of teeth. II. Histological study of 22 replanted anterior teeth in humans. *Acta odont. Scand.* **24**, 287–306.

ANDREASEN, J. O., REINHOLDT, J., RIIS, I., DYBDAHL, R., SÖDER, P.-O. & OTTESKOG, P. (1978) Periodontal and pulpal healing of monkey incisors preserved in tissue culture before replantation. *Int. J. oral Surg.* **7**, 104–112.

AUSTEN, K. F. (1974) Reaction mechanisms in the release of mediators of immediate hypersensitivity from human lung tissue. *Fed. Proc.* **33**, 2256–2262.

AZUMA, M., ENLOW, D. H., FREDRICKSON, R. G. & GASTON, L. G. (1975) A myofibroblastic basis for the physical forces that produce tooth drift and eruption, skeletal displacement of sutures, and periosteal migration. In: *Determinants of mandibular form and growth*, J. A. McNAMARA (ed.), pp. 179–207. Ann Arbor, University of Michigan.

BARNETT, M. L. (1973) The fine structure of human epithelial mast cells in periodontal disease. *J. periodont. Res.* **8**, 371–380.

BASSETT, C. A. L. (1971) Biophysical principles affecting bone structure. In: *The biochemistry and physiology of bone*, Vol. III (2nd ed.), G. H. BOURNE (ed.), pp. 1–76. London, Academic Press.

BEERTSEN, W. & EVERTS, V. (1977) The site of remodelling of collagen in the periodontal ligament of the mouse incisor. *Anat. Rec.* **189**, 479–498.

BEERTSEN, W., EVERTS, V. & HOUTKOOPER, J. M. (1975) Frequency of occurrence and position of cilia in fibroblasts of the periodontal ligament of the mouse incisor. *Cell. Tiss. Res.* **163**, 415–431.

BEERTSEN, W., EVERTS, V. & VAN DEN HOOFF, A. (1974) Fine structure of fibroblasts in the periodontal ligament of the rat incisor and their possible role in tooth eruption. *Archs. oral Biol.* **19**, 1087–1098.

BÉLANGER, L. F. (1971) Osteocytic resorption. In: *The biochemistry and physiology of bone*, Vol. III (2nd ed.), G. H. BOURNE (ed.), pp. 240–270. London, Academic Press.

BIENKOWSKI, R. S., BAUM, B. J. & CRYSTAL, R. G. (1978) Fibroblasts degrade newly synthesised collagen within the cell before secretion. *Nature* **276**, 413–416.

BINGHAM, P. J., BRAZELL, I. A. & OWEN, M. (1969) The effect of parathyroid extract on cellular activity and plasma calcium levels *in vivo*. *J. Endocrinol.* **45**, 387–400.

BIRKDAL-HANSEN, H., COBB, C. M., TAYLOR, R. E. & FULLMER, H. M. (1976) *In vivo* and *in vitro* stimulation of collagenase production by rabbit alveolar macrophages. *Archs. oral Biol.* **21**, 21–25.

BRUNETTE, D. M., KANOZA, R. J. J., MARMARY, Y., CHAN, J. & MELCHER, A. H. (1977) Interactions between epithelial and fibroblast-like cells in cultures derived from monkey periodontal ligament. *J. Cell. Sci.* **27**, 127–140.

BRUNETTE, D. M., MELCHER, A. H. & MOE, H. K. (1976) Culture and origin of epithelium-like and fibroblast-like cells from porcine periodontal ligament explants and cell suspensions. *Archs. oral Biol.* **21**, 393–400.

CHO, M. & GARANT, P. R. (1978) Effects of colchicine on periodontal ligament fibroblasts of the mouse: 1. Cytoplasmic changes. *J. dent. Res.* **57**, Special issue A, 139.

COHN, S. A. (1965) Disuse atrophy of the periodontium in mice. *Archs. oral Biol.* **10**, 909–920.

COHN, S. A. (1966) Disuse atrophy of the periodontium in mice following partial loss of function. *Archs. oral Biol.* **11**, 95–105.

COMBS, J. W. (1966) Maturation of rat mast cells. An electron microscope study. *J. Cell. Biol.* **31**, 563–575.

DEPORTER, D. A. & TEN CATE, A. R. (1973) Fine structural localisation of acid and alkaline phosphatase in collagen-containing vesicles of fibroblasts. *J. Anat.* **114**, 457–461.

DOREY, C. K. & BICK, K. L. (1977) Ultrahistochemical analysis of glycosaminoglycan hydrolysis in the rat periodontal ligament. II. Aryl sulfatose and bone resorption. *Calcif. Tiss. Res.* **24**, 143–149.

DOTY, S. B., SCHOFIELD, B. H. & ROBINSON, R. A. (1967) The electron microscopic identification of acid phosphatase and adenosinetriphosphatase in bone cells following parathyroid extract or thyrocalcitonin administration. In: *Parathyroid hormone and thyrocalcitonin (calcitonin)*, R. V. TALMAGE and L. F. BÉLANGER (eds.), pp. 169–181. Amsterdam, Excerpta Medica.

EHRLICH, H. P. & BORNSTEIN, P. (1972) Microtubles in transcellular movement of procollagen. *Nature* **238**, 257–260.

ELEY, B. M. & HARRISON, J. D. (1975) Intracellular collagen fibrils in the periodontal ligament of man. *J. periodont. Res.* **10**, 168–170.

FRANK, R. M., FELLINGER, E. & STEUER, P. (1976) Ultrastructure du ligament alvéolo-dentaire du rat. *J. biol. Buccale* **4**, 295–313.

FREILICH, L. S. (1971) Ultrastructure and acid phosphatase cytochemistry of odontoclasts: Effects of parathyroid extract. *J. dent. Res.* **50**, 1047–1055.

FULLMER, H. M. (1967) Connective tissue components of the periodontium. In: *Structural and chemical organisation of teeth*, Vol. 2, A. E. W. MILES (ed.), pp. 349–414. London, Academic Press.

FURTH, R. van (1975) Modulation of monocyte production. In: *Mononuclear phagocytes in immunity infection and pathology*, R. VAN FURTH (ed.), pp. 161–174. Oxford, Blackwell.

GABBIANI, G. (1979) The role of contractile proteins in wound healing and fibrocontractive diseases. *Meth. Achiev. exp. Pathol.* **9**, 187–206.

GARANT, P. R. (1976) Collagen resorption by fibroblasts. *J. Periodont.* **47**, 380–390.

GOLDBERG, B. & RABINOVITCH, M. (1977) Connective tissue. In: *Histology* (4th ed.), L. WEISS & R. O. GREEP (eds.), pp. 145–178. New York, McGraw-Hill.

GOTHLIN, G. & ERICSSON, J. L. E. (1973a) Electron microscopic studies on the uptake and storage of thorium dioxide molecules in different cell types of fracture callus. *Ácta Path. Microbiol. Scand.* A: **81**, 523–543.

GOTHLIN, G. & ERICSSON, J. L. E. (1973b) On the histogenesis of the cells in fracture callus. Electron microscopic autoradiographic observations in parabiotic rats and studies on labelled monocytes. *Virchows Archs. Zellpathol.* **12**, 318–329.

GOTHLIN, G. & ERICSSON, J. L. E. (1976) The osteoclast. *Clin. Orthop. Rel. Res.* **120**, 201–231.

GOULD, T. R. L., MELCHER, A. H. & BRUNETTE, D. M. (1977) Location of progenitor cells in periodontal ligament of mouse molar stimulated by wounding. *Anat. Rec.* **188**, 133–142.

GRANT, D. A. & BERNICK, S. (1969) A possible continuity between epithelial rests and epithelial attachment in miniature swine. *J. Periodont.* **40**, 87–95.

GRANT, D. A. & BERNICK, S. (1972) The periodontium of ageing humans. *J. Periodont.* **43**, 660–667.

GRANT, M. A., HARWOOD, R. & SCHOFIELD, J. D. (1975) Recent studies on the assembly, intracellular processing and secretion of procollagen. In: *Dynamics of connective tissue macromolecules*, P. M. C. BURLEIGH & A. R. POOLE (eds.), pp. 1–29. Amsterdam, North-Holland.

GRUPE, H. E., TEN CATE, A. R. & ZANDER, H. A. (1967) A histochemical and radiobiological study of *in vitro* and *in vivo* human epithelial cell rest proliferation. *Archs. oral Biol.* **12**, 1321–1329.

HALL, B. K. (1975) The origin and fate of osteoclasts. *Anat. Rec.* **183**, 1–12.

HANCOX, N. M. (1972) The osteoclasts. In: *The biochemistry and physiology of bone*, Vol. I (2nd ed.), G. H. BOURNE (ed.), pp. 45–69. New York, Academic Press.

HEERSCHE, J. N. M. & DEPORTER, D. A. (1979) The mechanism of osteoclastic bone resorption: a new hypothesis. *J. periodont. Res.* **14**, 266–267.

HOLTROP, M. E. & WEINGER, J. M. (1972) Ultrastructural evidence for a transport system in bone. In: *Calcium parathyroid hormone and the calcitonins*, R. V. TALMAGE & P. L. MUNSON (eds.), pp. 365–374. Amsterdam, Excerpta Medica.

JEE, W. S. S. & NOLAN, P. D. (1963) Origin of osteoclasts from the fusion of phagocytes. *Nature* **200**, 225–226.

JENSEN, J. L. & TOTO, P. D. (1968) Radioactive labelling index of the periodontal ligament in ageing rats. *J. dent. Res.* **47**, 149–153.

JOTEREAU, F. V. & LE DOUARIN, N. M. (1978) The developmental relationship between osteocytes and osteoclasts: A study using the quail-chick nuclear marker in endochondral ossification. *Develop. Biol.* **63**, 253–265.

JOWSEY, J., KELLY, P. J., RIGGS, B. L., BIANCO, A. J., SCHOLZ, D. A. & GERSHON-COHEN, J. (1965) Quantitative microradiographic studies of normal and osteoporotic bone. *J. Bone Joint Surg. Amer.* **47A**, 785–806.

KALLIO, D. M., GARANT, P. R. & MINKIN, C. (1971) Evidence of coated membranes in the ruffled border of the osteoclast. *J. Ultrastruct. Res.* **37**, 169–177.

KANOZA, R. J. J., BRUNETTE, D. M., PURDON, A. D. & SODEK, J. (1978) Isolation and identification of epithelial-like cells in culture by a collagenase-separation technique. *In Vitro* **14**, 746–752.

KEMBER, N. F. (1960) Cell division in endochondral ossification. A study of cell proliferation in rat bones by the method of tritiated thymidine autoradiography. *J. Bone Joint Surg. Amer.* **42B**, 824–839.

KLINGSBERG, J. & BUTCHER, E. O. (1960) Comparative histology of age changes in oral tissues of rat, hamsters and monkey. *J. dent. Res.* **39**, 158–169.

LEESON, T. S. & LEESON, C. R. (1970) *Histology* (2nd ed.), p. 95. Philadelphia, Saunders.

LEIBOVICH, S. J. & ROSS, R. (1976) A macrophage-dependent factor that stimulates the proliferation of fibroblasts *in vitro*. *Amer. J. Pathol.* **84**, 501–513.

LESTER, K. S. (1969) The incorporation of epithelial cells by cementum. *J. Ultrastruct. Res.* **27**, 63–87.

LEVY, B. M., DREIZEN, S. & BERNICK, S. (1972) Effect of ageing on the marmoset periodontium. *J. oral Path.* **1**, 61–65.

LIMEBACK, H. F., SODEK, J. & BRUNETTE, D. M. (1978) Nature of collagens synthesised by monkey periodontal ligament fibroblasts *in vitro*. *Biochem. J.* **170**, 63–71.

LISTGARTEN, M. A. (1973) Intracellular collagen fibrils in the periodontal ligament of the mouse, rat, hamster, guinea pig and rabbit. *J. periodont. Res.* **8**, 335–342.

LISTGARTEN, M. A. (1975) Cell rests in the periodontal ligament of mouse molars. *J. periodont. Res.* **10**, 197–202.

LITWIN, J., LUNDQUIST, G. & SÖDER, P.-O. (1971) Studies on long term maintenance of teeth and viable associated cells *in vitro*. *Scand. J. Dent. Res.* **79**, 536–539.

LUK, S. C., NOPAGAROONSRI, C. & SIMON, G. T. (1974) The ultrastructure of endosteum. A topographic study in young adult rabbits. *J. Ultrastruct. Res.* **46**, 165–183.

MALKANI, K., LUXEMBOURGER, M. M. & REBEL, A. (1973) Cytoplasmic modifications at the contact zone of osteoclasts and calcified tissue in the diaphyseal growing plate of foetal guinea pig tibia. *Calcif. Tiss. Res.* **11**, 258–264.

MARMARY, Y., BRUNETTE, D. M. & HEERSCHE, J. N. M. (1976) Differences *in vitro* between cells derived from periodontal ligament and skin of *Macaca irus*. *Archs. oral Biol.* **21**, 709–716.

McHUGH, W. H. & ZANDER, H. A. (1965) Cell division in the periodontium of developing and erupted teeth. *Dent. Pract.* **15**, 451–457.

MELCHER, A. H. (1978) Biological process in resorption, deposition and regeneration of bone. In: *Periodontal surgery – Biological basis and technique*, S. S. STAHL (ed.), pp. 99–120. Springfield, Charles Thomas.

MELCHER, A. H., CHAN, J. & SVOBODA, E. (1978) Collagen phagocytosis by fibroblasts *in vivo*: a study of serial sections. *J. Cell Biol.* **79**, 151a.

MELCHER, A. H., REIMERS, S., BRUNETTE, D. M., FENG, J. & CHAN, J. (1978) A comparison between osteoclasts *in vitro* and *in vivo* in the periodontal ligament of the adult mouse. *Archs. oral Biol.* **23**, 1121–1125.

MELCHER, A. H. & TURNBULL, R. S. (1976) Organ culture in studies on the periodontium. In: *Organ culture in biomedical research*, M. BALLS & M. A. MONNICKENDAM (eds.), pp. 149–163. Cambridge, Cambridge University Press.

NYLEN, M. W. & GRUPE, H. E. (1969) Ultrastructure of epithelial cells in human periodontal ligament explants. *J. periodont. Res.* **4**, 248–258.

ORLOWSKI, W. A. (1978) Biochemical study of collagen turnover in rat incisor periodontal ligament. *Archs. oral Biol.* **23**, 1163–1165.

OWEN, M. (1970) The origin of bone cells. *Int. Rev. Cytol.* **28**, 213–238.

OWEN, M. (1971) Cellular dynamics in bone. In: *The biochemistry and physiology of bone,* Vol. III (2nd ed.), G. H. BOURNE (ed.), pp. 271–298. London, Academic Press.

OWEN, M. & SHETLAR, M. R. (1968) Uptake of ^{3}H-glucosamine by osteoclasts. *Nature* **220**, 1335–1336.

PARAKKAL, P. F. (1969) Involvement of macrophages in collagen resorption. *J. Cell Biol.* **41**, 345–354.

RAO, L. F., MOE, H. K. & HEERSCHE, J. N. M. (1978) *In vitro* culture of porcine periodontal ligament cells: response of fibroblast-like and epithelial-like cells to prostaglandin E_1, parathyroid hormone and calcitonin and separation of a pure population of fibroblast-like cells. *Archs. oral Biol.* **23**, 957–964.

RASMUSSEN, H. & BORDIER, P. (1974) *The physiological and cellular basis of metabolic bone disease.* Baltimore, Williams & Wilkins Co.

REEVE, C. M. & WENTZ, F. M. (1962) The prevalence, morphology and distribution of epithelial rests in the human periodontal ligament. *J. Oral Med. Oral Surg. Oral Path.* **15**, 785–793.

REINHOLDT, J., ANDREASEN, J. O., SÖDER, P.-O., OTTESKOG, P., DYBDAHL, R. & RIIS, I. (1977) Cultivation of periodontal ligament fibroblasts on extracted monkey incisors. A histological study of three culturing methods. *Int. J. Oral Surg.* **6**, 215–225.

REITAN, K. (1961) Behaviour of Malassez epithelial rests during orthodontic tooth movement. *Acta Odont. Scand.* **19**, 443–468.

RIPPIN, J. W. (1976) Collagen turnover in the periodontal ligament under normal and altered functional forces. I: Young rat molars. *J. periodont. Res.* **11**, 101–107.

ROBERTS, W. E. (1975) Cell population dynamics of periodontal ligament stimulated with parathyroid extract. *Amer. J. Anat.* **143**, 363–370.

ROBERTS, W. E. & CHAMBERLAIN, J. G. (1978) Scanning electron microscopy of the cellular elements of rat periodontal ligament. *Archs. oral Biol.* **23**, 587–589.

ROSE, G. G., YAJIMA, T. & MAHAN, C. J. (1978) Microscopic assay for the phagocytotic-collagenolytic performance (PCP Index) of human gingival fibroblast *in vitro. J. dent. Res.* **57**, 1003–1015.

ROSS, R. (1968) The connective tissue fiber forming cell. In: *Treatise on collagen.* Vol. 2: *Biology of collagen,* Part A. B. S. GOULD (ed.), pp. 2–82. London, Academic Press.

ROSSMAN, L. E., ROSENBLOOM, J. & ROBINSON, P. (1975) Biosynthesis of collagen in isolated periodontal ligament. *J. dent. Res.* **54**, 1115–1119.

SCHROEDER, T. E. (1973) Actin in dividing cells: contractile ring filaments bind heavy meromyosin. *Proc. Natl. Acad. Sci. USA* **70**, 1688–1692.

SCOTT, B. L. (1967) Thymidine-^{3}H electron microscope radioautography of osteogenic cells in fetal rat. *J. Cell Biol.* **35**, 115–126.

SELYE, H. (1965) *The mast cell.* Washington, Butterworths.

SHORE, R. C. & BERKOVITZ, B. K. B. (1979) An ultrastructural study of periodontal ligament fibroblasts in relation to their possible role in tooth eruption and intracellular collagen degradation in the rat. *Archs. oral Biol.* **24**, 155–164.

SHORE, R. C., BERKOVITZ, B. K. B. & MOXHAM, B. J. (in press). Intercellular contacts between fibroblasts in the periodontal connective tissues of the rat. *J. Anat. Lond.*

SODEK, J. (1976) A new approach to assessing collagen turnover by using a microassay. *Biochem. J.* **160**, 243–246.

SODEK, J. (1977) A comparison of the rates of synthesis and turnover of collagen and non-collagenous protein in adult rat periodontal tissues and skin using a microassay. *Archs. oral Biol.* **22**, 655–665.

SODEK, J. (1978) A comparison of collagen and non-collagenous protein metabolism in rat molar and incisor periodontal ligaments. *Archs. oral Biol.* **23**, 977–982.

SÖDER, P.-O. & LUNDQUIST, G. (1972) Autotransplantation of teeth with use of cell cultivation technique. *Int. dent. J.* **22**, 327–340.

SUTTON, J. S. & WEISS, L. (1966) Transformation of monocytes in tissue culture into macrophages, epitheloid cells and multi-nucleate giant cells. An electron microscopic study. *J. Cell Biol.* **28**, 303–332.

SVOBODA, E. L. A., BRUNETTE, D. M. & MELCHER, A. H. (1979) *In vitro* phagocytosis of exogenous collagen by fibroblasts from the periodontal ligament: an electron microscopic study. *J. Anat.* **128**, 301–314.

TEN CATE, A. R. (1965) The histochemical demonstration of specific oxidative enzymes and glycogen in the epithelial cell rests of Malassez. *Archs. oral Biol.* **10**, 207–213.

TEN CATE, A. R. (1967) The formation and function of the epithelial cell rests of Malassez. In: *The mechanisms of tooth support,* D. J. ANDERSON, J. E. EASTOE, A. H. MELCHER & D. C. A. PICTON (eds.), pp. 80–83. Bristol, Wright & Sons.

TEN CATE, A. R. (1972) Morphological studies of fibrocytes in connective tissue undergoing rapid remodelling. *J. Anat.* **112**, 401–414.

TEN CATE, A. R. & DEPORTER, D. A. (1975) The degradative role of the fibroblast in the remodelling and turnover of collagen in soft connective tissue. *Anat. Rec.* **182**, 1–14.

TEN CATE, A. R., DEPORTER, D. A. & FREEMAN, E. (1976) The role of fibroblasts in the remodelling of the periodontal ligament during physiologic tooth movement. *Amer. J. Orthod.* **69**, 155–168.

TEN CATE, A. R. & FREEMAN, E. (1974) Collagen remodelling by fibroblasts in wound repair – preliminary observations. *Anat. Rec.* **179**, 543–546.

TEN CATE, A. R. & SYRBU, S. (1974) Relationship between alkaline phosphatase activity and the phagocytosis and degradation of collagen by the fibroblasts. *J. Anat.* **117**, 351–359.

TONNA, E. A. (1960) Osteoclasts and the aging skeleton: a cytological, cytochemical and autoradiographic study. *Anat. Rec.* **137**, 251–270.

TONNA, E. A. & CRONKITE, E. P. (1961) Use of tritiated thymidine for the study of the origin of the osteoclast. *Nature* **190**, 459–460.

TONNA, E. A. & STAHL, S. S. (1974) Comparative assessment of the cell proliferative activities of injured paradontal tissues in aging mice. *J. dent. Res.* **53**, 609–622.

TOTO, P. D. & BORG, M. (1968) Effect of age changes on the premitotic index in the periodontium of mice. *J. dent. Res.* **47**, 70–73.

TOTO, P. D. & KWAN, H. W. (1970) Doubling time of labelled periodontal cells of rats. *J. dent. Res.* **49,** 1017–1019.

TOTO, P. D., RUBENSTEIN, A. S. & GARGIULO, A. W. (1975) Labelling index and cell density of aging rat oral tissues. *J. dent. Res.* **54,** 553–556.

VALDERHAUG, J. P. (1974) Epithelial cells in the periodontal membrane of teeth with and without periapical inflammation. *Int. J. oral Surg.* **3,** 7–16.

VALDERHAUG, J. P. & NYLEN, M. V. (1966) Function of epithelial rests as suggested by their ultrastructure. *J. periodont. Res.* **1,** 69–78.

VALDERHAUGH, J. & ZANDER, H. (1967) Relationship of 'epithelial rests of Malassez' to other periodontal structures. *J. Am. Soc. Periodont.* **5,** 254–258.

WALKER, D. G. (1961) Citric acid cycle in osteoblasts and osteoclasts. A histochemical study of normal and parathormone-treated rats. *Bull. Johns Hopkins Hosp.* **108,** 80–99.

WEINSTOCK, M. & LEBLOND, C. P. (1974) Formation of collagen. *Fed. Proc.* **33,** 1205–1218.

WEISS, R., STAHL, S. S. & TONNA, E. A. (1968) Functional demands on the cell proliferative activity of the rat periodontium studied autoradiographically. *J. dent. Res.* **47,** 1153–1157.

WENTZ, F. M., WEINMANN, J. P. & SCHOUR, I. (1950) The prevalence distribution and morphologic changes of the epithelial remnants in the molar region of the rat. *J. dent. Res.* **29,** 637–646.

WHITTLE, B. J. R. (1977) Prostaglandins and mast cell histamine. In: *Prostaglandins and thromboxanes,* F. BERTI, B. SAMUELSSON & G. P. VELO (eds.), pp. 345–352. New York, Plenum Press.

WONG, G. & COHN, D. V. (1974) Separation of parathyroid hormone and calcitonin-sensitive cells from non-responsive bone cells. *Nature* **252,** 713–714.

YAEGER, J. A. & KRAUCUNAS, E. (1969) Fine structure of the resorptive cells in the teeth of frogs. *Anat. Rec.* **164,** 1–14.

YAJIMA, T. & ROSE, G. G. (1977) Phagocytosis of collagen by human gingival fibroblasts *in vitro. J. dent. Res.* **56,** 1271–1277.

YEN, H. E. K. & MELCHER, A. H. (1978) A continuous-flow culture system for organ culture of large explants of adult tissue: Effect of oxygen tension on mouse molar periodontium. *In Vitro* **14,** 811–818.

YOUNG, R. W. (1962) Cellular proliferation and specialization during endochondrial osteogenesis in young rats. *J. Cell Biol.* **14,** 357–370.

YOUNG, R. W. (1963) Nucleic acids, protein synthesis and bone. *Clin. Orthop. and rel. Res.* **26,** 147–160.

YOUNG, R. W. (1964) Specialisation of bone cells. In: *Bone biodynamics,* H. M. FROST (ed.), pp. 117–139. Boston, Little, Brown & Co.

Chapter 3

STRUCTURAL ORGANIZATION OF THE FIBRES OF THE PERIODONTAL LIGAMENT

P. Sloan

TYPES OF FIBRES

The fibres make up a considerable part of the extra-cellular substance of connective tissues and are believed to be largely responsible for their physical properties. Water, ground substance and in some cases mineral are closely associated with the fibres in varying amounts and diverse structural arrangements are found according to the mechanical function required of the tissue (Eastoe, 1976; Jackson, 1976). In common with most connective tissues, the most abundant fibre type in the periodontal ligament is collagen.

Collagen and reticulin

The collagen of the periodontal ligament is mostly Type I though some Type III is present (Butler *et al.*, 1975). The periodontal collagen is formed into fibrils at an early stage in the ligament's development, by the process of extracellular fibrillogenesis (Freeman and Ten Cate, 1971). It would appear from all published electron micrographs that, in the

mammalian periodontal ligament, the individual collagen fibrils comprising fibre bundles tend to be of a fairly uniform width of approximately 55 nm (Fig. 1a). This is a small diameter compared to, for example, tendon, where the fibrils are 100–250 nm in diameter. This large size may be related to a relatively high content of side chains or non-collagenous macromolecules in the tissue (Spiro, 1972; Jackson, 1976). Large fibril diameters have been associated with ageing of tissue (Torp, Baer and Friedman, 1975), suggesting that the small fibril diameter in the periodontal ligament could be related to the high rate of collagen turnover. Fibrils having a diameter of up to 250 nm have been found in association with 55 nm fibrils in the periodontal ligament of a non-mammalian vertebrate *Caiman sclerops,* in which turnover may be slower than in mammals (Berkovitz and Sloan, 1979: Fig. 1b). Although the cross-banding period of the individual fibrils is typically 65 nm (Fig. 2), few systematic surveys of the fibril dimensions of any periodontal ligament have been published. Recently, Berkovitz, Weaver, Shore and Moxham (in press) have shown that, for the rat mandibular dentition, the fibril diameters range from 17–70 nm with a mean of about 45 nm. No

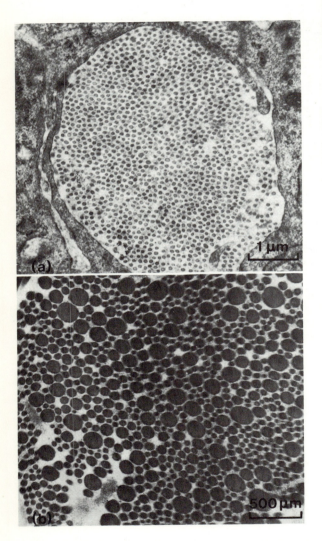

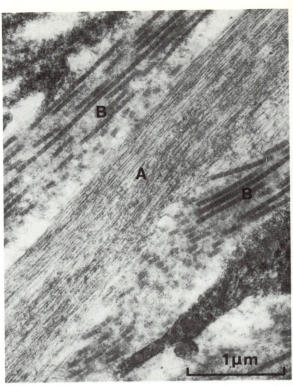

FIG. 2. Transmission electron micrograph showing a longitudinally sectioned oxytalan fibre (A) comprised largely of a parallel assemblage of microfibrils, and some collagen fibrils (B) which exhibit periodic crossbanding at 65 nm intervals.

FIG. 1. (a) Transmission electron micrograph showing a transversely sectioned collagen bundle in the rat periodontal ligament. The collagen fibrils have a uniform diameter of approximately 55 nm and exhibit a punctate appearance. (b) Transmission electron micrograph showing a transversely sectioned collagen bundle in the Caiman periodontal ligament. Collagen fibrils having a range of diameters of approximately 55–250 nm are present. (From Berkovitz and Sloan, 1979.)

significant differences were observed between the fibrils in the periodontal ligament of the continuously growing incisor, the periodontal ligament of the non-continuously growing molar and the enamel-related connective tissue of the incisor. Whilst Parry and Craig (1979) claimed that collagen fibrils have diameters which are multiples of 8 nm, such characteristics were not seen for the periodontal tissues.

The vast majority of collagen fibrils in the periodontal ligament are believed to be grouped together to form bundles (Melcher and Eastoe, 1969; Figs. 1a, 3), though their precise arrangement is controversial.

Cross-banded collagen fibrils also occur in a non-aggregated form. Such fibrils are probably composed of Type III collagen and are associated with abundant

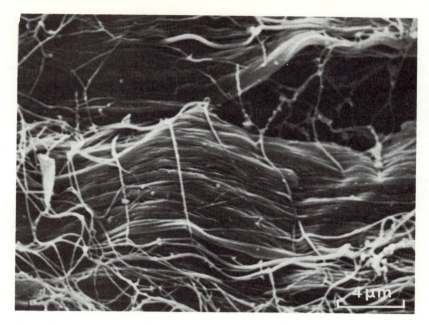

FIG. 3. Scanning electron micrograph of a sheet of α-amylase treated collagen in the rabbit periodontal ligament. Individual collagen fibrils, some exhibiting a periodic beaded structure, can be resolved.

ground substance forming the material known as reticulin (Melcher and Eastoe, 1969; Eastoe, 1976). Though reticulin forms a supporting framework in the lympho-reticular system, its mechanical properties are likely to be inferior to those of aggregated collagen fibres. It is therefore unlikely that reticulin plays a supportive role in the periodontal ligament. Reticulin is often confused with developing collagen, as both materials are argyrophilic and often occur in the same site. Melcher (1966) has suggested that in the developing periodontal ligament reticulin may form a lattice-work in which the highly orientated principal fibres develop. Persistence of such a lattice-work would account for the presence of reticulin in the formed periodontal ligament.

Oxytalan

Special connective tissue fibres, termed by Fullmer and Lillie (1958) oxytalan fibres, have been found in the periodontal ligaments of man, monkeys, guinea pigs, rats and mice (Fullmer, 1959, 1961; Lieberman,

1960; Carmichael and Fullmer, 1966; Simpson, 1967; Sims, 1973, 1975; Sheetz, Fullmer and Narkates, 1973; Fullmer, Sheetz and Narkates, 1974; Edmunds *et al.*, 1979). These fibres have a similar distribution to the elastin fibres which occur in the periodontal ligaments of deer, swine, cattle and dogs and are believed to be related to elastin fibres (Fullmer, Sheetz and Narkates, 1974). They have never been isolated, however, and therefore very little is known of their composition or properties. The available data concerning oxytalan fibres has, perforce, been obtained using histochemical and ultrastructural techniques.

Oxytalan fibres are characterized by their ability to stain with aldehyde fuchsin only after their oxidation with a suitable oxidizing agent (Fullmer, 1960; Rannie, 1963). As this is also a property of pre-elastin fibres, it is impossible to distinguish between the two fibre types histochemically. Also, oxytalan and pre-elastin fibres have a similar ultrastructural appearance in that they both consist of an organized assemblage of fibrils 5–15 nm in diameter arranged parallel to the long axis of the fibre and with variable amounts of amorphous interfibrillar material (Fig.

2). It seems impossible therefore, at the present time, to know whether oxytalan fibres are modified pre-elastin fibres which do not become infilled with elastin (Ross, 1973), or whether they represent a completely different type of fibre.

Sims (1977) found that oxytalan fibres retained their histochemical properties and could be distinguished from elastin fibres in experimental lathyrism. In prolonged lathyrism, when the collagen and elastin in the mouse periodontium exhibited marked changes, the oxytalan fibre network persisted and retained its histochemical properties. Thus, it seems that although there may be some relationship between oxytalan and elastin fibres, the two types are metabolically distinct in character.

Elastin

Elastin fibres are composed of a glycoprotein microfibrillar component and an amorphous component which is a protein rubber, elastin (Ross, 1973). Early in their formation elastin fibres appear as aggregates of microfibrils. With maturation, elastin forms in the interstices of the microfibrils. When fully formed, the fibres consist largely of elastin surrounded by an envelope of microfibrils, though some microfibrils remain embedded in the elastin core (Ross, 1973; Kadar, 1974). On the basis of biochemical characterization studies, Gray, Sandberg and Foster (1973) proposed that the elementary units of elastin were rod-like in shape and a rod-like structure has been observed by Gotte et al. (1974) using high-resolution ultrastructural techniques. The elementary units are probably aggregated into globular protein masses with free solvent in the intervening spaces (Partridge, 1967; Kadar, 1974). Such a model, in which the globular protein masses are compressed or restrained by their hydrophobic tendency, is in accord with the thermodynamic behaviour of elastin (Wainwright et al., 1976). Elastin usually occurs in association with collagen and may function as a static elastic element in a pliant composite or as a resilient material (Wainwright et al., 1976; Serafini-Fracassini et al., 1977).

Prominent elastin fibres are present in the coronal one-third of the periodontal ligaments of the rabbit, dog, sheep, swine and deer (Fullmer, 1960; Fullmer, Sheetz and Narkates, 1974). In the herbivorous mammals, the pronounced nature and arrangement of the fibres suggest that they may play a role in damping lateral masticatory stresses. In this situation the low modulus and long-range reversible extensibility of elastin would seem to be more important than resilience as a physical property.

Elastin fibres are not present in the periodontal ligaments of man and many other mammals. However, oxytalan fibres are usually present where elastin fibres are absent. A phylogenetic relationship between the two fibre types may exist, which is connected with differing mechanical requirements for tooth support. Further comparative studies are needed to shed light on this problem.

ARRANGEMENT OF FIBRES

Unless otherwise stated, the descriptions given in this section relate to teeth of limited growth.

Collagen

The standard textbook picture of the fibrous architecture of the periodontal ligament collagen (Fig. 4) is derived from studies published around the turn of the century. Black (1887, 1899) described the organization of the collagen into bundles termed principal fibres and the arrangement of the bundles into gingival, crestal, horizontal, oblique and apical groups (Figs. 4 and 5). Other fibres were described interspersed between the principal fibre bundles, termed indifferent fibres. The principal fibre bundles were considered to pass directly from tooth to bone, thus supporting the tooth in the manner of a sling. More recent studies (Sloan, 1979 a, b) have questioned certain aspects of this arrangement.

In the light microscope, the bundles appear to split into smaller branches within the ligament, forming a continuous network with narrow meshes (Zwarych and Quigley, 1965; Grant et al., 1972). Such histological investigations into the arrangement of the periodontal fibres are, however, limited by the lack of specific stains for differentiating collagen

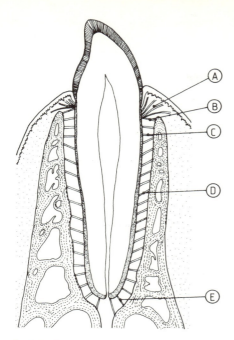

FIG. 4. Diagram to show the arrangement of the periodontal collagen into groups of principal fibre bundles as follows: A = gingival, B = crestal, C = horizontal, D = oblique, E = apical.

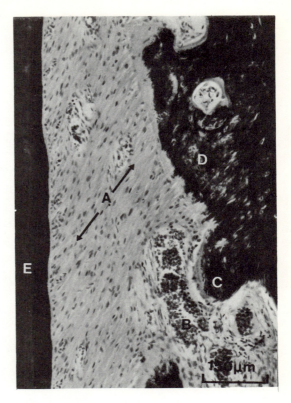

G. 5. Photomicrograph showing the orientation of the lique fibres (A) in the human periodontal ligament. A neurovascular bundle (B) is present in the ligament close to alveolar bone (C). The principal fibres are continuous with Sharpey fibres in bone (D) and cementum (E). Masson's trichrome.

fibres and ground substances and the difficulty of deducing the three-dimensional arrangement of the fibres from two-dimensional sections.

In the transmission electron microscope (TEM), collagen fibrils can be identified by their dimensions and cross-banding (Figs. 1, 2), though in extremely thin sections a granular appearance which can be confused with resorbing collagen may be seen (Melcher and Chan, 1978). The majority of the collagen appears to be organized into bundles in all regions of the periodontal ligament (Bevelander and Nakahara, 1968; Ten Cate, 1972; Frank, Fellinger and Steuer, 1976). The usefulness of TEM in deducing the three-dimensional arrangement is limited, however, by the extreme thinness of the sections used. The use of scanning electron microscopy (SEM) overcomes this problem.

In the SEM, the appearance of the tissue varies greatly with the preparation technique used (Sloan, Shellis and Berkovitz, 1976). When an abrasive disc was used on undecalcified tissue a markedly different

tissue organization was seen compared with tissues which had been decalcified and carefully cut with a razor blade or with freeze-fractured surfaces (Fig. 6). Using material prepared by discing, Shackleford (1971, 1973) and Svejda and Skach (1973) claimed that the majority of the ligament collagen is randomly orientated, producing the appearance of an indifferent fibre plexus. However, since this view cannot be correlated with light and transmission electron microscope studies, the arrangement seems unlikely. In other SEM studies using macaque and human periodontal ligaments which were prepared by slicing demineralized jaws, Sloan (1978b, 1979b) found that the majority of the collagen fibrils were organized into bundles. It is likely, therefore, that the indifferent fibre plexus is an artefact produced by the method of preparation.

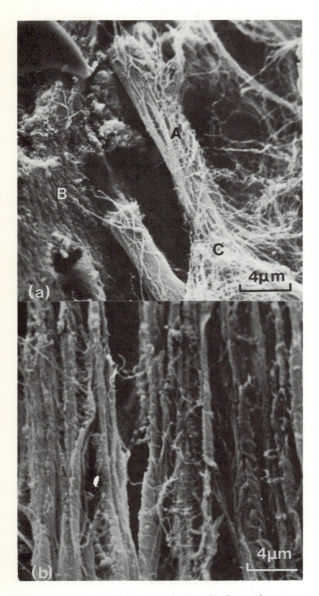

FIG. 6. (a) Scanning electron micrograph of a rat jaw transversely sectioned in the molar region with an abrasive disc. Principal fibre bundles (A) are present adjacent to alveolar bone (B) and merge with the 'indifferent plexus' (C) which makes up the main bulk of the periodontal ligament. (b) Scanning electron micrograph of a demineralized rat jaw, transversely sectioned with a razor blade. A branching network of principal fibre bundles is present throughout the entire width of the molar ligament.

The following description of the arrangement of the collagen fibres of the periodontal ligament, as seen in SEM, is derived from the reports of Sloan (1978b, 1979b). The macaque or human periodontal ligament appears as a fibrous band, 100–150 μm in width, which contains many large blood vessels which run mainly longitudinally (Fig. 7). At high magnifications, in both transversely and longitudinally sectioned specimens, the regions between the blood vessels are composed of profiles of fibre bundles which have been sectioned in a variety of planes. The bundle profiles are often curved, suggesting that the bundles pursue a complex wavy course. Fibroblasts, often possessing extensive flattened cytoplasmic processes, can be seen lying between the bundles (Fig. 8). The individual collagen fibrils which make up the bundle can also be seen and the arrangements of bundles and cells is such as to allow close contact between the fibrils and the cytoplasmic extensions. This arrangement would facilitate remodelling of these fibrils by intracellular degradation (as discussed in Chapters 2 and 4).

The collagen fibre bundles form branching networks which course around the neurovascular bundles. Close to cementum, the bundles are 3–10 μm in diameter, whilst close to the alveolar wall they are 10–20 μm in diameter. The majority of the remaining bundles in the ligament are 1–4 μm in diameter. Because of the frequent branching and anastomosing and the wavy course pursued by these bundles, it is impossible to trace an intact network of bundles across the periodontal space. Polarizing microscopy has shown that the networks of bundles have a complex arrangement relative to each other (Sloan, 1979b). In transverse sections viewed between crossed polars, the birefringence of the collagen is greatest in the 45° position suggesting a predominance of radially orientated fibres. When such regions are examined in the 90° position, individual networks of bundles can be seen crossing each other and curving around the neurovascular bundles. Overlapping bundle networks can also be seen in longitudinal sections within the horizontal, oblique and apical groups. The bundles often pursue a wavy course and crimping is frequently seen in both section planes. Overlapping layers of highly orientated bundle networks can also be seen in the SEM in specimens prepared by tearing critical-point dried material (Sloan, 1978b).

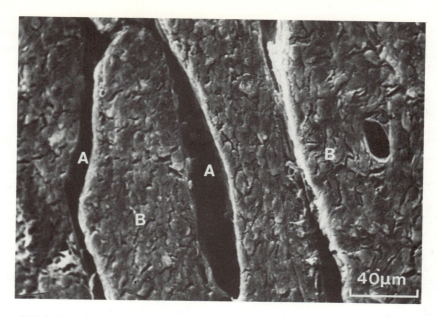

FIG. 7. Scanning electron micrograph of macaque periodontal ligament lying between cementum (left) and bone (right of field), longitudinally sectioned in the mid-root region. The blood vessels (A) are mostly longitudinally orientated and are surrounded by profiles of densely packed collagen bundles (B).

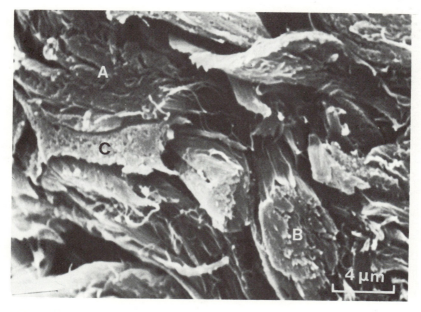

FIG. 8. Scanning electron micrograph of macaque periodontal ligament showing a curved collagen bundle sectioned in two places (A, B) and a fibroblast (C).

Using this method, the individual bundles also appear to be 1–4 μm in diameter and branch and anastomose frequently within the networks. The networks are obliquely orientated to the long axis of the tooth and descend apically from the alveolar surface (Fig. 9).

Thus, the periodontal fibres are grouped into highly organized bundles which are arranged into networks having a complex three-dimensional overlapping arrangement. However, a different arrangement of the collagen fibres is present in the periodontal tissues of some continuously growing teeth. For example, in the rabbit incisor the collagen is arranged into sheets (Sloan, 1978a).

The continuously growing incisor has been used extensively to study the appearance of the 'structure' termed the intermediate plexus. The collagen fibres in these teeth appear to be arranged into three layers (Fig. 10) (Sicher, 1923; Hunt, 1959; Ness and Smale, 1959; Eccles, 1964; Ciancio, Neiders and Hazen, 1967, Beertsen and Snijder, 1969, Beertsen, Everts and van den Hooff, 1974; Beertsen and Everts, 1977). All are agreed that, in the bone-related and tooth-related layers, the collagen is organized into bundles which are continuous with mineralized Sharpey fibres. Until recently, the fibrous arrange-

ment of the middle layer was less clear. Sicher (1923, 1942) proposed that in the middle layer the fibres were spliced together to form an intermediate plexus. This arrangement seemed to provide an explanation accounting for the mechanism whereby remodelling of the ligament occurred during eruption. It is now thought that the intermediate plexus is a histological artefact. While the three layers can be seen clearly in axial sections, in certain transverse sections the fibres form a continuous branching network (Ciancio et al., 1967; Hindle, 1967). However, from observations of the periodontal ligament of the rabbit incisor, Sloan (1978a) proposed a model (Fig. 11) which accounts for these histological appearances. The model is based on direct examination of the ligament using SEM. In this model, the collagen in the bone-related (alveolar) and tooth-related (cemental) layers is organized into approximately circular bundles (Fig. 12), the alveolar layer bundles being larger than the cemental layer bundles. The collagen fibres are orientated radially and those in the middle layer are arranged into thin sheets. These sheets form a series of flattened compartments which run in the long axis of the tooth (Fig. 13). A fibrous arrangement such as this is in accord with the histological obser-

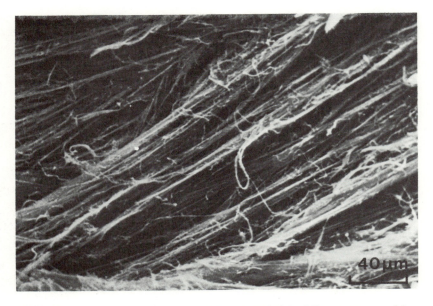

FIG. 9. Scanning electron micrograph of human periodontal ligament prepared by tearing critical-point dried material, showing overlapping networks of bundles.

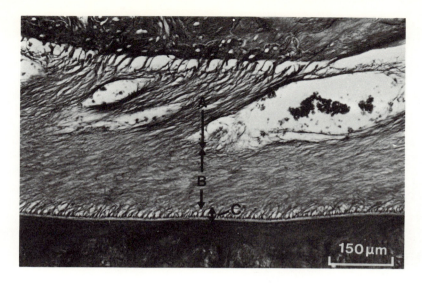

FIG. 10. Photomicrograph of a longitudinal section of rabbit incisor showing the arrangement of the periodontal ligament into three layers. The alveolar layer collagen (A) is arranged into groups of circular bundles separated by blood vessels. The middle layer collagen (B) is arranged into sheets, whilst that in the cemental layer (C) is organized into more evenly distributed bundles. Gordon and Sweets silver impregnation.

vations of Sicher (1923), Hindle (1967) and Ciancio *et al.* (1967), that the appearance of three distinct fibrous layers is more evident in axial than in transverse sections of continuously growing teeth. From the SEM observations it would seem that the appearance is due to the fact that, in axial section, the sheets of collagen lie in the section plane and do not appear as bundles as they do in transverse section. Arrangement of the middle layer fibres into sheets may also be in accord with the observation of Ness and Smale (1959) that the fibroblasts centrally in the rabbit incisor ligament seem to possess cytoplasmic extensions flattened in the longitudinal plane.

Attempts have been made to determine whether the collagen fibres in the middle layer differ from those of the other layers using polarizing microscopy and histochemistry. Hindle (1967), using polarizing microscopy, concluded that the collagen fibres in the middle layer were less mature than those of the alveolar and cemental layers, on account of their relatively low birefringence. However, the lower birefringence can be explained by the spatial distribution of the collagen fibres occurring as a result of their arrangement in sheets. The polarizing properties

of the ligament have recently been reinvestigated and the birefringence of the middle layer was found to vary with the plane of section whilst that of the other layers remained constant (Sloan, 1979a). In transverse section the middle layer collagen appeared as a network of birefringement bundles, whereas in longitudinal section the middle layer collagen showed only patchy birefringence. This effect could be explained entirely by the arrangement of the middle layer collagen into sheets proposed on the basis of the SEM findings. The highly orientated collagen fibres which make up a sheet would produce measurable birefringence when the sheet was transversely sectioned. A longitudinal section, however, would include several sheets or parts of sheets, separated by intervening cells. This separation, together with a variation in the orientation of fibrils between adjacent sheets, would produce a generally lowered and patchy birefringence.

On the basis of a polychrome staining technique, Kraw and Enlow (1967) concluded that the middle layer was composed of precollagenous fibres. The polychrome stain used (Herovici, 1963 a, b) is based on methylene blue staining of young collagen fibres

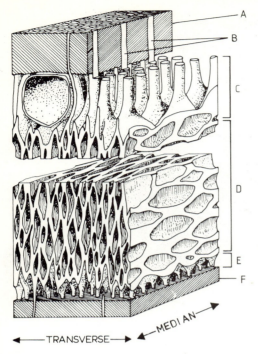

FIG. 11. Model representing the arrangement of the collagen in the periodontal ligament of the continuously growing incisor, showing alveolar bone (A) with mineralized Sharpey fibres (B) which are continuous with ligament bundles in the alveolar layer (C). The middle layer collagen (D) is arranged into sheets running in the median longitudinal plane, whilst that in the cemental layer (E) is arranged into bundles which are inserted into cementum (F).

and is supposed to differentiate between precollagenous (stained blue) and collagenous (stained red) fibres. The stain was also used by Van Bladeren (1972) to study the distribution of collagenous and precollagenous fibres in the developing rat periodontal ligament. In the incisor, both during development and with function, three layers were present. In direct contradiction to the findings of Kraw and Enlow (1967), the fibres of the middle layer appeared more mature than those of the alveolar or cemental layers. Such contradictory results emphasize the 'idiosyncratic' nature of the staining method. Currently, histochemical techniques have failed to localize any special layer of fibre remodelling within the periodontal ligament which could act as a zone of shear.

It is apparent that histological studies have not solved the problem of where the periodontal ligament collagen remodels. Several workers have used autoradiography to investigate the periodontal ligament collagen directly, as it has been shown that many apparently stable structures turn over at the molecular level (Lapiere, 1967). A high turnover rate of periodontal collagen has been reported in studies based on measurement of uptake of tritiated proline (Stallard, 1963; Crumley, 1964; Carneiro and Leblond, 1966; Ramos and Hunt, 1967; Anderson, 1967; Magnusson, 1968; Skougaard, Levy and Simpson, 1970; Robins, 1972) and tritiated glycine (Carneiro and Fava de Moraes, 1965; Carneiro and Leblond, 1966; Thomas, 1967). The half-life of the collagen was reported as varying between 3 and 23 days. At best, such results are only semi-quantitative, as uptake of the labelled amino acid precursor alone was measured. These studies failed to demonstrate any layer within the ligament where collagen turnover was localized, or higher than elsewhere, though differences were noted between apical and crestal regions. However, the proportions of labelled amino acid precursor taken up specifically into the collagen was not measured. Orlowski (1976), using microchemical techniques for the determination of hydroxyproline, found that most proline was incorporated into non-collagenous proteins in rat molar ligament after 24 hours. This finding was disputed by Sodek et al. (1977) and Sodek (1977) who, using a more refined microassay technique, found hydroxyproline incorporation into collagen to be high. In all three studies, the collagen turnover was estimated to be several times greater in the periodontal ligament than in skin or oral mucosa.

Recently, an autoradiographic technique which allows more accurate measurement of collagen turnover from histological sections has been used to investigate the rat molar ligament (Rippin, 1976 a, b). Tritiated proline was administered by intraperitoneal injection and groups of animals were killed at intervals over a 12-day period. Following autoradiography, grain densities were determined in various regions of the ligament and regression lines of log grain density were plotted against time after administration of the label. Because the log activity/time curves were linear, they were almost certainly related to a single proline-containing protein (probably collagen) in

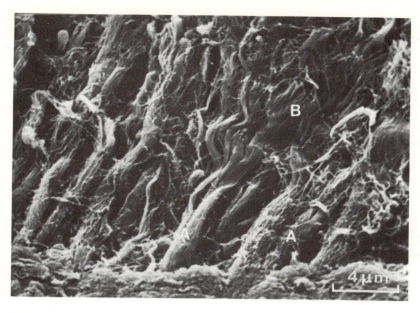

FIG. 12. Scanning electron micrograph showing collagen bundles (A) in the cemental layer of the rabbit periodontal ligament which fan out into the middle layer (B).

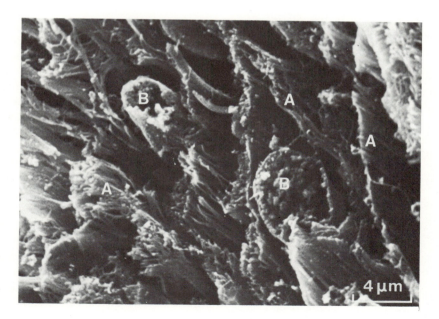

FIG. 13. Scanning electron micrograph showing transversely sectioned sheets of collagen (A) in the middle layer of the rabbit periodontal ligament. Fibroblast nuclei (B) are present within compartments formed by the sheets.

each region studied. Half-lives calculated from the regression lines showed that collagen turnover varied. For example, in the crestal region, rates varied from 2.45 to 6.47 days. However, in all the regions studied a high turnover seemed to occur over the whole width of the ligament. This finding does not support the concept of a localized layer of rapid remodelling in the middle of the ligament. Baumhammers and Stallard (1968) studied the turnover of ground substance using labelled sulphated glycosaminoglycans, and found no region or layer within the ligament where turnover was localized.

Beertsen and Everts (1977) claimed that a zone of shear exists towards the mid-region of the periodontal ligament, the inner dental zone moving with the tooth, the outer alveolar zone remaining behind. Their evidence is derived from studies of the pattern of uptake and subsequent loss of tritiated proline. Initially, grain densities were found to be highest in the basal region but with time there was a shift of the peak of labelling occlusally at a rate comparable with that of tooth eruption, this shift being interpreted as evidence for the movement of the inner dental zone of the periodontal ligament. The outer alveolar zone was assumed to remain stationary. However, a model has been presented based upon differential rates of turnover of collagen, which explains these observations without requiring any movement of the extracellular protein (Shore and Berkovitz, 1979).

The absence of a zone of shear in the mid-region of the periodontal ligament is also indicated by the results of an ultrastructural study of the rat incisor ligament following root resection (Berkovitz, Shore and Sloan, 1980). Following resection, it was found that the periodontal ligament persisted for a short distance beneath the erupting tooth fragment lining the vacated socket. Almost the entire width of the ligament was present and its fibrous architecture was maintained. Such evidence places the zone of shear close to the tooth surface. These results also suggest that remodelling is not specifically related to a zone of shear, and favour the concept of piecemeal remodelling.

In teeth of limited growth, the presence of three layers within the periodontal ligament has been described during development and eruption using light microscopy (Eccles, 1959; Kerebel and Balouet, 1967; Levy and Bernick, 1968; Levy, Dreizen and Bernick, 1972; Grant et al., 1972) and SEM (Sloan, 1978b). By the time functional occlusion is reached, the collagen fibres which are attached to bone and cementum are organized as bundles continuous with the mineralized parts of Sharpey fibres.

Examination of the periodontal ligament fibres in polarized light and by SEM has shown that the collagen fibre bundles having a wavy course have a crimped structure. The crimping is thought to be important in conferring certain physical properties to the ligament and is discussed in Chapter 5.

At their insertions, the collagen bundles of the periodontal ligament are embedded into cementum and alveolar bone in a fashion similar to tendon inserting into bone — that is, in the form of mineralized Sharpey fibres. On the basis of ultrastructural and microradiographic observations, Dreyfuss and Frank (1964) and Selvig (1965) stated that most of the Sharpey fibres have unmineralized cores and are separated from each other by mineralized fibres which run parallel to the mineral surface or are randomly arranged. The orientation of the Sharpey fibres in bone is similar to that of the adjacent ligament bundles (Melcher and Eastoe, 1969) while a variety of orientations are seen in cementum (Selvig, 1964, 1965). The light microscope observations of Quigley (1970) and Cohn (1972 a, b, 1975) suggested that in mice, hamsters, monkey and man some Sharpey fibres pass right through alveolar bone. This indicates that there may be continuity between the collagen fibres of the periodontal ligaments of adjacent teeth. The existence of these transalveolar fibres has been disputed on histological grounds as many Sharpey fibres do not pass completely through bone (Atkinson, 1978).

Boyde (1968, 1972), Boyde and Jones (1968) and Jones and Boyde (1972, 1974) studied the surface of alveolar bone and cementum using SEM after removing the soft covering connective tissue by enzymatic or chemical means. They found that Sharpey fibres may be mineralized to a level above (Fig. 14) or below the level of the mineralized bone matrix (Fig. 15), depending on their state of development. Where the fibres insert obliquely, the bone surface exhibits a stepped appearance and it has been suggested (Jones and Boyde, 1972) that mineralization occurs at approximately right angles to the long axis of the fibre, the mineralized periphery possibly

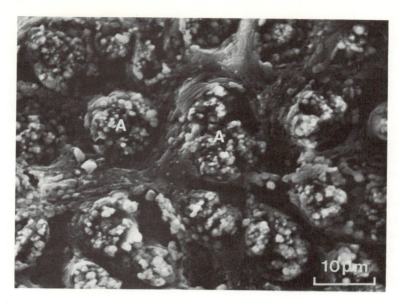

FIG. 14. Scanning electron micrograph of hypochlorite-treated alveolar bone. The mineralized parts of the Sharpey fibres (A) appear as projecting stubs covered with mineral clusters.

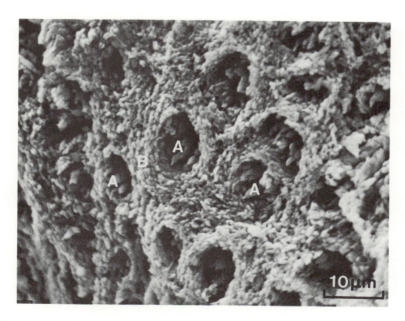

FIG. 15. Scanning electron micrograph of human alveolar bone treated with hypochlorite to expose the mineral surface. The mineralized parts of the Sharpey fibres (A) are concave relative to the matrix (B) and are studded with mineral clusters.

conferring some local mechanical advantage for transmitting axially-directed forces. Ultrastructural examination of the alveolar and cemental surfaces of undemineralized specimens of rat and of human alveolus (Fig. 16) has confirmed the SEM view. The mineral 'surface' of each Sharpey fibre is concave and mineral clusters associated with individual fibrils may be present (Fig. 15). The occurrence of mineralization at approximately right angles to the long axis of the fibre suggests that in function the fibres are subjected to tensional forces. The concave mineralization pattern would confer maximum strength to the mineral/collagen interface, which would be expected to be the weakest part of the fibre bundle (Jones and Boyde, 1972).

Kardos and Simpson (1979) have suggested that the periodontal ligament behaves as a thixotropic gel. The evidence for this theory is based on a re-interpretation of the tooth support data of Parfitt (1967) as well as on reports on the properties of other connective tissues. Kardos and Simpson (1979) suggested that, until ageing occurs, only the transseptal fibres of the ligament are polymerized, the remainder persisting as a gel. Application of a force to such a system could cause changes which would result in flow. In order to satisfy the requirements of the theory, the fibres seen in histological preparations must be considered as artefacts. It is difficult to reconcile this view with the observations of Mashouf and Engel (1975) who found highly organized bi-refringent collagen fibres in the rat periodontal ligament in unfixed and undemineralized sections. The appearance of the collagen in this untreated material can also be correlated with optical micro-scopical and ultrastructural findings. It would seem that the theory proposed by Kardos and Simpson (1979) could be tested experimentally by applying loads to a tooth *in situ* where the transseptal fibres had been severed. It would be expected that the recoil effect noted by Parfitt (1967) would be abolished. Another possibility might be to investigate the state of polymerization of the periodontal ligament collagen directly by examining small samples under physiological conditions using polarizing microscopy. Thus, the hypothesis proposed by Kardos and Simpson (1979) awaits experimental verification.

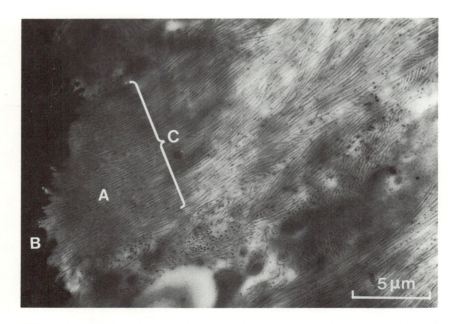

FIG. 16. Transmission electron micrograph of human alveolar bone and periodontal ligament. The interface between the unmineralized (A) and mineralized (B) parts of a Sharpey fibre (C) is concave and covered with minute mineral clusters.

FUNCTIONAL CONSIDERATIONS RELATING TO THE ARRANGEMENT OF PERIODONTAL COLLAGEN FIBRES

The collagen fibres of the periodontal ligament have been implicated in bringing about the forces required to produce tooth eruption, though it seems that there is little evidence to support this view (see Chapter 10). Two hypotheses have been postulated to account for the development of tension within the periodontal ligament, one involving collagen contraction (Shrimpton, 1960; Thomas, 1967), the other fibroblast movement or contraction (Ness, 1967; Beertsen et al., 1974). The basis of the collagen contraction hypothesis is that tractional forces could be set up within the oblique fibres of the periodontal ligament as a result of cross-linking and aggregation during collagen maturation (Thomas, 1967, 1976). These hypotheses are discussed in Chapter 10.

Current theories of tooth support envisage a multiphasic system involving fibres, ground substance, blood vessels and fluid acting together to resist mechanical forces, and it seems that there is both tension and compression of the tissues (see Chapter 11). The crimping which occurs in periodontal ligament fibres may confer special mechanical properties on the ligament. Examination of a typical stress—strain curve for rat-tail tendon shows that there is an early, easily extensible, non-linear region due to straightening out of the crimp (Diamant et al., 1972; Keller and Gathercole, 1976). In their work on several collagenous connective tissues, Minns, Soden and Jackson (1973) showed that the internal orientation of collagen fibres influenced the mechanical properties of a tissue and suggested that in general collagenous bundles could best resist axially-directed forces. The arrangement of the majority of the periodontal ligament collagen fibres into horizontal and obliquely directed groups may be related to resisting axial forces, which would involve straightening the crimp. The overlapping arrangement of the bundle networks seen in the SEM and by polarizing microscopy may be of importance in resisting rotational forces. Such an arrangement has mechanical advantages over a simple radial arrangement and is often used in engineering (e.g. in arranging the wire spokes of a wheel). The overlapping arrangement of the bundles may also be advantageous in resisting intrusive forces, as axial displacement of the tooth would tend to straighten out the fibre bundles and compress the blood vessels. The complex three-dimensional arrangement of the fibres also means that, irrespective of the direction of an applied force, some bundles would always be placed in tension. This would enable local areas of the periodontal ligament to resist compressive forces, a property which might otherwise be impossible on account of the anisotropic properties of the collagenous bundles (Minns et al., 1973). In continuously growing teeth, no overlapping arrangement of the bundles is seen and crimping occurs only in the transverse plane. This parallel arrangement of fibres may reflect the mainly intrusive nature of the forces to which rodent teeth are subjected. Thus, the organization of the periodontal ligament collagen may reflect the magnitude and direction of masticatory forces.

COMPARISONS BETWEEN PERIODONTAL AND GINGIVAL COLLAGEN FIBRES

The organization of the gingival connective tissue has been extensively studied (Goldman, 1951; Arnim and Hagerman, 1953; Melcher, 1962; Schroeder, 1969; Glenwright, 1970; Page et al., 1974), and thus no detailed description need be given here. However, the fibres of the transseptal group of gingival collagen merge directly into the periodontal ligament and possess a similar orientation to periodontal fibres. This group, in conjunction with the periodontal ligament, may play an important role in tooth support and movement (Picton and Moss, 1973; Moss and Picton, 1974). The other gingival fibres form a highly complex, three-dimensional arrangement, unlike that seen in the periodontal ligament where there are no circularly disposed fibres. Interweaving of the gingival fibre groups is a prominent feature (Page et al., 1974), and it seems likely that this arrangement is related to maintaining gingival tone and conferring strength to the soft tissue/tooth interface (Arnim and Hagerman, 1953), rather than contributing greatly to tooth support or movement. The turnover rate of gingival collagen is estimated to be two to five times slower than that of periodontal collagen (Orlowski, 1976; Sodek, 1977; Rippin, 1978). This difference in activity between gingival and periodontal collagen is further supported by some histochemical data (Beynon, A. D. G., personal communication; Fig. 17) and is the basis of a clinical treatment where gingival fibres are severed to prevent the relapse of orthodontically treated teeth (e.g. Edwards, 1970).

Oxytalan

Considerable interweaving of oxytalan and collagen fibre bundles has been demonstrated (Simpson, 1967). Oxytalan fibres lie parallel to the root surface except where they turn to be attached to cementum

(Fullmer *et al.*, 1974; Fig. 18). Sims (1975, 1976) found that oxytalan fibres in human premolar and mouse molar teeth formed a three-dimensional meshwork extending from the dentine-cementum junction to the peripheral periodontal blood vessels. Within the ligament, the meshwork exhibited a predominantly apico-occlusal orientation, with a laterally interconnecting system of fine fibrils.

Oxytalan fibres can be identified on the basis of their ultrastructure (Fullmer *et al.*, 1974; Fig. 2). However, in the TEM the fibres identified are relatively scarce and narrow compared to those seen in the light microscope. In transmission electron micrographs (Fig. 19), the two types of bundle often appear orientated at right angles to each other. Recently, Edmunds *et al.* (1979) have demonstrated

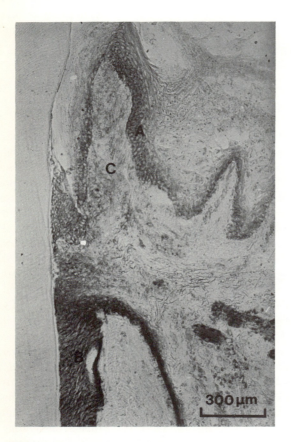

FIG. 17. Rat molar periodontium stained for alkaline phosphatase and succinic dehydrogenase activity. Succinic dehydrogenase is present in all the soft tissues and is most marked in the gingival epithelium (A). Alkaline phosphatase activity (dark appearance) is greater in the periodontal ligament (B) than in the gingival collagen (C).

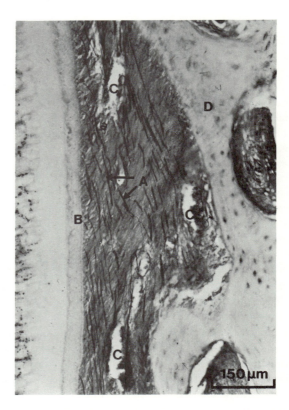

FIG. 18. Photomicrograph of macaque periodontal ligament in the mid-root region of an incisor. Oxytalan fibres (A) are inserted into cementum (B) but for the greater part of their length lie parallel to the root surface. They are closely related to blood vessels (C) but are not inserted into alveolar bone (D). Monopersulphate-thionine stain.

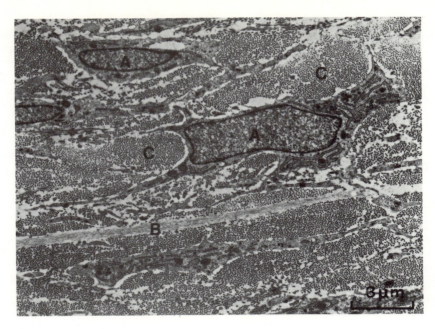

FIG. 19. Transmission electron micrograph of rabbit incisor periodontal ligament showing fibroblasts (A), a longitudinally sectioned oxytalan fibre (B) and many transversely sectioned collagen bundles (C).

interweaving of individual oxytalan filaments and collagen fibrils, again occurring at right angles. Similar relationships are known to exist in elastic ligaments (such as *ligamentum nuchae*) where individual collagen fibrils and elastin filaments are closely associated near the site of insertion of the ligament (Serafini-Fracassini *et al.*, 1977). In the centre of such ligaments, the collagen fibrils form separate bundles which weave about the elastin bundles in a spiral or crimped fashion. If oxytalan fibres were to act in the same fashion as elastin fibres, an attachment of the fibres would be necessary, perhaps to collagen as proposed by Edmunds *et al.* (1979). Further work needs to be done to establish the ultrastructural relationship between collagen and oxytalan fibrils. Oxytalan fibres have not yet been identified in the SEM, though this technique seems to offer the possibility of investigating their three-dimensional arrangement with respect to the networks of collagenous bundles.

With regard to their function, oxytalan fibres have been implicated in both the tooth eruption and support mechanisms. Beertsen *et al.* (1974) have suggested

that oxytalan fibres may serve to guide the fibroblasts in their apico-occlusal migration, the cells generating the eruptive force. This hypothesis is discussed in Chapter 10. With respect to the tooth support mechanism, it may be that the considerable interweaving of collagen and oxytalan helps to stabilize the tooth. The observation of Fullmer *et al.* (1974), that more numerous and large oxytalan fibres are found in the periodontal ligaments of teeth subjected to heavy occlusal stress than in normal or non-functional teeth, tends to confirm this view. Sims (1975, 1976) demonstrated that oxytalan fibres often terminate around blood vessels and suggested that they may be concerned with their support. Equally it could be argued that the blood vessels, themselves anchored by collagen, may provide attachment for the oxytalan fibres. Sims (1978) showed that forced extrusion of the mouse molar produced straightening, whereas forced intrusion produced waviness of the fibres. This finding suggests that the oxytalan fibres may act in the same way as elastin fibres. Oxytalan fibres could also influence blood flow, which might itself influence the tooth support mechanism. Further information concerning a haemodynamic hypothesis of tooth support is discussed in Chapter 11. In view of the fact that oxytalan fibres have not been isolated and are therefore enigmatic in character, the functional concepts proposed for these fibres remain hypothetical.

AGEING OF FIBRES

Comparatively few studies have been carried out on the effects of ageing on the fibres of the periodontium. Grant and Bernick (1972), in a histological study of four post-mortem aged human specimens, found that the main age changes to the periodontal ligament were collagen fibrosis and decreased cellularity. The fibre bundles appeared thicker and the fibre groups seemed to be broader, and more highly organized. Areas of hyalinization were present. There was decreased argyophilia, increased fuchsinophilia and a reduction in alcian blue-positive areas. Sporadic mineralization of the fibres was also seen. A decrease in the number of periodontal fibres, however, has been reported in aged galagos primates (Grant, Chase and Bernick, 1973), and in human post-mortem specimens (Severson et al., 1978), where there was also an increase in the size of interstitial spaces. The decrease in collagen fibre content may be associated with the decrease in cellularity (Klingsberg and Butcher, 1960; Grant and Bernick, 1972; Severson et al., 1978). A decrease in the number of synthesizing connective tissue cells has been found in the ageing periodontal ligament of the mouse and rat using DNA synthesis tracers (Toto and Borg, 1968; Jensen and Toto, 1968). An age-dependent decrease in the rate of collagen synthesis in the palatal ante-molar mucosa of the rat has been reported (Schneir, Furuto and Berger, 1976). A similar decrease in collagen synthesis with age has been found in the mouse molar periodontal ligament (Stahl and Tonna, 1977). Other age changes associated with the biochemistry of collagen and with fibril diameters are discussed in Chapters 4 and 5.

Severson et al. (1978) found that in young adults the periodontal alveolar bone surface was smooth and regular and the insertions of the ligament fibres were fairly evenly distributed. In older specimens, the corresponding surfaces were jagged and uneven and an irregular insertion of fibres was seen. Cementum was thicker in aged specimens and the cemental surface also became irregular with time. This irregularity of the fibre insertions, together with replacement of some of the ligament space by interstitial areas and fat cells, suggests that the structural organization of the ligament degenerates with age.

The recognition of the dividing line between age change and pathological change poses one of the fundamental problems in studying the pathogenesis of periodontal disease. Using gnotobiotic rats, Socransky, Hubersak and Propas (1970) found that age-related changes, including recession of the alveolar crest, occurred within the periodontium in the absence of inflammatory periodontal disease. It has been shown that in rodents the response of connective tissues to injury is affected by ageing (Holm-Pedersen and Viidik, 1972) and age-related changes to collagen fibres both in structure (Torp et al., 1975) and composition (Bailey and Robins, 1976) have been reported. Amstad-Jossi and Schroeder (1978) also found that there was a gradual recession of alveolar bone in the gnotobiotic rat with increasing age. Using morphometric techniques, they found that the volume density of gingival connective tissue occupied by collagen fibrils remained fairly constant with age, while the size and numerical density of the fibroblasts varied greatly. This may be compared to studies of early inflammatory periodontal disease where collagen loss is a prominent feature (Schroeder, Munzel-Pedrazzoli and Page, 1973; Garant, 1976). The later stages of periodontal disease, however, involve the deeper structure of the ligament and ultimate failure involves the breakdown of the tooth support mechanism. It seems likely that alteration to the collagen fibres of the ligament plays a prominent role in the breakdown. Greater understanding of the part played by the fibres in normal tooth support would therefore contribute greatly to the understanding of periodontal disease.

REFERENCES

AMSTAD-JOSSI, M. & SCHROEDER, H. E. (1978) Age-related alterations of periodontal structures around the cemento-enamel junction and of the gingival connective tissue composition in germ-free rats. *J. periodont. Res.* **13**, 76–90.

ANDERSON, A. A. (1967) The protein matrixes of the teeth and periodontium in hamsters: a tritiated proline study. *J. dent. Res.* **46**, 67–78.

ARNIM, S. S. & HAGERMAN, D. A. (1953) The connective tissue fibres of the marginal gingiva. *J. Amer. dent. Assoc.* **47**, 271–282.

ATKINSON, M. E. (1978) The development of transalveolar periodontal ligament fibres in the mouse. *J. dent. Res.* **57**, 151 (Abst.).

BAILEY, A. J. & ROBINS, S. P. (1976) Current topics in the biosynthesis, structure and function of collagen. *Sci. Prog.* **63**, 419–444.

BAUMHAMMERS, A. & STALLARD, R. E. (1968) S³⁵-sulfate utilization and turnover by the connective tissues of the periodontium. *J. periodont. Res.* **13**, 187–193.

BEERTSEN, W. & SNIJDER, J. (1969) A comparative study on the histological structure of the periodontal membranes of teeth with a continuous and non-continuous eruption. *Nederl. T. Tandheelk.* **76**, 542–569.

BEERTSEN, W., EVERTS, V. & VAN DEN HOOFF, A. (1974) Fine structure of fibroblasts in the periodontal ligament of the rat incisor and their possible role in tooth eruption. *Archs. oral Biol.* **19**, 1087–1098.

BEERTSEN, W. & EVERTS, V. (1977) The site of remodelling of collagen in the periodontal ligament of the mouse incisor. *Anat. Rec.* **189**, 479–498.

BERKOVITZ, B. K. B. & SLOAN, P. (1979) Attachment tissues of the teeth in *Caiman sclerops* (Crocodilia). *J. Zool., Lond.* **187**, 179–194.

BERKOVITZ, B. K. B., SHORE, T. C. & SLOAN, P. (1980) An histological study of the periodontal ligament of rat mandibular incisor following root resection with special reference to the zone of shear. *Archs. oral Biol.* **25**, 235–244.

BERKOVITZ, B. K. B., WEAVER, M. E., SHORE, R. C. & MOXHAM, B. J. (in press) Fibril diameters in the extracellular matrix of the periodontal connective tissues of the rat. *Conn. Tiss. Res.* **8**, 127–132.

BEVELANDER, G. & NAKAHARA, H. (1968) The fine structure of the human peridental ligament. *Anat. Rec.* **162**, 313–326.

BLACK, G. V. (1887) Periosteum and peridental membrane. *Dent. Rev. (Wien)* **1**, 289–302.

BLACK, G. V. (1899) The fibres and glands of the periodontal membrane. *Dental Cosmos. Philad.*, Vol. XLI, 101–162.

BOYDE, A. (1968) Scanning electron microscopy of collagen free calcified connective tissue. *Beitr. elektronmikroskop. Direktabb. Oberfl.* **1**, 213–222.

BOYDE, A. & JONES, S. J. (1968) Scanning electron microscopy of cementum and Sharpey fibre bone. *Z. Zellforsch.* **92**, 536–548.

BOYDE, A. (1972) Scanning electron microscope studies of bone. In: *The biochemistry and physiology of bone.* G. H. BOURNE (ed.) (2nd ed.), Vol. 1, pp. 259–309. London, Academic Press.

BUTLER, W. T., BIRKEDAL-HANSEN, H., BEAGLE, W. F., TAYLOR, R. E. & CHUNG, E. (1975) Proteins of the periodontium. Identification of collagen with the $[\alpha 1 \text{ (I)}]_2 \alpha 2$ and $[\alpha 1 \text{ (III)}]_3$ structures in the

bovine periodontal ligament. *J. Biol. Chem.* **250**, 8907–8912.

CARMICHAEL, G. G. & FULLMER, H. M. (1966) The fine structure of the oxytalan fiber. *J. Cell Biol.* **28**, 33–36.

CARNEIRO, J. & FAVA DE MORAES, F. (1965) Radioautographic visualization of collagen metabolism in the periodontal tissues of the mouse. *Archs. oral Biol.* **10**, 833–848.

CARNEIRO, J. & LEBLOND, C. P. (1966) Suitability of collagenase treatment for the autoradiographic identification of newly synthesised collagen labelled with ³H-glycine or ³H-proline. *J. Histochem. Cytochem.* **14**, 334–344.

CIANCIO, S. C., NEIDERS, M. E. & HAZEN, S. P. (1967) The principal fibres of the periodontal ligament. *Periodontics* **5**, 76–81.

COHN, S. A. (1972a) A re-examination of Sharpey's fibres in alveolar bone of the mouse. *Archs. oral Biol.* **17**, 255–260.

COHN, S. A. (1972b) A re-examination of Sharpey's fibres in alveolar bone of the marmoset. *Archs. oral Biol.* **17**, 261–269.

COHN, S. A. (1975) Transalveolar fibres in the human periodontium. *Archs. oral Biol.* **20**, 257–259.

CRUMLEY, P. J. (1964) Collagen formation in the normal and stressed periodontium. *Periodontics* **2**, 53–61.

DIAMANT, J., KELLER, A., BAER, E., LITT, M. & ARRIDGE, R. G. C. (1972) Collagen; ultrastructure and its relation to mechanical properties as a function of ageing. *Proc. R. Soc. Lond.* B. **180**, 293–315.

DREYFUSS, F. & FRANK, R. (1964) Microradiographie et microscopie électronique du cément humain. *Bull. Grp. int. Rech. sci. Stomat.* **7**, 167–181.

EASTOE, J. W. (1976) Collagen chemistry and tissue organization. In: *The eruption and occlusion of teeth,* D. F. G. POOLE & M. V. STACK (eds.), pp. 247–249. London, Butterworths.

ECCLES, J. D. (1959) Studies on the development of the periodontal membrane. The principal fibres of the molar teeth. *Dent. Prac.* **10**, 31–35.

ECCLES, J. D. (1964) The development of the periodontal membrane in the rat incisor. *Archs. oral Biol.* **9**, 127–133.

EDMUNDS, R. S., SIMMONS, T. A., COX, C. F. & AVERY, J. K. (1979) Light and ultrastructural relationship between oxytalan fibres in the periodontal ligament of the guinea-pig. *J. oral Path.* **8**, 109–120.

EDWARDS, J. G. (1970) A surgical procedure to eliminate rotational relapse. *Amer. J. Orthodont.* **57**, 35–46.

FRANK, R. M., FELLINGER, E. & STEUER, P. (1976) Ultrastructure du ligament alvéolo-dentaire du rat. *J. Biol. Buccal.* **4**, 295–313.

FREEMAN, E. & TEN CATE, A. R. (1971) Development of the periodontium: an electron microscope study. *J. Periodontol.* **42**, 387–395.

FULLMER, H. M. & LILLIE, R. D. (1958) The oxytalan fiber: a previously undescribed connective tissue fiber. *J. Histochem. Cytochem.* **6**, 425–430.

FULLMER, H. M. (1959) Observations on the development of oxytalan fibres in the periodontium of man. *J. dent. Res.* **38**, 510–516.

FULLMER, H. M. (1960) A comparative histochemical study of elastic, pre-elastic and oxytalan connective tissue fibres. *J. Histochem. Cytochem.* **8**, 290–295.

FULLMER, H. M. (1961) A histochemical study of periodontal disease in the maxillary alveolar processes of 135 autopsies. *J. Periodontol.* **32**, 206–218.

FULLMER, H. M., SHEETZ, J. H., & NARKATES, A. J. (1974) Oxytalan connective tissue fibers: A review. *J. oral Path.* **3**, 291–316.

GARANT, P. R. (1976) An electron microscopic study of the periodontal tissues of germ free rats and rats mono-infected with *Actinomyces naeslundii*. *J. periodont. Res. Supp.* **15**.

GLENWRIGHT, H. D. (1970) Observations on circular and longitudinal gingival collagen fibres in the rhesus monkey. *Dent. Prac.* **20**, 337–341.

GOLDMAN, H. (1951) The topography and role of the gingival fibres. *J. dent. Res.* **30**, 331–336.

GOTTE, L., GIRO, G., VOLPIN, D. & HORNE, R. W. (1974) The ultrastructural organization of elastin. *J. Ultrastruct. Res.* **46**, 23–34.

GRANT, D. & BERNICK, S. (1972) The periodontium of ageing humans. *J. Periodontol.* **43**, 660–667.

GRANT, D., BERNICK, S., LEVY, B. M. & DREIZEN, S. (1972) A comparative study of periodontal ligament development in teeth with and without predecessors in marmosets. *J. Periodontol.* **43**, 162–169.

GRANT, D., CHASE, J. & BERNICK, S. (1973) Biology of the periodontium in primates of the Galago species. I. The normal periodontium in young animals. II. Inflammatory periodontal disease. III. Lability of cementum. IV. Changes in ageing. Ankylosis. *J. Periodontol.* **44**, 540–550.

GRAY, W. R., SANDBERG, L. B. & FOSTER, J. A. (1973) Molecular model for elastin structure and function. *Nature* **246**, 461–466.

HEROVICI, C. (1963a) Le picropolychrome. Technique de coloration histologique destinée à l'étude du tissu conjonctif, normal et pathologique. *Rev. franç. Etud. Clin. Biol.* **8**, 88–89.

HEROVICI, C. (1963b) A polychrome stain for differentiating precollagen from collagen. *Stain Technol.* **38**, 204–205.

HINDLE, M. O. (1967) The intermediate plexus of the periodontal membrane. In: *The mechanisms of tooth support*, D. J. ANDERSON, J. E. EASTOE, A. H. MELCHER & D. C. A. PICTON (eds.), pp. 66–67. Bristol, Wright.

HOLM-PEDERSEN, P. & VIIDIK, A. (1972) Tensile properties and morphology of healing wounds in old and young rats. *Scand. J. plast. reconst. Surg.* **6**, 24–35.

HUNT, A. M. (1959) A description of the molar teeth and investing tissues of normal guinea pigs. *J. dent. Res.* **38**, 216–243.

JACKSON, D. S. (1976) Biochemical aspects of collagen in relation to biological function. In: *The eruption and occlusion of teeth*, D. F. G. POOLE & M. V. STACK (eds.), pp. 252–261. London, Butterworths.

JENSEN, J. L. & TOTO, P. D. (1968) Radioactive labelling index of the periodontal ligament in ageing rats. *J. dent. Res.* **47**, 149.

JONES, S. J. & BOYDE, A. (1972) A study of human root cemental surfaces as prepared for and examined in the SEM. *Z. Zellforsch.* **130**, 318–337.

JONES, S. J. & BOYDE, A. (1974) The organization and

gross mineralization patterns of the collagen fibres in Sharpey fibre bone. *Cell Tiss. Res.* **148**, 83–96.

KADAR, A. (1974) The ultrastructure of elastic tissue. *Path. Europe* **9**, 133–146.

KARDOS, T. B. & SIMPSON, L. O. (1979) A theoretical consideration of the periodontal membrane as a collagenous thixotropic system and its relationship to tooth eruption. *J. Periodont. Res.* **14**, 445–451.

KELLER, A. & GATHERCOLE, L. J. (1976) Biophysical and mechanical properties of collagen in relation to function. In: *The eruption and occlusion of teeth*, D. F. G. POOLE & M. V. STACK (eds.), pp. 262–266. London, Butterworths.

KEREBEL, B. & BALOUET, G. (1967) Observations sur le plexus intermédiaire du ligament paradontal. *Actualités Odontostomat.* **80**, 395–409.

KLINGSBERG, J. & BUTCHER, E. O. (1960) Comparative histology of age change in oral tissues of rat, hamster and monkey. *J. dent. Res.* **39**, 158.

KRAW, A. G. & ENLOW, D. H. (1967) Continuous attachment of the periodontal membrane. *Amer. J. Anat.* **120**, 133–148.

LAPIERE, Ch. M. (1967) Mechanism of collagen fibre remodelling. In: *The mechanisms of tooth support*, D. J. ANDERSON, J. E. EASTOE, A. H. MELCHER & D. C. A. PICTON (eds.), pp. 20–24. Bristol, Wright.

LEVY, B. M. & BERNICK, S. (1968) Development and organization of the periodontal ligament of deciduous teeth in marmosets. *J. dent. Res.* **47**, 27–33.

LEVY, B. M., DREIZEN, S. & BERNICK, S. (1972) *The marmoset periodontium in health and disease*. Basel, Karger.

LIEBERMAN, M. A. (1960) The oxytalan fibre in the periodontal ligament of the rat incisor. M.S. Thesis. University of Illinois.

MAGNUSSON, B. (1968) Tissue changes during molar tooth eruption. *Trans. R. Schs Dent. Stockh. Umea*, No. 13, 1–122.

MASHOUF, K. & ENGEL, M. B. (1975) Maturation of periodontal connective tissue in the newborn rat incisor. *Archs. oral Biol.* **20**, 161–166.

MELCHER, A. H. (1962) The interpapillary ligament. *Dent. Pract.* **12**, 461–462.

MELCHER, A. H. (1966) Gingival reticulin: Identification and role in the histogenesis of collagen fibres. *J. dent. Res.* **45**, 426–439.

MELCHER, A. H. & EASTOE, J. E. (1969) The connective tissues of the periodontium. In: *Biology of the periodontium*, A. H. MELCHER & W. H. BOWEN (eds.), pp. 167–343. London, Academic Press.

MELCHER, A. H. & CHAN, J. (1978) The relationship between section thickness and the ultrastructural visualization of collagen. *Archs. oral Biol.* **23**, 231–233.

MINNS, R. J., SODEN, P. D. & JACKSON, D. S. (1973) The role of the fibrous components and ground substance in the mechanical properties of biological tissues: A preliminary investigation. *J. Biomechanics* **6**, 153–165.

MOSS, J. P. & PICTON, D. C. A. (1974) The effect of approximal drift of cheek teeth of dividing mandibular molars of adult monkeys (*Macaca irus*). *Archs. oral Biol.* **19**, 1211–1214.

NESS, A. R. & SMALE, D. E. (1959) The distribution of

mitoses and cells in the tissues bounded by the socket wall of the rabbit mandibular incisor. *Proc. R. Soc. B.* **151**, 106–128.

NESS, A. R. (1967) Eruption – a review. In: *The mechanisms of tooth support*, D. A. ANDERSON, J. E. EASTOE, A. H. MELCHER & D. C. A. PICTON (eds.), pp. 84–88. Bristol, Wright.

ORLOWSKI, W. A. (1976) The incorporation of H³-proline into the collagen of the periodontium of a rat. *J. periodont. Res.* **11**, 96–100.

PAGE, R. C., AMMONS, W. F., SCHECTMAN, L. R. & DILLINGHAM, L. A. (1974) Collagen fibre bundles of the normal marginal gingiva in the marmoset. *Archs. oral Biol.* **19**, 1039–1043.

PARFITT, G. J. (1967) The physical analysis of the tooth supporting structures. In: *The mechanisms of tooth support*, D. J. ANDERSON, J. E. EASTOE, A. H. MELCHER & D. C. A. PICTON (eds.), pp. 154–156. Bristol, Wright.

PARRY, D. A. D. & CRAIG, A. S. (1979) Electron microscopic evidence for an 80Å unit in collagen fibrils. *Nature*, **282**, 213–215.

PARTRIDGE, S. M. (1967) Diffusion of solutes in elastin. *Biochim. Biophys. Acta* **140**, 132–141.

PICTON, D. C. A. & MOSS, J. P. (1973) The part played by the trans-septal fibre system in experimental approximal drift of the cheek teeth of monkeys (*Macaca irus*). *Archs. oral Biol.* **18**, 669–680.

QUIGLEY, M. B. (1970) Perforating (Sharpey's) fibres of the periodontal ligament and bone. *Ala. J. med. Sci.* **7**, 336–342.

RAMOS, A. B. & HUNT, A. M. (1967) Remodelling of the periodontal ligament of guinea pig molars. In: *The mechanisms of tooth support*, D. J. ANDERSON, J. E. EASTOE, A. H. MELCHER & D. C. A. PICTON (eds.), pp. 107–112. Bristol, Wright.

RANNIE, I. (1963) Observations on the oxytalan fibres of the periodontal membrane. *Trans. Euro. orthodont. Soc.* **39**, 127–136.

RIPPIN, J. W. (1976a) Collagen turnover in the periodontal ligament under normal and altered functional forces. 1. Young rat molars. *J. periodont. Res.* **11**, 101–107.

RIPPIN, J. W. (1976b) Collagen turnover in rat molar periodontal ligament. In: *The eruption and occlusion of teeth*, D. F. G. POOLE & M. V. STACK (eds.), pp. 304–305. London, Butterworths.

RIPPIN, J. W. (1978) Collagen turnover in the periodontal ligament under normal and altered functional forces. II Adult rat molars. *J. periodont. Res.* **13**, 149–154.

ROBINS, M. W. (1972) Collagen metabolism in the periodontal ligament of the rat incisor. *J. dent. Res.* **51**, 1246.

ROSS, R. (1973) The elastic fibre, a review. *J. Histochem. Cytochem.* **21**, 199–208.

SCHNEIR, M., FURUTO, D. & BERGER, K. (1976) Collagens of oral soft tissues, 1. The influence of age on the synthesis and maturation of collagen in rat palatal mucosa as determined *in vitro. J. periodont. Res.* **11**, 235–241.

SCHROEDER, H. E. (1969) Struktur und Ultrastruktur des normalen marginalen Paradonts. *Paradontalogie* **23**, 159–176.

SCHROEDER, H. E., MUNZEL-PEDRAZZOLI, S. & PAGE, R. C. (1973) Correlated morphometric and biochemi-

cal analysis of gingival tissue in early chronic gingivitis in man. *Archs. oral Biol.* **18**, 899–923.

SELVIG, K. A. (1964) An ultrastructural study of cementum formation. *Acta odont. Scand.* **22**, 105–120.

SELVIG, K. A. (1965) The fine structure of human cementum. *Acta odont. Scand.* **23**, 423–441.

SERAFINI-FRACASSINI, A., FIELD, J. M., SMITH, J. W. & STEPHENS, W. G. S. (1977) The ultrastructure and mechanics of elastic ligaments. *J. Ultrastruc. Res.* **58**, 244–251.

SEVERSON, J. A., MOFFETT, B. C., KOKICH, V. & SELIPSKY, H. (1978) A histologic study of age changes in the adult human periodontal joint (ligament). *J. Periodontol.* **49**, 189–200.

SHACKLEFORD, J. M. (1971) Scanning electron microscopy of the dog periodontium. *J. periodont. Res.* **6**, 45–54.

SHACKLEFORD, J. M. (1973) The indifferent fibre plexus and its relationship to principal fibres of the periodontium. *Amer. J. Anat.* **131**, 427–442.

SHEETZ, J. H., FULLMER, H. M. & NARKATES, A. J. (1973) Oxytalan fibers: Identification of the same fibre by light and electron microscopy. *J. oral Path.* **2**, 254–263.

SHORE, R. C. & BERKOVITZ, B. K. B. (1979) Model to explain apparent occlusal movement of extracellular protein of periodontal ligament of the rat incisor. *Archs. oral Biol.* **24**, 861–862.

SHRIMPTON, B. A. (1960) Dynamics of eruption. *N.Z. dent. J.* **56**, 122–124.

SICHER, H. (1923) Über die Fixation und das Wachstum dauernd wachsender Zähne. *KorrespBl. Zahnärzte* **49**, 332–343.

SICHER, H. (1942) Tooth eruption: The axial movement of continuously growing teeth. *J. dent. Res.* **21**, 201–210.

SIMPSON, H. E. (1967) A three-dimensional approach to the microscopy of the periodontal membrane. *Proc. R. Soc. Med.* **60**, 537–542.

SIMS, M. R. (1973) Oxytalan fibre of molars in the mouse mandible. *J. dent. Res.* **52**, 797–803.

SIMS, M. R. (1975) Oxytalan-vascular relationships observed in histologic examination of the periodontal ligaments of man and mouse. *Archs. oral Biol.* **20**, 713–717.

SIMS, M. R. (1976) Reconstitution of the human oxytalan system during orthodontic tooth movement. *Amer. J. Orthod.* **70**, 38–58.

SIMS, M. R. (1977) The oxytalan fiber system in the mandibular periodontal ligament of the lathyritic mouse. *J. oral Path.* **6**, 233–250.

SIMS, M. R. (1978) Oxytalan fibre response to tooth intrusion and extrusion in normal and lathyritic mice. A statistical analysis. *J. periodont. Res.* **13**, 199–206.

SKOUGAARD, M. R., LEVY, B. M. & SIMPSON, J. (1970) Collagen metabolism in skin and periodontal membrane of the marmoset. *Scand. J. dent. Res.* **78**, 256–262.

SLOAN, P., SHELLIS, R. P. & BERKOVITZ, B. K. B. (1976) Effect of specimen preparation on the appearance of the. rat periodontal ligament in the scanning electron microscope. *Archs. oral Biol.* **21**, 633–635.

SLOAN, P. (1978a) Scanning electron microscopy of the collagen fibre architecture of the rabbit incisor periodontium. *Archs. oral Biol.* **23**, 567–572.

SLOAN, P. (1978b) Microanatomy of the periodontal liga-
ment in some animals possessing teeth of continuous
and limited growth. Ph.D. Thesis, University of
Bristol.
SLOAN, P. (1979a) Polarising microscopy of the rodent
periodontal ligament. *J. dent. Res.* **53**, 118.
SLOAN, P. (1979b) Collagen fibre architecture in the periodontal ligament. *J. R. Soc. Med.* **72**, 188–191.
SOCRANSKY, S. S., HUBERSAK, C. & PROPAS, D. (1970)
Induction of periodontal destruction in gnotobiotic
rats by a human oral strain of *Actinomyces naeslundii*.
Archs. oral Biol. **15**, 993–995.
SODEK, J. (1977) A comparison of the rates of synthesis
and turnover of collagen and non-collagen proteins in
adult rat periodontal tissues and skin using a micro-
assay. *Archs. oral Biol.* **22**, 655–665.
SODEK, J., BRUNETTE, D. M., FENG, J., HEERSCHE,
J. N. M., LIMEBACK, H. F., MELCHER, A. H. &
NG, B. (1977) Collagen synthesis is a major component of protein synthesis in the periodontal ligament
of various species. *Archs. oral Biol.* **22**, 647–653.
SPIRO, R. G. (1972) Basement membranes and collagens.
In: *Glycoproteins,* A. GOTTSCHALK (ed.), 2nd
ed. Amsterdam, Elsevier.
STAHL, S. S. & TONNA, E. A. (1977) H^3-proline study of
ageing periodontal ligament matrix formation. Com-
parison between matrices adjacent to either cemental
or bone surfaces. *J. periodont. Res.* **12**, 318–322.
STALLARD, R. E. (1963) The utilization of ^{3}H-proline by
the connective tissue elements of the periodontium.
Periodontics **1**, 185–188.
SVEJDA, J. and SKACH, M. (1973) The periodontium of

the human tooth in the scanning electron microscope.
J. Periodontol. **44**, 478–484.
TEN CATE, A. R. (1972) Morphological studies of fibrocytes
in connective tissue undergoing rapid remodelling.
J. Anat. **112**, 401–414.
THOMAS, N. R. (1967) The properties of collagen in the
periodontium of an erupting tooth. In: *Mechanisms
of tooth support,* D. J. ANDERSON, J. E. EASTOE,
A. H. MELCHER & D. C. A. PICTON (eds.), pp. 102–
106. Bristol, Wright.
THOMAS, N. R. (1976) Collagen as the generator of tooth
eruption. In: *The eruption and occlusion of teeth,*
D. F. G. POOLE & M. V. STACK (eds.), pp. 290–
301. London, Butterworths.
TORP, S., BAER, E. & FRIEDMAN, B. (1975) Effects of
age and of mechanical deformation on the ultrastructure of tendon. In: *Structure of fibrous biopoly-
mers,* E. D. T. ATKINS & A. KELLER (eds.), pp.
223–250. London, Butterworths.
TOTO, P. D. & BORG, M. (1968) Effect of age changes on
the premitotic index in the periodontium of mice.
J. dent. Res. **47**, 70.
VAN BLADEREN, T. P. (1972) Tooth eruption and the
development of the periodontal fibres. *Trans. Euro.
Orthodont. Soc.* **48**, 427–437.
WAINWRIGHT, S. A., BIGGS, W. D., CURREY, J. D. &
GOSLINE, J. M. (1976) *Mechanical design in
organisms,* pp. 116–119. London, Edward Arnold
Ltd.
ZWARYCH, P. D. & QUIGLEY, M. B. (1965) The inter-
mediate plexus of the periodontal ligament; History
and further observations. *J. dent. Res.* **44**, 383–391.

Chapter 4

BIOCHEMISTRY OF THE FIBRES OF THE PERIODONTAL LIGAMENT

D. J. Carmichael

INTRODUCTION

The periodontal ligament is a connective tissue consisting of a complex of cells and blood vessels embedded in an extracellular matrix. The basic constituents of the matrix are the proteins collagen and oxytalan (the fibres of the tissue) and an association of proteoglycans and glycoproteins. With the possible exception of oxytalan, which only forms a minor component of the tissue, the fibrillar elements are not elastic. The presence of elastin in the periodontal ligament is restricted to the walls of the small blood vessels in humans, but may be more widespread in some animals.

Functionally, the periodontal ligament has been adapted for the support of the tooth in the jaw. In many non-mammalian vertebrates the tooth is attached to the jaw bone by means of osseous cylinders, each termed a pedicel. The periosteum of the jaw bone may give rise to these cylinders (but see Chapter 1). In mammals, a fibrous tissue, the periodontal ligament, has evolved between the tooth and the cylindrical bone of attachment which has grown up as a sleeve to surround the tooth. Thus, the periodontal ligament can be regarded as an adaptation of the periosteum lining the inside of the bony sleeve. To date, no comparative studies of the biochemistry of these two tissues have been reported.

COLLAGEN

This review is written with the knowledge that in recent years a number of specialist reviews of collagen biochemistry (Ramachandran and Reddi, 1976; Hall and Jackson, 1976; Pearson, 1979) have been published. Nevertheless, the need remains for a description of the biochemistry of the extracellular matrix of the periodontal ligament directed to the oral biologist. That much of the substance of this review is derived from fundamental studies of the collagen molecule and comparatively less from investigations of the periodontal ligament is an accurate reflection of the fact that this tissue has only recently begun to receive the attention from biochemists which is its due.

Structure and composition

Collagen is arranged in the tissues as a precisely ordered aggregate of many similar molecules. The molecule is composed of three polypeptide chains (designated α-chains), each chain having a molecular weight of 95,000 to 100,000 daltons and containing about 1050 amino acids. The α-chains are assembled in a three-stranded helical form resulting in a rod-like molecule 290 nm long and 1.5 nm in diameter. The collagen fibres of the tissues are then formed by assembly of the individual molecules. The features of collagen structure at the various orders of size are depicted in Fig. 1.

The amino acid composition of collagen is distinctive. One-third of the amino acids are glycine, while the amino acids proline and hydroxyproline constitute a further 20 to 25%. The major portion of the sequence of each polypeptide consists of repeating tripeptides, represented as (-gly-x-y-), in which the

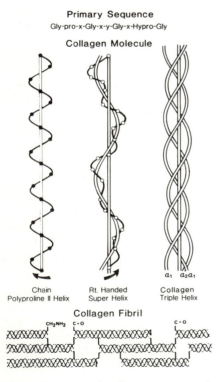

Primary Sequence
Gly-pro-x-Gly-x-y-Gly-x-Hypro-Gly

Collagen Molecule

| Chain | Rt. Handed | Collagen |
| Polyproline II Helix | Super Helix | Triple Helix |

Collagen Fibril

FIG. 1. Features of collagen structure at various orders of size.

first position is occupied by glycine and the other two positions by any of several amino acids (Fietzek and Kuhn, 1976). A number of amino acids demonstrate a marked preference for one or other of the two possible positions, x and y. Thus, proline frequently occurs at the x position and hydroxyproline at y. Glutamic acid is found more commonly at x and arginine at y. However, lysine and aspartic acid are detected in either position. The significance of the non-random distribution of certain amino acid residues is not understood. Possibly, intramolecular interactions between side chain groups of specific amino acids may contribute to the stability of the molecule. Such interactions would require a defined distribution of the appropriate side chain groups and would be of importance in the formation of covalent links between individual chains as well as for electrostatic and hydrophobic interactions. With the detailed knowledge of the full sequence of the amino acid residues for the α_1 chain, certain of these interactions can now be identified (see, for example, Fietzek and Kuhn, 1975). Such interactions can obviously be expected to be of importance in the self-assembly process whereby the collagen molecule (and ultimately the fibril) is formed. At both the amino and carboxy terminal ends of the polypeptide chain short regions exist that do not have the tripeptide (-gly-x-y-) sequence but are enriched in acidic and basic amino acids. These terminal regions do not form a part of the regular helical structure of the molecule. The amino acid composition of vertebrate collagen is shown in Table 1.

The secondary structure of the collagen molecule results from the steric restrictions imposed by the presence of glycine and the imino acids proline and hydroxyproline in the triplet structure (Ramachandran and Ramakrishnan, 1976). The rigid structure of the pyrrolidone ring of the proline and hydroxyproline residues results in the polypeptide chain forming a left-handed polyproline-II helix (Ramachandran, 1967; Traub and Piez, 1971). The three chains are supercoiled into a right-handed helix around a common axis so that a translation of 0.29 nm and a rotation of $110° \pm 2°$ is established. The compact size of the glycine residue permits it to pack tightly into the centre of the structure while the bulky rings of proline and hydroxyproline are positioned on the exterior. Rigidity is conferred on the structure

TABLE 1. *Amino acid composition of collagen from various species*

Amino Acid	Human [1]	Chick [2]	Carp [3]	Sea Anemone [4]	Ascaris [5]
3-Hydroxyproline	1	1	1	19	
4-Hydroxyproline	92	102	76	78	16
Aspartic acid	42	45	47	71	69
Threonine	17	19	28	36	19
Serine	36	28	37	39	19
Glutamic acid	69	73	71	95	67
Proline	128	119	116	68	296
Glycine	336	327	333	322	274
Alanine	113	120	125	62	72
Valine	25	19	18	29	18
Methionine	6	8	16	9	5
Isoleucine	9	10	10	21	10
Leucine	24	24	20	30	19
Tyrosine	3	2	3	4	4
Phenylalanine	12	13	13	8	10
Hydroxylysine	6	7	7	25	—
Histidine	5	4	4	2	8
Lysine	27	27	26	16	45
Arginine	50	50	52	66	29
Cysteine	—	—	—	—	27
Total acidic	111	118	118	166	136
Total imino	221	222	192	165	312

Residues/1000 residues

1. Epstein et al (1971)
2. Kang, Piez & Gross (1969)
3. Piez, Eigner & Lewis (1963)
4. Nordwig, Nowack & Hieber-Rogall (1973)
5. McBride and Harrington (1967)

by hydrogen bonding between the carboxyl groups of the peptide bonds of one chain and the amino groups of the peptide bonds of the adjacent chain.

The triple helical structure was originally proposed by Ramachandran and Kartha (1954, 1955) based on X-ray diffraction studies. Rich and Crick (1958, 1961) suggested two collagen models — collagen I and collagen II — derived from a consideration of the two possible systems of hydrogen bonding obtained from the two non-equivalent placings of a third chain relative to two parallel hydrogen bonded chains. Both these structures allow only one hydrogen bond per triplet repeat. Subsequently, Ramachandran *et al.* (1965) proposed a further alternative collagen structure involving two hydrogen bonds per triplet which required an initial glycine in the triplet but could not form hydrogen bonds if the sequence gly-pro-hypro was present in two chains at the same level. Present evidence on hydrogen bonding would seem to favour the latter model (for review see Ramachandran and Ramakrishnan, 1976).

Recently, there has been some speculation that fairly regularly spaced regions of the molecule might be 'soft' and depart from the helical structure. Certainly, model polytripeptides of the more polar triplets do not form the collagen structure (Anderson,

Rippon and Walton, 1970; Walton, 1975). In the native collagen such ideas are based on the appearance of a meridional lattice spacing of 13.5 nm in rat-tail tendon collagen following fixation, heavy phospho-tungstate staining and stretching (e.g. Nemetschek and Hosemann, 1973). This spacing is one-fifth of the repeat period of the native collagen fibril, although the significance of this distance has not yet been determined.

Genetic types of collagen

It has been demonstrated that several genetically distinct types of molecule exist in different tissues (Bailey, Robins and Balian, 1974; Martin, Byers and Piez, 1975). These various collagen species have been shown to differ in amino acid sequence and α-chain distribution. In addition, there are variations in the degree of hydroxylation of proline and lysine, glyco-sylation of hydroxylysine, aldehyde content, antigenic determinants and the size of amino and carboxy-terminal non-helical peptides. On this basis, four well-characterized main polymorphic genetic variants of collagen have been described (Fig. 2) and evidence for several further minor types has been reported. The nomenclature employed for the identification of each type reflects the order in which it was described.

Type I collagen (the major protein component of skin, bone, dentine, ligament and several other

Type	Distribution	Chain Composition	Chemical Characteristics
I	Bone, tendon, dentine, dermis Most connective tissues	$[\alpha_1(I)]_2\,\alpha_2$	Hybrid of two chain types; low in hydroxylysine and glycosylated hydroxylysine
II	Hyaline cartilage	$[\alpha_1(II)]_3$	Relatively high in hydroxylysine and glycosylated hydroxylysine
III	Reticulin fibres, smooth muscle, foetal connective tissue	$[\alpha_1(III)]_3$	High in hydroxyproline and low in hydroxlysine. Contains cysteine
IV	Basement membranes.	$[\alpha_1{}^{IV}]_2\,\alpha_2{}^{IV}$	High in hydroxylysine and glycosylated hydroxylysine. Carbohydrate content not limited to glucose and galactose. Contains cysteine.
V	Basement membranes and perhaps other tissues	$\alpha A\ \alpha B\ \alpha C$	Similar to Type IV

FIG. 2. Structurally and genetically distinct collagens.

tissues) contains two identical chains α_1 and a chemically different third chain α_2. The molecule was then represented by the formula $[(\alpha_1 I)_2 \alpha_2]$. A small amount of collagen containing three $\alpha_1 I$ chains has also been detected, generally in experimental conditions (Benya, Padilla and Nimmni, 1977; Little *et al.*, 1977; Wohllebe and Carmichael, 1978; Uitto, 1979). Type II collagen, which consists of three identical $(\alpha_1 II)$ chains, was first shown to be present in hyaline cartilage. Recently, this collagen species has been found in the cornea, vitreous body and neural retinal tissues (Linsenmeyer, Smith and Hay, 1977; von der Mark *et al.*, 1977). However, the presence of Type II collagen in the cornea has been disputed (Panjwani and Harding, 1978). Type III collagen, consisting of three identical $(\alpha_1 III)$ chains, occurs in skin, arteries, lung, liver and uterine tissue (Miller, Epstein and Piez, 1971; Gay *et al.*, 1975; Remberger, Gay and Fietzek, 1975).

The collagen from basement membranes has been designated Type IV but is probably more complex than the simple numerical identification would imply. Present data indicate that basement membrane collagen is not a single collagen species but most likely a group of related proteins similar to the mesodermally derived collagens (Glanville, Rauter and Fietzek, 1979; Kresina and Miller, 1979; Timpl, Risteli and Bachinger, 1979).

Most models of Type IV collagen propose that it is a procollagen-like molecule with significant non-collagenous segments that are retained in the matrix. While some studies have suggested that this molecule contains three identical polypeptide chains (Minor *et al.*, 1976; Heathcote *et al.*, 1978; Timpl, Bruchner and Fietzek, 1979), recent works indicate the presence of two genetically distinct chains in Type IV procollagen (Crouch, Sage and Bornstein, 1980; Tryggvason, Robey and Martin, 1980) which in one cell type has been observed to be in the form $[\text{pro } \alpha_1(IV)]_2 \text{ pro } \alpha_2(IV)$.

A further type of collagen that may arise from basement membranes has been isolated from skin, placenta and some other tissues (Brown, Shuttleworth and Weiss, 1978; Rhodes and Miller, 1978; von der Mark and von der Mark, 1979). This collagen is composed of polypeptides termed αA and αB chains and is designated variously AB collagen and Type V collagen. There are at present two molecular

structures for this collagen. The first proposes that the molecule is formed by the assembly of the two peptide chain types $[\alpha A (\alpha B)_2]$ (Burgeson *et al.*, 1976; Chung, Rhodes and Miller, 1976; Bentz *et al.*, 1978) while the alternate view holds that two distinct molecular species are formed $(\alpha A)_3$ and $(\alpha B)_3$ (Rhodes and Miller, 1978). More recently, a peptide chain αC has been identified (Brown, Shuttleworth and Weiss, 1978; Sage and Bornstein, 1979) which would form the molecule $(\alpha C)_3$. Kresina and Miller (1979) have reported the presence of a chain αD in some tissues. It has been suggested that each of the species $(\alpha A)_3$, $(\alpha B)_3$ and $(\alpha C)_3$ are all modifications of the same basic molecule (Brown and Weiss, 1979). However, this view is at variance with that of Sage and Bornstein (1979) and Kresina and Miller (1979), the latter authors having tentatively reported the presence of collagen molecules with the structure $(\alpha C)_2 \alpha D$.

The chemical structure of the mesodermally derived Type I, II and III collagens has now been largely established (Traub and Piez, 1971; Miller, 1973; Chung and Miller, 1974; Epstein, 1974; Butler *et al.*, 1975; Rauterberg and von Bassevitz, 1975; Birkedal-Hansen, Butler and Taylor, 1977; Timpl, Wick and Gay, 1977; Wohllebe and Carmichael, 1979) but the structure of Type IV collagen, which is associated with basement membranes, and is in part derived from the adjacent epithelial cells, is still open to question.

The structure and function of the various connective tissues are apparently related to the genetic species of collagen of which they are composed (Fietzek *et al.*, 1979). The periodontal ligament is composed primarily of Type I collagen with a lesser proportion of Type III collagen (for further details see p. 90). In most adult connective tissues the content of Type III collagen is normally low, but in foetal tissues it is present in significant amounts. The fibres in tissues containing a high proportion of Type III collagen are finer than those in tissues composed solely of Type I collagen (Lapiere, Nusgens and Pierard, 1977). In human foetal skin the proportion of Type I and III collagens in the dermis changes during development from a large proportion of Type III (approximately 30%) to increasing amounts of Type I collagen with simultaneous changes in mechanical properties and coarsening of the fibre bundles (Epstein, 1974; Pierard and Lapiere, 1976). *In vitro* studies have demonstrated that reconstituted Type I collagen develops a network of thick bundles of fibres whereas Type III collagen forms isolated thin fibres and tends to inhibit the association of Type I collagen to thicker fibres (Lapiere, Nusgens and Pierard, 1977).

Collagen biosynthesis

In recent years, the process of collagen synthesis has been studied extensively and several comprehensive reviews of the subject have been published (Prockop *et al.,* 1976; Fessler and Fessler, 1978; Jackson, 1978). The synthesis of each of the different types of collagen is thought to occur by the same mechanisms and is shown schematically in Fig. 3. As for many other extracellular proteins, each of the collagen

types is synthesized in a precursor form which undergoes post-translational modification prior to its secretion and aggregation to the microfibril. The precursor form, known as procollagen, contains additional peptide extensions called propeptides at both the amino and carboxy terminal ends of each of the three constituent polypeptide chains (referred to as pro α chains) of the molecule. The propeptides are surprisingly large, making up approximately 50% of the length of the pro α chains. They fulfil a number of important functions in the biosynthetic process. During conversion of procollagen to collagen, the propeptides are removed by peptidases which are specific either for the amino or carboxy terminal extensions.

The amino terminal propeptide of Type I procollagen has a molecular weight of about 20,000 daltons and contains three structurally distinct domains: a globular, amino terminal domain, a

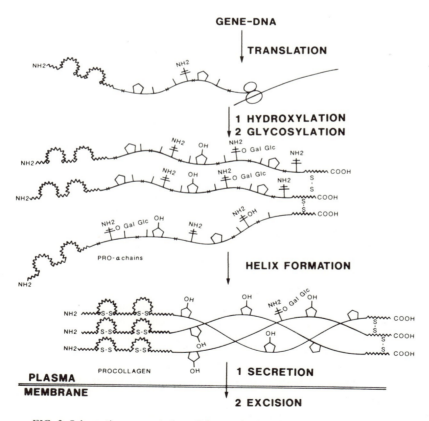

FIG. 3. Schematic representation of the synthesis and secretion of procollagen.

central, collagen-like domain and an additional short globular domain (Becker *et al.*, 1976; Horlein, Fietzek and Kuhn, 1978; Dixit *et al.*, 1979; Horlein *et al.*, 1979). The α_2 procollagen chain also contains an amino-terminal propeptide with a collagen-like domain that matches the same region of the pro α_1, Type I propeptide (Becker, Helle and Timpl, 1977; Smith, McKenney and Lustberg, 1977). The size of the pro α_2 amino terminal propeptide has not been conclusively determined, some reports suggesting that it is smaller than the pro α_1 amino terminal propeptide (Becker, Helle and Timpl, 1977; Tuderman, Kivirikko and Prockop, 1978). However, Smith, McKenney and Lustberg (1977) suggest that it is the same size. The amino acid sequence of the amino terminal pro α_1 Type I procollagen has recently been reported (Horlein *et al.*, 1979) but the equivalent data for the pro α_2 propeptide are not yet available. The carboxy terminal propeptides of both the pro α_1 and pro α_2 chains are globular in conformation without collagen-like domains (Olsen *et al.*, 1977). The molecular weights are 30,000 and 35,000 respectively and the primary structures of the two carboxy terminal propeptides are different (Hoffmann *et al.*, 1976; Olsen *et al.*, 1977).

The amino terminal Type I propeptide initially was thought to contain carbohydrate residues (Furthmayr *et al.*, 1972; Clark and Kefalides, 1978) although the recently reported sequence data for this propeptide do not present any evidence for an attached carbohydrate moiety (Horlein *et al.*, 1979). In the carboxy terminal Type I propeptides, on the other hand, N-acetyl glucosamine is present at a low level and while galactosamine may be present, firm evidence is lacking (Olsen *et al.*, 1977; Tanzer *et al.*, 1977; Clark and Kefalides, 1978). Mannose is the dominant sugar in the carboxy terminal propeptides (Olsen *et al.*, 1977). Clark (1979) has suggested that each carboxy terminal propeptide in Type I procollagen contains an oligosaccharide unit composed of 8–9 units of mannose. Inter- and intrachain disulphide bonds have been identified in the carboxy terminal Type I propeptides (Harwood *et al.*, 1977) while in the amino terminal propeptides of Type I collagen only intrachain disulphide bonds are found.

The propeptides of Type II and Type III procollagens bear a close similarity to those of Type I procollagen (Harwood *et al.*, 1975; Nowack, Olsen and Timpl, 1976; Uitto, Hoffmann and Prockop, 1977; Uitto, 1977; Fessler and Fessler, 1979). The amino terminal propeptide of Type II procollagen is smaller than the corresponding propeptide of the pro α_1 propeptide of Type I procollagen (Tuderman, Kivirikko and Prockop, 1978). Mannose has been identified in both amino and carboxy terminal propeptides of Type II procollagen, and possibly in the carboxy terminal propeptide of Type III procollagen (Smith *et al.*, 1977). Interchain disulphide bonds are formed in both the amino and carboxy terminal propeptides of Type III procollagen but only in the carboxy terminal propeptides of Type II procollagen (Nowack, Olsen and Timpl, 1976; Uitto, Hoffmann and Prockop, 1977).

Studies on basement membrane biosynthesis employing organ cultures of parietal yolk sac endoderm (Minor *et al.*, 1976) and lens capsule (Heathcote *et al.*, 1978) indicate that these tissues synthesize an apparent procollagen molecule composed of three identical procollagen chains each with a molecular weight in the range 160,000 to 180,000 daltons. This procollagen species does not, however, undergo a subsequent conversion to a smaller molecular weight molecule during incorporation into the basement membrane structure (Kresina and Miller, 1979).

There has been considerable speculation concerning the function of the procollagen propeptides. At least five separate functions have been proposed and are currently being investigated (Prockop *et al.*, 1979). The propeptides may serve to prevent premature fibril formation (Grant and Prockop, 1972), organize protein assembly into fibrils (Veis *et al.*, 1973), provide the specificity necessary for correct chain association in the monomer (Prockop *et al.*, 1976), direct the folding of the pro α chains into a triple helical conformation (Becker *et al.*, 1976; Engel *et al.*, 1977; Bruckner *et al.*, 1978), and, following scission from the parent molecule, the propeptides may function in some form of feedback inhibition (Lichtenstein *et al.*, 1973; Grant and Jackson, 1976; Paglia *et al.*, 1979; Wiestner *et al.*, 1979). Which function (or combination of functions) does operate has yet to be determined, although there is evidence in support of each.

While collagen may be synthesized by any of several different cell types, within the periodontal ligament this protein is synthesized primarily by the fibroblasts. It is possible, however, that the epithelial cell rests (of Malassez) may secrete a minor collagen component, probably Type IV collagen (Brunette *et al.,* 1979). The process of collagen synthesis is initiated in the nucleus of the cell, following transcription of the specific regions of DNA coded for each of the types of collagen. The messenger RNA for each procollagen α-chain is now generally accepted to be monocistronic and translated on membrane-bound ribosomes. In the early studies it was unclear whether the individual α chains were assembled from short peptides or as single chains. However, biosynthetic studies (Vuust and Piez, 1972) and sequence analysis (Bornstein, 1970) showed that synthesis occurred as the single polypeptide chain. It was then appropriate to question how the cell synthesizing Type I collagen could translate two α_1 chains for one α_2 chain so that the correct amount of each polypeptide was produced. The most sensitive control would be effected through a polycistronic messenger RNA with independent initiation of the pro α_1 and α_2 chains. However, studies of the collagen synthesizing polysomes indicated a size appropriate to monocistronic messenger RNA (Lazarides and Lukens, 1971) coding for a peptide of the length of the α_1 procollagen chain (pro α_1). Other investigations by Fessler, Morris and Fessler (1975), principally with chick embryo calvaria, demonstrated the presence of messenger RNA for pro α_1, and pro α_2 in the cells in a 2:1 ratio; the rate of synthesis of the two chains was then identical on each polysome. The assembly of pro α_1 chains *in vivo* takes approximately 6–7 minutes (Vuust and Piez, 1972; Miller, Woodall and Vail, 1973) which is nearly three times longer than expected from a comparison with the rates of translation for β-galactosidase and haemoglobin from mRNA. The reason for this slow rate of assembly has not been determined. The pathway for the synthesis and secretion of procollagen is essentially the same as for other extracellular proteins, although it is unusual in the number and variety of post-translational modifications which it undergoes. At least seven such reactions have been identified in procollagen, four of which occur intracellularly and are the hydroxylation of proline and lysine and glycosylation of specific hydroxylysine residues with galactose and glucose. Subsequent extracellular reactions consist of enzymatic cleavage of the procollagen propeptides, oxidative deamination and formation of crosslinks.

The polysomes, on which the assembly of the amino acids to form the pro α-chain occurs, are bound to the membranes of the rough endoplasmic reticulum (Goldberg and Green, 1967; Diegelmann, Bernstein and Peterkofsky, 1973; Olsen *et al.,* 1973). As the chain is formed the amino terminal extension passes through the membrane into the cisternae of the endoplasmic reticulum where the post-translational modifications are initiated. It is not known how the procollagen chains enter the cisternae, although in some proteins a hydrophobic amino terminal leader sequence, or prepeptide, has been detected which is believed to initiate transfer through the endoplasmic reticulum membrane. This observation has led to the formation of a 'signal hypothesis' by Blobel and Dobberstein (1975) in which the prepiece following synthesis on the ribosome is recognized by a multimeric, intrinsic, membrane protein which binds to the ribosome and forms a tunnel through the membrane. A unidirectional transfer of the nascent polypeptide into the cisternae of the endoplasmic reticulum then occurs (Habener *et al.,* 1978; Thibodeau, Lee and Palmiter, 1978). A sequence, apparently of this type, has been identified in chick procollagen (Palmiter *et al.,* 1979) synthesized in the reticulocyte system. To date, however, no tunnel-forming protein intrinsic to the membrane and essential to the 'signal hypothesis' has been demonstrated. As a consequence, an alternative hypothesis has been proposed (von Heijne and Blomberg, 1979) that does not require such a tunnel-forming protein but only a ribosomal binding site. This latter model is based upon a consideration of the thermodynamic interactions of ribosome and membrane and growing polypeptide chain. Once the prepeptide, which is strongly hydrophobic, has bound in an α-helical conformation to the lipophilic core of the membrane and the ribosome has bound to the surface of the membrane, energy is generated by this interaction such that the growing polypeptide chain is extruded through the membrane. After discharge of the completed chain, the ribosome dissociates from the endoplasmic reticulum membrane and the prepeptide is cleaved from the polypeptide chain. At present, however, it is not known which (or even if either) hypothesis is correct.

While the procollagen is within the lumen of the endoplasmic reticulum the processes of hydroxylation, interchain disulphide bonding and helical folding are completed (Brownell and Veis, 1975; Harwood, Grant and Jackson, 1975; Oikarinen, Anttinen and Kivirikko, 1976 a, b). The rate of passage through the endoplasmic reticulum appears to be inversely related to the degree of glycosylation, being most rapid for Type I procollagen (Brownell and Veis, 1975; Oikarinen et al., 1976b; Harwood et al., 1977).

The hydroxylation of both prolyl and lysyl residues is carried out by at least three enzymes: prolyl 4 hydroxylase, prolyl 3 hydroxylase and lysyl hydroxylase. These enzymes are mixed function oxygenases and require as cofactors molecular oxygen, ferrous iron, α-ketoglutarate and a reducing agent such as ascorbate (Abbott and Udenfriend, 1974). Although the predominant form of hydroxyproline in collagen is trans-4-hydroxyproline, 3-hydroxyproline can also be detected. A separate enzyme is apparently involved in the hydroxylation at the 3 position (Prockop et al., 1976) but this enzyme has been characterized only partially (Risteli, Tryggvason and Kivirikko, 1977). The subcellular location of the hydroxylases has been a matter for considerable debate. Recent analyses indicate that the enzymes are bound to the internal face of the cisternae of the endoplasmic reticulum (Harwood et al., 1975).

The hydroxylated amino acids (hydroxyproline and hydroxylysine) have been the focus of considerable study. Although initially considered to be specific to collagen, both hydroxyproline and hydroxylysine are now known to be more widespread (though still very restricted in distribution). Within the structure of the collagen molecule, hydroxyproline is found only in the helical regions. Hydroxylysine, on the other hand, occurs in both the helical and non-helical regions where it has an important function in the formation of intermolecular cross-links (Tanzer, 1973; Bailey, Robins and Balian, 1974). The important physical properties of the collagen fibres depend, to a large extent, on the stability imparted to the fibre structure by the system of covalent intermolecular crosslinks.

The presence of galactose and glucose has been demonstrated in all vertebrate collagens that have been examined. Both galactosyl-O-β-hydroxylysine and O-α-D-glycosyl $(1 \rightarrow 2)$ -O-β-D galactosyl hydroxylysine have been identified in the helical region and a more complex mixture of carbohydrate residues has been reported in the propeptide region (Furthmayr et al., 1972; Fessler et al., 1973; Oohira, Kusakabe and Suzuki, 1975; Olsen et al., 1977). The synthesis of the galactosyl and glucosyl-galactosyl residues has been shown to involve the enzymes collagen UDP galactosyl transferase and collagen UDP glycosyl transferase (Spiro, 1972). It appears probable that the enzymes responsible for post-translational modifications may constitute a multi-enzyme system bound to the inner membrane of the cisternae of the endoplasmic reticulum.

Both the hydroxylase and transferase enzymes require their substrate to be in the non-helical form (Berg and Prockop, 1973; Kivirikko et al., 1973; Risteli, Myllyla and Kivirikko, 1976; Myllyla, Risteli and Kivirikko, 1975). Tissue-labelling studies (Oohira et al., 1979) have revealed that proline hydroxylation closely follows peptide synthesis, commencing prior to the release of the nascent peptide from the polysome. Synthesis is envisaged as a coordinated progression involving peptide assembly on membrane-bound polysomes followed by passage into the lumen of the endoplasmic reticulum. Hydroxylation of both proline and lysine residues is followed by glycosylation of the hydroxylysine residues beginning shortly after the N-terminal ends pass into the cisternae of the rough endoplasmic reticulum (Brownell and Veis, 1975; Harwood, Grant and Jackson, 1975; Oikarinen, Anttinen and Kivirikko, 1976a). Although sugars may continue to be added after the chains have been released from the ribosomes, glycosylation ceases when the collagen domains fold into a triple helix (Oikarinen, Anttinen and Kivirikko, 1976a).

The sugars in the propeptides of procollagen are also added when the pro α-chains are non-helical, probably occurring in the cisternae of the rough endoplasmic (Anttinen, Oikarinen, Ryhanen and Kivirikko, 1978; Guzman, Graves and Prockop, 1978). It is probable that the mechanism by which the propeptide sugars are added is different to that in the collagen domain (Prockop et al., 1979).

The extent of hydroxylation in the newly synthesized Type I collagen appears to be decreased in older animals (Barnes *et al.*, 1974; Pearson and Ainsworth, 1978). In particular, the hydroxylation of lysine of the N-terminal non-helical region of both α_1 and α_2 chains is decreased, which may have important consequences for the stability of the covalent intermolecular crosslinks. In the periodontal ligament, the total hydroxylysine content has been observed to decrease in older animals (Pearson *et al.*, 1975; Pearson and Ainsworth, 1978). However, whether this decrease is reflected in the important extrahelical terminal region has not been determined. If such a decrease is confirmed in the human periodontal ligament this could well be of clinical significance, reflecting on the tensile strength of this tissue in the older patient.

Although the secretory route of procollagen has been the subject of considerable discussion, it is now generally accepted that the procollagen molecule passes from the cisternae of the endoplasmic reticulum through the Golgi complex to the cell membrane (Kishida *et al.*, 1975; Olsen *et al.*, 1975). Autoradiographic studies of highly polarized odontoblast cells have provided evidence that the procollagen molecules are packed into vacuoles (Trelstad and Coulombre, 1971; Weinstock and Leblond, 1974; Weinstock *et al.*, 1975) prior to secretion by exocytosis. That the microtubule system of the cell is probably involved in intracellular transport is indicated by the fact that colchicine (which inhibits microtubule formation) delays secretion of procollagen (Diegelmann and Peterkofsky, 1972). Details of the secretory route of procollagen remain to be determined.

The precise form of the procollagen molecule as it is secreted is open to question. Although it has been suggested by Dehm and Prockop (1971), Jimenez *et al.* (1974), Uitto and Prockop (1974) and Uitto *et al.* (1975) that non-helical procollagen is not secreted but accumulates in the cells, other work has demonstrated that the helical conformation is not an absolute requirement for secretion but that cells can secrete non-helical procollagen (Bates *et al.*, 1972; Muller *et al.*, 1973; Muller *et al.*, 1974). Recently, kinetic experiments have indicated that the secretion of procollagen is not a single first-order process, but approximates at least two first-order processes with half-times of 14 and 115 minutes (Kao, Prockop and Berg, 1979). Kao *et al.* (1979) proposed that the slower rate probably reflects the

secretion of a non-helical procollagen fraction. This suggests that although the formation of the triple helix favours secretion it is not an essential precursor to secretion.

Formation of the collagen fibril

Following secretion of the procollagen molecule, conversion to the collagen monomer is initiated. Isotopic labelling experiments show that the initial cleavage occurs in the amino terminal propeptide (Morris *et al.*, 1975), while the carboxy terminal propeptide is removed later (Davidson, McEneany and Bornstein, 1975). It is believed that the removal of the amino terminal propeptide is associated with the cell whereas cleavage of the carboxy terminal propeptide is entirely extracellular (Morris *et al.*, 1975; Fessler, Greenberg and Fessler, 1978). The state of aggregation of procollagen following exocytosis and prior to the appearance of fibrils has not been determined. It has frequently been assumed that, following secretion of procollagen, the propeptides are removed and the dispersed monomers self-assemble to form native fibrils (Warshawsky, 1972; Veis and Brownell, 1975; Leung *et al.*, 1979). However, prior removal of the propeptides is not essential for association of procollagen molecules to occur, although it is a precondition for the formation of wide, native Type I fibres (Fessler *et al.*, 1978). Alternatively, it is possible that procollagen is secreted as small molecular aggregates, that are not disrupted by processing, and assemble into fibrous arrays, undergoing intermolecular rearrangement to native fibrils (Trelstad, Hayashi and Gross, 1976). Current data by Leung *et al.* (1979) indicate that the procollagen peptidases can act on either the molecules in solution or when present as molecular aggregates. Bruns *et al.* (1979), on the other hand, have obtained evidence for the secretion of segment-long-spacing aggregates that then apparently assemble in linear arrays. The assembly takes place either following the removal of the propeptides or possibly during their scission in a specific sequence. This work is of special interest in that it also suggests a mechanism for control of the location and orientation of the collagen molecules during fibrillogenesis. The situation in the basement membrane differs in that the propeptides of Type IV collagen are apparently not removed (Minor *et al.,* 1976; Heathcote, Sear and Grant, 1978) but are preserved within the tissue. This presumably has important effects on the fibre structure of this collagen type.

Within the connective tissue, collagen molecules aggregate to form a network of insoluble fibrils. On the basis of electron microscopic studies, Hodge and Schmitt (1960) concluded that the long asymmetric collagen molecules were packed into fibrils in a polarized, parallel fashion, giving rise to a periodic cross-striation of 60—70 nm characteristic of the native fibril. The repeat period has been interpreted as a consequence of the staggered arrangement of the molecules which are displaced axially relative to one another by 67 nm, corresponding to 234 residues. This model was extended subsequently by Petruska and Hodge (1964) to include the concept of gap regions, necessitated by the fact that since each molecule is 4.4 times the length of the fundamental repeat distance, it was impossible to have end-to-end contact between molecules and maintain the periodicity of the structure. In two-dimensional representation, this structure works very well. However, it is not applicable to a three-dimensional packing of collagen molecules.

In three dimensions, only two-thirds of the lateral contacts between molecules can be staggered to yield 1 D periodic shifts with regard to all nearest neighbours. A number of models have been postulated to explain the lateral arrangement of the collagen molecules in the smallest fibrillar unit termed a microfibril (Katz and Li, 1973; Hosemann, Dreissig and Nemetschek, 1974; Woodhead-Galloway, Hukins and Wray, 1975; Veis and Yuan, 1975; Golub and Katz, 1977). Other models not structured on microfibrillar arrangements have also been proposed (Ross and Benditt, 1961; Ramachandran, 1967). A more detailed discussion of microfibrillar organization is included in Chapter 5. Among the microfibril models that have been proposed, those gaining the widest degree of acceptance appear to be an assembly of 4 molecules arranged in a square space group (Veis *et al.,* 1967; Veis and Yuan, 1975) and a 5-molecule aggregate in the form of a closed cylinder (Smith, 1968). The latter model appears to fit the X-ray

diffraction data of Miller and Wray (1971) and Miller and Parry (1973) most closely. On the basis of this evidence, a five-stranded microfibril related to the closed-cylinder model previously proposed by Smith (1968) is favoured. Other studies (Trus and Piez, 1976; Piez and Trus, 1978; Traub, 1978) have examined the primary structure of the molecule to identify those residues whose interactions could be of importance in determining the ordered molecular assembly to fibrils. Nevertheless, the complete three-dimensional molecular arrangement cannot yet be said to have been determined and the microfibril remains a hypothetical, though plausible, structure. Electron microscopic examination of fibrils undergoing some form of physical disruption has indicated the presence of thinner fibrillar structures very possibly corresponding to the microfibril.

The mechanism by which microfibrils are aggregated extracellularly to form the tissue fibril is not yet understood. Some insights have been obtained through *in vitro* studies (Williams *et al.,* 1978; Gelman, Williams and Piez, 1979; Veis *et al.,* 1979). These indicate that fibril formation requires at least three steps: nucleation, linear growth and lateral association. To the physical chemist these terms have precise meaning. The formation of nuclei is called nucleation, and in the present context the nuclei are the earliest aggregation of collagen microfibrils to produce a crystalline form. This is an energy related step. Linear growth refers to an increase in length of the crystalline structure while lateral association is a subsequent increase in diameter. In the third step, covalent crosslinking may well be of importance in preserving the stability of the fibril. Collagen fibres are formed through aggregation of the fibrils. Such fibres are found in a wide variety of patterns in various tissues. The highly specific arrangement of the collagen fibres imparts the characteristic weave to each of the connective tissues by which each tissue type may be recognized.

A system of covalent crosslinks is formed extracellularly after the molecules have aggregated to form fibres (Fig. 4). Both intermolecular and intra-molecular crosslinks are formed. The intra-molecular crosslink does not add stability to the collagen molecule or fibre and its function (if any) is unclear. However, the suggestion has been made that it may participate in the formation of a trifunctional inter-

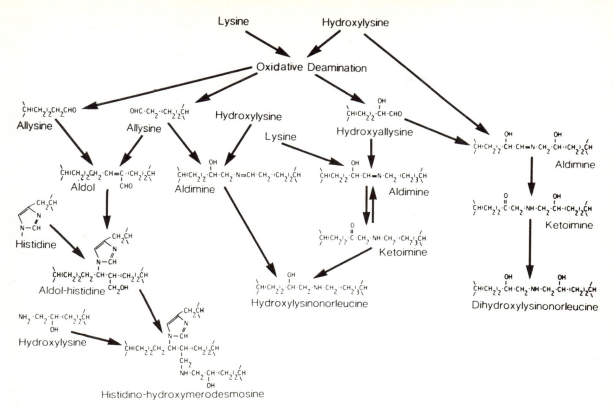

FIG. 4. Biosynthesis of lysine-derived crosslinks.

molecular crosslink. The intermolecular crosslink is physiologically important (Bailey and Robins, 1973). The initial step in the formation of both types of crosslink is identical and involves an enzymatically mediated oxidative deamination of specific lysyl and hydroxylysyl residues. The intramolecular crosslinks then arise as aldol condensation products between suitably positioned allysine residues on adjacent α-chains of the molecule. The more important intermolecular crosslink occurs through aldimine bond formation between allysyl or hydroxyallysyl residues with the ε-amino group of other suitably positioned lysyl or hydroxylysyl residues (Swann, Caulfield and Broadhurst, 1976). Alternatively, an intermolecular crosslink may be formed through a further reaction of the intramolecular aldol with histidine or hydroxylysine to form trifunctional

aldol histidine or hydroxymerodesmosine (Tanzer, 1976). The physiological significance of this latter type of crosslink has been questioned, however, by Robins and Bailey (1973). They have suggested that these structures may be artefactual, arising as a result of the basic conditions present during borohydride reduction which is used to stabilize the crosslink during chemical determination. Within the collagen molecule, certain of the hydroxylysyl residues are glycosylated and thus both glycosylated and non-glycosylated crosslinks may be identified.

It has been suggested that the Schiff base forms of the intermolecular crosslinks are intermediates which are transformed to non-reducible crosslinks on maturation (Gallop, Blumenfeld and Seifter, 1972). Robins, Shimokomaki and Bailey (1973) proposed the migration of the double bond of the intermolecular aldimine crosslinks to form a keto form by spontaneous Amadori rearrangement. Alternatively, *in vivo* reduction of the aldimine bond has been suggested as a possible method of stabilization, and a condensation product, hydroxyaldolhistidine, has been proposed by Housley *et al.* (1975) in which reduction is involved. Davis *et al.* (1975) have proposed stabilization through the formation of a gem-diamine (by addition across the aldimine bond), although this type of compound is usually considered to be unstable.

Evidence has been presented for an oxidative pathway for the maturation of the collagen structure (Bailey *et al.,* 1977; Robins and Bailey, 1977). It was proposed that the maturation of the reducible crosslinks and changes in solubility during ageing are independent processes. The degree of solubility of a collagenous matrix is generally regarded as inversely related to the number and type of crosslinks in the collagen. If the recent proposal is correct, then it is possible that a secondary age-dependent system might operate which would account for the changes in physical characteristics of the collagen fibrils.

Consideration of the mechanism for intermolecular crosslinking in collagen also involves the problem of the molecular packing in collagenous tissues and the location of crosslinkages in the fibril system. Based on the known primary structure together with a detailed knowledge of the axial staggered organization of molecules within the fibrils, the positions of the possible intermolecular sites connecting α_1 chains of adjacent molecules may be deduced (Fietzek and Kuhn, 1976). Some of the bonds predicted in this way have been experimentally verified by identification of the corresponding crosslinked peptides (Kang, 1972; Becker, Furthmayr and Timpl, 1975; Scott, Veis and Mechanic, 1976). The experimental procedure employed has generally involved reduction of the aldimine crosslinks followed by cleavage of the polymeric collagen with specific reagents or enzymes (Dixit and Bensusan, 1973; Scott *et al.,* 1976; Kang, 1972). The major problem has been the selection from the complex mixture of the specific peptides that contain an intermolecular crosslink joining two or more polypeptide chains (Tanzer, 1976).

Several reports have established the role of both N-terminal non-helical peptides (Kang, 1972; Volpin and Veis, 1973; Stimler and Tanzer, 1979) and the C-terminal non-helical peptides (Eyre and Glimcher, 1973 a, b) in crosslink formation. Crosslinks have been identified between the non-helical peptides on adjacent chains (Kang, 1972; Volpin and Veis, 1973) and between the helical region and the amino and carboxy terminal non-helical peptides (Eyre and Glimcher, 1973b; Stimler and Tanzer, 1979; Light and Bailey, 1980). The existence of intermolecular crosslinks between helical regions has also been proposed. Although no indication has been obtained for the existence of crosslinks between the molecules of adjacent fibres, intermolecular crosslinks between and within microfibrils have been suggested. Alignment of the microfibrils would then occur in a regular linear manner such as that within the fibril, the molecules along each edge being in a non-staggered array with those of the adjacent microfibril. This would allow the formation of crosslinks between adjacent carboxy terminal non-helical peptides. During the ageing process, additional crosslinks of this type could then be found conferring increased stability on the fibrillar structure. Evidence supportive of this hypothetical pattern of maturation has been reported by Veis and Schleuter (1964).

To date, detailed consideration of the location of crosslinkages in the fibril system are restricted by the fact that the sequence has been completely established only for the α_1 chain. In the longer term, structural studies of this type must also consider the primary structure of the α_2 chain and the triple helical conformation of the collagen molecule.

Collagen catabolism

The catabolism of the collagen matrix is fundamental to the process of remodelling which is involved in maintenance of tissue morphology and wound repair. In spite of considerable study of these processes, the mechanisms by which they operate have not yet been made clear. It is generally accepted, however, that catabolism is a multistep, enzymatically mediated process. The collagen fibrils may be first depolymerized by a depolymerase or 'crosslinkase' and then fragmented extracellularly by secreted collagenase and neutral proteinases (Woessner, 1973); the residual material is removed by phagocytosis and digestion then completed intracellularly by lysosomal enzymes (Parakkal, 1969; Deporter and Ten Cate, 1973). The probable steps necessary for complete collagen degradation are depicted in Fig. 5.

Under normal physiological conditions, mature collagens are unusually resistant to attack by most proteolytic enzymes. Indeed, it was not until 1962 that the first vertebrate collagenase was discovered (Gross and Lapiere, 1962), with subsequent purification and mode of action characterized (Gross and Nagai, 1965). Extensive study since has resulted in the identification of only a small group of enzymes that have the potential to be involved in the degradation of native collagen.

COLLAGENASE

Collagenase has been defined as an enzyme capable of degrading native collagen at physiologic pH and temperature (Gross, 1970). With the recent demonstration of collagen attack by at least one of the cathepsins, however, this definition needs to be modified to indicate cleavage of a particular peptide bond (or bonds) in the triple helix of native collagen at physiologic pH and temperature. The detection of specific collagenolytic activity requires native collagen as the substrate under conditions at which denaturation does not occur. In the early studies, collagenase could not be isolated directly from the tissue, but required the maintenance of an implant in culture.

More recently, the enzyme has been obtained by direct extraction from various tissues including embryonic chick bones (Sakamoto *et al.*, 1973), involuting mouse uterus and mouse skin (Wirl, 1975) and rat dermis (Nagai and Hori, 1972).

While certain properties of the collagenase enzyme (such as molecular weight and sensitivity to specific inhibitors) vary according to the tissue of origin, its action on the collagen molecule does not vary. Vertebrate collagenases cleave all of the three α-chains at one specific site in the native collagen molecule, giving two fragments. The larger fragment consists of three-quarters of the α chain and includes the amino terminal end. The smaller piece (one-quarter of the α-chain) contains the carboxy terminal end. The specificity of mammalian collagenases (Gross, 1976; Highberger, Corbett and Gross, 1979) is directed to the peptide bond between residues 775 and 776 of the helical region of the collagen molecule. In the α_1 chain, this bond is between a glycyl and an isoleucyl residue. In the α_2 chain, it is between glycyl and leucyl residues.

Although the major site of cleavage is known to be the same for each of Types I, II and III collagen (Gross, 1976), there are significant differences in the degradation of each of the genetically distinct species. Comparison of the relative susceptibilities (Harris *et al.*, 1975 a, b) of Types I, II and III collagens to vertebrate collagenase has indicated the order of susceptibility to be III > I > II. However, with rabbit tumour collagenase (Harris *et al.*, 1975a) Type III and Type I collagens are cleaved at the same rate. Skin collagenase, although able to cleave Type I, II and III collagens, has been reported to be incapable of degrading Type IV collagen (Woolley *et al.*, 1978; Liotta *et al.*, 1979) whereas collagenase prepared from a metastatic murine tumour could only degrade Type IV collagen (Liotta *et al.*, 1979, 1980). This variation in susceptibility to enzymic attack is probably due to sequence differences in portions of the α chain adjacent to the site of cleavage and may well have important biological and structural

Process	Enzyme
1. Depolymerization, or disruption of intermolecular cross-links within collagen fibrils. An enzyme active at the pH of the extracellular matrices is required.	A 'depolymerase' or 'cross-linkase'
2. Cleavage through the helical portion of individual collagen molecules	Specific neutral collagenases (extracellular)
3a Fragmentation of fibril with subsequent phagocytosis and intracellular (lysosomal) digestion of fibril fragments, and/or	Specific neutral collagenases (extracellular) followed by lysosomal hydrolases (e. g. cathepsin B and/or 'collagenolytic cathepsins') acting within phagolysosomes (intracellular)
3b Thermal denaturation of single molecular fragments produced by specific collagenase and degradation within or outside of cells to polypeptides of ≤ 10,000 molecular weight	Neutral gelatin-specific proteinase (extracellular) Non-specific neutral proteinases
4. Further cleavage to peptides small enough to be excreted in urine or completely catabolized intracellularly	Unknown enzymes. Pz - peptidase ?

FIG. 5. Steps involved in collagen degradation.

implications. Thus, although the digestive enzyme trypsin is not able to degrade native Type I collagen, under physiological conditions it can rapidly cleave Type III collagen α-chains at a single site close to that of collagenase cleavage (Miller *et al.*, 1976). Conceivably, therefore, degradation of Type III collagen *in vivo* could proceed through neutral proteinases rather than collagenase. This is an important consideration in the case of the periodontal ligament in which approximately 20% of the collagen matrix is in the Type III form. In addition to the initial or primary site of cleavage, collagenases isolated from a number of tissues have been reported to cleave the collagen molecule at further points (Jeffrey and Gross, 1970; Tokoro, Eisen and Jeffrey, 1972; Werb and Reynolds, 1975; Woolley *et al.*, 1975). Whether more extensive purification of the collagenase would eliminate the additional collagenolytic activity has not been determined.

Although both of the major fragments resulting from collagenase cleavage are able to retain the helical form at low temperatures, at physiological temperature spontaneous denaturation occurs. The denatured products would then be susceptible to further proteolytic attack by a variety of proteinases (probably both intra- and extracellularly).

It has proved to be particularly difficult to establish a physiological role for the vertebrate collagenases. Indeed, doubt has been expressed as to the ability of collagenase to attack the intact native collagen fibre (Leibovich and Weiss, 1970; Weiss, 1976). Vater, Harris and Siegel (1979) have demonstrated a significant resistance to collagenase action in the intermolecularly limited collagen fibril. Nevertheless, the direct extraction of collagenase from leucocytes (Lazarus *et al.*, 1972; Wirl, 1975; Weeks *et al.*, 1976) and the identification of collagenase in homogenates of fresh tissue (Chesney *et al.*, 1974; Dabbous *et al.*, 1974; Fujiwara *et al.*, 1974; Takahashi and Seifter, 1974; Highberger, Corbett and Gross, 1979) do point to a significant physiological function for this enzyme. Because of the strictly limited capacity of mammalian collagenase to cleave collagen except at the one specific locus, the presence of additional enzymes could well be essential for efficient collagenolysis.

Further speculation has concerned the form in which the collagenase is secreted within the mammalian tissues and fluids. It is generally accepted that

inactive intracellular forms of collagenase exist (e.g. Harris and Cartwright, 1977), but whether these latent enzymes represent true zymogens of collagenase or enzyme–inhibitor complexes has not been decided. That collagenase is secreted as a zymogen requiring activation by a specific mild proteolysis has been claimed (Birkedal-Hansen *et al.*, 1971; Harper, Bloch and Gross, 1971; Kruze and Wojtecka, 1972; Vaes, 1972; Mainardi *et al.*, 1976; Dayer, Russell and Krane, 1977; Eeckhout and Vaes, 1977; Woessner, 1977). Possible proteolytic activators were shown to include plasmin, cathepsin B, trypsin and kallikrein. The alternative proposal, that all latent collagenases are enzyme–inhibitor complexes, has also received considerable attention. In this case, activation would be accomplished by dissociation of the bound enzyme (Reynolds *et al.*, 1977; Sellers *et al.*, 1977 a, b). Recently, a latent substrate-bound collagenase has been identified in normal animal tissues (Montfort and Perez-Tamayo, 1975; Pardo and Perez-Tamayo, 1975; Vater, Mainardi and Harris, 1978).

A number of extracellular inhibitors to collagenase activity have been identified. In early studies of vertebrate collagenases, inhibition by EDTA, cysteine and serum was demonstrated (Lapiere and Gross, 1963; Nagai *et al.*, 1966). The action of EDTA is believed to be by chelation of the calcium ions which function both as an enzyme activator and to stabilize the tertiary structure of the enzyme at physiological temperatures. Similarly, cysteine may induce a conformational change in the enzyme (Daniels, Lian and Lazarus, 1969). Strong chelating agents also remove zinc, an essential cofactor (Seltzer *et al.*, 1977).

The collagenase inhibitors naturally present in serum are of particular importance. Included in this category are the high molecular weight α_2 macroglobulin (Werb *et al.*, 1974) and a β_1 serum protein, designated β_1-anticollagenase (Woolley *et al.*, 1976). Because of its smaller size, it has been suggested that the β_1 anticollagenase might diffuse through capillary walls and act as a collagenase inhibitor in tissue locations from which the large α_2 macroglobulin would be excluded (Woolley and Evanson, 1977a; Woolley *et al.*, 1978). A series of inhibitory components ranging in molecular weight from approximately equivalent to the β_1 anticollagenase (40,000) to considerably smaller (6000) have been identified. These inhibitors have been shown to occur in such sites as embryonic chick skin explants (Shinkai *et al.*, 1977), cartilage and aortic tissue (Kuettner *et al.*, 1976), bone cultures (Sellers *et al.*, 1977 a, b), and tumour extracts and fibroblast cultures (Bauer *et al.*, 1975; McCroskery *et al.*, 1975). Whether these inhibitors are chemically related to one another or are associated with the β_1 anticollagenase has not been determined.

In addition to the regulation of the initiation of the collagenolytic activity, the limitation of action of the enzyme is also of crucial importance. It has been postulated that the destruction of collagen in tissues distant from the immediate site of enzyme action is prevented by the circulating α_2 macroglobulin (Barrett and Starkey, 1973; Werb *et al.*, 1974). The recent identification of β_1 anticollagenase and other naturally occurring collagenase inhibitors provides a further sensitive mechanism for the extracellular regulation or limitation of collagenase action. Thus, inhibition of collagenolytic activity could occur both prior to the initiation of the degradative process and as a mechanism to limit the extent of collagen breakdown.

Of similar physiological importance is the possible inhibition of collagenase activity by proteoglycan or glycoprotein fractions. The suggestion was made by Gnadinger *et al.* (1969) that proteoglycans might have a protective function in relation to the collagen matrix. If such is the case then degradation of the non-collagen components of the matrix would be an essential first step to collagen breakdown. Woolley and Evanson (1977b) have concluded that cartilage proteoglycans do not have a direct inhibitory effect on human collagenase *in vitro*. Nevertheless, *in vivo* proteoglycans might provide a physical barrier restricting contact of the enzyme with its substrate.

The fundamental importance of this discussion is that, with several forms of latency or inhibition of the collagenase enzyme, a number of regulatory mechanisms are possible. Before a full understanding of collagenase action can be achieved, therefore, the form in which the latent enzyme is present in the tissue at any time must be determined. In addition to the identification of the inhibitory components, the synthesis of a number of activating substances has been reported (Oronsky, Perper and Schroder, 1973; Werb *et al.*, 1977; Deshmukh-Phadka, Lawrence and Nanda, 1978). Thus, physiological

control of collagenase activity may also be possible through regulation of the synthesis of activators of the enzyme. Other potential regulatory parameters could include hormonal control (see Harris and Cartwright (1977) for review), pH and oxygen tension (Yen, 1978). Clearly, more than one form of enzyme regulation could operate *in vivo* to provide a very close control of enzyme activity and, indeed, current evidence is for the existence of more than one mechanism in several different systems.

NON-SPECIFIC PROTEINASES

The group of enzymes termed neutral proteinases plays an important role in the degradation of collagen. These enzymes possess activity against denatured collagen and the non-helical terminal peptides of collagen. However, with the possible exception of neutrophil elastase, since they will not cleave native collagen they are distinguished from the true collagenases. Many of the neutral proteinases are capable of proteolytic activity on substrates other than collagen. The unique primary structure of collagen (in which proline, hydroxyproline and glycine residues are each at a high level) makes even the denatured protein a poor substrate except in those areas of the molecule that are low in amino acid content but high in polar or non-polar amino acids. Even in this case, however, large peptides are produced that remain resistant to further degradation.

To date, despite the fact that the factors affecting collagenase activity have been extensively studied and are becoming increasingly understood, much less is known of the role of neutral proteinases. In combination, collagenase and the neutral proteinases are known to be effective in degrading the extracellular matrix collagens. Neutral proteinases that have been identified include the synovial enzyme secreted by human tissue (Harris and Krane, 1972) and rabbit fibroblast cells (Werb and Reynolds, 1974), the rabbit bone enzyme (Sellers, Reynolds and Meikle, 1978; Sellers *et al.*, 1979) and the human granulocyte enzyme (Sopata and Dancewicz, 1974). Neutrophil proteinases have been identified in inflamed articular cartilage (Barrett, 1978), while cathepsin D has also been identified extracellularly in connective tissues (Poole *et al.*, 1976). Both act as cross-linkases (Barrett,

1978; Scott and Pearson, 1978 a, b) by cleaving the non-helical terminal peptides of collagen and so effectively solubilizing the fibres.

Most of the neutral proteinases which have been found to be active against denatured collagen are inhibited by chelating agents, reducing agents that contain sulphydryl groups and serum (as are the mammalian collagenases). Activation of certain of these systems can be achieved by the same agents that activate collagenase (Harris and Krane, 1972; Werb and Reynolds, 1974; Woessner, 1979). In rabbit bone explants, a collagenase inhibitor has been isolated that also blocks the activity of other neutral proteinases including collagenase (Sellers et al., 1979). The collagenase and other neutral proteinases may act together to degrade the collagen matrix. It would appear, therefore, that a group of metalloproteinases (collagenase and neutral proteinases) are synthesized and secreted in a co-ordinate fashion. In addition, activation and regulation are likely to be accomplished through similar mechanisms.

P-z PEPTIDASES

In certain of the studies of bacterial collagenase, synthetic oligopeptides which resemble the collagen molecule have been employed for the measurement of activity. Cleavage of such synthetic oligopeptides is not evidence for specific animal collagenase activity, however, since other peptidases in animal tissues can degrade these peptides yet not affect native collagen. Nevertheless, the synthetic substrate 4 phenylazo-benzylcarboxyl-α-proline-α-leucylglycine-α-proline D arginine has been employed to detect a series of vertebrate proteinases with collagenase-like specificity (Harris and Krane, 1972; Weiss, 1976). This substrate (termed P-z peptide) has a repeating sequence analogous to the repeating sequence of gelatin. Although some neutral proteinases are able to cleave the P-z peptide, other enzymes that are able to degrade denatured collagen (such as that from human polymorphonuclear leucocytes (Sopata and Dancewicz, 1974)) are not (Wunsch and Heidrich, 1963). The term gelatinase as suggested by Weiss (1976) as a preferable alternative to P-z peptidase is not entirely appropriate since both the neutral proteinases and collagenase will also cleave gelatin.

P-z peptidases have been identified in several tissues, including cultured rheumatoid synovial tissue, fibrotic liver, cornea, rat uterine, lung and liver homogenates, granuloma tissue, human tumour cell lines (Weiss, 1976) and human polymorphonuclear leucocytes (Sopata and Dancewicz, 1974). Several of these peptidases can also be classed as neutral proteinases. Tissue levels of the P-z peptidases appear to correlate closely with the rate of collagen degradation in the mouse tissue, indicating an active physiological role for this series of enzymes. The suggestion has been made that the P-z peptidase might have a role in the continued degradation of collagen after the molecule has been partially degraded by collagenase (Nordwig, 1971; Morales and Woessner, 1977).

CROSS-LINKASES

Tissue collagens that are stabilized by intermolecular crosslinks are not readily degraded by collagenase. Whether a depolymerase or cross-linkase functions to cleave the crosslink regions of the fibril prior to specific cleavage of the helical regions has not been determined. Certainly, the occurrence of such an enzyme system would facilitate the degradation of the fibrillar structure. Enzymes known to attack the non-helical crosslink region in vitro include a neutral proteinase (Steven et al., 1975), elastase (see Burleigh, 1977), cathepsin G (Starkey, 1977), cathepsin B (Burleigh, Barrett and Lazarus, 1974), a collagenolytic cathepsin separate from cathepsin B (Etherington, 1974, 1976) and cathepsin D (Scott and Pearson, 1978 a, b).

INTRACELLULAR DEGRADATION

Partially degraded collagen fibrils have been observed in phagolysosomes of fibroblasts and other cells (Harris and Krane, 1972; Montfort and Perez-Tamayo, 1975; Iijima et al., 1978; Pettigrew, 1978). Fibroblasts of the periodontal ligament have been shown to be capable of actively ingesting and degrading collagen fibrils (see Chapter 2, page 29), perhaps while also synthesizing new collagen fibrils. However, whether the collagen molecule undergoing catabolism in a particular fibroblast has been endogenously or exogenously synthesized cannot be determined readily in the tissue. That fibroblasts do ingest exogenously synthesized collagen has been demonstrated convincingly by *in vitro* studies (Ryan and Woessner, 1971). The significance of intracellular collagen profiles is considered further in Chapter 2.

The assumption has been made that for phagocytosis to be possible the ends of the collagen fibril must be free. Thus, preliminary partial cleavage by extracellular enzymes was thought to be an essential prerequisite. *In vitro* studies have led to the suggestion that sections along an intact fibril can be segmented by a fibroblast and subjected to lysosomal digestion (Deporter and Ten Cate, 1973). If this is correct, fibrils that form part of a network structure could be remodelled even though still anchored at each end. That this process could occur entirely in the absence of any extracellular enzyme or cross-linkase is questionable. Depolymerization of the fibril resulting from cross-linkase activity would at least facilitate the phagocytic process and may prove to be an essential step in the degradative process. The isolation of the ingested fibril within the lysosomal vacuole is apparently an essential step in the intracellular degradation of the collagen molecule. Although the proteases of lysosomal origin have been investigated extensively, of this class of enzyme (which functions optimally at an acid pH) only the endopeptidases cathepsins B, D and collagenolytic cathepsin (a thiol proteinase identified in bovine spleen by Etherington, 1974, 1976) have been shown to cleave the extrahelical terminal peptide regions. Cathepsin D and the collagenolytic cathepsin will not act on the helical region of native collagen while cathepsin B may do so (Burleigh, Barrett and Lazarus, 1974). Both cathepsin B and collagenolytic cathepsin require activation by thiol compounds and may act synergistically together (Etherington, 1976). Cathepsin D has been identified extracellularly (Poole *et al.*, 1976) and has been shown to function as a cross-linkase (Scott and Pearson, 1978 a, b). Both elastase and cathepsin G (which are classified as lysosomal enzymes (Starkey, 1977)) have also been shown to cleave the non-helical peptides of collagen, although the action of cathepsin G is apparently restricted to Type II collagen.

ENZYMES OF THE ORAL TISSUES

In the oral tissues, collagenase has been isolated in culture from the implant media of gingiva (Birkedal-Hansen *et al.*, 1974), dental follicle (Iijima *et al.*, 1978) and dental pulp (Kishi *et al.*, 1979). The collagenases of the dental follicle and gingiva, although initially in a latent form, are released as the active enzyme after a period of culture as an implant. The collagenase identified in the implant medium of the dental pulp, on the other hand, remained in the latent form during all stages of culture. Explants of rodent periodontal ligament obtained following experimental tooth movement have also been shown, *in vitro*, to produce collagenase (Ozaki, 1971). In the normal tissue, however, a collagenase has not been detected under either *in vivo* or *in vitro* conditions. Although an inhibitor of collagenase has been demonstrated in the media from periodontal ligament cell cultures, no evidence has been obtained for either an active or latent collagenase (Ryan and Woessner, 1971; Pettigrew, 1978). Nevertheless, the presence of an inhibitor in this tissue does suggest that a collagenase might be produced within the periodontal ligament under the appropriate conditions.

Ageing of collagen

The general, and often subtle, changes that take place in the structure of organ systems with resulting functional deterioration are classified as the ageing process. With the improved life expectancy of the population, this phenomenon has been increasingly studied in recent years.

Age changes in the periodontal ligament closely parallel those observed in the connective tissues elsewhere in the body (Courtney, 1972). Of particular importance is a decrease in the thickness of the periodontal ligament in the aged (Coolidge, 1938) implying a reduced masticatory function (Courtney, 1972). This modification is associated with an increase in the diameter of collagen fibres, a reduction in the cellular component, and a decreased solubility and increased resistance to chemical and enzymic attack of the collagen fibres (e.g. Courtney, 1972).

The major chemical change that can be detected in the collagen molecules of the aged tissue concerns the covalent crosslinks that are essential to the stability of the fibre. Several changes take place in the crosslinks. Following formation of the aldimine crosslink, stabilization by rearrangement to the keto derivative occurs relatively rapidly. Subsequently, there is a slow transformation to a more stable non-reducible form. In addition, a recent study (Robins and Bailey, 1977) has suggested that decreased solubility in ageing connective tissue may occur independently in the crosslinking process. As yet, this solubility change mechanism has not been identified, although it is an oxygen-dependent process (Bailey et al., 1977; Robins and Bailey, 1977). Excepting pathological change, there is no firm evidence of further chemical modification to the collagen molecule during the ageing process.

Collagen of the periodontal ligament

Only in recent years has the periodontal ligament received the concentrated biochemical study that is appropriate to a tissue of fundamental importance to dental science. Previously, technical difficulties associated with the small size of this tissue and its dissection from the surrounding mineralized tissues have discouraged a detailed analysis. Although the number of individual laboratories engaged in the study of this tissue remains small, our understanding of the biochemistry of the periodontal ligament is now expanding rapidly.

In an early study of the rat periodontal ligament, Eastoe and Melcher (1971) reported a total protein content of approximately 50% of which some 30% was thought to be non-collagenous glycoprotein. Subsequently, Butler et al. (1975) demonstrated that the major component of bovine periodontal ligament collagen was Type I with a smaller proportion (up to 20%) of Type III collagen. To date, the significance of the occurrence of Type III collagen in the periodontal ligament has not been explained. The fibre identified as reticulin which occurs in the periodontal ligament has long been studied by histologists. Good evidence is now available that this fibre is composed of Type III collagen (Fietzek and Kuhn, 1976). Re-

cent data (Brunette et al., 1979) suggest that epithelial cells derived from the rests of Malassez secrete small amounts of Type IV collagen.

Isotope incorporation studies have indicated that the turnover of collagen in the mature rodent molar ligament is approximately the same for both Type I and Type III collagens (Sodek, 1978). Immuno-histochemical studies (Rao et al., 1979) suggested a greater concentration of Type I collagen adjacent to alveolar bone than to the cementum in some regions, whereas in other areas there was no apparent difference. Although a relationship is thought to exist between the collagenous fibre diameter and its constituent collagen type in some tissues, in the periodontal ligament fibre diameters are approximately uniform (see also Chapter 3).

It is well known that the solubility of collagen varies in different tissues and that this property is generally considered to be related to the degree of intermolecular crosslinking of the collagen in each tissue. For example, the collagen matrix of dentine is formed as a densely woven network of very fine, relatively uniform fibrils. This collagen is characterized by a very high degree of insolubility in both neutral and distinct buffers, little detectable swelling in acid and no apparent swelling on denaturation in strong denaturing agents (Veis and Schleuter, 1964). These properties are thought to be due to a combination of the close fibre weave and the high degree of intermolecular crosslinking. The collagen fibrils of the ligament are likewise strengthened by the formation of a series of intermolecular crosslinks (Fig. 5). The major reducible crosslink of periodontal ligament is dehydrodihydroxylysinonorleucine (aldimine-linked hydroxyallysyl and hydroxylysyl residues) and dehydrohydroxylysinonorleucine (aldimine-linked allysyl and hydroxylysyl residues) forms a minor component (Pearson et al., 1975). Although the proportion of reducible crosslinks relative to the total collagen content of the matrix of some tissues decreases with age (Veis, Anesey and Mussell, 1967; Bailey and Shimokamoki, 1971), no such change could be observed in the periodontal ligament. Rather, the content of reducible crosslinks was observed to be consistently high in the ligament of the bovine molar both before and after eruption (Pearson et al., 1975). This may reflect a very high rate of turnover of the collagen in this tissue such that the normal process of maturation to non-reducible crosslinks is not completed.

At present, although considerable data have been obtained concerning the content of reducible crosslinks of this tissue, little is known about the mature, non-reducible crosslink components. This is because, although procedures have been devised to permit semiquantitative estimation of the latter crosslink (Scott and Veis, 1976; Light and Bailey, 1979), quantitative analysis is not yet possible. Thus, in the mature tissue only a partial quantitation of the actual number of crosslinks is possible with present techniques. Moreover, as these crosslinks are probably only transitory in nature, the value of such studies for improving our understanding of the structure and stability of the tissue is severely limited.

Various studies have indicated that protein metabolism in the ligament is rapid (Stallard, 1963; Crumley, 1964; Carneiro and Fava de Moraes, 1965; Skougaard, Frandsen and Baker, 1970; Skougaard, Levy and Simpson, 1970; Kivirikko, 1971; Rippon, 1976; Sodek, 1976, 1977, 1978; Sodek et al., 1977). The greater part of this activity is attributed to the collagen fraction of the tissue (Sodek et al., 1977). The half-life for the turnover of mature collagen in the periodontal ligament of the rodent has been reported by Sodek et al. (1977) to be approximately 1 day in the molar and 3 days in the incisor, although Orlowski (1978) has suggested up to 9.5 days in the latter tooth. In either case, however, it is clear that the turnover of collagen in the periodontal ligament is unusually rapid.

No immediate explanation is apparent for the exceptionally high metabolic turnover of the structural proteins of the periodontal ligament. Much has been made of the turnover of this tissue in terms of the process of tooth eruption (see Chapter 10). That there is no simple relation to the process of eruption is indicated by the fact that, in spite of the rate of collagen synthesis being similar, the rate of turnover of mature collagen in the periodontal ligament of the non-continuously growing rat molar is approximately three-fold faster than in the ligament of the continuously growing incisor (Sodek et al., 1977). Much of the collagen of the incisor ligament may not be incorporated, therefore, in the extracellular matrix in an insoluble form, but is degraded soon after synthesis while still readily soluble. That a portion of the total collagen pool is degraded within hours of synthesis has been demonstrated in other tissues (Bienkowski, Baum and Crystal, 1978; Sakamoto et al., 1979), and in rabbit lung explants 30–40% of newly synthesized collagen is degraded within minutes of synthesis (Bornstein, 1974). A similar system might exist in the incisor ligament, whereas in the molar ligament, although turnover is rapid, the collagen does form a mature molecular structure first. In contrast to the collagen fraction, the metabolic activities of the non-collagenous proteins in both incisor and molar ligaments are closely similar (Sodek, 1978). To date, however, no study has been undertaken to determine the metabolic activity of the molar periodontal ligament both during eruption and at maturity.

The rate of synthesis is apparently uniform along the length of the periodontal ligament (e.g. Beertsen and Everts, 1977) and the turnover of both Type I and Type III collagens within the ligament is also similar (Sodek, 1978). Several studies have been directed to establishing the site of remodelling of collagen in the periodontal ligament. Initially it was believed that the fibres of the periodontal ligament that originated within the cementum and bone were joined at the mid-region of the periodontal space to form an histologically distinct 'intermediate plexus'. This was thought to be the region where rapid remodelling of the fibrillar structure occurred. Employing radioautographic procedures, Beertsen and Everts (1977) observed that synthesis and turnover of total protein occurred across the width of the rodent incisor ligament though the remodelling of collagen (as assessed by the number of intracellular collagen profiles) appeared to occur primarily in the intermediate area of the ligament. In the mature molar, on the other hand, remodelling of the collagen matrix was observed to be evenly distributed across the width of the ligament (Beertsen, Brekelmans and Everts, 1978), although some have suggested that a remodelling activity is increased adjacent to the alveolar bone (e.g. Stallard, 1963; Crumley, 1964). Other ultrastructural studies (e.g. Sloan, 1978, 1979) have failed to provide firm evidence for the occurrence of intermediate plexus. A more detailed discussion of the concept of the intermediate plexus is contained in Chapter 3.

The apparent identification of an intermediate

plexus was convenient in that it provided a zone within the periodontal ligament where a system of collagen fibres could be sliced and separated from the anchoring Sharpey's fibres. Nevertheless, regardless of the presence or absence of an histologically demonstrable intermediate plexus, the question of the mechanism by which fibrillar structure of the periodontal ligament can be separated during such processes as eruption and orthodontic movement remains highly significant and must be answered before these phenomena can be said to be fully understood. In particular, the process of eruption has attracted the attention of many investigators, but without the evolution of a universally acceptable explanation for the eruption mechanism. The generation of a tensile force by the connective tissue of the periodontal ligament has been postulated. As originally proposed, the maturing collagen fibres of the periodontal ligament were required to contract (Thomas, 1967). This hypothesis has been seriously questioned, however. An alternative hypothesis by Beertsen, Everts and van den Hooff (1974) (subsequently developed by Garant and Cho (1979 a, b)) has associated the movement of the teeth during eruption to fibroblast contraction and migration. For this hypothesis, the meshwork of collagen fibres attached into the cementum would provide the base from which the fibroblast could anchor in order to achieve movement of the tooth. It is reasonable to speculate that the attachment of the fibroblast to the collagen matrix might be through a recently characterized high molecular weight glycoprotein termed fibronectin (Bornstein et al., 1978; see also Chapter 6). Indeed, it is possible that the fibronectin component is involved both in adhesion to the collagen fibril and in mediating the absorption and subsequent degradation of the collagen by the fibroblast. For further information concerning the theories of eruption the reader is referred to Chapter 10.

It has been proposed that one step in the degradation of the collagen matrix involves the phagocytosis of collagen segments by fibroblasts (Kivirikko, 1971) or other cells (Azuma et al., 1975). Studies of the site of collagen resorption in the periodontal ligament have in several cases been based on the observation of periodontal ligament fibroblasts containing intracellular collagen fibrils (e.g. Deporter and Ten Cate, 1973). An unequivocal interpretation of

these experimental data is difficult, however, because of the recent demonstration that fibroblasts can degrade newly synthesized collagen within the cell before secretion (Bienkowski et al., 1978). Thus, although the evidence for collagen phagocytosis by fibroblasts is strong, whether the intracellular collagen segments observed in a periodontal ligament fibroblast represent a degraded collagen that has never been secreted or a matrix collagen in the process of degradation is not known. The answers to these problems must await a more detailed knowledge of the mechanism for the control of collagen metabolism in the periodontal ligament.

In normal circumstances, it may be assumed that the rates of synthesis and degradation are carefully synchronized. That fibroblasts can modulate and synchronize these opposing functions is indicated by the work of Beertsen and Everts (1977). They showed that the rates of collagen secretion and degradation were proportionally increased in response to a doubling in the eruption rate in the rat incisor. Similarly, Rippon (1976) has shown that when mandibular rat molars are allowed to over-erupt following extraction of the opposing maxillary teeth, the half-life of collagen in the alveolar crest region is shortened. Collagen turnover is also increased on the 'tension' side of the ligament during orthodontic movement (Freeman and Ten Cate, 1978).

Although considerable knowledge exists concerning the pathways of synthesis and degradation of collagen and many substances are known to affect these processes (for review see Harris and Cartwright (1977)), the factors ultimately responsible for synchronizing collagen turnover in the functional tissues have not been defined. Nevertheless, current studies are rapidly advancing our understanding of specific aspects of these processes.

While the ultimate control of protein synthesis is at the level of gene expression by selective transcription, regulation of collagen production could also be initiated at translation or at any step prior to secretion (Paglia et al., 1979). One form of regulation has been shown to be through mRNA limited control in which the rate of synthesis of certain proteins is restricted by the mRNA content of the cell (Gelinas and Kafatos, 1977; Moen, Rowe and Palmiter, 1979). In collagen synthesis a further method of control has been extensively studied whereby regulation is effected through enzymes that modify the peptide chains of the protein. Limitation of the post-translational hydroxylation of the peptides reduces both stability and secretion of collagen. Thus, regulation of the hydroxylase could control the amount of collagen reaching the extracellular matrix (Berg and Prockop, 1973; Jimenez *et al.*, 1974). Recently, it has been demonstrated that amino terminal propeptides removed during the conversion of procollagen to collagen are able to inhibit collagen synthesis whereas peptides from other regions of the collagen chain have no effect (Krieg *et al.*, 1978; Paglia *et al.*, 1979; Wiestner *et al.*, 1979). The synthesis of other proteins was not inhibited by the presence of amino terminal collagen propeptides.

Fundamental studies such as these are contributing much to our knowledge of the processes by which the synthesis of collagen and other proteins is controlled. Other studies are directed to the regulation of collagen degradation. However, as yet, little is known of the mechanism by which the two processes are interrelated.

OXYTALAN

A fibre termed oxytalan has been found in the periodontal and gingival tissues of a number of mammalian species (Fullmer, 1967). Following oxidation of the tissue section, oxytalan fibres can be detected in the light microscope by the staining techniques used for visualization of elastin fibres (Fullmer and Lillie, 1958). Indeed, in the electron microscope these fibres resemble immature elastin fibres (Melcher, 1976). Sodek (1978), on the basis of amino acid analysis data, has suggested a closer similarity to collagenous fibrilloproteins. The detailed composition and origin of oxytalan is yet to be defined and requires the application of more precise biochemical and histological studies.

SUMMARY

Our understanding of the synthesis, structure and function of the collagen molecule and fibre is now extensive. That several genetically distinct types of

collagen molecules exist in different tissues has been documented. There are at least two species present in the periodontal ligament, and the majority of tissues appear to be formed from more than one collagen type. It is possible that the collagen of the basement membrane might be composed of a further group of related collagens, as is the case for the interstitial connective tissues. To date, no interrelationship has been established between collagen type identity and physiological function of the tissue. Nevertheless, a collagen type/function interdependence is to be expected.

Studies of the amino acid sequence of collagen have revealed the complete sequence of the $\alpha_1 I$ chain and partial sequences for the α_2 chain, the $\alpha_1 II$ chain and the $\alpha_1 III$ chain. Such investigations are providing the basis for a detailed understanding of the stability of the triple helix, its crosslinking capabilities and microfibril—fibre formation and structure.

The complex field of enzymatic degradation of the periodontal ligament proteins and specifically of the collagenous matrix is still only partially understood. Several types of enzyme, including collagenases, gelatinases, neutral and acidic proteases, have been identified and the potential for both intra- and intercellular degradation of the collagen molecule established. The precise pathway by which the collagen of the periodontal ligament is catabolized has not been defined and remains an exciting and important challenge.

The origin and composition of oxytalan fibres in the periodontal ligament remain unknown.

REFERENCES

ABBOTT, M. R. & UDENFRIEND, S. (1974) α Ketoglutarate-coupled dioxygenases, *Molecular mechanisms of oxygen activation,* O. HAYASHI (ed.), 167–214. New York, Academic Press.

ANDERSON, J. M., RIPPON, N. B. & WALTON, A. G. (1970) Model tripeptides for collagen. *Biochem. Biophys. Res. Commun.* 39, 802–808.

ANTTINEN, H., OIKARINEN, A., RYHANEN, L. & KIVIRIKKO, K. (1978) Evidence for the transfer of mannose to the extension peptides of procollagen within the cisternae of the rough endoplasmic reticulum. *FEBS Lett.* 87, 222–226.

AZUMA, M., ENLOW, D. H., FREDERICKSON, R. G. & GASTON, L. G. (1975) *Determination of mandibular growth* (J. A. MacNAMARA), Monograph No. 4 Craniofacial Growth Series, Centre for Human Growth and Development, The University of Michigan, 179–207.

BAILEY, A. J., RANTA, M. H., NICHOLLS, A. C., PARTRIDGE, S. M. & ELSDEN, D. F. (1977) Isolation of α aminoadipic acid from mature dermal collagen and elastin. Evidence for an oxidative pathway in the maturation of collagen and elastin. *Biochem. Biophys. Res. Commun.* **78**, 1403–1410.

BAILEY, A. J. & ROBINS, S. P. (1973) In: *Frontiers in matrix biology*, L. ROBERT (ed.), I, pp. 130–156. Basle, Karger.

BAILEY, A. J., ROBINS, S. P. & BALIAN, G. (1974) Biological significance of intermolecular crosslinks of collagen. *Nature (Lond.)* **251**, 105–109.

BAILEY, A. J. & SHIMOKAMOKI, M. (1971) Age related changes in the reducible crosslinks of collagen. *FEBS Lett.* **16**, 86–88.

BARNES, M. J., CONSTABLE, B. J., MORTON, L. F. & ROYCE, P. M. (1974) Age-related variations in hydroxylation of lysine and proline in collagen. *Biochem. J.* **139**, 461–468.

BARRETT, A. J. (1978) The possible role of neutrophil proteinases in damage to articular cartilage. *Agents & Actions* **8**, 11–18.

BARRETT, A. J. & STARKEY, P. M. (1973) The interaction of α$_2$-macroglobulin with proteinases. Characteristics and specificity of the reaction and a hypothesis concerning its molecular mechanism. *Biochem. J.* **133**, 709–724.

BATES, C. J., PRYNNE, C. J. & LEVENE, C. I. (1972) The synthesis of underhydroxylated collagen by $_3$T6 mouse fibroblasts in culture. *Biochim. Biophys. Acta* **263**, 397–405.

BAUER, E. A., STRICKLIN, G. P., JEFFREY, J. J. & EISEN, A. Z. (1975) Collagenase production by human skin fibroblasts. *Biochem. Biophys. Res. Commun.* **64**, 232–240.

BECKER, U., FURTHMAYR, H. & TIMPL, R. (1975) Tryptic peptides from the cross-linking regions of insoluble calf skin collagen. *Hoppe-Seyler's Z. Physiol. Chem.* **356**, 21–32.

BECKER, U., HELLE, O. & TIMPL, R. (1977) Characterization of the amino-terminal segment in procollagen pα2 chain from dermatosparactic sheep. *FEBS Lett.* **73**, 197–200.

BECKER, U., TIMPL, R., HELLE, O. & PROCKOP, D. J. (1976) NH$_2$-terminal extensions on skin collagen from sheep with a genetic defect in conversion of procollagen into collagen. *Biochemistry* **15**, 2853–2862.

BEERTSEN, W., BREKELMANS, M. & EVERTS, V. (1978) The site of collagen resorption in the periodontal ligament of the rodent molar. *Anat. Rec.* **192**, 305–318.

BEERTSEN, W. & EVERTS, V. (1977) Site of remodeling of collagen in periodontal ligament of mouse incisor. *Anat. Rec.* **189**, 479–498.

BEERTSEN, W., EVERTS, V. & VAN DEN HOOFF, W. (1974) Fine structure of fibroblasts in periodontal ligament of rat incisor and their possible role in tooth eruption. *Archs. oral Biol.* **19**, 1087–1098.

BENTZ, H., BACKINGER, H. P., GLANVILLE, R. & KUHN,

K. (1978) Physical evidence for the assembly of A and B chains of human placental collagen in a single triple helix. *Eur. J. Biochem.* **92**, 563–567.

BENYA, P. D., PADILLA, S. R. & NIMMNI, M. E. (1977) The progeny of rabbit articular chondrocytes synthesize collagen Types I and III and Type I trimer but not Type II. Verification of cyanogen bromide peptide analysis. *Biochemistry* **16**, 865–872.

BERG, R. A. & PROCKOP, D. J. (1973) Purification of ^{14}C protocollagen and its hydroxylation by prolylhydroxylase. *Biochemistry* **12**, 3395–3401.

BIENKOWSKI, R. S., BAUM, B. J. & CRYSTAL, R. G. (1978) Fibroblasts degrade newly synthesized collagen within the cell before secretion. *Nature* **276**, 413–416.

BIRKEDAL-HANSEN, H., BUTLER, W. T. & TAYLOR, R. E. (1977) Proteins of the periodontium. Characterization of the insoluble collagens of bovine dental cementum. *Calc. Tiss. Res.* **23**, 39–44.

BIRKEDAL-HANSEN, H., COBB, C. M., TAYLOR, R. E. & FULLMER, H. M. (1971) Activation of latent bovine gingival collagenase. *Archs. oral Biol.* **20**, 681.

BIRKEDAL-HANSEN, H., COBB, C. M., TAYLOR, R. E. & FULLMER, H. M. (1974) Bovine gingival collagenase: demonstration and initial characterization. *J. oral Path.* **3**, 232–238.

BLOBEL, G. & DOBBERSTEIN, B. (1975) Transfer of proteins across membranes. *J. Cell Biol.* **67**, 835–851.

BORNSTEIN, P. (1970) Structure of α1-CB8, a large cyanogen bromide produced fragment from the α-1 chain of rat collagen. The nature of a hydroxylamine-sensitive bond and composition of tryptic peptides. *Biochemistry* **9**, 2408–2421.

BORNSTEIN, P. (1974) Biosynthesis of collagen. *Ann. Rev. Biochem.* **43**, 567–603.

BORNSTEIN, P., DUKSIN, D., BALIAN, G., DAVIDSON, J. M. & CROUCH, E. (1978) Organization of extracellular proteins on the connective tissue cell surface: relevance to cell-matrix interactions *in vitro* and *in vivo*. *Ann. N.Y. Acad. Sci.* **312**, 93–105.

BROWN, R. A., SHUTTLEWORTH, C. A. & WEISS, J. B. (1978) Three new α-chains of collagen from a nonbasement membrane source. *Biochem. Biophys. Res. Commun.* **80**, 866–872.

BROWN, R. A. & WEISS, J. B. (1979) Type V collagen possible shared identity of αA αB αC chains. *FEBS Lett.* **106**, 71–75.

BROWNELL, A. G. & VEIS, A. (1975) Intracellular location of glycosylation of hydroxylysine of collagen. *Biochem. Biophys. Res. Commun.* **63**, 371–377.

BRUCKNER, P., BACHINGER, H. P., TIMPL, R. & ENGEL, J. (1978) Three conformationally distinct domains in the amino-terminal segment of Type III procollagen and its rapid helix coil transition. *Eur. J. Biochem.* **90**, 595–603.

BRUNETTE, D. M., LIMEBACH, R., PETTIGREW, D., MELCHER, A. H. & SODEK, J. (1979) Proteins secreted *in vitro* by epithelial cells cultured from porcine periodontal ligament. *J. dent. Res.* **58**, Spec. Iss. A. Abstr. No. 246.

BRUNS, R. R., HOLMES, D. J. S., THERRIEN, S. F. & GROSS, J. (1979) Procollagen segment-long-segment crystallites: their role in collagen fibrillogenesis. *Proc. Natl. Acad. Sci. USA* **76**, 313–317.

BURGESON, R. E., EL ADLI, F. A., KAITILA, I. I. &

HOLLISTER, D. W. (1976) Fetal membrane collagens: identification of two new collagen alpha chains. *Proc. Nat. Acad. Sci. USA* 73, 2579–2583.

BURLEIGH, M. C. (1977) Degradation of collagen of non-specific proteinases. In: *Proteinases in mammalian cells and tissues*, A. J. BARRETT (ed.); *Research monographs in cell and tissue physiology*, J. T. DINGLE, (ed.), 2, 285–309. New York, North-Holland.

BURLEIGH, M. C., BARRETT, A. J. & LAZARUS, G. S. (1974) Cathepsin B1: a lysosomal enzyme that degrades native collagen. *Biochem. J.* 137, 387–398.

BUTLER, W. F. (1975) Fragility of skin in a cat. *Res. in Vet. Sci.* 19, 213–216.

BUTLER, W. T., BIRKEDAL-HANSEN, H., BEEGLE, W. R., TAYLOR, R. E. & CHUNG, E. (1975) Proteins of periodontium – identification of collagens with $\alpha(I)_2$, $\alpha 2$ and $\alpha(III)_3$ structures in bovine periodontal ligament. *J. Biol. Chem.* 250, 8907–8912.

CARNEIRO, J. & DE MORAES, F. (1965) Radioautographic visualization of collagen metabolism in the periodontal tissues of the mouse. *Archs. oral Biol.* 10, 833–834.

CHESNEY, C., McI. HARPER, E. & COLMAN, R. W. (1974) Human platelet collagenase. *J. Clin. Invest.* 53, 1647–1654.

CHUNG, E. & MILLER, E. J. (1974) Collagen polymorphism – characterization of molecules with chain composition [αI(III)3] in human tissues. *Science* 183, 1200–1201.

CHUNG, E., RHODES, R. K. & MILLER, E. J. (1976) Isolation of three collagenous components of probable basement membrane origin from several tissues. *Biochem. Biophys. Res. Commun.* 71, 1167–1174.

CLARK, C. C. (1979) The distribution and initial characterization of oligosaccharide units on the COOH-terminal propeptide extensions of the pro-α_1 and pro-α_2 chains of Type I procollagen. *J. Biol. Chem.* 254, 1798–1802.

CLARK, C. C. & KEFALIDES, N. A. (1978) Localization and partial composition of the oligosaccharide units on the propeptide extensions of Type I procollagen. *J. Biol. Chem.* 253, 47–51.

COOLIDGE, E. D. (1938) Traumatic and functional injuries occurring in supporting tissues of human teeth. *J. Am. dent. Ass.* 25, 343–357.

COURTNEY, R. M. (1972) Age changes in the periodontium and oral mucous membranes. *J. Mich. dent. Assoc.* 54, 335–344.

CROUCH, E., SAGE, H. & BORNSTEIN, P. (1980) Structural basis for apparent heterogeneity of collagens in human basement membranes type IV procollagen containing two distinct chains. *Proc. Natl. Acad. Sci. USA*, 77, 745–749.

CRUMLEY, P. J. (1964) Collagen formation in the normal and stressed periodontium. *Periodontics* 2, 53–61.

DABBOUS, M. K., YAMANISHI, Y., MAEYENS, E. E., HASHIMOTO, K. & HARDISON, H. (1974) Collagenolytic activity in rheumatoid nodules. I. Effect on acid-soluble tropocollagen. *Acta Derm. Venereol.* 54, 265–269.

DANIELS, J. R., LIAN, J. & LAZARUS, G. (1969) Polymorphonuclear leukocyte collagenase: isolation and kinetic characteristics. *Clin. Res.* 17, 154.

DAVIDSON, J. M., McENEANY, L. S. G. & BORNSTEIN, P. (1975) Intermediates in the limited proteolytic conversion of procollagen to collagen. *Biochemistry* 14, 5188–5194.

DAVIS, N. R., RISEN, O. M. & PRINGLE, G. A. (1975) Stable non-reducible crosslinks of mature collagen. *Biochemistry* 14, 2031–2036.

DAYER, J. M., RUSSELL, R. G. G. & KRANE, S. M. (1977) Collagenase production of rheumatoid synovial cells, stimulation by a human lymphocyte factor. *Science* 195, 181–183.

DEHM, P. & PROCKOP, D. J. (1971) Synthesis and extrusion of collagen by freshly isolated cells from chick embryo tendon. *Biochem. Biophys. Acta* 240, 358–369.

DEPORTER, D. A. & TEN CATE, A. R. (1973) Fine structural localization of acid and alkaline phosphatase in collagen-containing vesicles of fibroblasts. *J. Anat.* 114, 457–461.

DESHMUKH-PHADKA, K., LAWRENCE, M. & NANDA, S. (1978) Synthesis of collagenase and neutral proteases by articular chondrocytes: stimulation by a macrophage-derived factor. *Biochem. Biophys. Res. Commun.* 85, 490–496.

DIEGELMANN, R. F., BERNSTEIN, L. & PETERKOFSKY, B. (1973) Cell-free collagen synthesis on membrane-bound polysomes of chick embryo connective tissue and localization of prolyl hydroxylase on polysome membrane complex. *J. Biol. Chem.* 248, 6514–6521.

DIEGELMANN, R. F. & PETERKOFSKY, B. (1972) Inhibition of collagen secretion from bone and cultured fibroblasts by micro-fibrillar disruptive drugs. *Proc. Natl. Acad. Sci. USA* 69, 892–896.

DIXIT, S. N. & BENSUSAN, H. (1973) The isolation of crosslinked peptides of collagen involving αI-CB6. *Biochem. Biophys. Res. Commun.* 52, 1–8.

DIXIT, S. N., MAINARDI, C. L., SEYER, J. M. & KANG, A. H. (1979) Covalent structure of collagen: amino acid sequence of αCB5 of chick skin collagen containing the animal collagenase cleavage site. *Biochemistry* 24, 5416–5422.

EASTOE, J. E. & MELCHER, A. H. (1971) Amino acid composition of whole periodontal ligament from rat incisors. *J. dent. Res.* 50, 675.

EECKHOUT, Y. & VAES, G. (1977) Further studies on activation of procollagenase, latent precursor of bone collagenase – effects on lysosomal cathepsin B, plasmin and kallikrein, and spontaneous activation. *Biochem. J.* 166, 21–31.

ENGEL, J., BRUCKNER, R., BECKER, U., TIMPL, R. & RUTSCHMANN, B. (1977) Physical properties of the amino terminal precursor-specific portion of Type I procollagen. *Biochemistry* 16, 4026–4033.

EPSTEIN, E. H. (1974) [αI(III)3] human skin collagen. Release by pepsin digestion and preponderance in fetal life. *J. Biol. Chem.* 249, 3225–3231.

EPSTEIN, E. H., SCOTT, R. D., MILLER, E. J. & PIEZ, K. A. (1971) Isolation and characterization of the peptides derived from soluble human and baboon skin collagen after cynogen bromide cleavage. *J. Biol. Chem.* 246, 1718–1724.

ETHERINGTON, D. J. (1974) The purification of bovine cathepsin B1 and its mode of action on bovine collagens. *Biochem. J.* 137, 547–557.

ETHERINGTON, D. J. (1976) Bovine spleen cathepsin B1

and collagenolytic cathepsin: a comparative study of the properties of the two enzymes in the degradation of native collagen. *Biochem. J.* 153, 199–209.

EYRE, D. R. & GLIMCHER, M. J. (1973a) Analysis of a crosslinked peptide from calf bone collagen: evidence that hydroxylysyl glycoside participates in the crosslink. *Biochem. Biophys. Res. Commun.* 52, 663–671.

EYRE, D. R. & GLIMCHER, M. J. (1973b) Collagen crosslinking. Isolation of crosslinked peptides from collagen of chicken bone. *Biochem. J.* 135, 393–403.

FESSLER, J. H. & FESSLER, L. I. (1978) Biosynthesis of procollagen. *Ann. Rev. Biochem.* 47, 129–162.

FESSLER, J. H., GREENBERG, D. B. & FESSLER, L. I. (1978) *Biology and chemistry of basement membranes,* N. A. KEFALIDES (ed.), pp. 373–382. New York, Academic Press.

FESSLER, L. I., BURGESON, R. E., MORRIS, N. P. & FESSLER, J. H. (1973) Collagen synthesis: A disulphide-linked collagen precursor in chick bone. *Proc. Natl. Acad. Sci. USA* 70, 2993–3001.

FESSLER, L. I. & FESSLER, J. H. (1979) Characterization of Type III procollagen from chick embryo blood vessels. *J. Biol. Chem.* 254, 233–239.

FESSLER, L. I., MORRIS, N. P. & FESSLER, J. H. (1975) Procollagen: Biological scission of amino and carboxyl extension peptides. *Proc. Natl. Acad. Sci. USA* 72, 4905–4909.

FIETZEK, P. P., ALLMANN, H., RAUTERBERG, J., HENKEL, W., WACHTER, E. & KUHN, K. (1979) The covalent structure of calf skin Type III collagen. *Hoppe Seyler's Z. Physiol. Chem.* 360, 809–810.

FIETZEK, P. P. & KUHN, K. (1975) Information contained in the amino acid sequence of the α_1 I chain of collagen and its consequences upon the formation of the triple helix of fibril and crosslinks. *Molec. Cell. Biochem.* 8, 141–157.

FIETZEK, P. P. & KUHN, K. (1976) The primary structure of collagen. *Int. Rev. Connect. Tiss. Res.* 7, 1–60.

FREEMAN, E. & TEN CATE, A. R. (1978) Early ultrastructural changes in the periodontal ligament during orthodontic tooth movement. *J. dent. Res.* 57, Special Issue A. Abst. 256.

FUJIWARA, K., SAKAI, T., ODA, T. & IGARASHI, S. (1974) Demonstration of collagenase activity in rat liver homogenate. *Biochem. Biophys. Res. Commun.* 60, 166–171.

FULLMER, H. M. (1967) In: *Structural and chemical organization of teeth,* Vol. II, A. E. W. MILES (ed.), pp. 349–414. New York, Academic Press.

FULLMER, H. M. & LILLIE, R. D. (1958) The oxytalin fiber: a previously undescribed connective tissue fiber. *J. Histochem. Cytochem.* 6, 425–430.

FURTHMAYR, H., TIMPL, R., STARK, M., LAPIERE, G. M. & KUHN, K. (1972) Clinical properties of peptide extension in α-1 chain of dermatosparatic skin procollagen. *FEBS Lett.* 28, 247–250.

GALLOP, P. M., BLUMENFELD, O. O. & SEIFTER, S. (1972) Structure and metabolism of connective tissue proteins. *Ann. Rev. Biochem.* 41, 617–672.

GARANT, P. R. & CHO, M. I. (1979a) Cytoplasmic polarization of periodontal ligament fibroblasts. *J. Periodont. Res.* 14, 95–106.

GARANT, P. R. & CHO, M. I. (1979b) Autoradiographic

evidence of the co-ordination of the genesis of Sharpey's fibres with new bone formation in the periodontum of the mouse. *J. Periodont. Res.* 14, 107–114.

GAY, S., BALLEISEN, L., REMBERGER, K., FIETZEK, P. P., ADELMANN, B. C. & KUHN, K. (1975) Immunohistochemical evidence for the presence of collagen Type III in human arterial walls, arterial thrombosis and in leukocytes incubated with collagen *in vitro. Klin. Wschr.* 53, 899.

GELINAS, R. E. & KAFATOS, F. C. (1977) The control of chorion protein synthesis in silk moths. mRNA production parallels protein synthesis. *Devl. Biol.* 55, 179–190.

GLANVILLE, R. W., RAUTER, A. & FIETZEK, P. P. (1979) Isolation and characterization of a native placental basement-membrane collagen and its component α chains. *Eur. J. Biochem.* 95, 383–389.

GNADINGER, M. C., ITOI, M., SLANSKY, H. & DOHLMAN, C. H. (1969) The role of collagenase in the alkali burned cornea. *Amer. J. Ophthalmol.* 68, 478–483.

GOLDBERG, B. & GREEN, H. (1967) Collagen synthesis on polyribosomes of cultured mammalian fibroblasts. *J. molec. Biol.* 26, 1–18.

GOLUB, E. E. & KATZ, E. P. (1977) Nonequivalent intermolecular stagger states in collagen fibrils. *Biopolymers* 16, 1357–1361.

GRANT, M. E. & JACKSON, D. S. (1976) Biosynthesis of procollagen. *Essays in Biochem.* 12, 77–113.

GRANT, M. E. & PROCKOP, D. J. (1972) The biosynthesis of collagen. *N. Engl. J. Med.* 286, 194–199, 242–249, 291–300.

GROSS, J. (1970) In: *Chemistry and molecular biology of the intercellular matrix,* E. A. BALAZS (ed.), 3, 1623–1636. New York, Academic Press.

GROSS, J. (1976) Aspects of animal collagenases. In: *Biochemistry of collagen,* G. N. RAMACHANDRAN & A. H. REDDI (eds.), pp. 275–318. New York, Plenum Press.

GROSS, J. & LAPIERE, C. M. (1962) Collagenolytic activity in amphibian tissues: A tissue culture assay. *Proc. Natl. Acad. Sci. USA* 48, 1014–1022.

GROSS, J. & NAGAI, Y. (1965) Specific degradation of the collagen molecule by tadpole collagenolytic enzyme. *Proc. Natl. Acad. Sci. USA* 54, 1197–1204.

GUZMAN, N. A., GRAVES, P. N. & PROCKOP, D. J. (1978) Addition of mannose to both the amino and carboxy terminal propeptides of Type II procollagen occurs without formation of triple helix. *Biochem. Biophys. Res. Commun.* 84, 691–698.

HABENER, J. F., ROSENBLATT, M., KAMPER, B., KRONENBERG, H. M., RICH, A. & POTTS, J. T. Jr. (1978) Pre-parathyroid hormone: amino acid sequence, chemical synthesis and some biological studies of the precursor region. *Proc. Natl. Acad. Sci. USA* 75, 2616–2620.

HALL, D. A. & JACKSON, D. S. (eds.) (1976) *Int. Rev. Connect. Tiss. Res.* 7.

HARPER, E., BLOCH, K. J. & GROSS, J. (1971) The zymogen of tadpole collagenase. *Biochem. Amer. Chem. Soc.* 10, 3035–3041.

HARRIS, E. D. & CARTWRIGHT, E. C. (1977) Mammalian collagenases. In: *Proteinases in mammalian cells and tissues*, A. J. BARRETT (ed.); *Research monographs in cell and tissue physiology*, J. T. DINGLE (ed.), **2**, 249–283. Amsterdam, North-Holland.

HARRIS, E. D., FAULKNER, C. S. & BROWN, F. E. (1975a) Collagenolytic systems in rheumatoid arthritis. *Clin. Orthop. Rel. Res.* **110**, 303–316.

HARRIS, E. D. Jr. & KRANE, S. M. (1972) An endopeptidase from rheumatoid synovial tissue culture. *Biochim. Biophys. Acta* **258**, 566–576.

HARRIS, E. D., McCROSKERY, P. A., MILLER, E. J. & BUTLER, W. T. (1975b) Primary structure at the cleavage site of α,I(II) by a specific mammalian collagenase. *Proc. III Int. Congr. Rhem.*

HARWOOD, R., BHALLA, A. K., GRANT, M. E. & JACKSON, D. S. (1975) The synthesis and secretion of cartilage procollagen. *Biochem. J.* **148**, 129–138.

HARWOOD, R., GRANT, M. E. & JACKSON, D. S. (1975) Biosynthesis and subcellular localization of collagen galactosyltransferase and collagen glucosyltransferase in tendon and cartilage cells. *Biochem. J.* **152**, 291–302.

HARWOOD, R., MERRY, A. H., WOOLLEY, D. E., GRANT, M. E. & JACKSON, D. S. (1977) Disulfide bonded nature of procollagen and role of extension peptides in assembly of molecules. *Biochem. J.* **161**, 405–418.

HEATHCOTE, J. G., SEAR, C. H. J. & GRANT, M. E. (1978) Studies on the assembly of the rat lens capsule: biosynthesis and partial characterization of the collagenous components. *Biochem. J.* **176**, 283–294.

HIGHBERGER, J. H., CORBETT, C. & GROSS, J. (1979) Isolation and characterization of a peptide containing the site of cleavage of the chick skin collagen αI(I) chain by animal collagenases. *Biochem. Biophys. Res. Commun.* **89**, 202–208.

HODGE, A. J. & SCHMITT, F. O. (1960) The charge profile of the tropocollagen macromolecule and the packing arrangement in native-type collagen fibrils. *Proc. Natl. Acad. Sci. USA* **46**, 186–197.

HOFFMANN, H. P., OLSEN, B. R., CHEN, H. T. & PROCKOP, D. J. (1976) Segment-long-spacing aggregates and isolation of COOH-terminal peptides from Type I procollagen. *Proc. Natl. Acad. Sci. USA* **73**, 4304–4308.

HORLEIN, D., FIETZEK, P. P. & KUHN, F. (1978) PRO-GLN: the procollagen peptidase cleavage site in the α1(I) chain of dermatosparactic calf skin procollagen. *FEBS Lett.* **89**, 279–282.

HORLEIN, D., FIETZEK, P. P., WACHTER, E., LAPIERE, C. M. & KUHN, K. (1979) Amino acid sequence of the aminoterminal sequence of dermatosparactic calf-skin procollagen Type I. *Eur. J. Biochem.* **99**, 31–38.

HOSEMANN, R., DREISSIG, W. & NEMETSCHEK, T. (1974) Schachtelhalm – structure of the octafibrils in collagen. *J. Molec. Biol.* **83**, 275–280.

HOUSLEY, T. J., TANZER, M. L., HENSON, E. & GALLOP, P. M. (1975) Collagen crosslinking, isolation of hydroxyaldolhistidine, a naturally-occurring cross-link. *Biochem. Biophys. Res. Commun.* **67**, 824–830.

IIJIMA, K., KISHI, J., FUYAMADA, H., NAGATSU, T. & HAYAKAWA, T. (1978) Dental sac collagenase: demonstration and initial characterization. *J. dent. Res.* **57**, 724.

JACKSON, D. S. (1978) *Int. Rev. Biochem.* **18**, 233–259.

JEFFREY, J. J. & GROSS, J. (1970) Collagenase from rat uterus. Isolation and partial characterization. *Biochemistry* **9**, 268–273.

JIMENEZ, S. A., HANSCH, M., MURPHY, L. & ROSENBLOOM, J. (1974) Effects of temperature on conformation, hydroxylation and secretion of chick tendon procollagen. *J. Biol. Chem.* **249**, 4480–4486.

KANG, A. H. (1972) Studies on the location of intermolecular cross-links in collagen. Isolation of a CNBr peptide containing δ hydroxylysinonorleucine. *Biochemistry* **11**, 1828–1835.

KANG, A. H., PIEZ, K. A. & GROSS, J. (1969) Chains of chick skin collagen and the nature of the NH$_2$-terminal crosslink region. *Biochemistry* **8**, 3648–3655.

KAO, W. W. Y., PROCKOP, D. J. & BERG, R. A. (1979) Kinetics for the secretion of nonhelical procollagen by freshly isolated tendon cells. *J. Biol. Chem.* **254**, 2234–2243.

KATZ, E. P. & LI, S. T. (1973) Intermolecular space of reconstituted collagen fibrils. *J. Molec. Biol.* **73**, 351–369.

KISHI, J., IIJIMA, K. & HAYAKAWA, T. (1979) Dental pulp collagenase: initial demonstration and characterization. *Biochem. Biophys. Res. Commun.* **86**, 27–31.

KISHIDA, Y., OLSEN, B. R., BERG, R. A. & PROCKOP, D. J. (1975) Two improved methods for preparing ferritin-protein conjugates for electron microscopy. *J. Cell Biol.* **64**, 331–339.

KIVIRIKKO, K. I. (1971) Urinary excretion of hydroxyproline in health and disease. *Int. Rev. Connect. Tiss. Res.* **5**, 93–163.

KIVIRIKKO, K. I., RYHANEN, L., ANTTINEN, H., BORNSTEIN, P. & PROCKOP, D. J. (1973) Further hydroxylation of lysyl residues in collagen by procollagen lysyl hydroxylase *in vitro*. *Biochemistry* **12**, 4966–4971.

KRESINA, T. F. & MILLER, E. J. (1979) Isolation and characterization of basement membrane collagen from human placental tissue. Evidence for the presence of two genetically distinct collagen chains. *Biochemistry* **18**, 3089–3097.

KRIEG, T., HORLEIN, D., WEISTNER, M. & MULLEN, P. K. (1978) Aminoterminal extension peptides from Type I procollagen normalize excessive collagen synthesis of scleroderm fibroblasts. *Arch. Dermatol. Res.* **263**, 171–180.

KRUZE, D. & WOJTECKA, E. (1972) Activation of leucocyte collagenase proenzyme by rheumatoid synovial fluid. *Biochim. Biophys. Acta* **285**, 436–446.

KUETTNER, K. E., HITI, J., EISENSTEIN, R. & HARPER, E. (1976) Collagenase inhibition by cationic proteins derived from cartilage and aorta. *Biochem. Biophys. Res. Commun.* **72**, 40–46.

LAPIERE, C. M. & GROSS, J. (1963) In: *Mechanisms of hard tissue destruction*, R. F. SOGNNAES (ed.), No. 75, 663. Washington D.C. Amer. Assoc. Adv. Science.

LAPIERE, C. M., NUSGENS, B. & PIERARD, G. E. (1977) Interaction between collagen Type I and Type III in conditioning bundles organization. *Connect. Tiss. Res.* **5**, 21–29.

LAZARIDES, E. L. & LUKENS, L. N. (1971) Collagen synthesis on polysomes *in vivo* and *in vitro*. *Nature (New Biol.)* **232**, 37–40.

LAZARUS, G. S., DANIELS, J. R., LIAN, J. & BURLEIGH, M. C. (1972) Role of granulocyte collagenase in collagen degradation. *Amer. J. Pathol.* **68**, 565–578.

LEIBOVICH, S. J. & WEISS, J. B. (1970) Electron microscope studies of the effects of endo and exo-peptidase digestion on tropocollagen. *Biochim. Biophys. Acta* **214**, 445–454.

LEUNG, M. K. K., FESSLER, L. I., GREENBERG, D. B. & FESSLER, J. H. (1979) Separate amino and carboxyl procollagen peptidases in chick embryo tendon. *J. Biol. Chem.* **254**, 224–232.

LICHTENSTEIN, J. R., MARTIN, G. R., KOHN, L. D., BYERS, P. H. & McKUSICK, V. A. (1973) Defect in conversion of procollagen to collagen in a form of Ehlers–Danlos syndrome. *Science* **182**, 298–299.

LIGHT, N. D. & BAILEY, A. J. (1979) Changes in crosslinking during aging in bovine tendon collagen. *FEBS Lett.* **97**, 183–188.

LIGHT, N. D. & BAILEY, A. J. (1980) The chemistry of collagen cross-links. Purification and characterization of crosslinked polymeric peptide material from mature collagen containing unknown amino acids. *Biochem. J.* **185**, 323–381.

LINSENMAYER, T. F., SMITH, G. N. & HAY, E. D. (1977) Synthesis of two collagen types of embryonic chick corneal epithelium *in vitro. Proc. Natl. Acad. Sci. USA* **74**, 39–43.

LIOTTA, L. A., ABE, S., ROBEY, P. G. & MARTIN, G. R. (1979) Preferential digestion of basement membrane collagen by an enzyme derived from a metastatic murine tumour. *Proc. Natl. Acad. Sci. USA* **76**, 2268–2272.

LIOTTA, L. A., TRYGGVASON, K., GARBISA, S., HART, I., FOLTY, C. M. & SHABIE, S. (1980) Metastatic potential correlates with enzymatic degradation of basement membrane collagen. *Nature* **284**, 67–68.

LITTLE, C. D., CHURCH, R. L., MILLER, R. A. & RUDDLE, F. H. (1977) Procollagen and collagen produced by a teratocarcinoma-derived cell line TSD4: evidence for a new molecular form of collagen. *Cell* **10**, 287–295.

McBRIDE, O. W. & HARRINGTON, W. F. (1967) Ascaris cuticle collagen: on the disulphide crosslinkages and the molecular properties of the subunits. *Biochemistry* **5**, 1434.

McCROSKERY, P. A., RICHARDS, J. F. & HARRIS, E. D., Jr. (1975) Purification and characterization of a collagenase extracted from rabbit tumours. *Biochem. J.* **152**, 131–142.

MAINARDI, C. L., VATER, C. A., WERB, Z. & HARRIS, E. D. (1976) Rheumatoid synovial collagenase: A proposed mechanism for its release, activation and protection from inhibition *in vivo. Arthritis Rheum.* **19**, 809.

MARTIN, G. R., BYERS, P. H. & PIEZ, K. A. (1975) Procollagen. *Adv. Enzymol.* **42**, 167–191.

MELCHER, A. H. (1976) In: *Orban's oral histology and embryology* (8th ed.), S. R. BHASHKAR (ed.), pp. 206–233. St. Louis, Mosby.

MILLER, A. & PARRY, D. A. D. (1973) Structure and packing of microfils in collagen. *J. Molec. Biol.* **75**, 441–447.

MILLER, A. & WRAY, J. S. (1971) Molecular packing in collagen. *Nature* **230**, 437–439.

MILLER, E. J. (1973) A review of biochemical studies on the genetically distinct collagens of the skeletal system.

Clin. Orthop. Res. **92**, 260–280.

MILLER, E. J., EPSTEIN, E. H. Jr. & PIEZ, K. A. (1971) Identification of three genetically distinct collagens by cyanogen bromide cleavage of insoluble human skin and cartilage collagen. *Biophys. Res. Commun.* **42**, 1024–1029.

MILLER, E. J., FINCH, J. E., CHUNG, E., BUTLER, W. T. & ROBERTSON, P. B. (1976) Specific cleavage of the native Type III collagen molecule with trypsin. *Arch. Biochem. Biophys.* **173**, 631–637.

MILLER, E. J., WOODALL, D. L. & VAIL, M. S. (1973) Biosynthesis of cartilage collagen – use of pulse labelling to order cyanogen bromide peptides in [αI(II)] chain. *J. Biol. Chem.* **248**, 1666–1671.

MINOR, R. R., CLARK, C. C., STRAUSE, E. L., KOSZALKA, T. R., BRENT, R. L. & KEFALIDES, A. A. (1976) Basement membrane procollagen is not converted to collagen in organ cultures of parietal yolk sac endoderm. *J. Biol. Chem.* **251**, 1789–1794.

MOEN, R. C., ROWE, D. W. & PALMITER, R. D. (1979) Regulation of procollagen synthesis during the development of chick embryo calvaria. *J. Biol. Chem.* **254**, 3526–3530.

MONTFORT, I. & PEREZ-TAMAYO, R. (1975) The distribution of collagenase in normal rat tissues. *J. Histochem. Cytochem.* **23**, 910–920.

MORALES, T. I. & WOESSNER, C. J. (1977) PZ peptidase from chick embryos, *J. Biol. Chem.* **252**, 4855–4860.

MORRIS, N. P., FESSLER, L. I., WEINSTOCK, A. & FESSLER, J. H. (1975) Procollagen assembly and secretion in embryonic chick bone. *J. Biol. Chem.* **250**, 5719–5726.

MULLER, P. K., McGOODWIN, E. B. & MARTIN, G. R. (1973) In: *Biology of the fibroblast,* E. KULONEN and J. PIKKARAINEN (eds.), pp. 339–364. London, Academic Press.

MULLER, P. K., MEIGEL, W. N., PONTZ, B. R. & RAISCH, K. (1974) Influence of $\alpha\alpha^1$ dipyridyl on the biosynthesis of collagen in organ cultures. *Hoppe Seyler's Z. Physiol. Chem.* **355**, 985–996.

MYLLYLA, R., RISTELI, L. & KIVIRIKKO, K. I. (1975) Glucosylation of galactosylhydrocylysyl residues in collagen *in vitro* by collagen glycosyl transferase – Inhibition by triple helical conformation of substrate. *Eur. J. Biochem.* **58**, 517–521.

NAGAI, Y. & HORI, H. (1972) Vertebrate collagenase – direct extraction from animal skin and human synovial membrane. *J. Biochem.* **72**, 1147–1154.

NAGAI, Y., LAPIERE, C. M. & GROSS, J. (1966) Tadpole collagenase: preparation and purification. *Biochemistry* **5**, 3123.

NEMETSCHEK, T. & HOSEMANN, R. (1973) A kink model of native collagen. *Kolloid Z. und Z. Polymere* **251**, 1044–1056.

NORDWIG, A. (1971) Collagenolytic enzymes. *Adv. Enzymol.* **34**, 155–207.

NORDWIG, A., NOWACK, H. & HIEBER-ROGALL, E. (1973) Sea anemone collagen: further evidence for the existence of only one α-chain type. *J. Molec. Evol.* **2**, 175–180.

NOWACK, H., OLSEN, B. R. & TIMPL, R. (1976) Characterization of the amino-terminal segment in the Type III procollagen. *Eur. J. Biochem.* **70**, 205–216.

OIKARINEN, A., ANTTINEN, H. & KIVIRIKKO, K. I. (1976a) Hydroxylation of lysine and glycosylation of hydroxylysine during collagen biosynthesis in isolated chick embryo cartilage cells. *Biochem. J.* **156**, 545–551.

OIKARINEN, A., ANTTINEN, H. & KIVIRIKKO, K. I. (1976b) Effect of L-Azetidine-2-carboxylic acid on glycosylations of collagen in chick embryo tendon cells. *Biochem. J.* **160**, 639–645.

OLSEN, B. R., BERG, R. A., KISHIDA, Y. & PROCKOP, D. J. (1973) Collagen synthesis: localization of prolyl hydroxylase in tendon cells detected with ferrintin-labelled antibodies. *Science* **182**, 825–827.

OLSEN, B. R., BERG, R. A., KISHIDA, Y. & PROCKOP, D. J. (1975) Further characterization of embryonic tendon fibroblasts and use of immunoferritin techniques to study collagen biosynthesis. *J. Cell Biol.* **64**, 340–355.

OLSEN, B. R., GUZMAN, N. A., ENGEL, J., CONDIT, C. & AASE, S. (1977) Purification and characterization of a peptide from the carboxy terminal region of chick tendon procollagen Type I. *Biochemistry* **16**, 3030–3036.

OOHIRA, A., KUSAKABE, A. & SUZUKI, S. (1975) Isolation of a large glycopeptide from cartilage procollagen by collagenase digestion and evidence indicating the presence of glucose galactase and mannose in the peptide. *Biochem. Biophys. Res. Commun.* **67**, 1086–1092.

OOHIRA, A., NOGAMI, H., KUSAKABE, A., KIMATA, K. & SUZUKI, S. (1979) Structural differences among procollagens associated with rough and smooth microsomes from chick embryo cartilage. *J. Biol. Chem.* **254**, 3576–3583.

ORLOWSKI, W. A. (1978) Biochemical study of collagen turnover in rat incisor periodontal ligament. *Archs. oral Biol.* **23**, 1163–1165.

ORONSKY, A., PERPER, R. & SCHRODER, H. C. (1973) Phagocytic release and activation of human leukocyte procollagenase. *Nature* **246**, 417–418.

OZAKI, T. (1971) Collagenase activity during tooth movement in rabbits. *Bull. Tokyo Med. & Dent. Univ.* **18**, 319–337.

PAGLIA, L., WILCZEK, J., DELEON, L. D., MARTIN, G. R., HORLEIN, D. & MULLEN, P. (1979) Inhibition of procollagen cell-free synthesis by amino terminal extension peptides. *Biochemistry* **18**, 5030–5034.

PALMITER, R. D., DAVIDSON, J. M., GARNON, J., ROWE, D. W. & BORNSTEIN, P. (1979) NH$_2$-terminal sequence of the chick proα(I) chain synthesized in the reticulocyte lysate system. *J. Biol. Chem.* **254**, 1433–1436.

PANJWANI, N. A. & HARDING, J. J. (1978) Isolation and hydroxylysine glycoside content of some cyanogen bromide cleared fragments of collagen from bovine corneal stroma. *Biochem. J.* **171**, 687–695.

PARAKKAL, P. F. (1969) Role of macrophages in collagen resorption during hair growth cycle. *J. Ultrastruc. Res.* **29**, 210–217.

PARDO, A. & PEREZ-TAMAYO, R. (1975) Presence of collagenase in collagen preparations. *Biochim. Biophys. Acta* **392**, 121–130.

PEARSON, C. H. (1979) *Applied fibre science,* F. HAPPEY (ed.), **3**, 411–482. London, Academic Press.

PEARSON, C. H. & AINSWORTH, L. (1978) Variations in the hydroxylysyl glycoside contents of collagens in bovine periodontal ligament and dental pulp. *J. dent. Res.* **57**, 874.

PEARSON, C. H., WOHLLEBE, M., CARMICHAEL, D. J. & CHOVELON, A. (1975) Bovine periodontal ligament. An investigation of the collagen, glycosaminoglycan and insoluble glycoprotein components at different stages of tissue development. *Connect. Tiss. Res.* **3**, 195–206.

PETRUSKA, J. A. & HODGE, A. J. (1964) A subunit model for the tropocollagen macromolecule. *Proc. Natl. Acad. Sci. USA* **51**, 871–876.

PETTIGREW, D. W. (1978) Regulation of collagenolytic enzymes in periodontal tissue. Ph.D. Thesis, University of Toronto.

PIERARD, G. E. & LAPIERE, C. M. (1976) Microanatomy and mechanical properties of the dermis in bovine foetus and newborn calves. *Arch. Int. Physiol. Biochem.* **84**, Suppl. Fasc. 3, Abstr. 91.

PIEZ, K. A., EIGNER, E. A. & LEWIS, M. S. (1963) Chromatographic separation and amino acid composition of the subunits of several collagens. *Biochem.* **2**, 58–66.

PIEZ, K. A. & TRUS, B. L. (1978) Sequence regularities and packing of collagen molecules. *J. Molec. Biol.* **122**, 419–432.

POOLE, A. R., HEMBRY, R. M., DINGLE, J. T., PINDER, L., RING, F. F. J. & CASH, S. (1976) Secretion and localization of cathepsin D in synovial tissues removed from rheumatoid and traumatized joints. *Arth. Rheum.* **19**, 1295–1307.

PROCKOP, D. S., BERG, R. A., KIVIRIKKO, K. I. *et al.* (1976) In: *The biochemistry of collagen,* G. N. RAMA-CHANDRAN & A. H. REDDI (eds.), pp. 163–273. New York, Plenum Press.

PROCKOP, D. J., KIVIRIKKO, K. I., TUDERMAN, L. & GUZMAN, N. A. (1979) The biosynthesis of collagen and its disorders. *New Engl. J. Med.* **301**, 13–23, 77–85.

RAMACHANDRAN, G. N. (1967) *Treatise on collagen,* G. N. RAMACHANDRAN (ed.), pp. 103–183. New York, Academic Press.

RAMACHANDRAN, G. N. & KARTHA, G. (1954) Structure of collagen. *Nature* **174**, 269–270.

RAMACHANDRAN, G. N. & KARTHA, G. (1955) Structure of collagen. *Nature* **176**, 593–595.

RAMACHANDRAN, G. N. & RAMAKRISHNAN, C. (1976) *The biochemistry of collagen,* G. N. RAMACHAN-DRAN & A. H. REDDI (eds.), pp. 45–84. New York, Plenum Press.

RAMACHANDRAN, G. N. & REDDI, A. H. (1976) *The biochemistry of collagen,* G. N. RAMACHANDRAN & A. H. REDDI (eds.). New York, Plenum Press.

RAMACHANDRAN, G. N., SASISEKHARAN, V., LAK-SHMINARAYANAN, A. V. & RAMAKRISHNAN, C. (1965) In *Biochimie et physiologie du tissu conjonctif,* **81**, R. COMTE (ed.).

RAO, L. G., WANG, H. M., KALLIECHARAN, R., HEERSCHE, J. N. M. & SODEK, J. (1979) Specific immunohistochemical localization of Type I collagen in porcine periodontal tissues using the peroxidase-labelled antibody technique. *Histochem. J.* **11**, 73–82.

RAUTERBERG, J. & VON BASSEWITZ, D. (1975) Electron microscopic investigations of Type III collagen. Segment-long-spacing crystallites of Type III collagen from calf aorta and fetal calf skin. *Hoppe-Seyler's Z. Physiol. Chem.* **356**, 95–100.

REMBERGER, K., GAY, S. & FIETZEK, P. P. (1975) Immunohistochemische Untersuchungen zur Kollagencharakterisierung in Lebercirrhosen. *Virchows Arch. A. Path. Anat. Histol.* **367**, 231–240.

REYNOLDS, J. J., SELLERS, A., MURPHY, G. & CARTWRIGHT, E. (1977) New factors that may control collagen resorption. *Lancet* **2**, 333–335.

RHODES, R. K. & MILLER, E. J. (1978) Physiochemical characterization and molecular organization of the collagen A and B chains. *Biochemistry* **17**, 3442–3448.

RICH, A. & CRICK, F. H. C. (1958) *The structure of collagen in recent advances in gelatin and glue research*, G. STAINSBY (ed.). London, Pergamon.

RICH, A. & CRICK, F. H. C. (1961) The molecular structure of collagen. *J. Molec. Biol.* **3**, 483–506.

RIPPON, J. W. (1976) Collagen turnover in the periodontal ligament under normal and altered functional forces. 1. Young rat molars. *J. periodont. Res.* **11**, 101–107.

RISTELI, L., MYLLYLA, R. & KIVIRIKKO, K. I. (1976) Partial purification and characterization of collagen galactosyl-transferase from chick embryos. *Biochem. J.* **155**, 145–153.

RISTELI, J., TRYGGVASON, K. & KIVIRIKKO, K. I. (1977) Prolyl 3 hydroxylase: partial characterization of the enzyme from rat kidney cortex. *Eur. J. Biochem.* **73**, 485–492.

ROBINS, S. P. & BAILEY, A. J. (1973) The chemistry of the collagen crosslinks. The characterization of fraction C, a possible artifact produced during the production of collagen fibres with borohydride. *Biochem. J.* **135**, 657–665.

ROBINS, S. P. & BAILEY, A. J. (1973) The chemistry of the collagen crosslinks. The characterization of fraction *Biochim. Biophys. Acta* **492**, 408–414.

ROBINS, S. P., SHIMOKOMAKI, M. & BAILEY, A. J. (1973) The chemistry of the collagen crosslinks. Age-related changes in the reducible components of intact bovine collagen fibres. *Biochem. J.* **131**, 771–780.

ROSS, R. & BENDITT, E. P. (1961) Wound healing and collagen formation. *J. Biophys. Biochem. Cytol.* **11**, 677–700.

RYAN, J. N. & WOESSNER, J. F. (1971) Mammalian collagenase: direct demonstration in homogenates of involuting rat uterus. *Biochem. Biophys. Res. Commun.* **44**, 144–149.

SAGE, H. & BORNSTEIN, P. (1979) Characterization of a novel collagen chain in human placenta and its relation to AB collagen. *Biochemistry* **18**, 3815–3822.

SAKAMOTO, M., SAKAMOTO, S., BRICKLEY-PARSONS, D. & GLIMCHER, M. J. (1979) Collagen synthesis and degradation in embryonic chick bone explants. *J. Bone & Joint Surg.* **61**-A, 1042–1052.

SAKAMOTO, S., SAKAMOTO, M., GOLDHABER, P. & GLIMCHER, M. J. (1973) Isolation of tissue collagenase from homogenates of embryonic chick bones. *Biochem. Biophys. Res. Commun.* **53**, 1102–1108.

SCOTT, P. G. & PEARSON, C. H. (1978a) Cathepsin D: cleavage of soluble collagen and crosslinked peptides. *FEBS Lett.* **88**, 41–45.

SCOTT, P. G. & PEARSON, C. H. (1978b) Selective solubilization of Type I collagen from calf skin by cathepsin D. *Biochem. Soc. Trans.* **6**, 1197–1199.

SCOTT, P. G. & VEIS, A. (1976) Cyanogen bromide peptides of bovine soluble and insoluble collagens. II. Characterization of peptides from soluble Type I collagen by sodium dodecylsulfate polyacrylamide gel electrophoresis. *Connect. Tiss. Res.* **4**, 107–116.

SCOTT, P. G., VEIS, A. & MECHANIC, G. (1976) The identity of a cyanogen bromide fragment of bovine dentin collagen containing the site of an intermolecular crosslink. *Biochemistry* **15**, 3191–3198.

SELLERS, A., CARTWRIGHT, E., MURPHY, G. & REYNOLDS, J. J. (1977a) Evidence that latent collagenases are enzyme–inhibitor complexes. *Biochem. J.* **163**, 303–307.

SELLERS, A., CARTWRIGHT, E., MURPHY, G. & REYNOLDS, J. J. (1977b) An inhibitor of mammalian collagenase from foetal rabbit bone in culture. *Biochem. Soc. Trans.* **5**, 227.

SELLERS, A., MURPHY, G., MEIKLE, M. C. & REYNOLDS, J. J. (1979) Rabbit bone collagenase inhibitor blocks the activity of other neutral metalloproteinases. *Biochem. Biophys. Res. Commun.* **87**, 581–587.

SELLERS, A., REYNOLDS, J. J. & MEIKLE, M. C. (1978) Neutral metallo-proteinases of rabbit bone separation in latent forms of distinct enzymes that when activated degrade collagen, gelatin and proteoglycans. *Biochem. J.* **171**, 493–496.

SELTZER, J. L., JEFFREY, J. J. & EISEN, A. Z. (1977) Evidence for mammalian collagenases and zinc ion metalloenzymes. *Biochim. Biophys. Acta* **485**, 179–187.

SHINKAI, H., KAWAMOTO, T., HORI, H. & NAGAI, Y. (1977) A complex of collagenase with low molecular weight inhibitors in the culture medium of embryonic chick skin explants. *J. Biochem. (Tokyo)* **81**, 261–263.

SKOUGAARD, M. R., FRANDSEN, A. & BAKER, D. G. (1970) Collagen metabolism of skin and periodontal membrane in the squirrel monkey. *Scand. J. dent. Res.* **78**, 374–377.

SKOUGAARD, M. R., LEVY, B. M. & SIMPSON, J. (1970) Collagen metabolism in skin and periodontal membrane of the marmoset. *Scand. J. dent. Res.* **78**, 256–262.

SLOAN, P. (1978) Scanning electron microscopy of the collagen fibre architecture of the rabbit incisor periodontium. *Archs. oral Biol.* **23**, 567–572.

SLOAN, P. (1979) Collagen fibre architecture in the periodontal ligament. *J. R. Soc. Med.* **72**, 188–191.

SMITH, B. D., McKENNEY, K. H. & LUSTBERG, T. J. (1977) Characterization of collagen precursors found in rat skin and rat bone. *Biochemistry* **16**, 2980–2985.

SMITH, J. W. (1968) Molecular pattern in native collagen. *Nature* **219**, 157–158.

SODEK, J. (1976) A new approach to assessing collagen turnover by using a micro-assay: a highly efficient and rapid turnover of collagen in rat periodontal tissues. *Biochem. J.* **160**, 342–346.

SODEK, J. (1977) Comparison of rates of synthesis and turnover of collagen and non-collagen proteins in adult rat periodontal tissues and skin using a micro-assay. *Archs. oral Biol.* **22**, 655–665.

SODEK, J. (1978) A comparison of collagen and non-collagenous protein metabolism in rat molar and incisor periodontal ligaments. *Archs. oral Biol.* **23**, 977–982.

SODEK, J., BRUNETTE, D. M., FENG, J., HEERSCHE, J. N. M., LIMEBACK, H. F., MELCHER, A. H. & NG, B. (1977) Collagen synthesis is a major component of protein synthesis in the periodontal ligament in various species. *Archs. oral Biol.* **22**, 647–653.

SOPATA, I. & DANCEWICZ, A. M. (1974) Presence of a gelatine-specific proteinase and its latent form in human leucocytes. *Biochim. Biophys. Acta* **370**, 510–523.

SPIRO, R. G. (1972) *Glycoproteins – their composition, structure and function* (2nd ed.), A. GOTTSCHALK (ed.), pp. 964–998. Amsterdam, Elsevier.

STALLARD, R. (1963) The utilization of ^{3}H-proline by the connective tissue elements of the periodontium. *Periodontics* **1**, 185–188.

STARKEY, P. (1977) *Proteinases in mammalian cells and tissues*, A. J. BARRETT (ed.) 57. New York, North-Holland.

STEVEN, F. S., TORRE-BLANCO, A. & HUNTER, J. J. A. (1975) A neutral protease in rheumatoid synovial fluid capable of attacking the telopeptide regions of polymeric collagen fibrils. *Biochim. Biophys. Acta* **405**, 188–200.

STIMLER, H. & TANZER, M. L. (1979) Isolation and characterization of a double chain intermolecular crosslinked peptide from insoluble calf bone collagen. *J. Biol. Chem.* **254**, 666–671.

SWANN, D. A., CAULFIELD, J. B. & BROADHURST, J. B. (1976) The altered fibrous form of vitreous collagen following solubilization with pepsin. *Biochim. Biophys. Acta* **427**, 365–370.

TAKAHASHI, S. & SEIFTER, S. (1974) An enzyme with collagenolytic activity from dog pancreatic juice. *Israel J. Chem.* **12**, 557–571.

TANZER, M. L. (1973) Crosslinking collagen. Endogenous aldehydes in collagen reaction. Several ways to form a variety of unique covalent crosslinks. *Science* **180**, 561–566.

TANZER, M. L. (1976) Crosslinking. In: *Biochemistry of collagen*, G. A. RAMACHANDRAN & A. H. REDDI (eds.), pp. 137–162. New York, Plenum Press.

TANZER, M. L., ROWLAND, F. N., MURRAY, L. W. & KAPLAN, J. (1977) Inhibitory effects of tunicamycin on procollagen biosynthesis and secretion. *Biochim. Biophys. Acta* **500**, 187–196.

THIBODEAU, S. N., LEE, D. C. & PALMITER, R. D. (1978) Identical precursors for serum transferrin and egg white conalbumin. *J. Biol. Chem.* **253**, 3771–3774.

THOMAS, N. R. (1967) The properties of collagen in the periodontium of an erupting tooth. In: *The mechanisms of tooth support*, D. J. ANDERSON, J. E. EASTOE, A. H. MELCHER & D. C. A. PICTON (eds.), pp. 102–106. Bristol, Wright.

TIMPL, A., BRUCHNER, P. & FIETZEK, O. (1979) Characterization of pepsin fragments of basement membrane collagen obtained from a mouse tumour. *Eur. J. Biochem.* **95**, 225–263.

TIMPL, R., RISTELI, J. & BACHINGER, H. P. (1979) Identification of a new basement membrane collagen by the aid of a large fragment resistant to bacterial collagenase. *FEBS Lett.* **101**, 265–268.

TIMPL, R., WICK, G. & GAY, S. (1977) Antibodies to distinct types of collagens and procollagens and their application in immunohistology. *J. Immunol. Methods* **18**, 165–182.

TOKORO, Y., EISEN, A. Z. & JEFFREY, J. J. (1972) *Biochim. Biophys. Acta* **258**, 289–302.

TRAUB, W. (1978) Molecular assembly in collagen. *FEBS Lett.* **92**, 114–120.

TRAUB, W. & PIEZ, K. A. (1971) The chemistry and structure of collagen. *Adv. Prot. Chem.* **25**, 243–352.

TRELSTAD, R. L. & COULOMBRE, A. J. (1971) Morphogenesis of the collagenous stoma in the chick cornea. *J. Cell Biol.* **50**, 840–858.

TRELSTAD, R. L., HAYASHI, K. & GROSS, J. (1976) Collagen fibrillogenesis: intermediate aggregates and supra-fibrillar order. *Proc. Natl. Acad. Sci. USA* **73**, 4027–4031.

TRUS, B. L. & PIEZ, K. A. (1976) Molecular packing of collagen: three dimensional analysis of electrostatic interactions. *J. Molec. Biol.* **103**, 705–732.

TRYGGVASON, K., ROBEY, P. G. & MARTIN, G. R. (1980) Biosynthesis of Type IV procollagens. *Biochemistry* **19**, 1284–1289.

TUDERMAN, L., KIVIRIKKO, K. I. & PROCKOP, D. J. (1978) Partial purification and characterization of a neutral protease which cleaves the N-terminal propeptides from procollagen. *Biochemistry* **17**, 2948–2954.

UITTO, J. (1977) Biosynthesis of Type II collagen: removal of amino- and carboxy terminal extensions from procollagen synthesized by chick embryo cartilage cells. *Biochemistry* **16**, 3421–3429.

UITTO, J., HOFFMANN, H. P. & PROCKOP, D. J. (1975) Retention of nonhelical procollagen containing cis-hydroxyproline in rough endoplasmic reticulum. *Science* **190**, 1202–1204.

UITTO, J., HOFFMANN, H. P. & PROCKOP, D. J. (1977) Purification and partial characterization of the Type II procollagen synthesized by embryonic cartilage cells. *Arch. Biochem. Biophys.* **179**, 654–662.

UITTO, J. & PROCKOP, D. J. (1974) Incorporation of proline analogs into collagen polypeptides – effects on production of extracellular procollagen and on stability of triple helical structure of molecule. *Biochim. Biophys. Acta* **336**, 234–251.

VAES, G. (1972) Multiple steps in the activation of the inactive precursor of bone collagenase by trypsin. *FEBS Lett.* **28**, 198–200.

VATER, C. A., HARRIS, E. J. & SIEGEL, R. C. (1979) Native crosslinks in collagen fibrils induce resistance to human synovial collagenase. *Biochem. J.* **181**, 639–645.

VATER, C. A., MAINARDI, C. L. & HARRIS, E. D. (1978) Activation *in vitro* of rheumatoid synovial collagenase from cell cultures. *J. Clin. Invest.* **62**, 987–992.

VEIS, A., ANESEY, J. & MUSSELL, S. (1967) A limiting microfibril model for the three dimensional arrangement within collagen fibrils. *Nature* **215**, 931–934.

VEIS, A., ANESEY, J., YUAN, H. & LEVY, S. J. (1973) Evidence for an amino terminal extension in high molecular weight collagens from mature bovine skin. *Proc. Natl. Acad. Sci. USA* **70**, 1464–1467.

VEIS, A. & BROWNELL, A. (1975) Collagen biosynthesis. *Crit. Rev. Biochem.* **2**, 417–453.

VEIS, A., MILLER, A., LEIBOVICH, S. J. & TRAUB, W. (1979) The limiting collagen microfibril. The minimum structure demonstrating native axial periodicity. *Biochim. Biophys. Acta* **576**, 88–98.

VEIS, A. & SCHLEUTER, R. J. (1964) The macromolecular organization of dentine matrix collagen. I. The characterization of dentine collagen. *Biochemistry* **3**, 1650–1657.

VEIS, A. & YUAN, L. (1975) Structure of the collagen microfibril. A four strand of overlap model. *Biopolymers* **14**, 895–900.

VOLPIN, D. & VEIS, A. (1973) Cyanogen bromide peptides from insoluble skin and dentine bovine collagens. *Biochemistry* **12**, 1452–1464.

VON DER MARK, H. & VON DER MARK, K. (1979) Isolation and characterization of collagen A & B chains from chick embryos. *FEBS Lett.* **99**, 101–105.

VON DER MARK, K., VON DER MARK, H., TIMPL, R. & TRELSTAD, R. L. (1977) Immunofluorescent localization of collagen types I, II, & III in the embryonic chick eye. *Devl. Biol.* **59**, 75–85.

VON HEIJNE, G. & BLOMBERG, C. (1979) Trans-membrane translocation of proteins. (The direct transfer model.) *Eur. J. Biochem.* **97**, 175–181.

VUUST, J. & PIEZ, K. A. (1972) A kinetic study of collagen biosynthesis. *J. Biol. Chem.* **247**, 856–862.

WALTON, A. G. (1975) Synthetic polypeptide models for collagen structure and function. In: *Structure of fibrous biopolymers,* Colston Papers No. 26, E. D. T. ATKINS & A. KELLER (eds.), pp. 139–148. London, Butterworths.

WARSHAWSKY, H. (1972) Presence of atypical collagen fibrils in EDTA decalcified predentin and dentin of rat incisors. *Archs. oral Biol.* **17**, 1745–1754.

WEEKS, J. G., HALME, J. & WOESSNER, J. F., Jr. (1976) Extraction of collagenase from the involuting rat uterus. *Biochim. Biophys. Acta* **445**, 205–214.

WEINSTOCK, A., BIBB, C., BURGESON, R. E., FESSLER, L. I. & FESSLER, J. H. (1975) *Extracellular matrix influences on gene expression,* H. C. SLAVKIN & R. C. GREULICH (eds.), pp. 312–330. New York, Academic Press.

WEINSTOCK, H. & LEBLOND, C. P. (1974) Synthesis, migration and release of precursor collagen by odontoblasts as visualized by autoradiography after ^{3}H-Proline administration. *J. Cell Biol.* **60**, 92–127.

WEISS, J. B. (1976) Enzyme degradation of collagen. *Int. Rev. Connect. Tiss. Res.* **7**, 101–157.

WERB, Z., BURLEIGH, M. C., BARRETT, A. J. & STARKEY, P. M. (1974) The interaction of α_2-macroglobulin with proteinases (binding and inhibition of mammalian collagenases and other metal proteinases). *Biochem. J.* **139**, 359–368.

WERB, Z., MAINARDI, C. L., VATER, C. A. & HARRIS, E. D., Jr. (1977) Endogenous activation of latent collagenase by rheumatoid synovial cells. Evidence for a role of plasminogen activator. *N. Engl. J. Med.* **296**, 1017–1023.

WERB, Z. & REYNOLDS, J. J. (1974) Stimulation by endocytosis of the secretion of collagenase and neutral proteinase from rabbit synovial fibroblasts. *J. Exp. Med.* **140**, 1482–1497.

WERB, Z. & REYNOLDS, J. J. (1975) Purification and properties of a specific collagenase from rabbit synovial fibroblasts. *Biochem. J.* **151**, 645–653.

WIESTNER, M., KRIEG, T., HORLEIN, D., GLANVILLE, R. W., FIETZEK, P. P. & MULLEN, T. K. (1979) Inhibiting effect of procollagen peptides on collagen biosynthesis in fibroblast cultures. *J. Biol. Chem.* **254**, 7016–7023.

WILLIAMS, B. R., GELMAN, R. A., POPPKE, D. C. & PIEZ, K. A. (1978) Collagen fibril formation. Optimal *in vitro* conditions and preliminary kinetic results. *J. Biol. Chem.* **253**, 6578–6585.

WIRL, G. (1975) Extraction of collagenase from the 6000 times g sediment of uterine and skin tissues of mice. A comparative study. *Hoppe-Seyler's Z. Physiol. Chem.* **356**, 1289–1295.

WOESSNER, J. F., Jr. (1973) Mammalian collagenases. *Clin. Orthop. Relat. Res.* **96**, 310–376.

WOESSNER, J. F., Jr. (1977) A latent form of collagenase in the involuting rat uterus and its activation by a serine proteinase. *Biochem. J.* **161**, 535–542.

WOESSNER, J. F. (1979) Separation of collagenase and a metal dependent endopeptidase of rat uterus that hydrolyzes a heptapeptide related to collagen. *Biochim. Biophys. Acta* **571**, 313–320.

WOHLLEBE, M. & CARMICHAEL, D. J. (1978) Type I trimer and Type I collagen in neutral salt soluble lathyritic rat dentine. *Eur. J. Biochem.* **92**, 183–188.

WOHLLEBE, M. & CARMICHAEL, D. J. (1979) Biochemical characterization of guanidinium-chloride-soluble dentine collagen from lathyritic rat incisors. *Biochem. J.* **181**, 667–676.

WOODHEAD-GALLOWAY, J., HUKINS, D. W. L. & WRAY, J. S. (1975) Closest packing of two-stranded coiled coils as a model for the collagen fibril. *Biochem. Biophys. Res. Commun.* **64**, 1237–1244.

WOOLLEY, D. E. & EVANSON, J. M. (1977a) Collagenase and its natural inhibitors in relation to the rheumatoid joint. *Connect. Tiss. Res.* **5**, 31–35.

WOOLLEY, D. E. & EVANSON, J. M. (1977b) Effect of cartilage proteoglycans on human collagenase activities. *Biochim. Biophys. Acta* **497**, 144–150.

WOOLLEY, D. E., GLANVILLE, R. W., CROSSLEY, M. J. & EVANSON, J. M. (1975) Purification of rheumatoid synovial collagenase and its action on soluble and insoluble collagen. *Eur. J. Biochem.* **54**, 611–622.

WOOLLEY, D. E., GLANVILLE, R. W., ROBERTS, D. R. & EVANSON, J. M. (1978) Purification, characterization and inhibition of human skin collagenase. *Biochem. J.* **169**, 265–276.

WOOLLEY, D. E., ROBERTS, D. R. & EVANSON, J. M. (1976) Small molecular weight β_1 serum protein which specifically inhibits human collagenases. *Nature* **261**, 325–327.

WUNSCH, E. & HEIDRICH, H. G. (1963) Zur quantitativen Bestimmung der Kollagenase. *Hoppe-Seyler's Z. Physiol. Chem.* **333**, 149–151.

YEN, E. H. K. (1978) Organ cultures of adult mouse molar periodontium: effect of oxygen tension on protein synthesis. Ph.D. Thesis, University of Toronto.

Chapter 5

BIOPHYSICAL ASPECTS OF THE FIBRES OF THE PERIODONTAL LIGAMENT

L. J. Gathercole and A. Keller

INTRODUCTION

Most of this review will concern collagen fibres, not only because they comprise some 50% by weight of the periodontal ligament and because most is known about these fibres, but because we believe that models based on a knowledge of the upper hierarchic levels of collagen organization relate to the mechanics of tooth support, movement and possibly eruption.

While the fibres involved have been identified biochemically and by optical and electron microscopy, in approaching the biophysics of fibres of the periodontal ligament we are faced with the problem that most of what is known of the biophysics has been derived from their study in other connective tissues.

There have been numerous physical studies on collagen fibres and on reconstituted purified collagen. For instance, soluble collagens have an intrinsic viscosity of 11.5 to 20 dl g^{-1}, depending on the source. Phase transitions in collagen are characterized by at least two processes: a glass transition at $35-51°C$ and one associated with the helix-coil transformation at $50-60°C$. The melting temperature in water is $145°C$. Dry collagen can bind $100-120\%$ of its weight of water. It will not be our purpose here to elaborate

on such studies: there are several good reviews (e.g. Elden, 1968).

COLLAGEN FIBRE ORGANIZATION

That the collagen fibres have a hierarchical system is probably one of the most striking aspects of collagen structure and function. Order and organization exists on many levels — from the peptide bond to the anatomical functioning unit (the array of collagen fibres). However, these organizational levels are interdependent. Indeed, for the proper functioning of the anatomical unit correct organization at all levels is necessary. Figure 1 illustrates the hierarchy tree, as we see it. We shall have reason to refer to it throughout this article. Whilst the information presented in this part of the review refers to collagen in general, we are confident that most of it applies to the collagen of the periodontal ligament.

The first hierarchy — the molecular level

The triple helical collagen molecule, the so-called

tropocollagen, is a cylinder some 300 × 1.5 nm and consists of three polypeptide chains (α-chains), each consisting of just over 1000 residues in a unique triplet sequence in which every third amino acid is glycine. Details of the collagen structure at the molecular level have been given in the preceding chapter. Suffice it to say here that the intra- and intermolecular collagen crosslinking is accepted generally to contribute to strength and coherence in the collagen fibril (Bailey, 1975). However, mechanical strength depends equally on the type of higher level organization (see, for example, Gathercole *et al.*, 1980).

The microfibrillar and fibrillar hierarchy

The second level of hierarchy of collagen (Fig. 1) concerns the packing together of individual tropocollagen molecules. There is some disagreement about this (Fig. 2), mainly due to the diffuse and variable nature of the collagen X-ray diffraction patterns in the medium-angle region. It is thus possible to fit many geometrical or semi-geometrical solutions to the X-ray and electron microscopic evidence.

The first area of debate is whether the triple helices

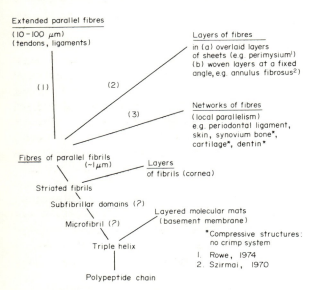

FIG. 1. Hierarchy 'tree' of collagen as it exists in various tissues, from molecular to macroscopic levels. All soft connective tissues show waveforms, rigid structures do not.

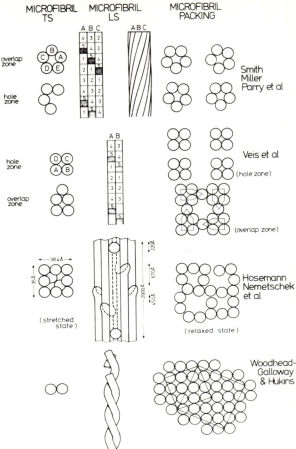

FIG. 2. Comparative scheme of microfibrillar models for collagen molecule packing, from the recent literature. Redrawn, with additions, from the various authors.

constitute a lattice as such or whether they form regular small aggregates or microfibrils first, the packing of the latter giving rise to a lattice. Either of these lattices would be within the collagen fibril — the familiar electron microscopic entity — a cylinder of length greater than 1 μm and between 10—500 nm in diameter (depending on age, tissue, etc.). The best general model of the collagen fibril is based on the stagger-with-hole array of triple helices devised by Hodge and Petruska (1963). This accounts for the banding patterns seen in the collagen fibril by electron microscopy with both positive and negative staining and generates the 68-nm axial period (often referred to as the D-period) revealed by these and low-angle diffraction techniques (e.g. Gathercole and Keller, 1978a). More recently, the model has been supported by comparison with the staining patterns of segmented, long spacing, collagen crystallites (which are parallel molecular arrays of precipitated collagen) and with other precipitated collagen forms (Hodge, 1967; Doyle *et al.*, 1974b). Also, knowledge of the collagen sequence has indicated the charge profile along the chain or molecule. This can be computer matched in interaction with itself in all overlap positions (Walton, 1975; Miller, 1976; Piez and Trus, 1978), the most lucid account being that of Cunningham, Davies and Hammonds (1976).

The general consensus is that the most advantageous energetic positions are at integer values of the D period (68 nm). There is also evidence from low-temperature electron beam etching of rat-tail tendon that hole regions exist at the periodicity (Gathercole *et al.*, 1978). In this context, the organization *within* the fibril may be discussed. The problem is that the Hodge—Petruska model is one-dimensional. The 68 nm spacing and low-to-medium-angle X-ray patterns must be accounted for in three dimensions. The simple stacking of arrays of staggered molecular layers does not lead to the large-scale order seen in the fibril in the electron microscope.

The pentafibril model proposed by Smith (1968) (Fig. 2) solved this problem neatly since the sum of the molecular length of 4.4D plus hole region of 0.6D means that a minimum of five molecules may be arranged to give the Hodge—Petruska pattern in three dimensions and a lattice of such in-register microfibrils will give the large-scale order seen in the fibril as a whole. This gives a microfibril 3.8 nm in diameter, and Miller and Wray (1971) reported X-ray evidence for such a unit. Their results indicated that the microfibril should have tetragonal symmetry and they proposed that slight twisting of the molecules achieved this. Miller and Parry (1973) suggested that the microfibrils lie on a tetragonal lattice probably 3.8 $\times$ 3.8 nm (Fig. 2).

Using electron microscopic evidence from reconstituted collagen, Veis *et al.* (1967) proposed a unit of similar size, based on four molecules in the gap hole region but five in the overlap region (Veis and Yuan, 1975). This may also be packed on a square lattice (Fig. 2).

A system based on an eight-membered microfibril has been proposed by Hosemann, Dreissig and Nemetschek (1974), in which the rather large space within the microfibril is occupied by 'tucked-in' ends of collagen molecules (allowed by having flexible regions in the helix). Such octafibrils would appear on stretching, the relaxed model for collagen being a paracrystalline array of molecules packed in a generally similar way but without crystalline register (Nemetschek and Hosemann, 1973).

A system requiring ten molecules per unit cell has been proposed by Woodhead-Galloway, Hukins and Wray (1975). The basic unit consists of two coiled, staggered helices which can be packed in two ways, of which the close-packed version is shown (Fig. 2). The same authors later proposed a liquid crystal model (Hukins and Woodhead-Galloway, 1977) in which molecular sheets in staggered arrangement are stacked in a liquid crystalline manner.

It seems that entities of a size consistent with the dimensions of most of the microfibril models are observable in disrupted collagen (Hosemann and Nemetschek, 1973; Torp, Baer and Friedman, 1975) and reconstituted collagen (Doyle *et al.*, 1974a). Oriented samples of such material may give rise to the 68-nm periodicity of X-ray diffraction while it remains unobservable in the electron microscope (Veis *et al.*, 1979).

Parry and Craig (1979) have analysed statistically the diameters of collagen fibrils from many sources, where these diameters are present in sharp unimodal distributions. They suggest that such diameters vary by quanta of 8 nm and that this may be achieved by the addition and removal of single layers of microfibrils onto the tetragonal lattice of Miller and Parry (1973). The findings of Nemetschek, Riedl and Jonak (1979), using collagen from rat-tail tendon, show evidence for a 8-nm unit outlined by phosphotungstic acid stain detectable in medium angle X-ray diffraction. Squire and Freundlich (1980) report direct observation of a lateral periodicity of 8 nm in collagen fibrils from tendon, detected by diffractometry of their longitudinal electron microscope images. For the periodontal tissues in the rat, however, Berkovitz *et al.* (in press) were unable to detect collagen fibrils diameters having multiples of 8 nm.

There are also models for the fibril packing not

dependent on microfibrillar arrangements based largely on hexagonal (Ross and Benditt, 1961; Burge 1963, 1965), pseudohexagonal (Ramachandran, 1967) or tetragonal (Ross and Benditt, 1961) packings. These assume a more extensive minimum fibril size. Similarly, hexagonal schemes involving pentafibrils have been devised (Katz, 1972; Petruska, 1972).

A hexagonal packing scheme of triple helices without recourse to intermediary microfibrils was proposed by MacFarlane (1971). This considered in detail the staggering of adjacent molecules by the 68 nm repeat, or multiples thereof. Renewed interest in such packing schemes has appeared with the quasi-hexagonal molecular lattice proposed by Hulmes and Miller (1979) (Fig. 3) as an alternative explanation of Miller and Wray's (1971) X-ray data. This packing is quasihexagonal, embodying both shears in two directions and a tilt of the tropocollagen accounting for the observed splittings of the equatorial reflections and row lines. The three closely packed planes are thus slightly unequal (1.33, 1.37 and 1.26 nm), arising from a unit cell of $a = 2.667$ nm, $b = 2.667$ nm and $\gamma = 104°58'$ containing five molecules. The 68 nm repeat is ensured by a $1D$ intermolecular shift along one direction (sequence 1,2,3,4,5 in Fig. 3) with different $n \times D$ staggers in the other two

crystallographic directions. Such schemes have the advantage that they lead to a higher calculated density for collagen than does the original pentafibril model. Since this work, Trus and Piez (1980) have shown that hexagonal packing schemes can be reconciled with the presence of 'collapsed' pentafibrils if near-neighbour molecules are in the 1,2,3,4,5 shift positions shown in Fig. 3. Bailey, Light and Atkins (1980) independently demonstrated the possibility of such arrangements. They also showed that the recovery from cyanogen bromide digests of tendon of polymeric peptides comprising the $1 \rightarrow 5$ intermolecular crosslink from more than one molecular pair argues strongly for several adjacent molecules in the 1,5 shift position. That is, the presence of 'runs' of 1,5,1,5 ... molecules would be an additional constraint on such models.

A further level of organization may exist at the subfibril level, at least in large fibrils. Units of the order of 15 nm have been reported in disrupted tendon (e.g. Torp, Baer and Friedman, 1975; Parry and Craig, 1977) and the streaking of 68 nm meridional reflections in low angle X-ray diffraction patterns of rat-tail tendon suggests that a limit of lattice coherence of this order may exist across the fibril (Baer, Gathercole and Keller, 1975). With reference to

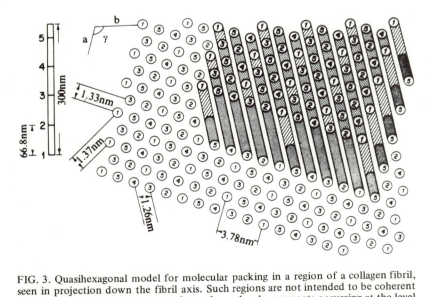

FIG. 3. Quasihexagonal model for molecular packing in a region of a collagen fibril, seen in projection down the fibril axis. Such regions are not intended to be coherent across the entire fibril. Numbers refer to the molecular segments occurring at the level of the section. Thick shaded lines show molecular tilt and connectivity between upper (bold type) and lower (regular type) surfaces. For further details see text.

periodontal ligament, however, this lower limit is the order of size of the fibrils themselves, and is a commonly found minimum size for striated fibrils in fully developed tissues. This will be further discussed.

The suprafibrillar hierarchy

The striated fibrils are arranged in a multitude of ways in the different tissues. They are the basic constituents of a further edifice of hierarchies leading from the electron microscopic dimensions to the macroscopic anatomy. As stated at the beginning, in order to understand the anatomical function or any macroscopically measured property of a tissue, a mapping of the hierarchical sequence and the appreciation of the role of each level within it is required. This is particularly evident in suprafibrillar regimes. Knowledge about the fibril arrangement is also insufficient. From the fibril level upwards, the collagen fibrils become associated with polysaccharides, proteoglycans, elastin, etc. Knowledge about the chemical characteristics, relative amounts, geometric arrangement and modes of mutual attachments as well as attachment to collagen of these substances are all needed for an ultimate appreciation. Our understanding of all these factors is very sketchy for collagenous material in general and for the periodontal ligament in particular. This is a kind of no-man's land between the traditional macroscopic and the more modern molecular—ultrastructural worlds, a gap which has close parallels in other fields of structural science. With the present scarcity of information, all we can do here is draw attention to the existence and importance of the hierarchical sequence together with a rough schematization, with a certain amount of detail added for the simplest case of the tendon.

Interfibrillar material plays a part in all higher level organizations of which the striated fibrils are the constituents. This material forms a matrix in which the fibrils are embedded, the whole tissue being a biological fibre-composite where the fibrils are the principal load-bearing elements and where the matrix (present in a highly swollen state) provides, amongst other functions, spacefilling and mechanical damping. The matrix—fibril ratio varies considerably between the tissues, and the amount of the fibrous

component usually increases with age. The principal matrix constituents are glycosaminoglycans and proteoglycans (see Chapter 6 and Scott, 1979). The existence of an intrafibrillar matrix has also been claimed (Pease and Bouteille, 1971), a point on which there is no consensus.

We may now return to the hierarchical tree in Fig. 1 and proceed from the striated fibrils onwards. From here upwards there are two branches. The small branch represents layer structures formed by these fibrils. It is noteworthy that if the directionality of the fibrils within the layer is to be removed (or looking at it in another way, if the layer is to benefit from the favourable directional properties of the collagen fibril in more than one direction), the fibrils need to be randomized in the plane of the layer. This is achieved not by arranging the fibrillar units in a haphazard fashion within the layer plane, but by laying sheets of parallel fibres on to each other in a regularly defined sequence. In the cornea, consecutive sheets lie orthogonally or near orthogonally (Trelstad and Coulombre, 1971). The Cuvierian tubule collagen of the sea cucumber (*Holothuria forskali*) provides an example of consecutive sheets rotated by small amounts always in the same direction leading to a helicoidal arrangement (Dlugosz, Gathercole and Keller, 1979). This is a small-scale analogue of cholesteric liquid crystals on a molecular level. The helical arrangement conforms to a much favoured building principle in nature for creating layers from fibres. This was first documented in the case of insect cuticles built of chitin fibres (see Neville, 1975). Current research indicates that such arrangements also exist in localized regions of the periodontal ligament (Gathercole *et al.,* unpublished results).

Returning to the second, major branch in Fig. 1, emanating from the striated fibril stage we come to the next level, the *fibre* unit containing the fibrils in a parallel array. There is no adequate definition of the fibre in terms of size. We define as fibres the minimal entities which can be readily seen as fibrous structures by optical microscopy and which, in soft tissues at least, display a characteristic banded appearance between crossed polars. These criteria place the fibres in the range of $1-2 \mu m$ diameter.

The fibres form a variety of further arrangements schematized by the outermost branches (1), (2), (3) of the hierarchical tree shown in Fig. 1.

1. Here, the fibres form large parallel bundles up to almost macroscopic dimensions. The main examples are tendons and ligaments. In these larger bundles, the polarizing optical banding of the constituent fibres is maintained (except for occasional distortions or disruptions) up to the macroscopic tendon level, i.e. the dark and bright bands remain essentially in phase (Fig. 4).

2. Here, the 1–2 μm fibres form sheets. In the simplest case, (a), the fibres are parallel throughout, the full sheet itself exhibiting the periodic banding when viewed under the polarizing microscope as, for example, in the pericardium (Fig. 5) or perimysium (Rowe, 1974). In more complicated cases, (b), the sheets have a woven tex—e where they contain the basic fibres in particular criss-cross arrangements (e.g. annulus fibrosus). Here, the polarizing optical banding is not apparent within the sheet, only in its constituent fibres.

3. Here, there is not displayed any identifiable overall arrangement of the fibres. The extreme case is complete (or near complete) randomness, giving rise to networks (as in the skin).

All the above arrangements can be identified within different localities of the periodontal ligament (illustrated by Figs. 6–8). Thus, these three arrangements become constituents of further structural hierarchies of still greater complexity. However, we are not yet in a position to organize these into any scheme.

In the majority of cases, the fibres are seen to be banded between crossed polars, regardless of their particular arrangement. Clearly, the nature of these fibres, and the origin of the banding in particular, can be studied most readily in the bundles where the fibres are all parallel. It is these tendons (rat-tail tendon in particular) we shall be primarily concerned with in order to provide some insight into the complex texture of the periodontal ligament.

The crimp morphology

The banding referred to above and illustrated by Fig. 4 reflects an underlying periodicity along the fibre. The wavy nature of fibrous collagen has long been noted, particularly in dissected or otherwise disrupted tissues. However, not until these were correlated with the banding detected by polarizing optics could this wave geometry be diagnosed as a representative feature, characterized quantitatively and used for correlation with the mechanical behaviour of the tendon as a whole.

It is important to realize that the polarizing optical evidence (as recognized and analysed first by Diamant *et al.* (1972)) does not rely on seeing shapes,

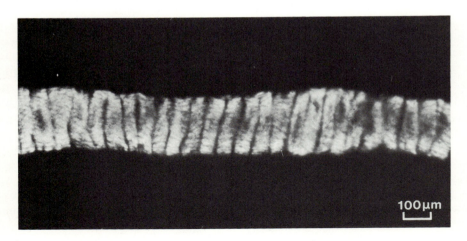

FIG. 4. Polarizing micrograph of a 3-month-old rat-tail tendon unit taken with the crossed polars, the polarizer parallel to the main fibre axis. The unit is smooth and elliptical in cross-section.

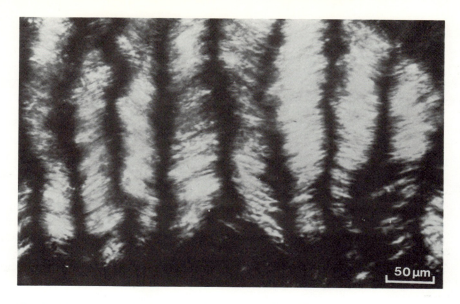

FIG. 5. Polarizing optical micrograph of a sheet of collagen fibres from human pericardium (87-year female) taken with crossed polars, polarizer parallel to the bulk fibre axis.

waves in particular. Indeed, the conventional tendons often used in such studies (e.g. Gathercole and Keller, 1975) do not appear wavy at all, and merely display alternating bands of dark and bright in an otherwise straight and smooth cylindrical fibre (Fig. 4). These bands shift and split in characteristic ways on appropriate rotations of the sample with respect to the optical system. This has led to the recognition that a wave form corresponding to a periodically varying orientation of the underlying birefringent units is the cause of the banding. Further analysis then revealed that this wave form is planar, close to a zig-zag (to be termed 'crimp') with a quantifiable periodicity (ℓ_0) and angular deflection (θ_0) from the fibre axis. Identification of this banding pattern with morphologically seen waves (where such were visible) then lent direct support to deductions from the polarizing optical observations based on the banding alone and served to relate these more recent rationalizations with the long-standing but sporadic records of observable waviness in collagenous tissues.

Subjected to mechanical tension, the wave form is gradually pulled out. This is most easily identified by observing the extinction bands between crossed polaroids as done first by Diamant *et al.* (1972) using rat-tail tendon with ℓ_0 about 100 μm and θ_0

of 10–15° (depending on age). The disappearance of the crimp is the first observable effect in the reversible low-strain region of the stress—strain curve. This is closely associated with the *in vivo* response (Gathercole and Keller, 1975; Keller and Gathercole, 1976), and is known as the 'toe' region in the corresponding stress—strain curve. A complete, idealized version of such a curve is shown in Fig. 9.

Using a model based on the elastica and assuming cantilever bending at rigid crimp sites, Diamant *et al.* (1972) were able to derive a relation between stress and strain which required measurement only of tendon unit cross-section, crimp length and crimp angle. All of these quantities were accessible experimentally and the relation fitted well with the tensile stress—strain curve actually observed in all but very young rats. (The reason for the difference in young animals is due to extension of the very compliant tendon occurring concurrently with crimp straightening; Diamant *et al.*, 1972.) Moreover, the basic load bearing unit diameters could be predicted and were approximately those of the mean *fibril* diameters at the various ages of rat-tail tendon investigated. In later work, Torp, Baer and Friedman (1975) measured these diameters in TEM directly and confirmed the relationship. The nature of crimp sites in rat-tail

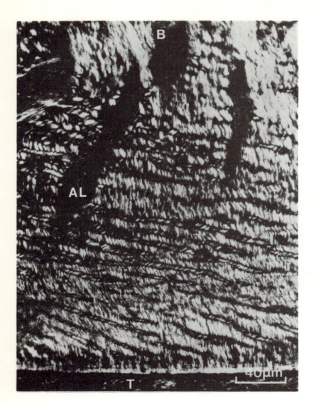

FIG. 6. Crimping in rabbit incisor periodontal ligament. Polarizing optical micrograph. Transverse section of central region; crossed polars. B: alveolar bone. T: tooth. Crimping with $1_0 \sim 16\ \mu m$ is evident, especially in the alveolar layers (AL).

tendon has been extended by relating the polarizing microscopy to information from SEM (Gathercole, Keller and Shah, 1974), low angle X-ray diffraction (Gathercole and Keller, 1975, 1978) and most strikingly by TEM (Dlugosz, Gathercole and Keller, 1978; Kastelic, Galeski and Baer, 1978). Indeed, once attention has been focused on them, crimp sites can be recognized easily in figures from many histological texts (e.g. Gersh, 1973; Craigmyle, 1975) and even popular biology texts (Nilsson, 1974).

Though small-scale waves may be observed in disrupted tendon (Torp, Baer and Friedman, 1975; Nemetschek et al., 1977; Meinel et al., 1977), these should not be confused with the non-artefactual crimp system. The latter is not due to the contraction of severed fibres and has been observed by incident light microscopy in intact bone—muscle systems (Gathercole and Keller, 1975).

THE PERIODONTAL LIGAMENT

The collagen structure hierarchies

As previously stated, the periodontal ligament contains virtually all the structure features within our hierarchy tree but each in specific anatomically distinct localities. Work in this area is not sufficiently advanced to attempt comprehensive mapping, though this is the ultimate aim. However, some guidelines can be given.

Fibres are clearly identifiable and display banding with polarizing microscopy. Consequently, the fibres are crimped in the sense referred to previously and, by the generalization stated there, they are likely to be exposed to tensile loading in both the developmental and functional stages of the teeth. While the fibre orientation varies greatly, there is an overall directionality: they run towards the apex obliquely between alveolar bone and cementum (apart from crestal and apical fibres). The textures illustrated in Figs. 4 and 5 are all broadly accommodated within this general directionality. In particular, they can form larger bundles (Fig. 8), uniaxial sheets (Fig. 7) or may cross to form a spoke-like arrangement (Sloan, 1978).

Fibre crimping in periodontal ligament

Though the effect of crimping on the mechanical behaviour has so far been investigated only for tendons and ligaments where the fibres are totally parallel (and inferences as regards the function of crimping all refer to such cases), it seems likely that crimping plays a similar role in the more complex textures here where crimping is strongly in evidence. In particular, locally parallel crimped regions have been noted by Sloan (1978) both by polarizing microscopy (Fig. 6) and SEM (Fig. 7). The period is about 16 μm and angle θ_0 in excess of $20°$. Similarly Berkovitz and Sloan's (1979) study of periodontal

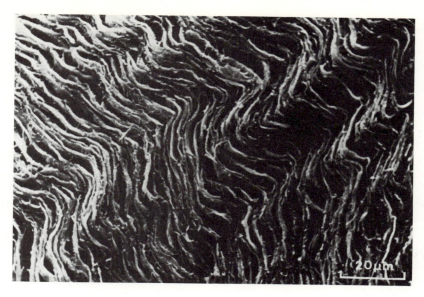

FIG. 7. Waveforms in a sheetlike arrangement in rabbit incisor periodontal ligament. Transverse section of middle layer of periodontal ligament in crestal region. The fibres are 1–3 μm thick. SEM.

ligament from a Cayman *Caiman sclerops* provides some evidence of crimped layers of collagen fibres in this reptile. Using polarizing microscopy we have observed wave forms associated with both permanent and deciduous human teeth (Fig. 8). In all cases, crimp parameters appear to vary with age (in this sample $\theta \simeq 25°$, $\ell_0 \simeq 16$ μm). Similarly, we have observed crimping in cat canine periodontal ligament, especially in the ascending fibres (cf. Schmidt and Keil, 1971) and in dog, pig and monkey periodontal ligament in histological sections (specimens kindly loaned by Professor A. I. Darling and Dr H. Levers) and in fresh pig and sheep periodontal ligament.

We have detected sinuous bend regions in human periodontal ligament by TEM (Fig. 10) but without the simultaneous polarizing microscopic confirmation we achieved in rat-tail tendon.

Fibril diameter related to age

Human adult periodontal ligament fibrils are of the order of 40 nm (dependent on age). This contrasts with ∼400 nm for adult rat-tail tendon. Furthermore, the crimp structure in adult periodontal ligament

seems to relate more closely to the situation in full-term foetal rat-tail tendon. Periodontal fibrils also resemble those from foetal rat-tail tendon in fibril diameter (Gathercole and Keller, 1978b) and in fibril diameter distribution, which remains very narrow (Parry and Craig, 1977).

The age changes in collagen fibril diameter in human periodontal ligament seem to set it in a unique place in connective tissues. As shown in Fig. 11, the mean fibril diameter in erupted teeth falls by more than 50% over the life span. This is in contrast with almost all other comparable soft connective tissues. Skin collagen fibril diameters are relatively constant over the life span, there being only a slight reduction with old age (Linke, 1955). Annulus fibrosus collagen fibrils from human intervertebral disc show a reduction in diameters through adolescence, but become almost constant in adult life, again falling with senility. The nucleus pulposus fibrils (which are much narrower and, together with a dominant mucopolysaccharide matrix, form a hydrostatic compressive shock absorber) show an almost opposite, mirror image variation with age (Happey *et al.*, 1974). Achilles tendon fibrils increase in diameter continually from birth

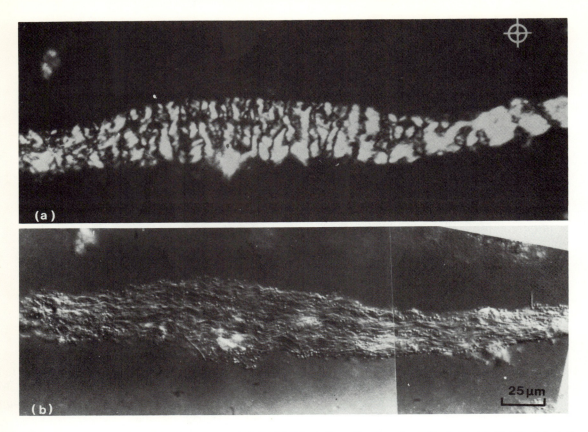

FIG. 8. A teased-out single fibre of human periodontal ligament (from 8-year male; unfixed; mounted in physiological saline), (a) under crossed polars, (b) Nomarski differential interference contrast of same field. The banding can be seen to be due to the wavy course of the fibril bundles.

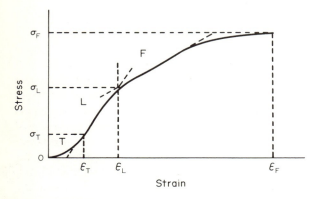

FIG. 9. Ideal tensile stress—strain curve of the type recorded for rat-tail tendon. The curve can conveniently be divided into three zones: the toe (T), linear (L) and yield-failure (F). The symbols σ and ϵ represent the limiting stress and strain respectively for the three zones. The limit of the toe region is identifiable with crimp straightening.

to maturity (Schwarz, 1957), as do fibrils in rat-tail tendon (Torp *et al.*, 1975; Parry and Craig, 1977).

This behaviour is probably related to the high turnover rate of periodontal ligament collagen (Sodek *et al.*, 1977; Sodek, 1978; Orlowski, 1978). This turnover is generally agreed to be a few days compared to weeks, months or years as in other tissues. Thus, periodontal ligament tissues must be laid down, crosslinked, degraded and resynthesized before fibril growth is initiated to any great extent. This, in turn, is related to the fact that periodontal ligament retains a high cellular content in the adult, erupted, state while the cell : fibre ratio in other connective tissues falls dramatically. In this context, recent work on the morphogenesis of crimping in chick digital tendon demonstrates an active role for the fibroblasts around day 15 of development (J. S. Shah,

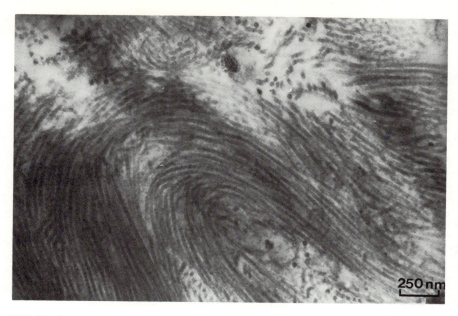

FIG. 10. Section of human periodontal ligament (Glutaraldehyde –OsO$_4$ fixed; uranyl acetate stained; male 72 years) showing local bending in a collagen fibril bundle. TEM.

E. L. Palacios-Prü and L. Palacios, personal communication). There is fibroblast bending at crimp sites, with fibroblast processes defining the linear fibril bundles. It is possible that periodontal ligament collagen fibres in their rapid turnover may be forming and re-forming crimps continually.

Implications from mechanical experiments

It is conceivable that crimping may be important in tooth support. For example, with regard to oblique principal fibres of the periodontal ligament, intrusive loads on the tooth may cause straightening of the crimp. However, the situation might be complicated by concurrent network straightening, especially around blood vessels and in the crestal regions.

We are conducting mechanical experiments on periodontal ligament in dissected pig mandibles, the results of which suggest that tensional modes predominate in periodontal ligament fibres. First and second deciduous premolars are bisected vertically to the level of the alveolar crest and intrusive load applied independently to the two roots in an Instron

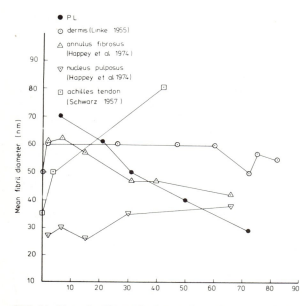

FIG. 11. Plot of collagen fibril mean diameter against age for various human tissues compared with periodontal ligament.

mechanical testing machine at crosshead speeds of 0.5 and 5.0 mm/min in an attempt to approach strain rates experienced in mastication. Intrusions of some 200 μm at a peak load of ~ 12 N are found to be completely reversible if left overnight between tests and almost completely reversible at a 30-minute interval between cycles. Non-linear, stress—strain curves of a form reminiscent of those of rat-tail tendon are obtained. This finding is consistent with the operation of a crimp flexing mechanism. Values found by us are in broad agreement with those reported for human periodontal ligament *in vitro* (Atkinson and Ralph, 1977). Destruction of alveolar bone at the apex does not grossly affect the mechanical response of the system. This further suggests a tensile suspension of the periodontal ligament fibres rather than a compressive upthrust from the narrowing apex (Gathercole *et al.,* unpublished results). This supports the findings of Picton (1976) that apicetomized teeth appear to function normally, and this would seem to be true in our *in vitro* system for intrusions of an order of magnitude larger than those mentioned by him during mastication *in vivo*. Chapter 11 describes the reactions of a tooth to loads *in vivo* and discusses further the mechanisms of tooth support.

Collagen crimping might be associated with the mechanism of tooth eruption if the force generated were a tractional one associated with collagen fibres in the periodontal ligament. Some ideas on collagen contraction have been debated (Thomas, 1976; Berkovitz, 1976) and are considered in detail in Chapter 10.

Non-collagen fibres

Both oxytalan and elastin fibres occur in that 20% of periodontal ligament protein that is non-collagenous. The distinction between elastin and oxytalan fibres is at histochemical level only; oxytalan fibres differ in that they stain with elastin stains only after oxidation (Fullmer and Lillie, 1958), though at the TEM level they resemble immature elastin fibres (Greenlee *et al.,* 1966). In human periodontal ligament, oxytalan fibres predominate and elastic fibres may be confined to blood-vessel walls (Page, 1972). In other mammalian periodontal ligaments (such as pig and deer), elastin fibres are the more abundant by 3 to 1 (Fullmer, 1960).

We have subjected thick transverse sections from the central region of pig premolars to the autoclave treatment of Tsuji, Lavker and Kligman (1979) to reveal elastin fibres. Following this, scanning electron microscopy revealed a fine branching network of ribbon-like fibres across the whole periodontal ligament space (Figs. 12 and 13). Thus, as in dermis (Tsuji *et al.,* 1979), the elastin network appears more extensive than might be thought on a weight-to-weight basis compared with collagen.

The biophysical function of the elastin and oxytalan fibres remains unclear, largely because they are difficult to isolate. They may interweave with collagen and enhance general tooth support (Simpson, 1967) and the observations above would seem to support this. In another view, based on human periodontal ligament, oxytalan fibres may be located mainly around blood vessels and form a network attaching these to the cementum without having an insertion

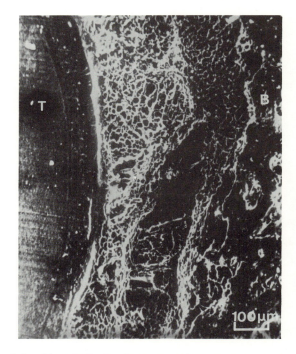

FIG. 12. Transverse section of central region of periodontal ligament of pig first deciduous premolar (autoclaved; shadowed with gold/palladium) showing elastin fibre network. SEM.

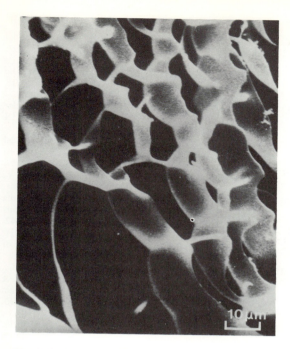

FIG. 13. Higher magnification of middle layer of Fig. 11 showing branching ribbonlike fibres.

in alveolar bone (Sims, 1975); their response to occlusal load may even be the reverse of collagen (Sims, 1975), with the oxytalan network relaxing rather than contracting under occlusal load.

Oxytalan fibres are more abundant in the gingival and apical regions than among the oblique collagen fibres in periodontal ligament. They are also found in non-periodontal connective tissues (reviews by Fullmer, 1960, 1967; Fullmer, Sheetz and Narkates, 1974).

Certainly there is a need for further investigation of elastin-containing fibres in the periodontal ligament, though the key to tooth support, movement and even eruption seems to lie in the collagen fibres.

REFERENCES

ATKINSON, H. F. & RALPH, W. J. (1977) *In vitro* strength of the human periodontal ligament. *J. dent. Res.* **56**, 48–52.

BAER, E., GATHERCOLE, L. J. & KELLER, A. (1975) Structure hierarchies in tendon collagen: an interim summary. In: *Structure of fibrous biopolymers*, Colston Papers No. 26, E. D. T. ATKINS & A. KELLER (eds.), pp. 189–196. London, Butterworths.

BAILEY, A. J. (1975) Collagen: general introduction. In: *Structure of fibrous biopolymers*, Colston Papers No. 26, E. D. T. ATKINS & A. KELLER (eds.), pp. 115–125. London, Butterworths.

BAILEY, A. J., LIGHT, N. D. & ATKINS, E. D. T. (1980) Chemical crosslinking restrictions on models for the molecular organization of the collagen fibre. *Nature* **288**, 408–410.

BERKOVITZ, B. K. B. (1976) Theories of tooth eruption. In: *The eruption and occlusion of teeth*, Colston Papers No. 27, D. F. G. POOLE & M. V. STACK (eds.), pp. 193–204. London, Butterworths.

BERKOVITZ, B. K. B. & SLOAN, P. (1979) Attachment tissues of the teeth in *Caiman sclerops* (Crocodilia). *J. Zool., Lond.* **187**, 179–194.

BERKOVITZ, B. K. B., WEAVER, M. E., SHORE, R. C. & MOXHAM, B. J. (1981) Fibril diameters in the extracellular matrix of the periodontal connective tissues of the rat. *Conn. Tissue Res.* **8**, 127–132.

BURGE, R. E. (1963) Equatorial X-ray diffraction by fibrous proteins: short range order in collagen, feather keratin and F-actin. *J. Molec. Biol.* **7**, 213–224.

BURGE, R. E. (1965) X-ray aspects of the structure of collagen and their comparison with other fibrous proteins. In: *Structure and function of connective and skeletal tissue*, S. FITTON-JACKSON et al. (eds.), pp. 2–7. London, Butterworths.

CRAIGMYLE, M. B. L. (1975) *A colour atlas of histology*, p. 30. London, Wolfe Medical Publications.

CUNNINGHAM, L. W., DAVIES, H. A. & HAMMONDS, R. G. (1976) An analysis of the association of collagen based on structural models. *Biopolymers* **15**, 483–502.

DIAMANT, J., KELLER, A., BAER, E., LITT, M. & ARRIDGE, R. G. C. (1972) Collagen: Ultrastructure and its relation to mechanical properties as a function of aging. *Proc. R. Soc. Lond.* B, **180**, 293–315.

DLUGOSZ, J., GATHERCOLE, L. J. & KELLER, A. (1978) Transmission electron microscope studies and their relation to polarizing optical microscopy in rat tail tendon. *Micron* **9**, 71–82.

DLUGOSZ, J., GATHERCOLE, L. J. & KELLER, A. (1979) Cholesteric analogue packing of collagen fibrils in the Cuvierian tubules of *Holothuria forskäli* (Holothuroidea, Echinodermata). *Micron* **10**, 81–87.

DOYLE, B. B., HULMES, D. J. S., MILLER, A., PARRY, D. A. D., PIEZ, K. A. & WOODHEAD-GALLOWAY, J. (1974a) A D-periodic narrow filament in collagen. *Proc. R. Soc. Lond.* B, **186**, 67–74.

DOYLE, B. B., HULMES, D. J. S., MILLER, A., PARRY, D. A. D., PIEZ, K. A. & WOODHEAD-GALLOWAY, J. (1974b) Axially projected collagen structures. *Proc. R. Soc. Lond.* B, **187**, 37–46.

ELDEN, H. R. (1968) Physical properties of collagen fibres. In: *International Review of Connective Tissue Research* **4**, D. A. HALL (ed.), pp. 283–348. New York, Academic Press.

FULLMER, H. M. (1960) A comparative histochemical study of elastic, pre-elastic and oxytalan connective tissue fibres. *J. Histochem. Cytochem.* **8**, 290–295.

FULLMER, H. M. (1967) Connective tissue components of the periodontium. In: *Structural and chemical organi-*

zation of teeth, Vol. 2, A. E. W. MILES (ed.), pp. 349–414. London, Academic Press.

FULLMER, H. M. & LILLIE, R. D. (1958) The oxytalan fiber: a previously undescribed connective tissue fiber. *J. Histochem. Cytochem.* **6**, 425–430.

FULLMER, H. M., SHEETZ, J. H. & NARKATES, A. J. (1974) Oxytalan connective tissue fibers: A review. *J. oral Path.* **3**, 291–316.

GATHERCOLE, L. J. & KELLER, A. (1975) Light microscopic waveforms in collagenous tissue and their structural implications. In: *Structure of fibrous biopolymers,* Colston Papers No. 26, E. D. T. ATKINS & A. KELLER (eds.), pp. 153–187. London, Butterworths.

GATHERCOLE, L. J. & KELLER, A. (1978a) X-ray diffraction effects related to superstructure in rat tail tendon collagen. *Biochim. Biophys. Acta* **535**, 253–271.

GATHERCOLE, L. J. & KELLER, A. (1978b) Early development of crimping in rat tail tendon collagen: a polarising optical and SEM study. *Micron* **9**, 83–89.

GATHERCOLE, L. J., KELLER, A. & SHAH, J. S. (1974) The periodic wave pattern in native tendon collagen: correlation of polarizing with scanning electron microscopy. *J. Microsc.* **102**, 95–106.

GATHERCOLE, L. J., BAILEY, A. J., DLUGOSZ, J. & KELLER, A. (1980) The Cuvierian tubules of Holothuria: design for successful failure in a collagenous system. In: *Mechanical properties of biological materials.* Symp. Soc. Exp. Biol. 28, J. F. V. VINCENT & J. CURREY (eds.), pp. 475–476. Cambridge University Press.

GATHERCOLE, L. J., BOOY, F. P., DLUGOSZ, J. & KELLER, A. (1978) Low temperature electron diffraction and beam effects in tendon collagen. *Connect. Tissue Res.* **5**, 201–204.

GERSH, I. (1973) Vascularity and protein-polysaccharide complex in tendons of young rats. In: *Submicroscopic cytochemistry,* Vol. 2, I. GERSH (ed.), pp. 206–212. New York, Academic Press.

GREENLEE, T. K., ROSS, R. & HARTMANN, J. (1966) The fine structure of elastin fibres. *J. Cell Biol.* **30**, 59–71.

HAPPEY, F., NAYLOR, A., PALFRAMAN, J., PEARSON, C. H. & TURNER, R. L. (1974) Variations in the diameter of collagen fibrils, bound hexose and associated glycoproteins in the intervertebral disc. In: *Connective tissues, biochemistry and pathophysiology,* R. FRICKE & F. HARTMANN (eds.), pp. 67–70. Berlin, Springer.

HODGE, A. J. (1967) Structure at the electron microscopic level, In: *Treatise on collagen,* Vol. 1, G. N. RAMACHANDRAN (ed.), pp. 187–205. London, Academic Press.

HODGE, A. J. & PETRUSKA, J. A. (1963) Recent studies with the electron microscope on ordered aggregates of the tropocollagen molecule. In: *Aspects of protein structure,* G. N. RAMACHANDRAN (ed.), p. 289. London, Academic Press.

HOSEMANN, R. F. & NEMETSCHEK, Th. (1973) Reaktionsabläufe zwischen Phosphorwolframsäure und Kollagen. *Kolloid Z. und Z. Polymere,* **251**, 53–60.

HOSEMANN, R., DREISSIG, W. & NEMETSCHEK, Th. (1974) Schachtelhalm – structure of the octafibrils in collagen. *J. Molec. Biol.* **83**, 275–280.

HUKINS, D. W. L. & WOODHEAD-GALLOWAY, J. (1977) Collagen fibrils as examples of smectic A biological fibres. *Molec. Cryst. Liq. Cryst.* **41**, 33–39.

HULMES, D. J. S. & MILLER, A. (1979) Quasi-hexagonal molecular packing in collagen fibrils. *Nature* **282**, 878–880.

KASTELIC, J., GALESKI, A. E. & BAER, E. (1978) The multicomposite structure of tendon. *Connec. Tiss. Res.* **6**, 11–23.

KATZ, E. P. (1972) Discussion. In: *The comparative molecular biology of extracellular matrices,* H. C. SLAVKIN (ed.), pp. 422–431. New York, Academic Press.

KELLER, A. & GATHERCOLE, L. J. (1976) Biophysical and mechanical properties of collagen in relation to function. In: *The eruption and occlusion of teeth,* Colston Papers No. 27, D. F. G. POOLE & M. V. STACK (eds.), pp. 262–266. London, Butterworths.

LINKE, K. W. (1955) Elektronmikroskopische Untersuchung über die Differenzierung der Interzellularsubstanz der menschlichen Lederhaut. *Z. Zellforsch.* **42**, 331–341.

MacFARLANE, E. F. (1971) Molecular packing structure of collagen. *Search* **2**, 171–172.

MEINEL, A., NEMETSCHEK-GANSLER, H., HOLZ, U., JONAK, R., KRAHL, H., NEMETSCHEK, Th. & RIEDL, H. (1977) Fibrilläre Gefügestörung bei Sehnenruptur. *Arch. orthop. Unfall – Chir.* **90**, 89–94.

MILLER, A. (1976) Molecular packing in collagen fibrils. In: *Biochemistry of collagen,* G. N. RAMACHANDRAN & A. H. REDDI (eds.), pp. 85–136. New York, Plenum.

MILLER, A. & PARRY, D. A. D. (1973) Structure and packing of microfibrils in collagen. *J. Molec. Biol.* **75**, 441–447.

MILLER, A. & WRAY, J. S. (1971) Molecular packing in collagen. *Nature* **230**, 437–439.

NEMETSCHEK, Th. & HOSEMANN, R. (1973) A kink model of native collagen. *Kolloid Z. und Z. Polymere* **251**, 1044–1056.

NEMETSCHEK, Th., JONAK, R., MEINEL, A., NEMETSCHEK-GANSLER, H. & RIEDL, H. (1977) Knickdeformationen an Kollagen. *Arch. orthop. Unfall – Chir.* **89**, 249–257.

NEMETSCHEK, Th., RIEDL, H. & JONAK, R. (1979) Topochemistry of the binding of phosphotungstic acid to collagen. *J. Molec. Biol.* **133**, 67–83.

NEVILLE, A. C. (1975) *Biology of the arthropod cuticle.* Berlin–Heidelberg, Springer.

NILSSON, A. (1974) In: *Behold man,* pp. 74, 121, 186. London, Harrap.

ORLOWSKI, W. A. (1978) Biochemical study of collagen turnover in rat incisor periodontal ligament. *Archs. oral Biol.* **23**, 1163–1165.

PAGE, R. C. (1972) Macromolecular interactions in the connective tissues of the periodontium. In: *Developmental aspects of oral biology,* H. C. SLAVKIN & L. A. BAVETTA (eds.), pp. 241–308. New York, Academic Press.

PARRY, D. A. D. & CRAIG, A. S. (1977) Quantitative electron microscope observation of the collagen fibrils in rat tail tendon. *Biopolymers* **16**, 1015–1031.

PARRY, D. A. D. & CRAIG, A. S. (1979) Electron microscope evidence for an 80Å unit in collagen fibrils. *Nature* **282**, 213–215.

PEASE, D. C. & BOUTEILLE, M. (1971) The tridimensional ultrastructure of native collagenous fibrils, cytochemical evidence for a carbohydrate matrix. *J. Ultrastruct. Res.* **35**, 339–358.

PETRUSKA, J. A. (1972) Discussion. In: *Comparative molecular biology of extracellular matrices*, H. C. SLAVKIN (ed.), pp. 431–434. New York, Academic Press.

PICTON, D. C. A. (1976) Tension and the periodontal ligament (discussion). In: *The eruption and occlusion of teeth*, Colston Papers No. 27, D. F. G. POOLE & M. V. STACK (eds.), pp. 224–225. London, Butterworths.

PIEZ, K. A. & TRUS, B. L. (1978) Sequence regularities and packing of collagen molecules. *J. Molec. Biol.* **122**, 419–432.

RAMACHANDRAN, G. N. (1967) Structure of collagen at the molecular level. In: *Treatise on collagen*, Vol. 1, G. N. RAMACHANDRAN (ed.), pp. 103–183. London, Academic Press.

ROSS, R. & BENDITT, E. P. (1961) Wound healing and collagen formation. I. *J. Biophys. Biochem. Cytol.* **11**, 677–700.

ROWE, R. W. D. (1974) Collagen fibre arrangement in intramuscular connective tissue. Changes associated with muscle shortening and their possible relevance to meat toughness measurements. *J. Food Technol.* **9**, 501–508.

SCHMIDT, W. J. & KEIL, A. (1971) In: *Polarising microscopy of dental tissues*, pp. 466–477. Oxford, Pergamon.

SCHWARZ, W. (1957) Morphology and differentiation of the connective tissue fibres. In: *Connective tissue*, R. E. TUNBRIDGE *et al.* (eds.), pp. 144–156. Oxford, Blackwell.

SCOTT, J. E. (1979) Hierarchy in connective tissues. *Chemistry in Britain* **15**, 13–18.

SIMPSON, H. E. (1967) A three-dimensional approach to the microscopy of the periodontal membrane. *Proc. R. Soc. Med.* **60**, 537–542.

SIMS, M. R. (1975) Oxytalan-vascular relationships observed in histologic examination of the periodontal ligaments of man and mouse. *Archs. oral Biol.* **20**, 713–717.

SLOAN, P. (1978) Microanatomy of the periodontal ligament in some animals possessing teeth of continuous and limited growth. Ph.D. thesis, University of Bristol.

SMITH, J. W. (1968) Molecular pattern in native collagen. *Nature* **219**, 157–158.

SODEK, J. (1978) A comparison of collagen and non-collagenous protein metabolism in rat molar and incisor periodontal ligaments. *Archs. oral Biol.* **23**, 977–982.

SODEK, J., BRUNETTE, D. M., FENG, J., HEERSCHE, J. N. M., LINEBACK, H. F., MELCHER, A. M. & NG, B. (1977) Collagen synthesis in a major component of protein synthesis in the periodontal ligament in various species. *Archs. oral Biol.* **22**, 647–653.

SQUIRE, J. M. & FREUNDLICH, A. (1980) Direct observation of a transverse periodicity in collagen fibrils. *Nature* **288**, 410–413.

SZIRMAI, J. A. (1970) Structure of the intervertebral disc. In: *Chemistry and molecular biology of the intercellular matrix*, vol. 3, E. A. BALASZ (ed.), pp. 1279–1303. London, Academic Press.

THOMAS, N. R. (1976) Collagen as the generator of tooth eruption. In: *The eruption and occlusion of teeth*. Colston Papers No. 27, D. F. G. POOLE & M. V. STACK (eds.), pp. 290–309. London, Butterworths.

TORP, S., ARRIDGE, R. G. C., ARMENIADES, C. D. & BAER, E. (1975) Structure–property relationships in tendon as a function of age. In: *Structure of fibrous biopolymers*, Colston Papers No. 26, E. D. T. ATKINS & A. KELLER (eds.), pp. 197–222. London, Butterworths.

TORP, S., BAER, E. & FRIEDMAN, B. (1975) Effects of age and of mechanical deformation on the ultrastructure of tendon. In: *Structure of fibrous biopolymers*, Colston Papers No. 26, E. D. T. ATKINS & A. KELLER (eds.), pp. 223–250. London, Butterworths.

TRELSTAD, R. L. & COULOMBRE, A. J. (1971) Morphogenesis of the collagenous stroma in the chick cornea. *J. Cell Biol.* **50**, 840–858.

TRUS, B. L. & PIEZ, K. A. (1980) Compressed microfibril model of the native collagen fibril. *Nature* **286**, 300–301.

TSUJI, T., LAVKER, R. M. & KLIGMAN, A. M. (1979) A new method for scanning electron microscopic visualization of dermal elastic fibres. *J. Microsc.* **115**, 165–173.

VEIS, A., ANESEY, J. & MUSSELL, S. (1967) A limiting microfibril model for the three-dimensional arrangement within collagen fibres. *Nature* **251**, 931–934.

VEIS, A., MILLER, A., LEIBOVICH, S. J. & TRAUB, W. (1979) The limiting collagen microfibril. The minimum structure demonstrating native axial periodicity. *Biochim. et Biophys. Acta* **576**, 88–98.

VEIS, A. & YUAN, L. (1975) Structure of the collagen microfibril. A four-strand of overlap model. *Biopolymers* **14**, 895–900.

WALTON, A. G. (1975) Synthetic polypeptide models for collagen structure and function. In: *Structure of fibrous biopolymers*, Colston Papers No. 26, E. D. T. ATKINS & A. KELLER (eds.), pp. 139–148. London, Butterworths.

WOODHEAD-GALLOWAY, J., HUKINS, D. W. L. & WRAY, J. S. (1975) Closest packing of two-stranded coiled coils as a model for the collagen fibril. *Biochem. Biophys. Res. Commun.* **64**, 1237–1244.

Chapter 6

THE GROUND SUBSTANCE OF THE PERIODONTAL LIGAMENT

C. H. Pearson

INTRODUCTION

There have been few studies of the ground substance of the periodontal ligament. Most of our ideas of it are derived from work on other connective tissues. The major components of ground substance are hyaluronic acid, proteoglycans (compounds containing anionic polysaccharides covalently attached to a protein core) and glycoproteins. Hyaluronic acid and the polysaccharide components of proteoglycans are glycosaminoglycans (subclasses: galactosaminoglycans and glucosaminoglycans) which are built up of repeating disaccharide units (Table 3). The carbohydrate components of glycoproteins have much less regular structures than glycosaminoglycans and are generally much smaller.

COMPONENTS DERIVED FROM SERUM

As other connective tissues (Anderson, 1976), the periodontal ligament will contain serum components. In addition to albumin, various glycoproteins probably originate from serum and some of these may be functionally important, e.g. as proteinase inhibitors (Twining and Brecher, 1977). However, normally the leakage of serum components into tissues is small (Shaw, 1978). The increase in permeability of blood vessel walls in inflammation will allow the passage of significant amounts of macromolecules. One of the most important is α_2-macroglobulin, an inhibitor of collagenase and other proteinases (Starkey and Barrett, 1977). In contrast with typical connective tissue glycoproteins, most of the components derived from serum are readily extracted with dilute salt solutions (Anderson, 1976).

NON-COLLAGEN GLYCOPROTEINS

General survey

Non-collagen glycoproteins are widely distributed in

connective tissues but they are not well characterized. There seems to be no evidence for the presence in soft connective tissues of the type of sialoglycoprotein which is an important component of bone (Andrews, Herring and Kent, 1969). However, a variety of glyco-proteins occur (the amino acid compositions of which are compared in Table 1), including compounds that appear to have a high affinity for collagen or proteo-glycans (Anderson, 1976; Herring, 1976).

The so-called structural glycoproteins (Wolf et al., 1971; Robert, Darrell & Robert, 1970; Robert and Robert, 1974, 1975; Anderson, 1976; Moczar, Moczar and Robert, 1977) are ubiquitously distri-buted in connective tissues. Their function is not

clear, but they interact with collagen (Moczar et al., 1977) and may be important organ and species-specific antigens (Robert et al., 1970; Robert and Robert, 1974; Anderson, 1976; Treffers and Broek-huyse, 1977). It has been suggested also that struc-tural glycoproteins act as a template for the orienta-tion of collagen fibrils (Robert and Robert, 1974, 1975).

The difficulty of isolating the structural glyco-proteins from tissues and their strong propensity for aggregation (Shipp and Bowness, 1975; Randoux et al., 1976; Moczar et al., 1977) has hampered their study, but a partially characterized glycoprotein has been isolated from the insoluble matrix of rabbit

TABLE 1. *Amino acid compositions (residues/1000 residues) of some connective tissue glycoproteins*

The cell surface glycoprotein (fibronectin) was isolated from chick embryo fibroblasts. Results are shown for only one (D_1) of the two similar chains of the structural glycoprotein (SGP) of rabbit skin and for only the major fraction (G) of the puppy rib cartilage SGP. Elastic fibre microfibrils (B) were isolated from arterial smooth muscle cell cultures and (A) were extracted from bovine ligamentum nuchae. The tendon glycoprotein (GP) was isolated from 3 M $MgCl_2$ extracts of bovine Achilles tendon and the link GP from bovine nasal cartilage. Bovine dental pulp was exhaustively extracted with 0.1 M NaCl and the insoluble residue treated with bacterial collagenase (Pearson, Ainsworth and Chovelon, 1978b) for 3 days at 37° under toluene and the residue lyophilized before hydrolysis and analysis by a previously described method (Pearson et al., 1975). These results were corrected for a small amount of collagen (11%) which was still present.

	Fibronectin[a]	Skin[b] SGP(D_1)	Aorta[c] SGP	Cartilage[d] SGP(G)	Elastic tissue[e] microfibrils A	B	Tendon[f] GP	Cartilage[g] link GP(1)	Dental pulp[h] collagenase-insoluble
Asp	94	108	95	104	114	88	128	135	94
Thr	100	69	54	50	55	75	32	52	52
Ser	74	84	66	51	59	101	70	62	56
Glu	117	138	136	124	111	130	105	76	116
Pro	77	54	62	54	70	70	98	48	62
Gly	106	80	104	86	120	131	64	104	60
Ala	48	92	79	76	59	66	41	80	52
Val	66	58	51	69	54	62	49	61	72
Met	13	8	4	14	16	11	10	3	28
Ile	37	50	55	51	45	36	47	29	53
Leu	55	88	91	96	57	58	137	80	107
Tyr	37	23	23	26	30	33	44	66	38
Phe	19	27	38	38	32	27	34	53	48
Lys	34	62	57	68	37	37	50	58	52
His	16	15	15	22	14	22	28	29	28
Arg	53	31	48	54	45	44	47	64	55
1/2 Cys	18*	15*	12*	16	80*	10*	16	†	26
Trp	36	ND	8	ND	ND	ND	ND	ND	ND

[a]Yamada et al. (1977); [b]Randoux et al. (1976); [c]Moczar et al. (1977); [d]Shipp and Bowness (1975); [e]Muir et al. (1976); [f]Anderson (1975); [g]Baker and Caterson (1979); [h]Pearson and Chovelon (unpublished work).

*Includes cysteine derivatives. † Other data indicated 23 residues/1000. ND, not determined.

dermis (Randoux *et al.,* 1976). Investigations of its effects on collagen biosynthesis and fibroblast morphology have begun (Randoux *et al.,* 1978). This glycoprotein remained insoluble when the skin collagen was removed by digestion with bacterial collagenase, but it dissolved subsequently in 8 M urea without the use of a reducing agent (which is usually required to effectively dissolve structural glycoproteins (Anderson, 1976)). Two glycoprotein chains finally were isolated, each having a molecular weight of 16,000 and differing only slightly in amino acid composition. However, one chain contained twice as much hexose and glucosamine as the other (Randoux *et al.,* 1976). Although the bacterial collagenase was purified, non-specific proteinase activity may not have been eliminated and proteolysis of the glycoprotein could have occurred during the collagen dissolution. Thus, the isolated glycoprotein may be smaller than the native molecule. However, Moczar *et al.* (1977) found that a 35,000 molecular weight structural glycoprotein of pig aorta (Table 1), isolated without using bacterial collagenase, seemed unaffected by incubation with a commercial preparation of the collagenase which has non-specific proteolytic activity.

We have observed that glycoproteins in collagenase-insoluble fractions of soft dental tissues are very resistant to cathepsin D, cathepsin B and leucocytic elastase (Pearson, C. H. and Lehocky, S., unpublished data). As these proteinases are prominent in the catabolism of proteins in normal or inflamed connective tissues, it seems likely that structural glycoproteins are persistent components of the matrix. If they are strongly antigenic, this could have important consequences. More needs to be known about the fate of these glycoproteins during tissue remodelling and inflammation.

A possibly different type of glycoprotein (more easily solubilized and having less tendency to self-associate or form aggregates) has been isolated from tendon (Anderson and Jackson, 1972; Anderson, 1975; Anderson and Labedz, 1977) and dermis (Anderson, Labedz and Brenchley, 1977). It is likely that this glycoprotein type occurs in other soft connective tissues, including the periodontal ligament. The tendon glycoprotein (molecular weight 60,000) appears to be quite different from the "link" glycoprotein (Table 1) associated with cartilage proteoglycans. Collagen fibrillogenesis is influenced

by the tendon glycoprotein *in vitro* (Anderson, Labedz and Kewley, 1977). They suggested that a weak binding of the glycoprotein to collagen would facilitate a control of collagen morphology. It is not clear to what extent this effect is specific to tendon glycoprotein, as many compounds can affect collagen fibrillogenesis (at least *in vitro*). Anderson (1978) has indicated that the glycoprotein could be an enzyme, e.g. prolyl hydroxylase (which occurs extracellularly). Neither the tendon glycoprotein nor the link glycoprotein of cartilage showed an aspartate : glutamate ratio of 1.0 or less which, as Shipp and Bowness (1975) suggest, may be characteristic of structural glycoproteins (see Table 1).

Another glycoprotein, fibronectin (LETS protein, CSP, galactoprotein a), has recently attracted considerable attention. Fibronectin has a high molecular weight (Fig. 1). It is associated with the surfaces of fibroblasts and some other cells (Hynes, 1976; Yamada and Olden, 1978; Dessau *et al.,* 1978; Furcht, Mosher and Wendelschafer-Crabb, 1978). Its distribution in the developing tooth germ has been reported by Thesleff *et al.* (1979). It has some characteristics in common with structural glycoproteins. Fibronectin forms intercellular fibrillary networks in early stages of tissue development. Indeed, it could be described as a primitive ground substance. This network may serve as the initial backbone for collagen fibrillogenesis (Chen *et al.,* 1978). The distribution of fibronectin is similar to that of reticulin fibres (Linder *et al.,* 1978) which contain Type III collagen (Nowack *et al.,* 1976; Pearson, 1979). In fibroblast cultures, collagen or procollagen was codistributed with fibronectin at the cell surface (Bornstein and Ash, 1977; Bornstein *et al.,* 1978; Vaheri *et al.,* 1978). Other evidence suggests that fibronectin mediates the adhesion of fibroblasts to collagen films (Yamada and Olden, 1978; Pena and Hughes, 1978; Kleinman *et al.,* 1978; Rouslahti *et al.,* 1979). The main functions of fibronectin appear to be expressed during active proliferation of connective tissue cells since it is not usually seen in the main matrices of mature connective tissues. However, collagen and proteoglycans could mask fibronectin, preventing its detection. Alternatively, fibronectin may have undergone proteolytic degradation, yielding fragments which could persist in the mature tissue as 'structural glycoproteins'.

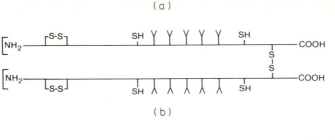

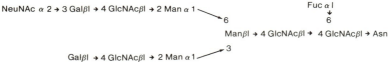

FIG. 1. Model of fibronectin structure. (a) The molecular weight of each poly-peptide chain is about 220,000. Aminotermini are blocked (Yamada *et al.,* 1977). Positions of disulphide bonds, –SH groups and oligosaccharide units (Y) are as proposed by Fukuda and Hakomori (1979a). (b) Structure of the major oligosaccharide unit of fibronectin (Fukuda and Hakomori, 1979b).

Proteolysis may expose antigenic sites, which would explain the potent antigenicity of structural glyco-proteins.

Bray (1978 a, b) demonstrated that structural glycoproteins from placenta and lung reacted with an antibody to a plasma form of fibronectin (cold-insoluble globulin) which is immunologically indis-tinguishable from cell surface fibronectin. Also, an antibody to a structural glycoprotein isolated from rib cartilage (Shipp and Bowness, 1975) gave a precipitin line with partially purified cold-insoluble globulin (Dr. M. Bowness, personal communication). Other similarities include the insolubility and aggre-gating tendency of cell surface fibronectin and struc-tural glycoproteins and the types of sugars present (with the possible exception of glucose (Yamada *et al.,* 1977; Fukuda & Hakomori, 1979a)). Differences in molecular weight and amino acid composition (Table 1) may be explained if structural glycoproteins are fragments of fibronectin. This proposal is consis-tent with suggestions that structural glycoproteins are related to components of cell membranes (Robert and Robert, 1974, 1975). An externally associated glycoprotein such as fibronectin seems to be a more likely normal precursor than a glycoprotein of the glycophorin type (Furthmayr, 1978) which is an integral part of some cell membranes. However, amino acid sequencing of the glycoproteins will be needed to answer these questions.*

Little is known about the biosynthesis of struc-tural glycoproteins. Assuming there are specific interactions between the structural glycoproteins and collagen, the observation that the relative rates of synthesis of these two molecules varied in dif-ferent tissues (Robert and Robert, 1975) could be important in understanding the adaptation of collagen morphology to specific tissue functions. Robert and Robert (1975) also concluded that the rate of syn-thesis of structural glycoproteins, proteoglycans, collagen and elastin were controlled independently and this was the main factor leading to changes in tissue composition during maturation and aging. Whilst catabolic rates must also be considered (par-ticularly for the proteoglycans), there have been no studies on the degradation of structural glycoproteins *in vivo.* Furuto and Schneir (1975) showed that a sialoglycoprotein in rat skin increased concomitantly with insoluble collagen during maturation. Since this sialoglycoprotein was dissolved with the collagen by incubating with bacterial collagenase, it is probably of a different type from the structural glycoproteins discussed previously. Structural glycoproteins usually decrease during maturation and aging (Robert and Robert, 1975), though a similar glycoprotein fraction

---

*The need for data on the primary structure is emphasized by recent evidence that some preparations of structural glycoproteins may consist largely of actin (Bach and Bentley, 1980).

in human nucleus pulposus increased after 40 years (Pearson *et al.*, 1972).

Glycoproteins in periodontal ligament and other soft dental tissues

There have been few attempts to study the non-collagen glycoproteins of the periodontal ligament except at the glycopeptide level. Non-collagen glycopeptides released from NaCl-insoluble matrices of the bovine ligament and other dental tissues by papain digestion were separated from the collagen glycopeptides (which are smaller) by chromatography on a column of Sephadex G-25. The neutral sugar composition of the non-collagen glycopeptides is shown in Table 2. In all cases, galactose predominated over

mannose and fucose occurred as a minor constituent. Glucose (a rare component of non-collagen glycoproteins) was always found. It is unlikely that the glucose was derived from the Sephadex gel used in isolating the compounds, as significant amounts of glucose have been detected also in similar non-collagen glycopeptides not exposed to Sephadex (Pearson, 1970). Another possible source of glucose, however, is contaminating glycolipids from cell membranes. The similarities between the glycopeptides of periodontal ligament and those of other connective tissues (Table 2) are remarkable, considering the different tissue sources, methods of isolation and also the fact that the glycopeptides of each tissue were derived almost certainly from a mixture of glycoproteins. However, the neutral sugar compositions of bacterial collagenase-insoluble fractions of the periodontal

TABLE 2.   *Neutral sugar compositions of non-collagen glycopeptides and glycoproteins*

Results shown for the soft dental tissues and bovine dermis refer to non-collagen glycopeptides isolated after papain digestion of the NaCl-insoluble matrices or the bacterial collagenase-insoluble residues (CR) of the latter. The glycopeptides of cementum and predentine were derived from decalcified matrices. In all these analyses neutral sugars were determined by ion-exchange chromatography of acid hydrolysates. Different methods were used by the various authors (see footnotes for references) in isolating and analysing purified structural glycoproteins (SGP) and the tendon glycoprotein (GP) but hexose values were obtained mainly by gas-liquid chromatography.

	% of total neutral sugar				g/14 g Hyp
	Gal	Man	Glc	Fuc	Total
Bovine periodontal ligament ⎰ Unerupted[a]	46	37	10	7	0.77
Erupted[a]	45	35	12	8	0.57
Occluded[a]	45	30	20	5	1.0
CR occluded[b]	25	28	44	3	—
Bovine dental pulp[b]	43	33	15	9	0.77
CR dental pulp[b]	33	34	27	6	—
Cementum[c]	45	29	18	8	0.9
Predentine[d]	38	27	23	12	2.2
Bovine dermis[a]	53	25	13	9	0.1
Rabbit skin SGP[e]	46	31	10	13	—
Pig aorta SGP[f]	39	52	9	—	—
Bovine tendon GP[g]	54	29	5	12	—

[a]Pearson *et al.* (1975).
[b]Pearson and Chovelon (unpublished work).
[c]Chovelon, Carmichael and Pearson (1975).
[d]Carmichael, Chovelon and Pearson (1975).
[e]Calculated from the data of Randoux *et al.* (1976) and Cornillet-Stoupy, Borel and Randoux (1978).
[f]Moczar *et al.* (1977).
[g]Anderson and Jackson (1972).

ligament (and dental pulp) were different, as mannose was approximately equal to galactose and glucose was significantly elevated. The mannose:galactose ratios were closer to that of the aortic structural glycoprotein, which, however, contained much less glucose and possibly no fucose (although this sugar was previously reported to be present (Robert and Robert, 1975)). The amino acid composition of the collagenase-insoluble residue of dental pulp (Table 1) had some features in common with structural glycoproteins, but further purification of these glycoproteins and those of the periodontal ligament is required.

The collagenase-insoluble residues contain a large part of the NaCl-insoluble glycoproteins of the bovine ligament (and pulp). Considerable dissolution of the residue occurs in 6 M urea – 0.1 M 2-mercaptoethanol, followed by aggregation and precipitation if the urea is removed by dialysis (even if the reducing agent is still present). This suggests the presence of structural glycoproteins (Moczar, Sepulchre and Moczar, 1975; Anderson, 1976). Like most connective tissue non-collagen proteins, these glycoproteins contain only small quantities of hexose and usually even less of other sugars. Generally, the hexose contents are in the range 4–10% (Anderson and Jackson, 1972; Robert and Robert, 1975; Francis and Thomas, 1975; Anderson, 1976; Randoux et al., 1976; Yamanishi and Sato, 1976).

We do not yet know the neutral sugar contents of pure glycoproteins of soft dental tissues, but they are unlikely to exceed greatly that of skin and tendon glycoproteins (especially as the bacterial collagenase-insoluble residues contained only 2–4% of hexose). We can infer from the neutral sugar values (Table 2) that the insoluble matrices of the dental tissues contained relatively large quantities of non-collagen glycoproteins (certainly more than in dermis), probably amounting to 10–20 g per 100 g collagen. This is supported by the finding that the dental pulp yielded more than five times as much collagenase-insoluble residue as the same wet weight of dermis. Even higher amounts of hexose were found in the whole periodontal ligament and gingiva (Michalites and Orlowski, 1977) and in dental pulp (Orlowski, 1974), presumably because serum glycoproteins were present as well as easily soluble connective tissue glycoproteins (Anderson, 1976; Anderson and

Labedz, 1977) which were removed by the NaCl solution prior to our own analyses.

Thus, non-collagen glycoproteins appear to be major components of the ground substance of soft dental tissues (quantitatively they may be more important than proteoglycans (page 129)). This is not apparent histologically because of the reliance on staining methods (such as PAS) which visualize only the small portions of the glycoprotein molecule containing carbohydrate. Furthermore, interactions with other tissue components may mask some of the carbohydrate. PAS-positive granules have been observed in most of the cells of developing rat incisor periodontal ligament (Mashouf and Engel, 1975). One interpretation of the high glycoprotein content is the large number of cells present in the dental tissues, the surfaces of which will contain glycoproteins. However, the distinction is difficult between cell surface glycoproteins and those occurring in the ground substance proper or those firmly associated with fibrous structures. Another complication is that the extrahelical regions of procollagen contain oligosaccharides and these glycopeptides have some resemblance to non-collagen glycoproteins, containing mannose and glucosamine (Olsen et al., 1977; Tanzer et al., 1977; Clark and Kefalides, 1978). The fate of these glycopeptides after cleavage from procollagen is uncertain, but it is likely that some persist in the tissue. Also, elastin fibres contain an apparently specific type of microfibrillar glycoprotein (Table 1) which has characteristics in common with other structural glycoproteins and fibronectin (Sear, Grant and Jackson, 1977). There is no evidence of such a glycoprotein in the periodontal ligament oxytalan fibres. Glycoproteins from basement membranes (Spiro, 1978; Rohde, Wick and Timpl, 1979) may also have to be taken into consideration.

In future work on the glycoproteins in soft dental tissues it will be essential to purify intact molecules and characterize the protein cores and the oligosaccharide units. As important is the need to locate different types of glycoproteins in situ. This should be possible using immunofluorescent methods once antibodies to purified glycoproteins are available. Attempts have been made to locate structural glycoproteins by electron-dense stains (e.g. phosphotungstate–alcian blue and ruthenium red (Shipp and

Bowness, 1975)). Because some proteoglycan occurs even in insoluble matrices, however, more specific stains are required. Only then will it be possible to study properly variations in periodontal ligament glycoproteins during tissue development (variations only tentatively suggested by the neutral sugar variations shown in Table 2).

GLYCOSAMINOGLYCANS

More is known about the glycosaminoglycans of the periodontal ligament and other soft dental tissues than about their non-collagen glycoproteins. For this reason, this section of the review deals mainly with soft dental tissues.

Glycosaminoglycans in the periodontal ligament have been investigated by autoradiographic (Baumhammers and Stallard, 1968), histochemical (Mashouf and Engel, 1975) and electron microscopic (Plecash, 1974) methods. However, there have been few attempts to isolate them from the tissue for full characterization. Munemoto *et al.* (1970) examined papain digests of bovine periodontal ligament of erupted molar teeth (without dissection) and identified hyaluronate, dermatan sulphate, chondroitin-4-sulphate and chondroitin-6-sulphate. Small amounts of heparan sulphate and undersulphated chondroitin

sulphate were also present. These glycosaminoglycans (see Table 3) have also been reported to occur in mammalian dental pulps (Linde, 1970, 1973; Embery, 1976) and gingiva (Munemoto, 1968; Kofoed and Bozzini, 1970). However, in other work chondroitin-6-sulphate was not detected in bovine, canine or human gingiva (Sakaki *et al.*, 1971; Tawa *et al.*, 1976; Sakamoto, Okamoto and Okuda, 1978; Embery, Oliver and Stanbury, 1979) or in dental pulp from human, bovine or rabbit teeth (Murakawa, 1974; Sakamoto, Okamoto and Okuda, 1979). This discrepancy is probably due to the different methods employed. Analyses based on digestion with chondroitinase AC or ABC (Saito, Yamagata and Suzuki, 1968) do not depend on the difficult separation of the polymeric chondroitin sulphates and can be applied to determine the relative amounts of chondroitin-4-sulphate (A periods) and -6-sulphate periods (C periods) when they occur in the same glycosaminoglycan chains (Rodén and Horowitz, 1978). It was with this method that most of the negative results for chondroitin-6-sulphate were obtained. Nevertheless, the absence of -6-sulphated periods from dental pulp and gingiva is surprising in view of its presence in periodontal ligament (Table 4). Functionally, the relative distribution of chondroitin-4- and -6-sulphate periods in dental tissues may be important in relation to calcification (see pp. 142–143).

TABLE 3.   *Glycosaminoglycan structures*

	Repeating disaccharide	Linkage region to protein
Hyaluronic acid	→4)GlcUA(β1→3)GlcNac(β1→	
Chondroitin sulphate	→4)GlcUA(β1→3)GalNAc4 or 6SO$_4$(β1→	→4)GlcUA(β1→3)Gal(β1→3)Gal(β1→4)Xyl→Ser
Dermatan sulphate[a]	→4)IdUA(α1→3)GalNAc4SO$_4$(β1→	as chondroitin sulphate
	→4)GlcUA(β1→3)GalNAc4 or 6SO$_4$(β1→	
Keratan sulphate (skeletal)	→4)GlcNAc6SO$_4$(β1→3)Gal[b](β1→	→4)GlcNAc6SO$_4$(β1→6)GalNAc[b]→Thr
		3
		↑
		1
		NeuAc(α1→4)Gal
Heparin and related compounds[c]	→4)IdUA(α1→4)GlcNAc(α1→	as chondroitin sulphate
including	→4)GlcUA(β1→4)GlcNSO$_3$(α1→	
	→4)GlcUA(β1→4)GlcNAc(α1→	
Heparan sulphate	→4)IdUA(α1→4)GlcNSO$_3$(α1→	

[a]Some of the L-iduronate residues are sulphated at C2 or C3 (Lindahl, 1976).
[b]An additional GalNAc residue may be present (Rodén and Horowitz, 1978).
[c]L-iduronate-2-SO$_4$ and GlcNAc-6- and -3-SO$_4$ also occur (Lindahl, 1976).

TABLE 4.   *Glycosaminoglycan contents of bovine periodontal ligament and their compositions*[a]

Glycosaminoglycan (GAG) fractions of mature ligaments of fully erupted bovine incisors were isolated by papain digestion, CPC precipitation and ethanol precipitation. Fraction weights were obtained from uronic acid analyses using previously determined conversion factors. Average values and standard deviations for μg uronate/mg hydroxyproline (Hyp), % GAG on dry weight and L-iduronate were from analyses of eight specimens of ligament or pooled ligaments, except for CPC fractions 3 and 4 (5 and 7 analyses, respectively). Dermatan sulphate contents and L-iduronate : uronate ratios were found from the results of analyses by the methods of Di Ferrante *et al.* (1971) and Bitter and Muir (1962). Determinations of hexosamines (and Hyp), ester sulphate and 4-SO_4/6-SO_4 ratios were carried out essentially as described by Pearson *et al.* (1978b), Terho and Hartiala (1971) and Saito *et al.* (1968) respectively. Molecular weights were obtained by gel chromatography on Sephadex G-200. (HA = hyaluronic acid, HS = heparan sulphate, GAG* = undersulphated GAG, CS = chondroitin sulphate, DS = dermatan sulphate, ND = not determined.)

Fraction	GAG	GAG % of dry wt	Uronate μg/mg Hyp	Iduronate μg/100 μg uronate	GlcNH$_2$ μg/mg Hyp	GalNH$_2$ μg/mg Hyp	Sulphate moles/mole GalNH$_2$	$\frac{4\text{-}SO_4}{6\text{-}SO_4}$	Mol.wt (M_r) $\times 10^{-3}$
CPC-4	HA	0.127 ± 0.013	7.1 ± 0.6	ND	5.61	0	ND	—	ND
CPC-3	HS + GAG*	—	0.61 ± 0.09	ND	0.13	0.25	ND	—	ND
CPC-2	CS periods[b]	0.26 ± 0.06	11.6 ± 3.0	0	—	—	—	—	—
	DS periods[b]	0.26 ± 0.05	10.0 ± 1.8	100[b]	—	—	—	—	—
18% EtOH	DS[b]	0.16 ± 0.02	6.8 ± 0.7	80 ± 4	0	6.5	1.1	98/2	28.8
25% EtOH	DS[b]	0.055 ± 0.004	2.2 ± 0.2	66 ± 3	ND	ND	ND	100/0	29.5
40% EtOH	CS(DS)[b]	0.11 ± 0.014	5.0 ± 0.7	14 ± 3	0	3.4	1.1	81/19	28.5
50% EtOH	(see text)	0.11 ± 0.014	5.2 ± 0.8	4 ± 3	0	3.4	0.95	52/48	18.2

[a] Adapted from Gibson (1979) and Gibson and Pearson (in press).
[b] As defined in the text.

As regards the periodontal ligament, the pioneering research of Munemoto *et al.* (1970) is open to criticism. Allowing papain to act on the ligament while still attached to the tooth does not permit the results to be related to the weight of the ligament. In addition, it may extract glycosaminoglycans from cementum. To overcome these difficulties, whole dissected specimens of mature bovine periodontal ligament were digested with papain before fractionation with cetyl pyridinium chloride (CPC) and ethanol (Table 4) (Gibson, 1979; Gibson and Pearson, in press). This approach was adopted instead of studying the compounds in NaCl-soluble and NaCl-insoluble fractions of the tissue (although such an investigation had indicated development-related variations in the glycosaminoglycans (Pearson *et al.*, 1975)). Table 4 shows that a high ratio of sulphated glycosaminoglycans (mainly galactosaminoglycans) to hyaluronate is a feature of mature bovine ligament (also see Fig. 2). A smaller difference between these fractions was reported for human ligament from subjects aged 35 years or less and in older people hyaluronate exceeded

sulphated glycosaminoglycans in amount (Paunio, 1969). Unfortunately, reliable quantitative data for dermatan sulphate and chondroitin sulphates were not obtained for the human tissue.

The total quantity of glycosaminoglycan in the bovine ligament is relatively small, less on a dry weight basis than in mammalian dental pulp (Sakamoto *et al.*, 1979) but rather similar to the amounts in bovine gingiva (Sakamoto *et al.*, 1978). However, because of the greater proportion of water in dental pulp (Sakamoto *et al.*, 1978, 1979) the concentrations of total glycosaminoglycans *in vivo* may be of the same order in these tissues. An interesting difference is that dermatan sulphate is a major component of the sulphated galactosaminoglycans of bovine ligament (Table 4 and Fig. 2) and gingiva (Sakamoto *et al.*, 1978), whereas at a comparable age it only comprises about a sixth of this fraction of the glycosaminoglycans of bovine dental pulp. It is also a minor component of rabbit dental pulp glycosaminoglycans (Sakamoto *et al.*, 1979). In contrast, dermatan sulphate is prominent in human dental pulp (Linde,

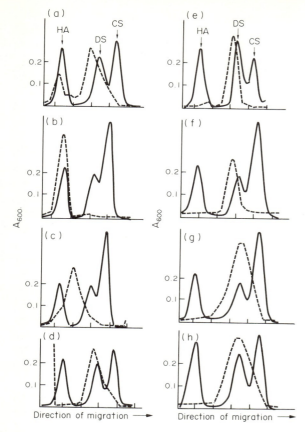

FIG. 2. Cellulose acetate electrophoresis of periodontal ligament glycosaminoglycans. Strips were scanned after staining with alcian blue. The broken lines represent the profiles of the ligament glycosaminoglycans and the solid lines show the positions of hyaluronic acid (HA), dermatan sulphate (DS) and chondroitin sulphate (CS) standards. (a) Total glycosaminoglycans, (b) CPC fraction 4, (c) CPC fraction 3, (d) CPC fraction 2 (sulphated galactosaminoglycans), (e) 18%, (f) 25%, (g) 40% and (h) 50% ethanol fractions of CPC fraction 2. For compositions of fractions see Table 4.

1973; Embery, 1976; Sakamoto *et al.,* 1979). It would be valuable to know whether there are other differences between human and bovine dental pulp (e.g. in the morphology of the collagen fibrils) which may relate to this difference in dermatan sulphate content.

Heparan sulphate occurs in only small amounts in connective tissues. Nevertheless, it may be important because of its association with cell surfaces (Lindahl and Höök, 1978). It was identified in the periodontal ligament from its infra-red spectrum (Munemoto *et al.,* 1970) and its susceptibility to degradation with nitrous acid (Gibson, 1979). It accounts for the glucosamine in CPC fraction 3 (Table 4 and see Fig. 2), whereas the galactosamine in this fraction is almost certainly a component of undersulphated galactosaminoglycans (Munemoto *et al.,* 1970; Pearson *et al.,* 1975).

It is not known whether keratan sulphate (Table 3) is present in the periodontal ligament (but it is unlikely to be a major glycosaminoglycan fraction) nor was it detected in gingiva or dental pulp (Sakamoto *et al.,* 1978, 1979). The failure to detect heparin (Table 3) in the periodontal ligament (Pearson *et al.,* 1975) is surprising as it occurs in mast cells which often surround blood vessels. Heparin was reported within rat gingiva (Kofoed and Bozzini, 1970) though not in rat dental pulp (Linde, 1973) or in the dental pulp of other mammalian species (Sakamoto *et al.,* 1979).

Hybrid sulphated galactosaminoglycans

When sulphated galactosaminoglycans of the periodontal ligament were separated from the glucosaminoglycans (hyaluronate and heparin-like molecules), repeating periods of chondroitin (-4- and -6-) sulphate and dermatan sulphate were demonstrated by infrared spectrometry, differential colorimetry and partial digestion by testicular hyaluronidase (Munemoto *et al.,* 1970; Pearson *et al.,* 1975). The latter enzyme cleaves β-hexosaminidic linkages to D-glucuronate residues as found in chondroitin sulphate, but not those formed with L-iduronate residues which typify dermatan sulphate (Table 3). Gibson (1979) obtained good agreement between quantitative estimations of dermatan sulphate from the fraction of the sulphated galactosaminoglycans that resisted testicular hyaluronidase and results obtained with the periodate–Schiff method of Di Ferrante, Donnelly and Berglund (1971). The difference between the dermatan sulphate content and the total sulphated galactosaminoglycans gave a measure of chondroitin sulphate periods. These were found in equal quantity to dermatan sulphate (Table 4). On further fractionation with ethanol in the presence of calcium acetate—

acetic acid, however, four fractions were recovered, all containing L-iduronate (Table 4) and therefore differing from chondroitin sulphate.

It was then demonstrated that L-iduronate as well as D-glucuronate was present in small oligosaccharides liberated by the action of testicular hyaluronidase on each of the ethanol fractions. This suggests that the two uronic acids were constituents of the same glycosaminoglycan chains. Support for this view was obtained from the results of a reaction with periodate followed by alkali which under controlled conditions selectively destroys L-iduronosyl bonds (Fransson, 1974). The most striking effect of this treatment was on the 40% ethanol fraction which was extensively degraded even though only a relatively small proportion of L-iduronate was present (Table 4). Thus, most (if not all) of the L-iduronate must have been a constituent of the major galactosaminoglycan chains in this fraction, rather than a part of a minor dermatan sulphate component present in admixture with chondroitin sulphate. Neither the 40% nor the 50% ethanol fraction yielded an electrophoretic band with the mobility of authentic chondroitin sulphate (Fig. 2). In the 50% ethanol fraction, the lower mobility may have been due to a small degree of undersulphation (Table 4). However, a similar fraction of ligament galactosaminoglycans isolated by Munemoto *et al.* (1970), which also had a lower mobility than chondroitin sulphate, was fully sulphated. These authors assumed that this difference was insignificant, but in view of other data (Gibson, 1979; Pearson and Gibson, 1979; Gibson and Pearson, in press) there is little justification for assuming that significant amounts of a classical chondroitin sulphate (containing no L-iduronate) occur in the periodontal ligament. In this connection, Fransson and Rodén (1967a) categorized only a small fraction of the total glycosaminoglycans in skin as authentic chondroitin sulphate. Furthermore, Toledo and Dietrich (1977) were unable to detect it in skin.

Notwithstanding the problems associated with the 50% ethanol fraction, it is clear that L-iduronate and D-glucuronate occur together in most of the periodontal ligament sulphated galactosaminoglycans. This type of molecule is described as a copolymer or hybrid.* Hybrid sulphated galactosaminoglycans are widely distributed in connective tissues (Fransson *et al.,* 1970; Lindahl, 1976). The sulphated glucos-

aminoglycan chains of heparin and heparin-like compounds (e.g. heparan sulphate) also contain both types of uronic acid (Lindahl, 1976; Rodén and Horowitz, 1978).

Hybrid sulphated galactosaminoglycans may be divided into two groups: (1) hybrids in which L-iduronate predominates .over D-glucuronate and (2) hybrids containing more D-glucuronate than L-iduronate. Dermatan sulphate (previously known as chondroitin sulphate B) is the archetype of group 1. However, some authors refer to hybrids of both classes as dermatan sulphates (e.g. Rodén and Horowitz, 1978). In what follows, group 1 hybrids (e.g. the 18% and 25% ethanol fractions isolated from the ligament) will be referred to as dermatan sulphates and those from group 2 (e.g. the 40% and 50% ethanol fractions) will be called CS(DS) hybrids in accordance with work on aortic glycosaminoglycans (Buddecke and von Figura, 1975). A homopolymeric dermatan sulphate does not seem to have been isolated, although fractions in which L-iduronate account for as much as 98% of the total uronate content have been reported (Stuhlsatz and Greiling, 1976). Also, it is not clear whether CS(DS) hybrids with low L-iduronate differ significantly in their properties *in vivo* from chondroitin sulphate. The biosynthesis of these two types of chains, however, must diverge (see pages 137–139) and it is likely that this is controlled by intracellular compartmentalization or by cells differing in degree of differentiation.

Sulphate distribution

Table 4 shows that little or no -6-sulphate was present in the dermatan sulphate fractions of periodontal ligament. The major repeating disaccharide in these fractions was L-iduronosyl-*N*-acetyl-galactosamine-4-sulphate, with a smaller proportion of D-glucuronosyl-*N*-acetyl-galactosamine-4-sulphate. Some of the L-iduronate residues may also be sulphated at carbon 2 or 3 (Lindahl, 1976). On the other hand, and in contrast with the other soft dental tissues (see page

---

*These terms are also used to indicate the occurrence of -4-sulphate and -6-sulphate in the same glycosaminoglycan chain. In the present article they refer to uronic acid composition.

125), the 40% and 50% fractions contained both -6- and -4-sulphated *N*-acetyl-galactosamine residues. Because of the low L-iduronate contents, it follows that most of these residues were linked to D-glucuronate, which is unlikely to be sulphated (Lindahl, 1976). It will be of interest to know whether in aging of the bovine tissue the proportion of galactosamine-6-sulphate increases and, more importantly, whether it occurs at all in human periodontal ligament.

Molecular sizes of the sulphated galactosaminoglycans

The molecular weights of sulphated galactosaminoglycans of bovine periodontal ligament have been studied by Gibson (1979), Pearson and Gibson (1979) and Gibson and Pearson (in press). A good agreement was found between results obtained for ethanol fractions of the galactosaminoglycans isolated from papain digests of the ligament (Table 4) and those found for fractions cleaved from purified proteoglycans of the ligament. It is difficult to compare the molecular weight of ligament dermatan sulphate (about 29,000) with that of the most widely studied dermatan sulphate (from pigskin) where values vary from about 17,000 to 27,000 (Tanford *et al.*, 1964; Fransson and Rodén, 1967 a, b; Öbrink, 1973; Gregory and Damle, 1979). Recently, a value of 17,500 was obtained for M_n of an 18% ethanol fraction of pigskin dermatan sulphate by end-group analysis and it was shown that it could undergo self-association, yielding dimers and even super aggregates (Fransson *et al.*, 1979). However, although the self-association may occur in gel chromatography, it was concluded that this could not have been an important factor in the work on the ligament dermatan sulphate (Gibson and Pearson, in press).

A more clear-cut comparison can be made between the molecular sizes of the predominant chains of the dermatan sulphate of ligament and bovine skin. The most prominent fraction of the skin dermatan sulphate (cleaved from a purified proteoglycan) was a 25% ethanol fraction which had a molecular weight of 16,000–17,000 (Gibson and Pearson, in press). The lower molecular weight of the bovine skin dermatan

sulphate is significant in relation to the relative molecular sizes of the parent proteoglycans (see pages 130–131).

The similarity in size of the ligament dermatan sulphates and the CS(DS) hybrids in the 40% ethanol fraction is consistent with a common synthetic pathway (see pages 137–139) whereas the much lower M_r (about 18,000) of the 50% ethanol fraction may indicate a different origin. The latter value, and the only slightly higher result of 20,000 obtained for the corresponding fraction of a purified ligament proteoglycan (PGl) (see page 133), were close to the average molecular weight of bovine nasal cartilage chondroitin sulphate determined by the same methods (Gibson and Pearson, in press). However, the 50% ethanol fraction contained sulphated galactosaminoglycan chains of much higher molecular weight than M_r and a precursor common to all the ethanol fractions is not ruled out.

PROTEOGLYCANS

Cartilage proteoglycans and aggregates have received more attention than any other kind of proteoglycan, partly because they occur in large amounts and their functional importance is undeniable and partly because they are less difficult to study than in many other tissues. Since this proteoglycan is not of particular relevance to the periodontal ligament, only the most important features are outlined here. For fuller details the reader is referred to Muir and Hardingham (1975), Hascall (1977) and Rosenberg *et al.* (1979).

Table 3 shows the sugars involved in linking the numerous chondroitin sulphate chains to serine or threonine residues in the protein core of cartilage proteoglycan 'subunits'. Distribution of the glycosaminoglycans along the protein core is uneven (Fig. 3) and one end of the core carries few polysaccharide chains and is free to associate noncovalently with hyaluronic acid. Thus, huge aggregates are formed from the polydisperse subunits (molecular weights $1-4 \times 10^6$) and stabilization occurs through interactions with 'link glycoproteins' (Fig. 3 and Table 1). These aggregates are probably essential for the functions of cartilaginous tissues but there is little evidence that they are important in more fibrous tissues.

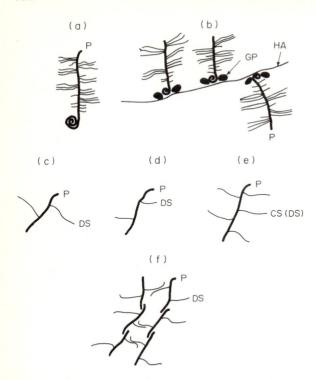

FIG. 3. Current models of proteoglycan subunits and aggregates. (a) Cartilage proteoglycan subunit. The longer chains represent chondroitin sulphate arranged in clusters along a protein core, P (probable molecular weight about 200,000) and the smaller side chains represent keratan sulphate. (b) An aggregate containing cartilage proteoglycan subunits, hyaluronate (HA) and link glycoprotein (GP). (c) and (d) Subunits of bovine periodontal ligament and skin proteodermatan sulphates respectively (Pearson and Gibson, 1979). Actual positions of the two or three dermatan sulphate (DS) chains on the protein core (P) are not known. (e) Scleral proteoglycan (I) containing CS(DS) hybrids (Cöster, 1979). (f) Possible structures assembled by self-association of proteodermatan sulphates in periodontal ligament or skin. Interactions may involve both the protein core (P) and the DS chains.

Much less is known about proteoglycans in non-cartilaginous tissues. From the periodontal ligament, two different proteoglycans have been isolated (Gibson, 1979; Pearson and Gibson, 1979, in press): a proteodermatan sulphate and a proteoglycan containing CS(DS) hybrids.

Proteodermatan sulphates

The most characteristic proteoglycan in non-cartila-

ginous connective tissues is proteodermatan sulphate, but it has been little studied at the macromolecular level. When bovine periodontal ligaments were extracted with 0.1 M NaCl (pH 7.6) containing several proteinase inhibitors (Pearson et al., 1978a; Pearson and Gibson, 1979), relatively little proteodermatan sulphate was removed but a different proteoglycan was isolated (see page 133). However, extractions of the NaCl-insoluble residue with 4 M guanidinium chloride gave a good yield of proteodermatan sulphate. The proteoglycan contained approximately equal amounts of dermatan sulphate and protein whereas bovine skin proteodermatan sulphate purified by the same methods (Pearson and Gibson, 1979, in press) contained about 60% protein. This confirms the results of Toole and Lowther (1968) who used more drastic extraction conditions (6 M urea at 60°).

The amino acid compositions of the ligament and bovine skin proteoglycans are almost identical (Table 5) and similar to that of bovine tendon (Table 5), pigskin (Gregory and Damle, 1979) and bovine sclera (Cöster, 1979) proteoglycans. Whilst the protein cores of proteodermatan sulphates are similar in bovine tissues at least, it remains to be seen whether there are larger variations in other species. The amino acid composition differs completely from that of cartilage proteoglycans and from proteoglycans isolated from aorta (Table 5). Because of purification problems, and the wide range of compounds found in the aorta, this comparison is less certain at present. Considering the role played by serine and threonine in the attachment of glycosaminoglycans to the protein core of proteoglycans, the relatively low values of these hydroxyamino acids in proteodermatan sulphate is of significance. However, other differences (such as the higher lysine, histidine, leucine and isoleucine) may greatly affect the properties of the core protein. A much larger amount of half-cystine is also present in proteodermatan sulphate, but the number of disulphide bonds is unknown.

The purified ligament and skin proteoglycans were essentially homogeneous in gel chromatography, or when stained for protein and glycosaminoglycan following electrophoresis in composite gels adapted to give high resolution for this type of molecule (Pearson et al., 1978a and see Fig. 4). In equilibrium sedimentation (particularly at low speeds) heterogeneity was observed, but possibly this arose from

TABLE 5.   *Amino acid compositions of proteoglycans of periodontal ligament and other tissues*
DSPG = Dermatan sulphate proteoglycans
PGl = NaCl − extracted proteoglycan

	Residues/1000 amino acid residues						
	Ligament[a] DSPG	Skin[a] DSPG	Tendon[b] DSPG	Ligament[a] PGl	Pigskin[c]	Cartilage[d]	Aorta[e]
Asp	125	126	110	74	57	77	103
Thr	39	39	43	59	51	58	86
Ser	74	68	79	168	136	123	90
Glu	108	108	104	174	150	145	140
Pro	67	69	87	51	97	92	93
Gly	80	81	89	135	151	136	67
Ala	49	49	53	72	58	77	61
Val	58	59	58	45	78	69	56
Met	9	9	10	4	f	9	11
Ile	57	60	54	28	35	38	40
Leu	123	122	119	43	86	78	88
Tyr	29	29	22	16	9	16	19
Phe	33	33	28	24	34	27	35
Lys	75	80	86	67	32	16	47
His	27	27	29	23	10	8	24
Arg	31	28	29	17	16	41	33
Cys	16	13	f	f	f	6	7

[a]Pearson and Gibson (in press). [b]Anderson (1975). [c]Damle *et al.* (1979). [d]Hardingham *et al.* (1976). [e]Oegema *et al.* (1979). [f]Not determined.

changes during ultracentrifugation. The whole cell averages at low speeds and at 8° were 1.2×10^5 for the skin proteodermatan sulphate and about 1.3×10^5 for the ligament proteoglycan. Mobilities in gel chromatography and gel electrophoresis both indicated that the ligament proteoglycan was somewhat larger than that of bovine skin (Pearson and Gibson, in press). However, it is clear that not more than an average of three dermatan sulphate chains are present in either proteoglycan and the earlier estimate of two chains per molecule (Pearson and Gibson, 1979) could be correct.

It has been postulated that the proteodermatan sulphates of pigskin (Gregory and Damle, 1979) and bovine sclera (Cöster, 1979) − both of which had protein contents of close to 60% − contained only two dermatan sulphate chains per molecule. (The great difference from a cartilage proteoglycan is illustrated in Fig. 3.) Further work is required before the sizes of the protein cores of these proteodermatan sulphates can be compared. In view of the very similar amino acid compositions, it seems unlikely that the

protein cores differ as much in size as present estimates suggest (viz. $6-7 \times 10^4$ for bovine periodontal ligament and skin proteoglycan cores, 1×10^5 for pigskin and 4.6×10^4 for sclera). In the case of the ligament and bovine skin proteoglycans at least (examined using the same methods), the small difference in size of the whole molecules is most likely due to the different lengths of the dermatan sulphate chains (page 129).

Oligosaccharides containing neutral sugars and hexosamine are attached to the protein cores of pigskin (Gregory and Damle, 1979) and sclera (Cöster, 1979) proteoglycans. The oligosaccharides of the pigskin proteoglycan also contain sialic acid. Similar oligosaccharides probably occur in periodontal ligament and bovine skin proteoglycans, accounting for the small amounts (1−2%) of glucosamine present. Thus, the protein core of a proteodermatan sulphate is one more type of glycoprotein to add to the growing list of these compounds in connective tissues.

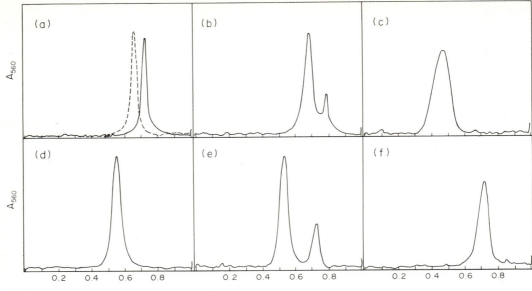

FIG. 4. Gel electrophoresis of proteodermatan sulphates: self-association of the proteoglycan. Electrophoresis in agarose-polyacrylamide gels, staining with coomassie blue, destaining and scanning were as described by Pearson *et al.* (1978a). (a) Purified proteodermatan sulphate of bovine skin (full line) and of periodontal ligament (broken line). These samples were not incubated at 37° before electrophoresis. (b–f) Before electrophoresis purified bovine skin proteodermatan sulphate (4 mg/ml) was treated as follows: (b) Incubated for 24 hours at 37° in 0.05 M tris-HCl − 0.02% sodium azide, pH 7.2 under chloroform vapour. (c) Incubated as in (b), but the buffer contained 10 mM PMSF. (d) Incubated as in (c), but in the presence of bacterial collagenase 40 units and 5 mM CaCl$_2$. (e) Pre-heated at 80° for 15 minutes and then incubated as in (b) (no PMSF). (f) Incubated as in (c), then urea was added to give a concentration of 6 M. The solution was allowed to stand for 4 hours at room temperature before gel electrophoresis. The small peak in (b) is a degradation of the proteoglycan which is usually more easily detected with toluidine blue staining. Peaks with relative mobilities of less than 0.6 (compared with the marker dye) are aggregated species.

Self-association of proteodermatan sulphates

Purified proteodermatan sulphates of pigskin (Gregory and Damle, 1979) or of sclera (Cöster, 1979) did not form aggregates with hyaluronate. The possibility that a modification of the proteoglycan molecule during isolation was responsible is difficult to exclude, but a significant association with hyaluronate *in vivo* seems unlikely. Experiments similar to those carried out with pigskin or scleral proteoglycans and hyaluronate have not been performed with periodontal ligament or bovine skin proteoglycans. However, although hyaluronate was not detected in purified bovine proteodermatan sulphates (Pearson and Gibson, in press), an aggregation phenomenon has been observed, first at pH values of 6 or less (Pearson *et al.*, 1978a) and later at physiological pH values. This

effect, which occurs with both periodontal ligament and bovine skin proteoglycans, has been examined mainly by gel electrophoresis (Fig. 4). Equilibrium sedimentation confirmed that aggregation rather than a change in conformation was occurring: species of apparent molecular weights of up to about 600,000 were observed (Pearson and Aarbo, unpublished work). However, there was no indication at physiological pH of the super-aggregates of apparent molecular weights of 3×10^6 (Obrink, 1972) and as high as 39×10^6 (Cöster, 1979), which have been reported in light scattering experiments.

The phenomenon appears to be one of self-association. Although dermatan sulphate chains themselves can self-associate (Fransson, 1976; Fransson *et al.*, 1979), it is possible that the protein core of the proteoglycan is involved also. Self-association is encouraged by incubation at 37°C but also seems to occur at lower temperatures. With long periods at 37°C, problems arise because a limited proteolysis occurs which significantly reduces or prevents self-association. Increased precautions to avoid bacterial contamination only partly solves the problem. The unlikely complication of a tissue proteinase not only surviving the denaturing solutions (4 M guanidine hydrochloride and 7 M urea) used in the isolation of the proteoglycan, but remaining with the latter throughout the purification, has to be considered (Gibson, 1979). From Fig. 4 it can be seen that a prior heating of the proteoglycan to 80° allowed self-association at 37°C, presumably because endogenous proteinase activity was destroyed. The presence of phenylmethanesulphonyl fluoride (PMSF) (1–10 mM) in the incubating buffer inhibited the enzyme activity, whereas EDTA or iodoacetate did not (Pearson and Davies, unpublished work). This suggests that the enzyme is a serine proteinase rather than metal or thiol-dependent.

Conclusions from the other experiments shown in Fig. 4 (and other data) may be summarized as follows. The aggregation is not dependent on the presence of small amounts of collagen that may have contaminated the preparations, even though hydroxyproline was not detected in highly purified preparations which were able to aggregate. Hydrophobic interactions (presumably involving the protein core) are probably important in the self-association, judging by the temperature dependence and the reversion of the association by 6 M urea. The aggregate is not stabilized by electrostatic interactions because 2 M NaCl does not cause dissociation. Reduction and alkylation of the proteoglycan did not prevent self-association, a significant difference from results obtained in the aggregation of cartilage proteoglycans with hyaluronate (Hardingham, Ewins and Muir, 1976) and also in the self-association of proteoglycans containing CS(DS) hybrids (Cöster, 1979, and see below).

Whether the self-association leads only to a moderate increase in size as we have observed, or to a marked one as found under some conditions in the work on pigskin and scleral proteodermatan sulphates, the effect could be important *in vivo*. For example, aggregation may occur at cell surfaces as well as in the matrix. It could also lead to the formation of a three-dimensional network (Fig. 3), or be responsible for end-to-end aggregation, giving orthogonal arrays of proteoglycan (probably proteodermatan sulphate) as observed on the surfaces of tendon collagen fibrils (Scott, 1980).

Proteoglycans containing CS(DS) hybrids

The major proteoglycan extracted with 0.1 M NaCl from bovine periodontal ligaments (PGl) was more heterogeneous than proteodermatan sulphate, of larger average molecular size, and of different composition (Pearson and Gibson, in press). The sulphated galactosaminoglycan component contained a small amount of L-iduronate (corresponding to about 7% of dermatan sulphate periods). Cellulose acetate electrophoresis of sulphated galactosaminoglycans present in the highest molecular fraction of the proteoglycan revealed only one broad band with a mobility similar to the CS(DS) hybrids isolated from the whole ligament (page 128 and Fig. 2). A fully sulphated, authentic chondroitin sulphate was not detected. The 40% and 50% ethanol subfractions isolated after alkaline cleavage of PGl, in the presence of tritiated borohydride, had molecular weights of 32,000 and 20,000 respectively (compare with Table 4). Undersulphated galactosaminoglycans and a smaller amount of heparan sulphate were also detected in PGl, but the latter GAG could be part of a distinct proteoglycan and further purification may also eliminate the hyaluronate that was present.

After purification by gel chromatography in 4 M guanidinium chloride, PGl contained about 20% protein. This is much less than in proteodermatan sulphates, but significantly more than has been found in purified cartilage proteoglycans (5–10%) or in a recently isolated D-glucuronate-rich proteoglycan of pigskin (about 5% protein, Damle *et al.,* 1979). Table 5 shows that there was some resemblance to the last two proteoglycans in terms of amino acid composition, but the differences were significant. There were even larger differences between the amino compositions of PGl and aortic proteoglycans, an example of which is included in Table 5. However, these proteoglycans resemble PGl both in protein content (16–20%, Oegema, Hascall and Eisenstein, 1979; McMurtrey *et al.,* 1979) and in the glycosaminoglycan components, which are CS(DS) hybrids containing 5–10% of DS periods (Oegema *et al.,* 1979; Radhakrishnamurthy *et al.,* 1977). Another proteoglycan containing CS(DS) hybrids (about 20% DS periods) was recently isolated from bovine sclera (Cöster, 1979). Its protein content of 45% was not much less than that of proteodermatan sulphates but it had a higher molecular weight (about 200,000) and different properties as well as a different amino acid composition.

Present data give little support to the idea that a core protein exists which is common to proteoglycans containing CS(DS) hybrids in different tissues and the relationship (if any) to the core proteins of proteodermatan sulphates or cartilage proteoglycans is obscure.

One might not expect a variety of protein cores if the prime function is to anchor the glycosaminoglycan chains. The separate role played by the polysaccharide-free region of the protein core of cartilage proteoglycans in binding to hyaluronate (Rosenberg *et al.,* 1979 and see Fig. 3) is an indicator of other possibilities. Protein cores of proteodermatan sulphates seem to lack the requisite features for this binding. However, they possess characteristics promoting self-association, which will also be more likely because the smaller number of attached anionic polysaccharide chains will cause less electrostatic repulsion than between cartilage proteoglycan molecules. It is conceivable that the protein core of a proteodermatan sulphate is adapted for self-association (and interaction with collagen (Scott, 1980)) rather than to allow the formation of larger aggregates with hyaluronate (this might be inappropriate to the functioning of the more fibrous connective tissues). Nevertheless, self-association is probably not restricted to proteodermatan sulphates. A similar phenomenon is seen with the scleral proteoglycan containing CS(DS) hybrids (Cöster, 1979) and cartilage proteoglycans (Sheehan *et al.,* 1978; Reihanian *et al.,* 1979; Serafini-Fracassini and Hinnie, 1979). However, Kitchen and Cleland (1978) concluded that impurities in cartilage proteoglycans were responsible for the aggregation.

There is little doubt that the various aggregates will differ in stability and importance *in vivo.* It can be assumed that self-association of proteodermatan sulphates is significant in tissues — even fragments of this proteoglycan produced by digestion with cathepsin D undergo aggregation (Pearson *et al.,* 1978a). This might explain why no glycosaminoglycan is *released* from the insoluble matrix of dermis by this enzyme (Pearson and Davies, unpublished work), although degradation almost certainly occurs. Conflicting data on the conditions that prevent or destroy self-association of proteoglycans have been reported. Sheehan *et al.* (1978) observed that self-association of cartilage proteoglycans was sensitive to small changes in salt concentration, whereas Serafini-Fracassini and Hinnie (1979) concluded that oligomeric species were stable even in 4 M guanidinium chloride. Obviously, such data are important not only for understanding function but also for assessing the true molecular weight of a proteoglycan subunit.

More optimistically, investigations of aggregation and self-association *in vitro* should help to elucidate the nature and formation of the granules and filaments observed ultrastructurally in ground substance (Hascall, 1980). Electron micrographs from one of the few studies of the periodontal ligament (Plecash, 1974) are shown in Fig. 5. Most of the ruthenium red-stained fine filaments and matrix granules were removed by extraction with saline before fixation. These structures therefore could consist of ligament PGI and/or hyaluronate, both of which can be extracted easily with 0.1 M NaCl (see page 133). However, the ruthenium red-stained material in close contact with collagen fibrils resisted extraction with saline. It is therefore more likely to be proteodermatan sulphate. The collagen-associated material was also largely resistant to testicular hyaluronidase (Fig. 5), whereas dermatan sulphate chains isolated from the ligament were degraded (Gibson and Pearson, in press). The effect on the dermatan sulphate attached to the protein core will depend on the positions of the D-glucuronate and L-iduronate residues. If a large block of periods rich in L-iduronate extended from the protein linkage region, much of the ruthenium red-staining would be retained after hyaluronidase digestion. This situation is unlikely, however, considering available hexuronate sequence data, especially on pigskin dermatan sulphate (reviewed by Lindahl, 1976 and Rodén and Horowitz, 1978). The efficiency of hyaluronidase digestion of protein-bound dermatan

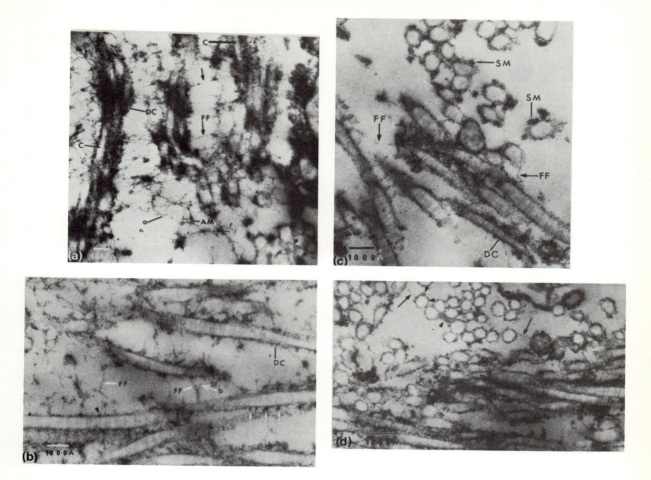

FIG. 5. Ultrastructure of periodontal ligament visualized with ruthenium red. Specimens of gingival periodontal ligament, from an area close to the cementum surface, were fixed in glutaraldehyde and osmium tetroxide solutions, both of which contained ruthenium red. Collagen fibres (c) were negatively stained. Ruthenium red-stained elements in the interfibrillary spaces consisted of fine filaments (FF) and granules. Some of the latter occurred at points of union of the fine filaments, as indicated (AM in specimen a). Ruthenium red-stained material also occurred as dense coats (DC) and spherical masses (SM) in close contact with the collagen fibrils and was particularly obvious when the fibrils were transverse sectioned (as in specimens c and d). (a) and (b), No pretreatment before fixation. (c) Preincubated in normal saline, 1 hour, 37°. (d) Preincubated with testicular hyaluronidase (Worthington, 1500 units/ml) in normal saline, 1 hour, 37°.

sulphate in tissue sections may be less than when the enzyme is acting on free chains, but alternative explanations for the results are possible. The hyaluronidase-resistant material observed in Fig. 5 may represent the glycoprotein core of proteodermatan sulphate containing sialic acid residues (see page 131) or it could be a distinct acidic structural glycoprotein (see pages 120–122). Shipp and Bowness (1975) reported that the latter type of glycoprotein stains with ruthenium red, although the presence of associated

proteoglycan complicated the interpretation. The specificity of ruthenium red staining is questionable and more specific, immunofluorescence techniques are required (Eisenstein and Kuettner, 1976).

Whether distinct proteoglycans containing chondroitin sulphate chains occur in the periodontal ligament (see page 128) or other collagen-rich tissues is questionable, although they have been claimed to occur in skin (Damle *et al.,* 1979) and aorta (Radhakrishnamurthy *et al.,* 1977). Improved methods are needed for distinguishing chondroitin sulphate from CS(DS) hybrids containing very small proportions of DS periods.

Quantitative variations of proteoglycans within the periodontal tissues during tooth eruption

Determinations have been made of hyaluronate, the different ethanol fractions of the sulphated galactosaminoglycans, and the quantities of collagen in the periodontal ligament of bovine incisors at various stages of tooth eruption (Gibson, 1979). Data obtained on the isolated proteoglycans show that the 18% + 25% ethanol fractions and the 40% + 50% ethanol fractions were representative of the trends in the contents of proteodermatan sulphate and PGl respectively. These results, and the hyaluronate values, are shown in Fig. 6. Group 1 specimens consisted of dental follicle. A recognizable periodontal ligament had developed in Group 2 specimens. Sharpey's fibres were discerned in Group 3 onwards. Average root length increased from Groups 2 to 4, but no significant lengthening was observed in Groups 5 or 6.

The typical obliquely oriented collagen fibres were first observed in Group 5 specimens (at which stage the tooth had just erupted into the oral cavity) and such fibres were predominant in Group 6 specimens from fully erupted teeth.

Hydroxyproline determinations showed that the collagen content increased greatly betweeen Group 1 and Group 2 and more gradually (but regularly) thereafter. Distinctive trends in the individual glycosaminoglycans were apparent whether the results were expressed on the dry weight or relative to the collagen contents. The marked decrease in hyaluronate from Group 1 to Group 2 is similar to that which occurs during embryonic development of other connective tissues, e.g. skin (Kawamoto and Nagai, 1976). This may be responsible for the decrease in water content and cell-free spaces during differentiation (Fisher and Solursh, 1977). The fall in hyaluronate, probably resulting from hyaluronidase activity, coincides with the onset of cytodifferentiation (Toole, 1979). Exogenous hyaluronate inhibited the synthesis of sulphated glycosaminoglycans by chondrocytes (Solursh *et al.,* 1980), but not by skin fibroblasts (Wiebkin and Muir, 1973). In bovine periodontal ligament, both types of sulphated galactosaminoglycan chains increased slightly on a dry basis

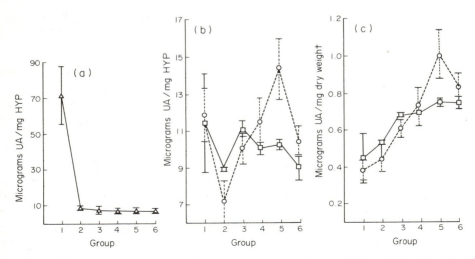

FIG. 6. Glycosaminoglycans in the developing periodontal ligament. Unerupted and erupted bovine incisors were divided into six groups according to size, wet weight, root formation, position in the jaw and attrition. Follicle (group 1) and ligaments were dissected for histological examination and for isolation of glycosaminoglycan fractions and determinations of hexuronate (UA) and hydroxyproline (Hyp) as in Table 4. Results are shown for (a) hyaluronate, (b) and (c) 18% + 25% ethanol fractions (□—□) and 40% + 50% ethanol fractions (○- -○).

between Groups 1 and 2 and more markedly between Groups 2 and 3. Subsequently, dermatan sulphate (and presumably proteodermatan sulphate) showed little change on a dry weight basis and decreased to some extent relative to collagen content. On the other hand, the sulphated galactosaminoglycans associated with PGl continued to increase over the whole period of eruption, only falling in the final stage (Group 6). This increase was most noticeable when expressed relative to the collagen content.

These results raise questions about the role of the proteoglycans in the mechanism of tooth eruption. If proteoglycan is involved, it seems more likely to be PGl than proteodermatan sulphate, not only because of the quantitative changes, but also on account of the probable locations of the proteoglycans in the tissues. An interfibrillar location of PGl would allow a fuller expression of its ability to influence the osmotic pressure and swelling of the tissue compared with proteodermatan sulphate which is more intimately associated with collagen fibrils. The latter association might partly 'tie up' the dermatan sulphate chains and reduce their effect on tissue swelling similar to that observed when glycosaminoglycans in umbilical cord or cornea were allowed to interact with polycations (Gelman and Silberberg, 1976; Comper and Laurent, 1978). Hyaluronate, like PGl, will be less affected by interactions with collagen. However, the content of this glycosaminoglycan was almost constant during eruption (Fig. 6).

Thus, PGl may have a controlling influence on the internal osmotic pressure of bovine periodontal ligament during tooth eruption. Because of the non-ideal behaviour of glycosaminoglycans and proteoglycans, the effects of small changes in concentration on osmotic pressure are amplified (Comper and Laurent, 1978; Urban *et al.*, 1979). An increase in osmotic pressure arising from an increasing concentration of PGl may be opposed by an osmotic pull on the interstitial water by the plasma proteins over the capillary wall and the physical swelling of the tissue will be opposed by the 'elastic contribution' of the collagen fibres (Comper and Laurent, 1978). However, the increase in collagen content from the stages represented by Groups 2 to 5 (or 6) was relatively small (from 40% to 50–55% on the dry weight) and its effects could be mitigated by the extensive remodelling during this period. The evidence

from physiological experiments that periodontal tissue hydrostatic pressure is implicated in the eruptive mechanism is reviewed in Chapter 10). However, caution must be taken in propounding views about a direct role of such pressures in eruption. For example, an increasing osmotic pressure might have important influences on the morphology and behaviour of the fibroblasts, as suggested for chondrocytes by Ogston (1970).

Some changes in proteoglycans with development have also been shown in pulp and gingiva. Sakamoto *et al.* (1979) found species differences in the quantitative changes observed in dental pulp glycosaminoglycans. Chondroitin sulphate increased in the pulp of bovine first molars during eruption and decreased sharply after the root apex was completed. No increase was observed, however, in the pulp of rabbit first premolars or incisors. The increase in the bovine pulp was relatively small compared with the ligament (Fig. 6) and, unfortunately, grading was mainly according to animal age rather than to defined stages of eruption. In a similar study, both chondroitin sulphate and dermatan sulphate (and to a less extent hyaluronate) were found to decrease with age in bovine gingiva (Sakamoto *et al.*, 1978).

THE BIOSYNTHESIS OF GLYCOSAMINO-GLYCANS AND PROTEOGLYCANS

The mechanism of hyaluronate biosynthesis is essentially unknown. However, knowledge of the monosaccharides present in the protein linkage region of sulphated galactosaminoglycans (Table 3) has led to advances in our understanding of the biosynthesis of these polysaccharides (Rodén and Horowitz, 1978). Chain initiation requires the transfer of xylose from UDP-xylose to a serine residue in the protein core or other acceptor. It is possible that one xylosyltransferase may be able to initiate the synthesis of a variety of sulphated galactosaminoglycans. The intracellular location and the timing of xylosylation in relation to the synthesis of core protein is unknown.

Xylosylation is followed by the sequential addition of monosaccharides from their UDP compounds. First, through the action of two galactosyltransferases and a glucuronosyltransferase the construction of the carbohydrate—protein linkage region (Table 3) is completed. This glucuronosyltransferase (I) is different from the enzyme (glucuronosyltransferase (II)) utilized in the addition of a D-glucuronate during the formation of the repeating disaccharide units (see below), showing that the D-glucuronate residue nearest to the (potential) reducing end of the chain must be regarded as part of the carbohydrate-protein linkage segment of the glycosaminoglycan.

The next step is probably the transfer of N-acetylgalactosamine to the linkage region, catalysed by a transferase of low specificity. Subsequently, the actions of the latter enzyme and of the second glucuronosyltransferase (II) complete the main body of the galactosaminoglycan chain, which also becomes sulphated. The synchronization of chain elongation and sulphation is not fully understood, but the action of a sulphotransferase (which is specific for the -4- position of N-acetylgalactosamine) probably lags behind chain elongation. On the other hand, glucuronosyltransferase II can act on the nonreducing terminal N-acetyl-galactosamine residues of chondroitin-6-sulphate oligosaccharides as well as on those of unsulphated oligosaccharides, indicating more latitude in the timing of -6-sulphation.

A definite chain termination mechanism has not been discovered, although -4-sulphation of N-acetyl-galactosamine is a possibility (Di Ferrante, 1976). It has been suggested also that lack of intracellular control over chain length explains the polydispersity of purified sulphated glycosaminoglycans. If so, the low degree of molecular dispersion shown by dermatan sulphates isolated from purified proteodermatan sulphate (Gibson and Pearson, in press) would suggest a new aspect of this question. In other ways, the biosynthesis is more tightly controlled (possibly by compartmentalization) than the specificities of some of the transferases suggest. For example, although chondrocytes synthesize hyaluronate as well as chondroitin sulphate, hybrids of these glycosamino-glycans are not formed.

The use of β-xylosides as exogenous chain initiators has been valuable in studying the biosynthesis of glycosaminoglycans and proteoglycans. With this, it is possible to divorce the polysaccharide synthesis from that of the protein core (Handley and Lowther, 1976; Schwartz, 1977). It seems that the synthesis of the core protein is independently controlled, but the requirement for core protein in the glycosamino-glycan chain initiation step has diverse effects which bring in the possibility of more than one kind of feed-back control of glycosaminoglycan synthesis (Rodén and Horowitz, 1978). Some ambiguities remain to be resolved. For instance, hyaluronate did not affect glycosaminoglycan biosynthesis in the presence of benzyl-β-D-xyloside, but a depression of proteoglycan synthesis occurred which could have been caused by inhibition of either protein core synthesis or the activity of xylosyltransferase (Handley and Lowther, 1976). Since general protein synthesis was unaffected, the second alternative is more likely. In any event, the xylosyl transfer step is of importance in the whole process.

With respect to the hybrid galactosaminoglycans, it is now evident that the biosynthesis of sulphated galactosaminoglycans containing L-iduronate occurs via the production of chondroitin sulphate — i.e. L-iduronate is not incorporated directly into a growing polysaccharide chain and UDP-L-iduronate is not required. Instead, C-5 inversion of D-glucuronate occurs at the polymer level (Malmström et al., 1975a) as for heparin and heparan sulphate (Lindahl, 1976; Rodén and Horowitz, 1978). In the biosynthesis of heparin, the coupling of C-5 inversion to sulphation of an adjacent hexosamine residue is absolute. Although this is not true for dermatan sulphate, 4-sulphation considerably promotes or stabilizes the epimerization, which may occur both internally and at the non-reducing end of the chain (Malmström et al., 1975a). The conversion of D-glucuronate to L-iduronate residues is catalysed by an epimerase. This enzyme has been demonstrated in a particulate, subcellular fraction of cultured fibroblasts (Malmström et al., 1975a). The epimerase has not been isolated, but a similar enzyme involved in heparin biosynthesis has been purified (Malmström et al., 1980).

It is possible that reversion of L-iduronate residues to D-glucuronate occurs. This was proposed to explain (i) the different hexuronate compositions of dermatan sulphates found in the medium and those remaining with the cells in fibroblast cultures (Fransson et al., 1973; Malmström et al., 1975b) and (ii) the apparent transformation of exogenous dermatan sulphate that occurred when it was incubated with the fibroblasts

(Fransson *et al.*, 1973). Little further work has been reported on this transformation, which was presumed to be mediated by a 'reverse epimerase'. Such an enzyme has not been isolated, but the idea of reverse epimerization is still promulgated (Cöster, 1979).

For further general information on biosynthesis, see reviews by Rodén and Schwartz (1975), Di Ferrante (1976), Rodén and Horowitz (1978) and Silbert (1978).

THE CATABOLISM OF GLYCOSAMINO-GLYCANS AND PROTEOGLYCANS

Less is known about the catabolic route of proteoglycans than the biosynthesis. Furthermore, more variability between tissues is likely, especially since at least part of the process is extracellular. Thus, in cartilage for example the disruption of the hyaluronate—proteoglycan aggregates is believed by some to be mediated by cartilage lysozyme (Kuettner *et al.*, 1974; Kuettner, Eisenstein and Sorgente, 1975; Howell and Pita, 1976) and by others to be part of a general process of degradation through proteolysis. Greenwald (1976) has claimed that at physiological concentrations lysozyme has no significant effect on either hyaluronate or aggregated proteoglycans. On the other hand, cartilage proteoglycans isolated from organ cultures undergo limited proteolysis which reduces their ability to aggregate with hyaluronate (Sandy, Brown and Lowther, 1978). However, the identity and cellular origin of the proteinases involved is uncertain. Though it is difficult to detect 'neutral' proteinase activity (significant at physiological pH values) in normal connective tissues, such proteinases have been isolated from skin (Hopsu-Havu, Fräki and Järvinen, 1977) and cartilage (Sapolsky *et al.*, 1976; Nagase and Woessner, 1977; Schwermann *et al.*, 1979). Significant neutral proteoglycanase activity is produced in cultures of various connective tissue cells (Barrett, 1975; Werb and Dingle, 1977; Sellers, Reynolds and Meikle, 1978; Malemud *et al.*, 1979), but much of it may be naturally inhibited or latent (Vaes *et al.*, 1978; Sellers *et al.*, 1978).

The lysosomal proteinase cathepsin D is able *in vitro* to degrade cartilage proteoglycans (Roughley, 1977; Roughley and Barrett, 1977), skin proteo-

dermatan sulphate (Pearson *et al.*, 1978a) and the two types of proteoglycan isolated from periodontal ligament (Gibson, 1979). Cathepsin D appears to be secreted by at least some connective tissue cells (Poole, Hembry and Dingle, 1973; Poole *et al.*, 1976), including odontoblasts (Nygren *et al.*, 1979), but as it has no activity at physiological pH values it is not usually believed to contribute to the extracellular degradation of proteoglycans. However, microenvironments in which the pH is low may occur (Dingle, 1973), e.g. around cell surfaces where cathepsin D has been located (Poole *et al.*, 1973; Poole *et al.*, 1976). Lysosomal cathepsin B (formerly Bl) also attacks the proteoglycans of cartilage (Roughley, 1977; Roughley and Barrett, 1977) and of periodontal ligament (Gibson, 1979). Although it has a low pH optimum, it retains some proteoglycanase activity at pH 7 (Morrison *et al.*, 1973). However, an extracellular occurrence of this proteinase in normal connective tissues has not yet been demonstrated.

The size of the degraded proteoglycans produced extracellularly *in vivo* may be important for their subsequent fate. Small fragments may enter the circulation, to be excreted or to be catabolized by liver cells (Wood *et al.*, 1976). Large fragments are more likely to be taken up by cells within the connective tissue itself. This has been studied in cultures of skin fibroblasts and fibroblast-like arterial cells (Kresse *et al.*, 1975b; Truppe and Kresse, 1978). The uptake of exogenous proteoglycans had the characteristics of adsorptive pinocytosis and exhibited specificity, e.g. dermatan sulphate-rich proteoglycan was internalized fastest (Kresse *et al.*, 1975b). It was shown also that structural integrity of the proteoglycan was necessary for optimal pinocytosis and subsequent degradation. Various receptors probably occur in the fibroblast surface and recognition sites on the proteoglycan molecules must be intact for rapid adsorption and internalization. Since intact proteoglycans were pinocytosed more rapidly than small fragments of proteoglycans (produced by trypsin digestion), extracellular degradation may actually hinder efficient catabolism. However, rates of pinocytosis of larger fragments of proteoglycans (such as those resulting from the action of cathepsin D (Roughley, 1977; Gibson, 1979) or cathepsin G (Roughley, 1977)) have not been determined.

The complete breakdown of the protein component of an internalized proteoglycan or peptidoglycan appears to present few problems considering the available battery of lysosomal proteinases and peptidases (Barrett, 1977; Patel, 1978). In relation to the glycosaminoglycan chains, it is usually assumed that the initial attack is by lysosomal hyaluronidase, although proof of its presence in a number of connective tissues is still lacking. However, it has been found in synovial tissue and fluid (Bollet, Bonner and Nance, 1963), in a lysosome-rich fraction of embryonic cartilage (Wasteson *et al.*, 1975), in human gingiva (Goggins, Fullmer and Steffek, 1968) and in the odontoblast—predentine region of rat incisors (Engström, Linde and Persliden, 1976). A 'mucopolysaccharidase' (perhaps hyaluronidase) was recently detected in the periodontal ligament of resorbing, human deciduous teeth (Alexander and Swerdloff, 1980). Two slightly different forms of hyaluronidase, one of which was secreted, were produced by cultured embryonic chick fibroblasts (Orkin and Toole, 1978). The secreted enzyme had a greater sialic acid content than the form found in the cell layer. As is always found for the lysosomal enzyme, however, it showed a low pH optimum (pH 3.7) which suggests that its action (like secreted cathepsin D) may be confined to the cell surface.

A large variety of exoglycosidases and sulphatases (Patel, 1978) are required for the complete breakdown of the full range of glycosaminoglycan chains. The specificities of some of these glycosidases and the stages in the degradation where their activities are most critical are still being investigated (Hayashi, 1977, 1978; Patel, 1978). Further, it is not clear whether all the enzymes necessary for the complete breakdown of dermatan sulphate periods and heparin-like molecules have been identified. The necessity for efficient catabolism is illustrated by the occurrence of rare, but often severe, storage disorders caused by deficiencies in various glycosidases (Neufeld, Lim and Shapiro, 1975; Dorfman and Matalon, 1976; von Figura, 1976; Patel, 1978).

The general metabolic heterogeneity of glycosaminoglycans and the occurrence of different intracellular, cell surface-associated and extracellular pools (Kresse *et al.*, 1975a; Gallagher, 1977) make turnover studies of these compounds difficult. Reported half-lives have varied from a few days

(Muir and Hardingham, 1975) to several years (Maroudas, Urban and Holm, 1976) and two pools with half-lives of 3 days and 60–70 days were found in one species of costal cartilage (Lohmander, 1977). The association of some proteoglycans with collagen is an important factor, as this can greatly reduce the rate of glycosaminoglycan degradation (David and Bernfield, 1979). Thus, although there are claims that the turnover of glycosaminoglycans in the periodontal ligament is particularly rapid (Baumhammers and Stallard, 1968; Orlowski, 1976), more extensive investigations are required.

FUNCTIONS OF GLYCOSAMINOGLYCANS AND PROTEOGLYCANS

Much has been written about this, often without sufficient knowledge of the nature and locations of the macromolecules in a given tissue and sometimes without regard to their concentrations.

The filtration and exclusion properties of hyaluronate and cartilage proteoglycans (Ogston, 1970) are well known. They prevent the diffusion of some large molecules (such as antibodies) and probably impose a directional bias to the movements of asymmetric molecules (such as procollagen) through the ground substance (Laurent, 1977). The restriction of a biologically active molecule (such as an enzyme) to a smaller extracellular space would result in a higher local concentration and activity. Steric restrictions are also to be expected in pericellular regions and other areas containing high local concentrations of glycosaminoglycans or proteoglycans, even when the total amounts in a tissue are low. Comper and Laurent (1978) have recently reviewed the exclusion effects in the more fibrous connective tissues. They concluded that the contribution of collagen fibres to exclusion phenomena in mature skin far exceeds that of the small concentrations of hyaluronate and proteoglycans. A considerable collagen contribution is also to be expected in the periodontal ligament, even from an early stage of development (see page 136).

With respect to the degree of hydration, osmotic swelling (Comper and Laurent, 1978) and functionally important properties such as viscoelasticity and lubrication, quite small concentrations of hyaluronate and proteoglycans will be significant. As indicated previously, these compounds exhibit non-ideal osmotic behaviour, arising mainly from their poly-anionic character (Gibbs—Donnan phenomena), with a smaller contribution from exclusion effects (Urban *et al.*, 1979). In a mixed system (e.g. one containing proteoglycans and serum components) osmotic pressures are higher than the sum of the contributions of the individual solutes at the same concentrations (Ogston, 1970; Wiederhielm, Fox and Lee, 1976). The collagen provides a resistance against internal swelling forces. This resistance will vary in different directions according to the orientation of the fibres (Comper and Laurent, 1978).

Recently, Bettelheim and Brady (1979) concluded that the most important component responsible for water uptake (and presumably a swelling pressure) in skin was hyaluronate, whereas water retention was greatly dependent on the sulphated proteoglycans. The methods used for measuring the sorption and retention of water have been criticized for not giving physiologically relevant values (Comper and Laurent, 1978) and further characterization of the proteoglycans involved is needed. However, it is likely that the roles of hyaluronate and sulphated proteoglycans differ considerably in relation to hydration, with resulting effects on the mechanical properties of the tissue.

The importance of the nature and concentration of a proteoglycan in the adaptation of a tissue to function has been illustrated in the rabbit flexor digitorum profundus tendon by Gillard *et al.* (1977). Most regions of this tendon are subject to tension and they contained less than 0.2% of total glycosaminoglycan (dry weight), mainly as proteodermatan sulphate. On the other hand, a sesamoid-like pad that was subject to friction and pressure contained about 3.5% of total glycosaminoglycan. The latter was considered to be chondroitin sulphate, but as a small amount of dermatan sulphate was present it is possible that these glycosaminoglycans occurred as CS(DS) hybrids, as in periodontal ligament. Although there is still debate about the relative importance of tension and compression for the dissipation of occlusal loads in the periodontal tissues (see Chapter 11), the nature and distribution of the ground substance components require more consideration. In general,

the requirement for hyaluronate and/or sulphated proteoglycans to dissipate mechanical shock (Ficat and Maroudas, 1975; Kopp, 1978) and protect not only bone surfaces but cells and delicate blood vessels seems clear, and the periodontal ligament and dental pulp (Linde, 1970) are probably good examples.

The most difficult problem in understanding the properties and functions of connective tissue matrices stems from the complex interactions between the various components, particularly those between the collagen and the ground substance. To date, most investigations have been confined to studying the collagen or proteoglycans in isolation. Knowledge of the individual components has now advanced to a stage where such problems can be tackled.

Studies on the effects of proteoglycans on fibrillogenesis provide contradictory data (reviewed by Lindahl and Höök, 1978), presumably because of problems of materials and techniques. Early *in vitro* investigations (Toole and Lowther, 1968) led to a belief that proteodermatan sulphate is more potent than other proteoglycans in precipitating soluble collagen, but this still awaits confirmation. There are formidable problems in extending this kind of experiment to 'in vivo-like' conditions, but a start may be made by employing procollagens instead of soluble, and often truncated, forms of collagen. Evidence of the marked influence of proteoglycans on the organization of collagen fibres *in vivo* includes the correlation between proteoglycan variations and collagen morphology in the transition from transparent cornea to opaque sclera (Borcherding *et al.*, 1975). A marked increase in fibre size and decrease in organization was accompanied by a large fall in total proteoglycan (mainly proteokeratan sulphate) concentration and the appearance of detectable amounts of dermatan sulphate. In cultures of embryonic limb cartilage, the presence of DON (6-diazo-5-oxonorleucine), which inhibits glycosaminoglycan synthesis, resulted in alterations of the width and arrangements of the collagen fibrils (Kochhar, Aydelotte and Vest, 1976). However, a full consideration of collagen morphology must take into account the influences of proteoglycans and possible non-collagen glycoproteins (Happey *et al.*, 1974) superimposed on the inherent differences between genetic forms of collagen, their hexose contents (Pearson, 1979) and extent of crosslinking (see Chapter 4).

Binding of glycosaminoglycans and proteoglycans to collagen has been investigated in various ways (Lindahl and Höök, 1978). Although the binding is electrostatic, it may be significant at physiological pH and ionic strength, especially with regard to proteoglycans rather than free glycosaminoglycans. Also, as neither hyaluronate nor keratan sulphate is bound, some specificity is indicated. Similar experiments with dermatan sulphate, CS(DS) hybrids and their proteoglycans may be rewarding, as light-scattering data indicated that L-iduronate in a glycosaminoglycan chain promoted interactions with soluble collagen (Öbrink, 1973). A firm binding to collagen *in vivo* might increase the influence of a proteoglycan on the fibres, not only in relation to organization but also in protecting them from enzymatic attack. There are numerous examples of glycosaminoglycans inhibiting various enzyme activities, including lysosomal proteinases as well as glycosidases (Avila and Convit, 1975, 1976; Avila, 1978). The possibility of proteoglycans retarding the extracellular breakdown of collagen has often been suggested, but evidence is still difficult to obtain.

The possible functions of glycosaminoglycans in unlikely locations, particularly the cell nucleus (reviewed by Rodén and Horowitz, 1978), has attacted attention. However, this must remain speculative until reliable techniques can confirm their presence *in vivo*.

With respect to the highly reactive heparin molecule, the physiological function of endogenous heparin is still debatable in spite of its known storage in mast cells and proved effectiveness *in vivo* as an anticoagulant (Rodén and Horowitz, 1978; Jacques, 1979). Other glycosaminoglycans containing L-iduronate have anticoagulant properties (Eisenstein, 1979; Oegema *et al.*, 1979). Their occurrence in blood vessel walls may therefore be significant.

There has been much discussion about the association of glycosaminoglycans and/or proteoglycans with the cell surface or coat, including a role as cell surface receptors (Lindahl and Höök, 1978; Comper and Laurent, 1978). Properties related to negative charge, hydration of the glycosaminoglycans and exclusion phenomena surely have functional significance, if only on account of spatial considerations. The domain occupied by a hydrated cell coat (glycocalyx) will prevent close contacts between glyco-

proteins that are more completely integrated with the cell membrane. This contrasts with exclusion from the territory occupied by proteoglycans in the matrix proper, which in some situations could encourage cell aggregation (Morris, 1979). On the other hand, more specific effects on cell adhesion have been proposed (Dietrich *et al.*, 1977; Lindahl and Höök, 1978). Interactions with cell surface fibronectin could also be significant in cell—cell and cell—substratum contacts (Jilek and Hörmann, 1979; Rollins and Culp, 1979). As previously indicated, heparan sulphate is prominent at cell surfaces (or in the 'undercellular' pool) (Kresse *et al.*, 1975a). This may correspond to the focal adhesion site or 'footpad' considered by Rollins and Culp (1979) to be a differentiated element of the cell surface. Proteoglycans may transmit electrical forces (Comper *et al.*, 1976; Comper and Laurent, 1978), a property which could be important in the mechanism by which cells communicate, or recognize changes in the extracellular matrix. For example, the fine filaments apparently extending from proteoglycan granules to cell surfaces (and to collagen and elastin fibres) could provide a means of communication, whether or not they are of structural importance (Wight and Ross, 1975).

This review has been primarily concerned with soft connective tissues, but some comments should be made about variations in chondroitin -4- and -6-sulphates in relation to calcification. Because the -6-sulphate has a higher affinity for calcium ions than the -4-sulphate, it is more likely to inhibit calcification (Sauk *et al.*, 1976; Di Ferrante, 1976; Mourao *et al.*, 1976). By the same reasoning, dermatan sulphate would be a more potent inhibitor than the chondroitin sulphates. It may therefore be significant that dermatan sulphate was prominent in the proliferation zone of cultured fracture callus cartilage, whereas almost none was present in hypertrophic regions (Dr. C. Arsenis, personal communication). Doubts have been expressed about whether the differences in calcium binding between any of these sulphated galactosaminoglycans have significance *in vivo*, but there is agreement that the catabolism of proteoglycans in the mineralizing zone of cartilage is a significant event (Howell and Pita, 1976). Howell and his colleagues believe that hyaluronate—proteoglycan aggregates (but not proteoglycan subunits) are able to shield embryonic mineral clusters. In their view, calcification will not proceed until the aggregates are dispersed (either by the action of lysozyme or because of proteolysis). Confirmation that aggregated proteoglycans are more potent inhibitors of calcification than proteoglycan monomers is still required, but different results could be related to technique. Howell *et al.* (1969) have employed a micropuncture fluid which lost its inhibitory properties simply on dilution. Whatever the basis of an inhibitory or even stimulatory (Bowness, 1968) influence of proteoglycans on calcification, they are not the only organic compounds affecting the process (Howell and Pita, 1976). As for the periodontal ligament, there is still no complete agreement on the most important factors which prevent calcification.

ACKNOWLEDGEMENTS

I am grateful for the cooperation of Dr. G. J. Gibson (present address, Department of Surgery, School of Medicine, University of Auckland, New Zealand) who carried out much of the experimental work on the proteoglycans of the periodontal ligament. Financial assistance was received from the Canadian Medical Research Council.

REFERENCES

ALEXANDER, S. A. & SWERDLOFF, S. A. (1980) Identification and localization of a mucopolysaccharidase in human deciduous teeth. *J. Dent. Res.* **59**, 594–601.

ANDERSON, J. C. (1975) Isolation of a glycoprotein and proteodermatan sulphate from bovine Achilles tendon by affinity chromatography on Concanavalin A-Sepharose. *Biochim. Biophys. Acta* **379**, 444–455.

ANDERSON, J. C. (1976) Glycoproteins of the connective tissue matrix. *Int. Rev. Connect. Tissue Res.* **7**, 251–322.

ANDERSON, J. C. (1978) Connective tissue glycoproteins. In: *Biochemistry of normal and pathological connective tissues* (6th Colloquium of the Federation of European Connective Tissue Clubs), Vol. 1, pp. 184–185. Paris. Editions du Centre National de la Recherche Scientifique.

ANDERSON, J. C. & JACKSON, D. S. (1972) The isolation of glycoproteins from bovine achilles tendon and their interaction with collagen. *Biochem. J.* **127**, 179–186.

ANDERSON, J. C. & LABEDZ, R. I. (1977) Extractability of connective-tissue glycoprotein from bovine tendon. *Biochem. Soc. Trans.* **5**, 434–435.

ANDERSON, J. C., LABEDZ, R. I. & BRENCHLEY, P. E. (1977) Connective-tissue glycoconjugates of bovine tendon and skin. *Biochem. Soc. Trans.* **5**, 431–433.

ANDERSON, J. C., LABEDZ, R. I. & KEWLEY, M. A. (1977) The effect of bovine tendon glycoprotein on the formation of fibrils from collagen solutions. *Biochem. J.* **168**, 345–351.

ANDREWS, A. T. DE B., HERRING, G. M. & KENT, P. W. (1969) The periodate oxidation of bovine bone sialoglycoprotein, and some observations on its structure. *Biochem. J.* **111**, 621–627.

AVILA, J. L. (1978) The influence of the type of sulphate bond and degree of sulphation of glycosaminoglycans on their interactions with lysosomal enzymes. *Biochem. J.* **171**, 489–491.

AVILA, J. L. & CONVIT, J. (1975) Inhibition of leucocytic lysosomal enzymes by glycosaminoglycans *in vitro*. *Biochem. J.* **152**, 57–64.

AVILA, J. L. & CONVIT, J. (1976) Physiochemical characteristics of the glycosaminoglycan–lysosomal enzyme interaction *in vitro*: a model of control of leucocytic lysosomal activity. *Biochem. J.* **160**, 129–136.

BACH, P. R. & BENTLEY, J. P. (1980) Structural glycoprotein, fact or artefact. *Connect. Tissue Res.* **7**, 185–196.

BAKER, J. R. & CATERSON, B. (1979) The isolation and characterization of the link proteins from proteoglycan aggregates of bovine nasal cartilage. *J. Biol. Chem.* **254**, 2387–2393.

BARRETT, A. J. (1975) The enzymic degradation of cartilage matrix. In: *Dynamics of connective tissue macromolecules*, M. C. BURLEY & A. R. POOLE (eds.), pp. 189–226. New York, North-Holland.

BARRETT, A. J. (1977) Introduction to the history and classification of tissue proteinases. In: *Proteinases in mammalian cells and tissues*, A. J. BARRETT (ed.), pp. 1–35. New York, North-Holland.

BAUMHAMMERS, A. & STALLARD, R. E. (1968) S³⁵-sulfate utilization and turnover by the connective tissues of the periodontium. *J. Periodont. Res.* **3**, 187–193.

BETTELHEIM, F. A. & BRADY, E. (1979) Hydration and proteoglycan content of rat skin. In: *Glycoconjugates*. R. SCHAUER *et al.* (eds.), pp. 662–664. Stuttgart, Georg Thieme.

BITTER, T. & MUIR, H. M. (1962) A modified uronic acid carbazole method. *Anal. Biochem.* **4**, 330–334.

BOLLET, A. J., BONNER, W. M. & NANCE, J. L. (1963) The presence of hyaluronidase in various mammalian tissues. *J. Biol. Chem.* **238**, 3522–3527.

BORCHERDING, M. S., BLACIK, L. J., SITTIG, R. A., BIZZELL, J. W., BREEN, M. & WEINSTEIN, H. G. (1975) Proteoglycans and collagen fibre organization in human corneoscleral tissue. *Exp. Eye Res.* **21**, 59–70.

BORNSTEIN, P. & ASH, J. F. (1977) Cell surface-associated structural proteins in connective tissue cells. *Proc. Natl. Acad. Sci. USA* **74**, 2480–2484.

BORNSTEIN, P., DUKSIN, D., BALIAN, G., DAVIDSON, J. M. & CROUCH, E. (1978) Organization of extracellular proteins on connective tissue cell surface: relevance to cell–matrix interactions *in vitro* and *in vivo*. *Ann. N.Y. Acad. Sci.* **312**, 93–105.

BOWNESS, J. M. (1968) Present concepts of the role of

ground substance in calcification. *Clin. Orthop. Rel. Res.* **59**, 233–244.

BRAY, B. A. (1978a) Cold-insoluble globulin (fibronectin) in connective tissues of adult lung and in trophoblast basement membrane. *J. Clin. Invest.* **62**, 745–752.

BRAY, B. A. (1978b) Presence of fibronectin in basement membranes and acidic structural glycoproteins from human placenta and lung. *Ann. N.Y. Acad. Sci.* **312**, 142–150.

BUDDECKE, E. & VON FIGURA, K. (1975) Different types of chondroitin sulfate-dermatan sulfate hybrids in arterial tissue. In: *Protides of the biological fluids*, H. PEETERS (ed.), pp. 219–226. Oxford, Pergamon.

CARMICHAEL, D. J., CHOVELON, A. & PEARSON, C. H. (1975) The composition of the insoluble collagenous matrix of bovine predentine. *Calcif. Tiss. Res.* **17**, 263–271.

CHEN, L. B., MURRAY, A., SEGAL, R. A., BUSHNELL, A. & WALSH, M. L. (1978) Studies on intercellular LETS glycoprotein matrices. *Cell* **14**, 377–391.

CHOVELON, A., CARMICHAEL, D. J. & PEARSON, C. H. (1975) The composition of the organic matrix of bovine cementum. *Archs. oral Biol.* **20**, 537–541.

CLARK, C. C. & KEFALIDES, N. A. (1978) Localization and partial composition of the oligosaccharide units on the propeptide extension of type I procollagen. *J. Biol. Chem.* **253**, 47–51.

COMPER, W. D. & LAURENT, T. C. (1978) Physiological function of connective tissue polysaccharides. *Physiol. Rev.* **58**, 255–315.

COMPER, W. D., LISBERG, W. & VEIS, A. (1976) Diffusion potentials of polyelectrolytes and their possible relationship to biological electrochemical phenomena. *J. Coll. Interf. Sci.* **57**, 345–352.

CORNILLET-STOUPY, J., BOREL, J. P. & RANDOUX, A. (1978) Reported at the 6th Colloquium of the Federation of European Connective Tissue Clubs, Université Paris – Val de Marne à Creteil, France.

CÖSTER, L. (1979) Dermatan sulphate proteoglycans. Thesis, University of Lund.

DAMLE, S. P., KIERAS, F. J., TZENG, W. K. & GREGORY, J. D. (1979) Isolation and characterization of proteochondroitin sulfate from pig skin. *J. Biol. Chem.* **254**, 1614–1620.

DAVID, G. & BERNFIELD, M. R. (1979) Collagen reduces glycosaminoglycan degradation by cultured mammary epithelial cells: possible mechanism for basal lamina formation. *Proc. Natl. Acad. Sci. USA* **76**, 786–790.

DESSAU, W., SASSE, J., TIMPL, R., JILEK, F. & VON DER MARK, K. (1978) Synthesis and extracellular deposition of fibronectin in chondrocyte cultures. Response to the removal of extracellular matrix. *J. Cell Biol.* **79**, 342–355.

DIETRICH, C. P., SAMPAIO, L. O., TOLEDO, O. M. S. & CASSARO, C. M. F. (1977) Cell recognition and adhesiveness: a possible biological role for the sulphated mucopolysaccharides. *Biochem. Biophys. Res. Commun.* **75**, 329–336.

DI FERRANTE, N. (1976) Carbohydrate components of teeth. In: *Dental biochemistry* (2nd edn.), E. P. LAZZARI (ed.), chapter 3. Philadelphia, Lea & Febiger.

DI FERRANTE, N., DONNELLY, P. V. & BERGLUND, R. K. (1971) Colorimetric determination of dermatan

sulphate. *Biochem. J.* **124**, 549–553.

DINGLE, J. T. (1973) The role of lysosomal enzymes in skeletal tissues. *J. Bone Joint Surg.* **55B**, 87–95.

DORFMAN, A. & MATALON, R. (1976) The mucopolysaccharidoses (a review). *Proc. Natl. Acad. Sci. USA* **73**, 630–637.

EISENSTEIN, R. (1979) Vascular extracellular tissue and atherosclerosis. *Artery* **5**, 207–221.

EISENSTEIN, R. & KUETTNER, K. (1976) The ground substance of the arterial wall. Part 2. Electron-microscopic studies. *Atherosclerosis* **24**, 37–46.

EMBERY, G. (1976) Glycosaminoglycans of human dental pulp. *J. Biol. Buccale* **4**, 229–236.

EMBERY, G., OLIVER, W. M. & STANBURY, J. B. (1979) The metabolism of proteoglycans and glycosaminoglycans in inflamed human gingiva. *J. periodont. Res.* **14**, 512–519.

ENGSTRÖM, C., LINDE, A. & PERSLIDEN, B. (1976) Acid hydrolases in the odontoblast–predentin region of dentinogenically active teeth. *Scand. J. Dent. Res.* **84**, 76–81.

FICAT, C. & MAROUDAS, A. (1975) Cartilage of the patella. Topographical variation of glycosaminoglycan content in normal and fibrillated tissue. *Ann. Rheum. Dis.* **34**, 515–519.

FISHER, M. & SOLURSH, M. (1977) Glycosaminoglycan localization and role in maintenance of tissue spaces in the early chick embryo. *J. Embryol. exp. Morph.* **42**, 195–207.

FRANCIS, G. & THOMAS, J. (1975) Isolation of acidic structural glycoproteins in pulmonary tissues. *Biochem. J.* **145**, 299–304.

FRANSSON, L. Å. (1974) Periodate oxidation of L-iduronic acid residues in dermatan sulphate. *Carbohyd. Res.* **36**, 339–348.

FRANSSON, L. Å. (1976) Interactions between dermatan sulphate chains. I. Affinity chromatography of copolymeric galactosaminoglycans on dermatan sulphate-substituted agarose. *Biochim. Biophys. Acta* **437**, 106–115.

FRANSSON, L. Å., ANSETH, A., ANTONOPOULOS, C. A. & GARDELL, S. (1970) Structure of dermatan sulphate. VI. The use of cetylpyridinium chloride-cellulose microcolumns for determination of the hybrid structure of dermatan sulphates. *Carbohyd. Res.* **15**, 73–89.

FRANSSON, L. Å., MALMSTRÖM, A., LINDAHL, U. & HÖÖK, M. (1973) In: *Biology of fibroblast*, E. KULONEN (ed.), pp. 439–448. New York, Academic Press.

FRANSSON, L. Å., NIEDUSZYNSKI, I. A., PHELPS, C. F. & SHEEHAN, J. K. (1979) Interactions between dermatan sulphate chains. III. Light scattering and viscometry studies of self-association. *Biochim. Biophys. Acta* **586**, 179–188.

FRANSSON, L. Å. & RODÉN, L. (1967a) Structure of dermatan sulfate. I. Degradation by testicular hyaluronidase. *J. Biol. Chem.* **242**, 4161–4169.

FRANSSON, L. Å., & RODÉN, L. (1967b) Structure of dermatan sulfate. II. Characterization of products obtained by hyaluronidase digestion of dermatan sulfate. *J. Biol. Chem.* **242**, 4170–4175.

FUKUDA, M. & HAKOMORI, S. (1979a) Proteolytic and chemical fragmentation of Galactoprotein A, a major transformation-sensitive glycoprotein released from hamster embryo fibroblasts. *J. Biol. Chem.* **254**, 5442–5450.

FUKUDA, M. & HAKOMORI, S. (1979b) Carbohydrate structure of galactoprotein A, a major transformation-sensitive glycoprotein released from hamster embryo fibroblasts. *J. Biol. Chem.* **254**, 5451–5457.

FURCHT, L. T., MOSHER, D. F. & WENDELSCHAFER-CRABB (1978) Immunocytochemical localization of fibronective (LETS protein) on the surface of L 6 myoblasts: light and electron microscopic studies. *Cell* **13**, 263–271.

FURTHMAYR, H. (1978) Structural comparison of glycophorins and immunochemical analysis of genetic variants. *Nature* **271**, 519–524.

FURUTO, D. & SCHNEIR, M. (1975) Concomitant tissue accumulation of 'collagen-associated' sialoglycoproteins and salt-insoluble collagen during rat skin maturation. *Mech. Age Dev.* **4**, 97–101.

GALLAGHER, J. T. (1977) Concepts of metabolic pools in the metabolism of proteoglycans and hyaluronic acid. *Biochem. Soc. Trans.* **5**, 402–410.

GELMAN, R. A. & SILBERBERG, A. (1976) The effect of a strongly-interacting macromolecular probe on the swelling and exclusion properties of loose connective tissue. *Connect. Tissue Res.* **4**, 79–90.

GIBSON, G. J. (1979) Proteoglycans of the periodontal ligament. Thesis, University of Alberta.

GIBSON, G. J. & PEARSON, C. H. (in press) Sulphated galactosaminoglycans of bovine periodontal ligament and skin: hybrid chains of different compositions and molecular sizes and occurrence in distinct proteoglycans.

GILLARD, G. C., MERRILEES, M. J., BELL-BOOTH, P. G., REILLY, H. C. & FLINT, M. H. (1977) The proteoglycan content and axial periodicity of collagen in tendon. *Biochem. J.* **163**, 145–151.

GOGGINS, J. F., FULLMER, H. M. & STEFFEK, A. J. (1968) Hyaluronidase activity of human gingiva. *Arch. Pathol.* **85**, 272–274.

GREENWALD, R. A. (1976) Lack of effect of lysozymes on cartilage proteoglycans. *Arch. Biochem. Biophys.* **175**, 520–523.

GREGORY, J. D. & DAMLE, S. P. (1979) Proteodermatan sulphate from pig skin. In: *Glycoconjugates,* R. SCHAUER *et al.* (eds.), pp. 65–66. Stuttgart, Georg Thieme.

HANDLEY, C. J. & LOWTHER, D. A. (1976) Inhibition of proteoglycan synthesis by hyaluronic acid in chondrocytes in cell culture. *Biochim. Biophys. Acta* **444**, 69–74.

HAPPEY, F., NAYLOR, A., PALFRAMAN, J., PEARSON, C. H., RENDER, R. M. & TURNER, R. L. (1974) Variations in the diameter of collagen fibrils, bound hexose and associated glycoproteins in the intervertebral disc. In: *Connective tissues: biochemistry and pathophysiology,* R. FRICKE & F. HARTMANN (eds.), pp. 67–70. New York, Springer-Verlag.

HARDINGHAM, T. E., EWINS, R. J. F. & MUIR, H. (1976) Cartilage proteoglycans. Structure and heterogeneity of the protein core and the effects of specific protein modifications on the binding to hyaluronate. *Biochem. J.* **157**, 127–143.

HASCALL, G. K. (1980) Cartilage proteoglycans: comparison of sectioned and spread whole molecules. *J. Ultrastruct. Res.* **70**, 369–375.

HASCALL, V. C. (1977) Interaction of cartilage proteoglycans with hyaluronic acid. *J. Supramol. Struct.* **7**, 101–120.

HAYASHI, S. (1977) Study on the degradation of glycosaminoglycans by canine liver lysosomal enzymes. I. The mode of contribution of hyaluronidase, β-glucuronidase and β-N-acetylhexosaminidase on hyaluronic acid. *J. Biochem.* **82**, 1287–1295.

HAYASHI, S. (1978) Study on the degradation of glycosaminoglycans by canine liver lysosomal enzymes. II. The contributions of hyaluronidase, β-glucuronidase, sulphatase and β-N-acetylhexosaminidase in the case of chondroitin-4-sulfate. *J. Biochem.* **83**, 149–157.

HERRING, G. M. (1976) A comparison of bone matrix and tendon with particular reference to glycoprotein content. *Biochem. J.* **159**, 749–755.

HOPSU-HAVU, V. K., FRÄKI, J. E. & JÄRVINEN, M. (1977) Proteolytic enzymes in the skin. In: *Proteinases in mammalian cells and tissues,* A. J. BARRETT (ed.), Chapter 13, New York, North-Holland.

HOWELL, D. S., PITA, J. C., MARQUEZ, J. F. & GATTER, R. A. (1969) Demonstration of macromolecular inhibitor(s) of calcification and nucleational factor(s) in fluid from calcifying sites in cartilage. *J. Clin. Invest.* **48**, 630–641.

HOWELL, D. S. & PITA, J. C. (1976) Calcification of growth plate cartilage with special reference to studies on micropuncture fluids. *Clin. Orthop. Relat. Res.* **118**, 208–229.

HYNES, R. O. (1976) Cell surface proteins and malignant transformation. *Biochim. Biophys. Acta* **458**, 73–107.

JACQUES, L. B. (1979) Heparin: an old drug with a new paradigm. *Science* **206**, 528–533.

JILEK, F. & HÖRMANN, H. (1979) Fibronectin (Cold-insoluble globulin), VI. Influence of heparin and hyaluronic acid on the binding of native collagen. *Hoppe-Seyler's Z. Physiol. Chem.* **360**, 597–603.

KAWAMOTO, T. & NAGAI, Y. (1976) Developmental changes in glycosaminoglycans, collagen and collagenase activity in embryonic chick skin. *Biochim. Biophys. Acta* **437**, 190–199.

KITCHEN, R. G. & CLELAND, R. L. (1978) Dilute solution properties of proteoglycan fractions from bovine nasal cartilage. *Biopolymers* **17**, 759–783.

KLEINMAN, H. K., McGOODWIN, E. B., MARTIN, G. R., KLEBE, R. J., FIETZEK, P. P. & WOOLLEY, D. E. (1978) Localization of the binding site for cell attachment in the $\alpha 1(I)$ chain of collagen. *J. Biol. Chem.* **253**, 5642–5646.

KOCHHAR, D. M., AYDELOTTE, M. B. & VEST, T. K. (1976) Altered collagen fibrillogenesis in embryonic mouse limb cartilage deficient in matrix granules. *Exp. Cell Res.* **102**, 213–222.

KOFOED, J. A. & BOZZINI, C. E. (1970) The effect of hydrocortisone on the concentration and synthesis of acid mucopolysaccharides in the rat gingiva. *J. periodont. Res.* **5**, 259–262.

KOPP, S. (1978) Topographical distribution of sulfated glycosaminoglycans in the surface layers of the human temperomandibular joint. *J. oral Path.* 7, 283–294.

KRESSE, H., VON FIGURA, K., BUDDECKE, E. & FROMME, H. G. (1975a) Metabolism of sulphated glycosaminoglycans in cultivated bovine arterial cells. I. Characterization of different pools of sulphated glycosaminoglycans. *Hoppe-Seyler's Z. Physiol. Chem.* 356, 929–941.

KRESSE, H., TEKOLF, W., VON FIGURA, K. & BUDDECKE, E. (1975b) Metabolism of sulphated glycosaminoglycans in cultivated bovine arterial cells. II. Quantitative studies on the uptake of $^{35}SO_4$-labelled proteoglycans. *Hoppe-Seyler's Z. Physiol. Chem.* 356, 943–952.

KUETTNER, K. E., EISENSTEIN, R. & SORGENTE, N. (1974) Lysozymes of cartilage and other connective tissues (a speculative review). In: *Lysozyme,* E. F. OSSERMAN, R. E. CRANFIELD & S. BEYCHOK (eds.). London, Academic Press.

KUETTNER, K. E., EISENSTEIN, R. & SORGENTE, N. (1975) Lysozyme in calcifying tissues. *Clin. Orthop. Relat. Res.* 112, 316–339.

LAURENT, T. C. (1977) Interaction between proteins and glycosaminoglycans. *Fed. Proc.* 36, 24–27.

LINDAHL, U. (1976) Structure and biosynthesis of iduronic acid-containing glycosaminoglycans. In: *Carbohydrates: International Review of Science, Organic Chemistry,* Series 2, G. O. ASPINALL (ed.), pp. 283–312. London, Butterworths.

LINDAHL, U. & HÖÖK, M. (1978) Glycosaminoglycans and their binding to biological macromolecules. *Ann. Rev. Biochem.* 47, 385–417.

LINDE, A. (1970) Glycosaminoglycans (mucopolysaccharides) of the porcine dental pulp. *Archs. oral Biol.* 15, 1035–1046.

LINDE, A. (1973) A study of the dental pulp glycosaminoglycans from permanent human teeth and rat and rabbit incisors. *Archs. oral Biol.* 18, 49–59.

LINDER, E., STENMAN, S., LEHTO, V. P. & VAHERI, A. (1978) Distribution of fibronectin in human tissues and relationship to other connective tissue components. *Ann. N.Y. Acad. Sci.* 312, 151–159.

LOHMANDER, S. (1977) Turnover of proteoglycans in guinea pig costal cartilage. *Arch. Biochem. Biophys.* 180, 93–101.

MALEMUD, C. J., WEITZMAN, G. A., NORBY, D. P., SAPOLSKY, A. I. & HOWELL, D. S. (1979) Metal-dependent neutral proteoglycanase activity from monolayer-cultured lapine articular chondrocytes. *J. Lab. Clin. Med.* 93, 1018–1030.

MALMSTRÖM, A., FRANSSON, L. Å., HÖÖK, M. & LINDAHL, U. (1975a) Biosynthesis of dermatan sulfate. I. Formation of L-iduronic acid residues. *J. Biol. Chem.* 250, 3419–3425.

MALMSTRÖM, A., CARLSTEDT, I., ÅBERG, L. & FRANSSON, L. Å. (1975b) The copolymeric structure of dermatan sulphate produced by cultured human fibroblasts. *Biochem. J.* 151, 477–489.

MALMSTRÖM, A., RODÉN, L., FEINGOLD, D. S., JACOBSSON, I., BÄCKSTRÖM, G. & LINDAHL, U. (1980) Biosynthesis of heparin: partial purification of the uronosyl C-5 epimerase. *J. Biol. Chem.* 255, 3878–3883.

MAROUDAS, A., URBAN, J. & HOLM, S. (1976) Collagen and glycosaminoglycan metabolism in articular cartilage and intervertebral disc. In: *Abstracts of proceedings of the European Federation of the Connective Tissue Clubs* (Vth meeting, Aug. 1976), pp. 25–26. University at Sart Tilman, Liège, Belgium.

MASHOUF, K. & ENGEL, M. B. (1975) Maturation of periodontal ligament connective tissue in new born rat incisor. *Archs. oral Biol.* 20, 161–166.

McMURTREY, J., RADHAKRISHNAMURTHY, B., DALFERES, E. R., BERENSON, G. S. & GREGORY, J. D. (1979) Isolation of proteoglycan–hyaluronate complexes from bovine aorta. *J. Biol. Chem.* 254, 1621–1626.

MICKALITES, C. & ORLOWSKI, W. A. (1977) Study of the noncollagenous components of the periodontium. *J. Dent. Res.* 56, 1023–1026.

MOCZAR, E., SEPULCHRE, C. & MOCZAR, M. (1975) Structural glycoproteins from connective tissues. In: *Protides of the biological fluids,* H. PEETERS (ed.), pp. 297–302. Oxford, Pergamon.

MOCZAR, M., MOCZAR, E. & ROBERT, L. (1977) Structural glycoprotein from the media of pig aorta. Aggregation of the S-carboxamidomethyl subunits. *Biochimie* 59, 141–151.

MORRIS, J. E. (1979) Steric exclusion of cells. A mechanism of glycosaminoglycan-induced cell aggregation. *Exp. Cell Res.* 120, 141–153.

MORRISON, R. I. G., BARRETT, A. J., DINGLE, J. T. & PRIOR, D. (1973) Cathepsins Bl and D. Action on human cartilage proteoglycans. *Biochim. Biophys. Acta* 302, 411–419.

MOURAO, P. A. S., ROSENFELD, S., LAREDO, J. & DIETRICH, C. P. (1976) The distribution of chondroitin sulfates in articular and growth cartilages of human bones. *Biochim. Biophys. Acta* 428, 19–26.

MUIR, H. & HARDINGHAM, T. E. (1975) Structure of proteoglycans. In: *Biochemistry of Carbohydrates:* MTP International Review of Science, Biochemistry Series, 1, Vol. 5. W. J. WHELAN (ed.), pp. 153–222. London, Butterworths.

MUIR, L. W., BORNSTEIN, P. & ROSS, R. (1976) A presumptive subunit of elastic fiber microfibrils secreted by arterial smooth muscle cells in culture. *Eur. J. Biochem.* 64, 105–114.

MUNEMOTO, K. (1968) A study of acid mucopolysaccharides in periodontal tissues. *J. Osaka Univ. Dent. Soc.* 13, 257–268.

MUNEMOTO, K., IWAYAMA, Y., YOSHIDA, M., SERA, M., AONO, M. & YOKOMIZA, I. (1970) Isolation and characterization of acid mucopolysaccharides of bovine periodontal membrane. *Archs. oral Biol.* 15, 369–382.

MURAKAWA, A. (1974) Acid mucopolysaccharides in the bovine dental pulp. *J. Osaka Dental University* 8, 19–32.

NAGASE, H. & WOESSNER, J. F. (1977) Neutral protease from bovine nasal cartilage that digests proteoglycan. *Clin. Res.* 25, (4), 644A.

NEUFELD, E. F., LIM, T. W. & SHAPIRO, L. J. (1975) Inherited disorders of lysosomal metabolism. *Ann. Rev. Biochem.* 44, 357–376.

NOWACK, H., GAY, S., WICK, G., BECKER, U. & TIMPL, R. (1976) Preparation and use in immunohistology of antibodies specific for type I and type III collagen and procollagen. *J. Immunol. Methods* 12, 117–124.

NYGREN, H., PERSLIDEN, B., HANSSON, H-A. &

LINDE, A. (1979) Cathepsin D: ultra-immunohisto-chemical localization in dentinogenesis. *Calcif. Tissue* **29**, 251–256.

ÖBRINK, B. (1972) Isolation and partial characterization of a dermatan sulphate proteoglycan from pig skin. *Biochim. Biophys. Acta* **264**, 354–361.

ÖBRINK, B. (1973) A study of the interactions between monomeric tropocollagen and glycosaminoglycans. *Eur. J. Biochem.* **33**, 387–400.

OEGEMA, T. R., HASCALL, V. C. & EISENSTEIN, R. (1979) Characterization of bovine aorta proteo-glycans extracted with guanidine hydrochloride in the presence of protease inhibitors. *J. Biol. Chem.* **254**, 1312–1318.

OGSTON, A. G. (1970) The biological functions of glycos-aminoglycans. In: *Chemistry and molecular biology of the intercellular matrix*, Vol. 3, E. A. BALAZS (ed.), pp. 1231–1240. London, Academic Press.

OLSEN, B. R., GUZMAN, N. A., ENGEL, J., CONDIT, C. & AASE, S. (1977) Purification and characterization of a peptide from the carboxyterminal region of chick tendon procollagen type I. *Biochemistry* **16**, 3030–3036.

ORKIN, R. W. & TOOLE, B. P. (1978) Chick embryo fibro-blasts produce two forms of hyaluronidase. *J. Cell Biol.* **79**, EM 819.

ORLOWSKI, W. A. (1974) Analysis of collagen, glycoproteins and acid mucopolysaccharides in the bovine and porcine dental pulp. *Archs. oral Biol.* **19**, 255–258.

ORLOWSKI, W. A. (1976) The incorporation of S^{35} sulfate and C^{14}-glucosamine into the gingiva and periodontal ligament of a rat. *J. Dent. Res.* **55** B, 67.

PATEL, V. (1978) Degradation of glycoproteins. In: *The glycoconjugates*, Vol. 2, M. I. HOROWITZ & W. PIGMAN (eds.), pp. 185–229. New York, Academic Press.

PAUNIO, K. (1969) Periodontal connective tissue: biochemi-cal studies of disease in man. *Suom. Hamasläak. Toim.* **65**, 249–290.

PEARSON, C. H. (1970) A study of the estimation and distribution of mucopolysaccharides in bovine skin. Thesis, University of Leeds.

PEARSON, C. H. (1979) Collagens and procollagens: molecu-lar aspects of collagen fibre polymorphism. In: *Applied fibre science*, Vol. 3, F. HAPPEY (ed.), chapter 10, London, Academic Press.

PEARSON, C. H., DAVIES, J. D., GIBSON, G. J., LEHOCKY, S. & SCOTT, P. G. (1978a) Degradation of skin der-matan sulphate proteoglycan by cathepsin D. *Biochem. Soc. Trans.* **6**, 1199–1202.

PEARSON, C. H., AINSWORTH, L. & CHOVELON, A. (1978b) The determination of small amounts of collagen hydroxylysyl glycosides. *Connect. Tissue Res.* **6**, 51–59.

PEARSON, C. H. & GIBSON, G. J. (1979) Proteoglycans of bovine periodontal ligament and dermis. In: *Glyco-conjugates*, R. SCHAUER *et al.* (eds.), pp. 559–560. Stuttgart, Georg Thieme.

PEARSON, C. H. & GIBSON, G. J. (in press) Proteoglycans of bovine skin and periodontal ligament: purification and characterization of the proteodermatan sulphates and first data on a second type of proteoglycan in the ligament. *Biochem. J.*

PEARSON, C. H., HAPPEY, F., NAYLOR, A., TURNER, R. L., PALFRAMAN, J. & SHENTALL, R. D. (1972) Collagens and associated glycoproteins in the human intervertebral disc. Variations in sugar and amino acid composition in relation to location and age. *Ann. Rheum. Dis.* **31**, 45–53.

PEARSON, C. H., WOHLLEBE, M., CARMICHAEL, D. J. & CHOVELON, A. (1975) Bovine periodontal liga-ment. An investigation of the collagen, glycosamino-glycan and insoluble glycoprotein components at different stages of tissue development. *Connect. Tissue Res.* **3**, 195–206.

PENA, S. D. J. & HUGHES, R. C. (1978) Fibronectin–plasma membrane interactions in the adhesion and spreading of hamster fibroblasts. *Nature* **276**, 80–83.

PLECASH, J. M. (1974) Proteoglycans of the rat periodon-tium. Thesis, University of Alberta, Edmonton, Alberta, Canada.

POOLE, A. R., HEMBRY, R. M. & DINGLE, J. T. (1973) Extracellular localization of cathepsin D in ossifying cartilage. *Calc. Tissue Int.* **12**, 313–321.

POOLE, A. R., HEMBRY, R. M., DINGLE, J. T., PINDER, I., RING, E. F. J. & COSH, J. (1976) Secretion and localization of cathepsin D in synovial tissues removed from rheumatoid and traumatized joints. *Arthritis Rheum.* **19**, 1295–1307.

RADHAKRISHNAMURTHY, B., RUIZ, H. A. Jr. & BERENSON, G. S. (1977) Isolation and characteri-zation of proteoglycans from bovine aorta. *J. Biol. Chem.* **252**, 4831–4841.

RANDOUX, A., CORNILLET-STOUPY, J., DESANTI, M. & BOREL, J. P. (1976) Isolement et caractéri-sation de deux subunités constitutives des glycopro-teines de structure du tissu cutane de lapin. *Biochim. Biophys. Acta* **446**, 77–86.

RANDOUX, A., MAQUART, F., CORNILLET-STOUPY, J., SZYMANOVICZ, G. & BOREL, J. P. (1978) Influence of structural glycoproteins on the biosyn-thesis of structural glycoproteins on the biosynthesis of collagen by fibroblasts in culture. In: *Biochemistry of normal and pathological connective tissues* (6th Colloquium of the Federation of European Connective Tissue Clubs), Vol. 1, pp. 257–258. Paris, Editions du Centre National de la Recherche Scientifique.

REIHANIAN, H., JAMIESON, A. M., TANG, L. H. & ROSENBERG, L. (1979) Hydrodynamic properties of proteoglycan subunit from bovine nasal cartilage. Self-association behaviour and interaction with hyalu-ronate studied by laser light scattering. *Biopolymers* **18**, 1727–1747.

ROBERT, L., DARRELL, R. W. & ROBERT, B. (1970) Immunological properties of connective tissue glyco-proteins. In: *Chemistry and molecular biology of the intercellular matrix*, Vol. 3, E. A. BALAZS (ed.), pp. 1591–1614. London, Academic Press.

ROBERT, L. & ROBERT, B. (1974) Structural glycoproteins of connective tissues: their role in morphogenesis and immunopathology. In: *Connective tissues: biochemistry and pathophysiology*, R. FRICKE & F. HARTMANN (eds.), pp. 240–256. New York, Springer-Verlag.

ROBERT, B. & ROBERT, L. (1975) Cellular differentiation and morphogenesis of the intercellular matrix. In: *Protides of the biological fluids*, H. PEETERS (ed.), pp. 15–21. Oxford, Pergamon.

RODÉN, L. & HOROWITZ, M. I. (1978) Structure and

biosynthesis of connective tissue proteoglycans. In: *The glycoconjugates*, Vol. 2, M. I. HOROWITZ & W. PIGMAN (eds.), pp. 3–71. New York, Academic Press.

RODÉN, L. & SCHWARTZ, N. B. (1975) Biosynthesis of connective tissue proteoglycans. In: *Biochemistry of carbohydrates*. MTP International Review of Science, Biochemistry Series I, Vol. 5, W. J. WHELAN (ed.), pp. 95–152. London, Butterworths.

ROHDE, H., WICK, G. & TIMPL, R. (1979) Immunochemical characterization of the basement membrane glycoprotein, Laminin. *Eur. J. Biochem.* **102**, 195–201.

ROLLINS, B. J. & CULP, L. A. (1979) Preliminary characterization of the proteoglycans in the substrate adhesion sites of normal and virus-transformed murine cells. *Biochemistry* **18**, 5621–5629.

ROSENBERG, L., CHOI, H., PAL, S. & TANG, L. (1979) Carbohydrate–protein interactions in proteoglycans. In: *Carbohydrate–protein interaction*, ACS Symposium Series, No. 88, I. J. GOLDSTEIN (ed.), pp. 186–216. American Chemical Society.

ROUGHLEY, P. J. (1977) The degradation of cartilage proteoglycans by tissue proteinases. Proteoglycan heterogeneity and the pathway of proteolytic degradation. *Biochim. J.* **167**, 639–646.

ROUGHLEY, P. J. & BARRETT, A. J. (1977) The degradation of cartilage proteoglycans by tissue proteinases. Proteoglycan structure and its susceptibility to proteolysis. *Biochim. J.* **167**, 629–637.

ROUSLAHTI, E., HAYMAN, E. G., KUUSELA, P., SHIVELY, J. E. & ENGVALL, E. (1979) Isolation of a tryptic fragment containing the collagen-binding site of plasma fibronectin. *J. Biol. Chem.* **254**, 6054–6059.

SAITO, H., YAMAGATA, T. & SUZUKI, S. (1968) Enzymatic methods for the determination of small quantities of isomeric chondroitin sulphates. *J. Biol. Chem.* **243**, 1536–1542.

SAKAKI, T., TSURUMI, N., MAEDA, J., HOUDA, T., KAWAKATSU, K., TAJIME, T. & KAMATA, Y. (1971) Studies on acid mucopolysaccharides in bovine normal gingiva. *J. Osaka Odont. Soc.* **34**, 333–340.

SAKAMOTO, N., OKAMOTO, H. & OKUDA, K. (1978) Qualitative and quantitative analyses of bovine gingival glycosaminoglycans. *Archs. oral Biol.* **23**, 983–987.

SAKAMOTO, N., OKAMOTO, H. & OKUDA, K. (1979) Qualitative and quantitative analyses of bovine, rabbit and human dental pulp glycosaminoglycans. *J. Dent. Res.* **58**, 646–655.

SANDY, J. D., BROWN, H. L. G. & LOWTHER, D. A. (1978) Degradation of proteoglycan in articular cartilage. *Biochim. Biophys. Acta* **543**, 536–544.

SAPOLSKY, A. I., KEISER, H., HOWELL, D. S. & WOESSNER, J. F. Jr. (1976) Metalloproteases of human articular cartilage that digest cartilage proteoglycan at neutral and acid pH. *J. Clin. Invest.* **58**, 1030–1041.

SAUK, J. J. Jr., BROWN, D. M., CORBIN, K. W. & WITKOP, C. J. Jr. (1976) Glycosaminoglycans of predentin, peritubular dentin and dentin: A biochemical and electron microscopic study. *Oral Surg.* **41**, 623–630.

SCHWARTZ, N. B. (1977) Regulation of chondroitin sulphate synthesis. Effect of β-xylosides on synthesis of chondroitin sulfate proteoglycan, chondroitin sulfate chains and core protein. *J. Biol. Chem.* **252**, 6316–6321.

SCHWERMANN, J., SCHMIDT, A., SCHMIDT, M. & BUDDECKE, E. (1979) A new proteoglycan degrading proteinase of cartilage. In *Glycoconjugates,* R. SCHAUER et al. (eds.), pp. 384–385. Stuttgart, Georg Thieme.

SCOTT, J. E. (1980) Collagen–proteoglycan interactions. Localization of proteoglycans in tendon by electron microscopy. *Biochem. J.* **187**, 887–891.

SEAR, C. H. J., GRANT, M. E. & JACKSON, D. A. (1977) Biosynthesis and release of glycoproteins by human skin fibroblasts in culture. *Biochem. J.* **168**, 91–103.

SELLERS, A., REYNOLDS, J. J. & MEIKLE, M. C. (1978) Neutral metalloproteinases of rabbit bone. Separation in latent forms of distinct enzymes that when activated degrade collagen, gelatin and proteoglycans. *Biochem. J.* **171**, 493–496.

SERAFINI-FRACASSINI, A. & HINNIE, J. (1979) Molecular weight distribution profile of cartilage proteoglycan in aqueous guanidinium chloride before and after carboxyl group modification. *Archs. Biochem. Biophys.* **192**, 364–370.

SHAW, J. H. (1978) Role of inflammation in disease. In: *Textbook of oral biology*, J. H. SHAW, E. A. SWEENEY, C. C. CAPPUCCINO & S. M. MELLER (eds.), Chapter 24, London, W. B. Saunders.

SHEEHAN, J. K., NIEDUSZYNSKI, I. A., PHELPS, C. F., MUIR, H. & HARDINGHAM, T. E. (1978) Self-association of proteoglycan subunits from pig laryngeal cartilage. *Biochem. J.* **171**, 109–114.

SHIPP, D. W. & BOWNESS, J. M. (1975) Insoluble non-collagenous cartilage glycoproteins with aggregating subunits. *Biochim. Biophys. Acta* **379**, 282–294.

SILBERT, J. E. (1978) Ground substance. In: *Textbook of oral biology,* J. H. SHAW, E. A. SWEENEY, C. C. CAPPUCCINO & S. M. MELLER (eds.), Chapter 13. London, W. B. Saunders.

SOLURSH, M., HARDINGHAM, T. E., HASCALL, V. C. & KIMURA, J. H. (1980) Separate effects of exogenous hyaluronic acid on proteoglycan synthesis and deposition in pericellular matrix by cultured chick embryo limb chondrocytes. *Develop. Biol.* **75**, 121–129.

SPIRO, R. G. (1978) Nature of the glycoprotein components of basement membranes. *Ann. N.Y. Acad. Sci.* **312**, 106–121.

STARKEY, P. M. & BARRETT, A. J. (1977) α_2-Macroglobulin, a physiological regulator of proteinase activity. In: *Proteinases in mammalian cells and tissues*, A. J. BARRETT (ed.), Chapter 16. New York, North-Holland.

STUHLSATZ, H. W. & GREILING, H. (1976) The preparation of dermatan sulphate. In: *The methodology of connective tissue research,* D. A. HALL (ed.), Chapter 14. Oxford, Joynson-Bruvvers.

TANFORD, C., MARLER, E., JURY, E. & DAVIDSON, E. A. (1964) Determination of the molecular weight distribution of chondroitin sulphate B by sedimentation equilibrium. *J. Biol. Chem.* **239**, 4034–4040.

TANZER, M. L., ROWLAND, F. N., MURRAY, L. W. & KAPLAN, J. (1977) Inhibitory effects of tunicamycin on procollagen biosynthesis and secretion. *Biochim.*

Biophys. Acta **500,** 187–196.

TAWA, T., HONDA, T., FUJITA, A., KIM, Y. B., CHUNG, T. Y., KUWAJIMA, S., MATSUMOTO, M. & MIKI, M. (1976) Studies on acid mucopolysaccharides in dog normal gingiva. *J. Osaka Odont. Soc.* **39,** 799–811.

TERHO, T. T. & HARTIALA, K. (1971) Method for the determination of the sulphate content of glycosaminoglycans. *Anal. Biochem.* **41,** 471–476.

THESLEFF, I., STENMAN, S., VAHERI, A. & TIMPL, R. (1979) Changes in the matrix proteins, fibronectin and collagen, during differentiation of mouse tooth germ. *Develop. Biol.* **70,** 116–126.

TOLEDO, O. M. S. & DIETRICH, C. P. (1977) Tissue specific distribution of sulfated mucopolysaccharides in mammals. *Biochim. Biophys. Acta* **498,** 114–122.

TOOLE, B. P. (1979) Morphogenetic role of glycosaminoglycans (acid mucopolysaccharides) in brain and other tissues. In: *Neuronal recognition,* S. BARONDES (ed.), pp. 275–329. New York, Plenum Press.

TOOLE, B. P. & LOWTHER, D. A. (1968) Dermatan sulfate-protein: isolation and interaction with collagen. *Archs. Biochem. Biophys.* **128,** 567–578.

TREFFERS, W. F. & BROEKHUYSE, R. M. (1977) Ocular antigens VII. The influence of Freund's complete adjuvant and corneal structural glycoprotein in xenogeneic keratoplasty. *Exp. Eye Res.* **25,** 289–295.

TRUPPE, W. & KRESSE, H. (1978) Uptake of proteoglycans and sulphated glycosaminoglycans by cultured fibroblasts. *Eur. J. Biochem.* **85,** 351–356.

TWINING, S. S. & BRECHER, A. S. (1977) Identification of α_1-acid glycoprotein, α_2-macroglobulin and antithrombin III as components of normal and malignant human tissues. *Clin. Chim. Acta* **75,** 143–148.

URBAN, J. P. G., MAROUDAS, A., BAYLISS, M. T. & DILLON, J. (1979) Swelling pressures of proteoglycans at the concentrations found in cartilaginous tissues. *Biorheol.* **16,** 447–464.

VAES, G., EECKHOUT, Y., LENAERS-CLAEYS, G., FRANCOIS-GILLET, C. & DRUETZ, J.-E. (1978) The simultaneous release by bone explants in culture and the parallel activation of procollagenase and of a latent neutral proteinase that degrades cartilage proteoglycans and denatured collagen. *Biochem. J.* **172,** 261–274.

VAHERI, A., ALITALO, K., HEDMAN, K., KURKINEN, M., LEHTO, V. P., LEIVO, I., STENMAN, S. & WARTIOVAARA, J. (1978) Fibronectin, a glyco-

protein present in connective tissues and in circulation. In: *Biochemistry of normal and pathological connective tissues,* 6th Colloquium of the Federation of European Connective Tissue Clubs, Vol. 1, pp. 198–200. Paris, Editions du Centre National de la Recherche Scientifique.

VON FIGURA, K. (1976) Biochemie und Funktion der Glykosaminoglykane der Haut. *Der Hautarzt* **27,** 206–213.

WASTESON, Å., AMADÒ, R., INGMAR, B. & HELDIN, C. H. (1975) Degradation of chondroitin sulphate by lysosomal enzymes from embryonic chick cartilage. In: *Protides of the biological fluids,* H. PEETERS (ed.), pp. 431–435, Oxford, Pergamon.

WERB, Z. & DINGLE, J. T. (1977) Lysosomes as modulators of cellular functions. Influence on the synthesis and secretion of non-lysosomal materials. In: *Lysosomes in biology and pathology,* vol. 5, J. T. DINGLE & R. T. DEAN (eds.), Chapter 5, Amsterdam, North-Holland.

WIEBKIN, O. E. & MUIR, H. (1973) The inhibition of sulphate incorporation in isolated adult chondrocytes by hyaluronic acid. *FEBS Lett.* **37,** 42–46.

WIEDERHIELM, C. A., FOX, J. R. & LEE, D. R. (1976) Ground substance mucopolysaccharides and plasma proteins: their role in capillary water balance. *Amer. J. Physiol.* **230,** 1121–1125.

WIGHT, T. N. & ROSS, R. (1975) Proteoglycans in primate arteries. I. Ultrastructural localization and distribution in the intima. *J. Cell. Biol.* **67,** 660–674.

WOLF, I., FUCHSWANS, W., WEISER, M., FURTHMAYR, H. & TIMPL, R. (1971) Acidic structural proteins of connective tissue. *Eur. J. Biochem.* **20,** 426–431.

WOOD, K. M., CURTIS, C. G., POWELL, G. M. & WUSTEMAN, F. S. (1976) The metabolic fate of intravenously injected peptide-bound chondroitin sulphate in the rat. *Biochem. J.* **158,** 39–46.

YAMADA, K. M. & OLDEN, K. (1978) Fibronectins-adhesive glycoproteins of cell surface and blood. *Nature* **275,** 179–184.

YAMADA, K. M., SCHLESINGER, D. H., KENNEDY, D. W. & PASTAN, I. (1977) Characterization of a major fibroblast cell surface glycoprotein. *Biochemistry* **16,** 5552–5559.

YAMANISHI, H. & SATO, Y. (1976) The removal of non-collagen components from newborn dermis with magnesium chloride solution. *J. Biochem.* **79,** 131–144.

Chapter 7

THE VASCULATURE OF THE PERIODONTAL LIGAMENT

L. G. A. Edwall

INTRODUCTION

It is often stated that, for a fibrous connective tissue, the periodontal ligament is highly vascular. However, data are not yet available to compare the density of vessels in the periodontal ligament against that in other fibrous tissues. Irrespective of whether the density is high or low, the vasculature clearly must be adequate to provide the physiological exchange of materials between the blood and the periodontal tissues. The periodontal vasculature also provides a significant exchange between the blood and dentine. A further possible function for the vasculature in the periodontal ligament concerns a role in the mechanisms of tooth support and eruption.

This review is concerned primarily with the basic morphology and physiology of the blood vessels in the periodontal ligament; for information concerning its part in the eruptive mechanism and tooth support, the reader is referred to Chapters 10 and 11 respect-

ively. Brief mention will also be made of age changes and the lymphatics. As will be shown, many diverse techniques have been employed to study the periodontal ligament vasculature. Indeed, much of this review has been written with reference to methodological considerations.

STRUCTURE AND ARRANGEMENT OF THE PERIODONTAL LIGAMENT VASCULATURE

Gross anatomy

The gross anatomy of the blood vessels which supply the periodontal ligament in man has been described by Hayashi (1932), Steinhardt (1935), Perint (1949), Waerhaug (1954), Cohen (1959) and Castelli (1963). For the common laboratory animals, the vasculature has been described by Kindlová and Matěna (1959,

1962), Cohen (1960), Boyer and Neptune (1962), Castelli and Dempster (1965), Kindlová (1965), Carranza *et al.* (1966), Turner *et al.* (1969), Khouw and Goldhaber (1970) and Matĕna (1973). Saunders and Röckert (1967) have written a review on the topic.

The above studies show that the vessels supplying the periodontal ligament are derived mainly from the superior alveolar arteries in the maxilla and the inferior alveolar artery in the mandible. These arteries are branches of the maxillary artery. However, there are sources in addition to this primary supply. In the mandible, periodontal ligament vessels may be derived from the sublingual branch of the lingual artery via the gingiva and also from branches of the buccal, inferior labial, masseteric and mental arteries. In the maxilla, periodontal ligament vessels may arise from the greater (anterior) palatine artery via the lingual gingiva and from the superior labial branches of the facial and infraorbital arteries. In *Macaca rhesus,* the blood supply to the periodontal ligament of most teeth resembles that in man. In contrast, Castelli and Dempster (1965) reported that the monkey maxillary incisor ligaments were supplied solely by a branch of the greater (anterior) palatine artery. Also, the mandibular incisor ligaments were said to be supplied by a branch of the sublingual artery (which enters the mandible at the symphysis). The observation that only one artery supplies certain periodontal ligaments is surprising. However, Kindlová (1965) found that the periodontal ligaments of the anterior teeth in the macaque monkey obtained their major, but not sole, blood supply from the palatine and lingual arteries. Thus, the general observation seems to be that the periodontal ligaments receive their arterial blood supply from several different sources. The existence of a rich accessory blood supply to the periodontal ligaments from intraosseal and periosteal sites has been noted by several investigators (Noyes, 1897; Waugh, 1904; Perint, 1949; Boyer and Neptune, 1962; Kindlová and Matĕna, 1962; Kindlová, 1965; Castelli and Dempster, 1965; Carranza *et al.,* 1966; Folke and Stallard, 1967; Turner *et al.,* 1969; Cutright and Hunsuck, 1970). Many of the periodontal vessels are derived from arterioles less than 100 μm in diameter which initially run in the marrow spaces of the alveolar bone and subsequently enter the perio-

dontal ligament at various levels (Kindlová and Matĕna, 1962; Castelli and Dempster, 1965; Carranza *et al.,* 1966; Folke and Stallard, 1967; Lenz, 1968).

The venous drainage from the periodontal ligament has been described by Castelli (1963) and Castelli and Dempster (1965). In monkey and man, both the veins in the alveolar bone and those from the periodontal ligament drain into veins in the interalveolar and interradicular septi. These veins do not follow the arteries, but instead join to form larger veins in the interalveolar septi which in turn are connected to a rich venous network surrounding the apex of each alveolus (Fig. 1). Anastomoses with veins in the gingiva also occur. Castelli and Dempster (1965) described a venous reservoir system linking the periodontal ligament with the bone marrow spaces. In the human mandible, one or several inferior alveolar veins accompany the inferior alveolar artery. These veins may drain anteriorly through the mental foramen into the facial vein, or posteriorly through the mandibular foramen into the pterygoid venous plexus. However, the main venous drainage of the mandible is via periosteal veins which themselves drain into the jugular veins (Cohen, 1959). In the maxilla, the veins accompany the superior alveolar arteries and drain either anteriorly into the facial vein or posteriorly into the pterygoid venous plexus.

Because of its frequent use as a model for studying the periodontal ligament, it is appropriate to mention here the vasculature of the continuously growing incisor. Such teeth have a more complicated vascular supply, due perhaps to the special requirement associated with the continuous formation of dental tissues by the proliferative odontogenic zone at its base. Kindlová and Matĕna (1959) and Matĕna (1973) studied the mandibular incisor of the rat using a variety of techniques: corrosive specimens, cleared jaws and histological sections. The arterial and venous vessels could be distinguished by comparing specimens obtained after intra-arterial and intravenous injections. Regarding the arterial system, Kindlová and Matĕna (1959) found two basic variations. In some animals, the mandibular artery was seen to supply the apical part of the incisor periodontal ligament, the central and incisal parts being supplied by the mental artery. In others, the mental artery supplied the incisal and apical parts of the

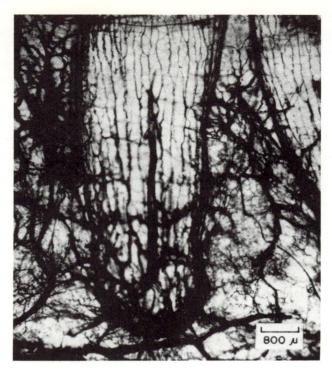

FIG. 1. Human mandibular periodontal ligament and surrounding alveolar bone. Delicate vessels arranged in palisades are seen in the ligament. A dense venous network surrounds the apex of alveolus. China ink injection, decalcified and cleared.

periodontal ligament, the mandibular artery running into the central part of the periodontal ligament. For both variants, the mandibular artery supplied the molars. As well as these main arteries, many small vessels from the periosteum were seen to perforate the bone to form a rich accessory supply for the periodontal ligament.

The venous outflow from the rat incisor periodontal ligament is collected into a rich venous network which is located close to the alveolus outside the continuous layer of supplying arteries (Kindlová and Matěna, 1959). Near the enamel organ, where the periodontal connective tissue is not attached into the tooth, the venous network is particularly dense. From this network, large veins ascend in the connective tissue close to the enamel. Similar observations have been made by Carranza *et al.* (1966).

Arrangement of vessels within the periodontal ligament

A variety of techniques have been used to investigate the structure and arrangement of the blood vessels within the periodontal ligament. Studies have been based upon routine histological and ultrastructural techniques, the inspection of perforations in the wall of the tooth socket, the use of microspheres to determine vessel diameters and, most commonly, various perfusion techniques.

THE VASCULAR ARRANGEMENT AS DEDUCED BY STUDYING THE PERFORATIONS IN THE WALLS OF THE TOOTH SOCKET

Following intravascular injection of indian ink to rats, Birn (1966) found a correlation between the number and size of perforations in the tooth socket and the vessels that they carried. It seems, therefore, that simply by examining a tooth socket reasonably reliable data about the periodontal ligament vasculature can be obtained. On this basis, Birn (1966) estimated the vascularity of the human periodontal ligament from the examination of eighty-four human tooth sockets (in dried specimens). He reported that generally the blood supply was greatest in the cervical part of the periodontal ligament and least marked in its middle third. Furthermore, the periodontal tissues of posterior teeth seemed to be more vascular than those for anterior teeth. However, different reports on the distribution of perforating vessels through the alveolar wall have been published. For example, Castelli and Dempster (1965) stated that perforating arterioles generally enter the periodontal ligament through the apical two-thirds of the alveolus. In view of such discrepancies, the assumption of a correlation between numbers and sizes of perforations and blood vessels awaits confirmation. It also should be mentioned that the number of wide-bore vessels per unit surface area reported gives little information about the blood flow. Instead, a high density of wide-bore blood vessels (i.e. veins) is simply indicative of the capacity of the tissue to hold blood.

BLOOD VESSELS STUDIED IN CORROSIVE SPECIMENS AND HISTOLOGICAL SECTIONS

To visualize the arrangement of blood vessels supplying the periodontal ligament it is possible to perfuse the vascular system with a radiopaque, coloured or particle-containing perfusion medium. The tissue may then be cleared (Boyer and Neptune, 1962; Castelli, 1963; Castelli and Dempster, 1965; Kennedy, 1969; Turner et al., 1969; Khouw and Goldhaber, 1970), serially sectioned (Hayashi, 1932; Waerhaug, 1954; Ishimitsu, 1960; Kennedy, 1969; Turner et al., 1969) or radiographed (Perint, 1949; Castelli and Dempster, 1965). Saunders (1966) combined radiography with microscopy. Alternatively, using material which congeals within the blood vessels, it is possible to dissolve the surrounding tissues to produce a corrosive specimen which can be studied with the stereomicroscope (Kindlová

and Matěna, 1959, 1962; Lenz, 1968) or with the scanning electron microscope (Lenz, 1968, 1974; Ichikawa, Watanabe and Yamamura, 1977). However, that significant dimensional changes occur with such techniques must be remembered when measuring vessel diameters. Brånemark, Lundskog and Lundström (1968) reported that vessel diameters in perfused specimens varied by as much as 10–15% from the values obtained using vital microscopy. Zweifach (1961) concluded that neither perfusion nor histological techniques should be used alone to measure vessels which are less than 30 μm in diameter. Another problem concerns the fact that corrosive specimens have the inherent disadvantage of not permitting the localization of the vessels in relation to other tissue elements. Care also must be taken when classifying fine vessels using these techniques. Knowledge of the direction of blood flow in a vessel and its connections with other vessels (in addition to data on width and structure) is essential for a proper classification.

The periodontal ligament vasculature has been studied using corrosive specimens and histological sections in a number of species. For example, it has been examined by Kindlová (1965) and Lenz (1968) in primates, by Ichikawa et al. (1977) in dogs and by Kindlová and Matěna (1959, 1962) in rats.

In the monkey, the main vessels of the ligament are arranged in palisades and run parallel to the long axis of the tooth. They are surrounded by loose connective tissue and pass between the principal fibre bundles of the ligament. These main vessels branch to form capillaries arranged in a flat network. In this way, a basket-like net of vessels surrounds the root surface. This is located nearer the alveolus than the root surface. Lenz (1968) estimated that the calibre of the vessels was between 15 μm and 100 μm, with the wider-bore vessels predominating. Kindlová (1965) found that arteries adjacent to the interradicular septi of multirooted teeth were fewer than in other parts of the ligament.

In the cervical region of the periodontal ligament, Kindlová (1965) observed that the vascular bed had a slightly different arrangement. Here, the rather flat main network was condensed into a narrow band from which single capillaries were given off to form structures resembling glomeruli. Near the junctional epithelium, slender, looped capillaries with markedly coiled arterial parts were observed. The main vessels of the periodontal ligament were seen to anastomose in this area with vessels from the gingiva (Fig. 2). (For further information regarding the glomeruli, see below.)

A vascular arrangement similar to that seen in the primates was observed in the ligament of the rat molar (Kindlová and Matěna, 1962). However, it was noted that there were no direct, fine anastomoses between periodontal and gingival arteries, though communicating capillaries were seen between gingival arterioles and periodontal ligament veins.

Kindlová and Matěna (1959) have described the vascular arrangement in the rat incisor periodontal ligament. They observed that the vasculature is different in the apical, middle and incisal parts of the ligament. Near the root base numerous capillaries arise separately from the afferent artery, forming a fine plexus. These capillaries drain independently into the rich venous net. In the middle region of the ligament the main afferent arteries run parallel to the long axis of the tooth and show few anastomoses with each other. From these vessels, branches pass out to supply the sides of the ligament where they form capillary networks. These capillaries lead into short venous channels (which also receive blood from the capillaries supplying the enamel organ). In the incisal area, the arteries again run parallel to the long axis of the tooth but are interconnected. At the margins of the periodontal ligament close to the enamel they form an irregular meshwork. The vascular supply associated with the enamel organ forms a more or less self-contained unit with a vascular arrangement different to that of the periodontal ligament proper.

Routine histological studies with light microscopy have produced results which generally agree with the above-mentioned observations obtained using corrosive specimens combined with histology. Carranza et al. (1966) described the periodontal blood vessels in rat, mouse, hamster, guinea pig, cat and dog using a histochemical technique to demonstrate adenosine-triphosphatase. In all species, a vascular plexus located close to the bone was seen running parallel to the long axis of the tooth. Vessels perforating the alveolar walls were most abundant in the middle and apical thirds of the alveolus. In areas close to the enamel in guinea-pig molar and rodent incisors, an increased density of vessels was observed. For the rat and mouse molars, communications were seen between periodontal and pulpal blood vessels. Similar communications have been reported in man (Hayashi, 1932; Sicher, 1966). The histological appearance of human periodontal ligament blood vessels is illustrated in Figs. 3 and 4. Note that the blood vessels (and nerves) are located in interstitial spaces (containing loose connective tissue) between the principal collagen fibres. Several blood vessels of different diameters are seen in each space.

Wedl (1881) was the first to mention the resemblance between the vascular formations in the periodontal ligament and renal glomeruli. He reported that 'periodontal glomeruli' were seen in several mammals (including man). Hayashi (1932) and Ishimitsu (1960) also reported on the 'glomeruli' in the human periodontal ligament. However, in studies where the

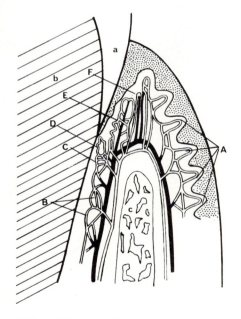

FIG. 2. Scheme of the blood supply of the marginal periodontium in monkey. A: Subepithelial capillary network of gingiva. B: Capillary network in the periodontal ligament. C: Band of denser capillary network in the periodontal ligament. D: Coiled capillaries resembling glomeruli. E: Capillary loops with the amply coiled arterial part. F: Simple capillary loops. a: Enamel. b: Dentine. c: Bone.

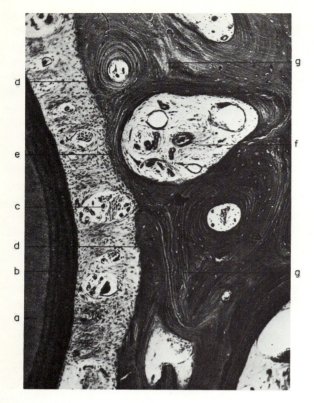

FIG. 3. Human periodontal ligament. Horizontal section. a: Dentine. b: Cementum. c: Interstitial space. d: Resorption lacunae on the wall of the alveolus. e: Narrow bone trabecula separating a marrow space (f) from the periodontal ligament. g: Lamellated bone.

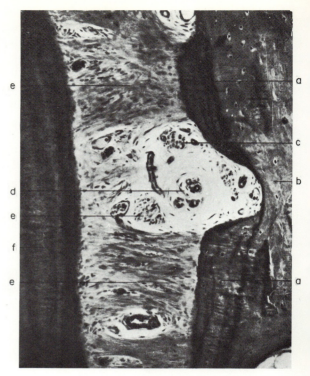

FIG. 4. Human periodontal ligament. Horizontal section. a: Bundle bone, on both sides of an interstitial space containing blood vessels (d) and bundles of nerve fibres (c). b: Lamellated bone. e: Principal fibres. f: Cementum.

tissue is perfused and then macerated, the 'glomeruli' have not been observed in the periodontal ligament. Kindlová (1965) has reported another site in the periodontal tissues containing glomeruli-like structures. She observed coiled capillaries resembling glomeruli between the alveolar crest and the junctional epithelium in the monkey (Fig. 2). At the corresponding location in the rat molar, Kindlová and Matěna (1962) also found coiling capillary loops. Combining the results from perfusion and histological studies in the monkey, Lenz (1968) did not observe any 'glomeruli' in the periodontal ligament proper. In a subsequent study on the monkey, however, Lenz (1974) confirmed Kindlová's observation on the presence of glomeruli-like structures coronal to the alveolar crest. Waerhaug (1954) interpreted the 'glomeruli' in the periodontal liga-

ment proper as being branching vessels which perforate the alveolar wall. Hayashi's (1932) claim that the 'glomeruli' are always located in recesses in the alveolar wall lends support to the idea that a 'glomerulus' is a bundle of branching vessels contained in an interstitial space. In this context, Ishimitsu (1960) reported the presence of many arterio-venous shunts in these areas. He also observed that the thickness of the arterial walls showed great variability in different sections, perhaps indicating a capacity to change lumen diameter actively.

STUDIES ON VESSEL DIAMETERS USING MICROSPHERES

Folke and Stallard (1967) studied periodontal ligament blood vessel diameters in the monkey following the injection of plastic microspheres into the external carotid artery. This technique relies upon the spheres being carried with the blood until they are trapped by vessels with a corresponding diameter. Folke and Stallard (1967) found that few 35 μm spheres were trapped in the periodontal tissues. They concluded, therefore, that the vessel diameters in the periodontal ligament and the gingiva were 30 μm or less. Using 15 ± 5 μm microspheres, they were unable to verify the presence of periodontal vessels running parallel to the root, which have often been described in perfusion studies. Instead, the microspheres were found most frequently within the branching vessels which resembled the 'glomeruli' described by Wedl (1881) and in which Ishimitsu (1960) found arterio-venous shunts (Fig. 5). Despite the lack of quantification, Folke and Stallard (1967) claimed that fewer microspheres were trapped in the periodontal ligament than in the other tissues of the periodontium. They suggested that the ligament vasculature 'consists of a greater number of either preferential channels or an overall increase in vessel diameter'. That most spheres in the ligament were trapped in the 'glomeruli' supports the view of Waerhaug (1954) that they are the branching points of perforating arterioles coming from the bone marrow. Folke and Stallard (1967) suggested that these branching points acted as sphincters to control blood flow in the ligament. However, data of this kind cannot answer the question whether arterio-venous shunting of blood really occurs at these sites.

In contrast to Folke and Stallard (1967), Vandersall and Zander (1967) reported that intra-arterial injection of 35 ± 5 μm microspheres resulted in trapping of spheres throughout the gingiva, alveolar bone and periodontal ligament. However, their results agree with respect to the relative distribution of spheres in the various tissues. Thus, the periodontal ligament trapped a much smaller number of spheres than the gingiva and the alveolar bone.

Kennedy and Zander (1969) injected 20 ± 7 μm microspheres into the external carotid arteries of monkeys and observed histopathological reactions. They found lesions in gingival epithelium 10 hours after injection as a result of the ischaemia produced by the trapped spheres. Necrosis of all epithelial layers of the gingiva was seen 24 hours after injection. However, the junctional epithelium was least affected. The authors suggested that this was due to the presence of a collateral circulation from the vessels in the periodontal ligament. In a subsequent study, Kennedy (1969) perfused the periodontal vascular beds bilaterally with India ink after a unilateral injection of microspheres. This technique enabled visualization of those vessels which remained patent after the microspheres injection. As for previous studies, spheres were seldom seen trapped in the vessels of the periodontal ligament and the alveolar bone. In contrast to periosteal and gingival vessels, most periodontal ligament and bone marrow vessels could be perfused with the indian ink after the injection of microspheres. Hence, it seems that the periodontal ligament (and the adjacent bone marrow) contains preferential channels and/or arterio-venous shunts which are wider than the corresponding vessels in the gingiva and the periosteum.

ULTRASTRUCTURAL STUDIES OF THE BLOOD VESSELS OF THE PERIODONTAL LIGAMENT

There is little information on the ultrastructure of the periodontal ligament vasculature. Bevelander and Nakahara (1968) studied the human ligament and reported that the vessels were thin-walled and showed marked variations in lumen calibre. They were seen to be surrounded by a thin coat of collagen fibres and scattered fibroblasts. The inner lining of endothelial cells rested upon a basement membrane. In the rat molar ligament, Frank, Fellinger and Steuer (1976) observed that, whilst most blood capillaries have a continuous epithelium, a few fenestrated capillaries may be seen. Since continuous and fenestrated capillaries possess markedly different permeability characteristics (e.g. Dresel, Folkow and Wallentin, 1966), a more detailed, and quantitative, ultrastructural study may contribute much to our understanding of the functioning of the periodontal ligament vasculature.

Griffin and Spain (1972) described in the human periodontal ligament blood vessels closely associated with nerves (myelinated and unmyelinated). They considered these complexes to be a type of mechano-receptor (see also Chapter 8). The complexes were vascularized by encapsulated terminal arterioles, metarterioles and capillaries. Veins (presumably collecting veins) formed arcades surrounding the

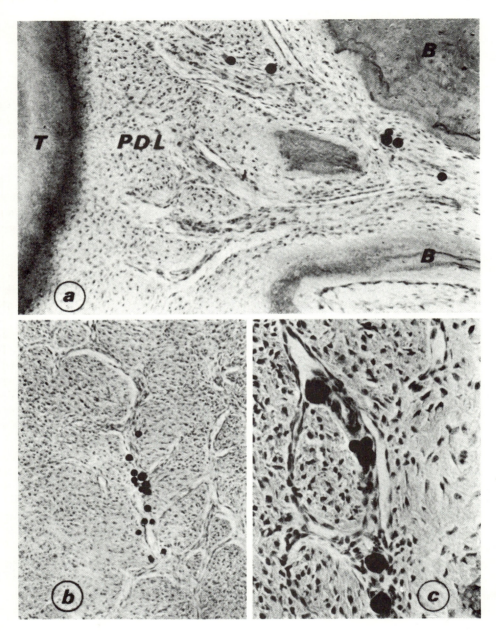

FIG. 5. Monkey periodontal ligament. Composite photomicrograph demonstrating the location of microspheres. (a) Note the emergence of the blood vessels from the alveolar bone (B) into the periodontal ligament (PDL) and their subsequent branching. T: Tooth. (b) Network of vessel within the ligament and trapped microspheres in association with them. (c) Higher magnification demonstrating the presence of microspheres within the vessel bundles called 'glomeruli' by Wedl.

neuro-vascular complexes. Griffin and Spain (1972) could not demonstrate any innervation of the terminal arterioles or metarterioles. Harris and Griffin (1974) further studied the neural complexes and reported that a metarteriole terminating in a capillary complex is encapsulated with the myelinated and unmyelinated nerve fibres.

Sims (1975, 1976) demonstrated that oxytalan fibres in the periodontal ligament often terminate around the blood vessels. This arrangement he implicated in the support of the blood vessels. Assuming that oxytalan fibres influence blood flow in the periodontal ligament during biting such fibres might also play a role in the tooth support mechanism (see Chapter 11 for information concerning the involvement of the vasculature in the tooth support mechanism). Whilst oxytalan fibres have been identified with the electron microscope, to date the relationship between the oxytalan fibres and the blood vessels has only been studied under the light microscope.

VASCULAR FUNCTION IN THE PERIODONTAL LIGAMENT

Blood flow as studied directly by vital microscopy

While intravital microscopic techniques for studying blood flow in bone and dental pulp have been established for more than two decades, only recently have they been used to study the microcirculation of the periodontal ligament. One of the major difficulties encountered relates to the fact that the blood supply of the periodontal ligament is derived from virtually all the neighbouring tissues. Consequently, a window cut for intravital observation of blood flow is likely to disturb detrimentally the periodontal blood supply. However, Gängler and Merte (1979a) have described a technique using the rat mandibular incisor which they claim minimizes this disturbance. The mandible is divided at the symphysis to allow alveolar bone, dentine and pulp to be removed from the lateral side until only a thin layer of dentine remains through which the periodontal ligament blood flow can be

observed under transmitted light (Fig. 6). Using this technique, Gängler and Merte (1979b) compared the resting blood flow in the periodontal ligament and gingival microcirculations. The linear flow velocity was measured in various types of vessels in both tissues and found to be about the same for each type. With respect to the structural arrangement of the ligament vasculature, they reported that numerous anastomoses between arterial and venous vessels which formed polygonal rings could be found (Figs. 7 and 8). However, they did not mention whether there were any short, wide-bore, arteriovenous shunts of the kind seen in the dental pulp. Also they could not see any sinusoidal, venous, capacitance vessels.

Since the periodontal ligament receives a major part of its blood supply from the alveolar bone marrow, it is pertinent to provide comparisons between the microcirculations in periodontal ligament and bone. It should be kept in mind, however, that, in contrast to periodontal ligament vessels, bone-marrow vessels are enclosed in a rigid bone capsule. Further, spacious thin-walled sinusoids are dominant in the marrow. Brånemark (1959) studied rabbit tibial blood flow, both in compact bone and in the marrow. For the vessels in compact bone, the flow was remarkably constant and resistant to environmental change. He reported that the linear flow rate in compact bone was 0.5—0.8 mm/s in capillaries

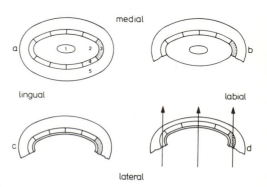

FIG. 6. Technique for vital microscopy of the rat incisor periodontal ligament. a: Transverse section in the middle of the root. 1: Pulp. 2: Dentine. 3: 'Perienamel' space. 4: 'Peridentine' space. 5: Alveolar bone. b, c and d show the stages of preparation of a window for vital microscopy with transmitted light.

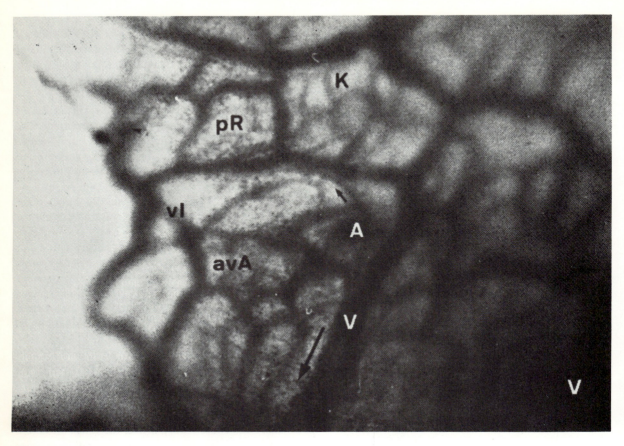

FIG. 7. Rat periodontal ligament vasculature seen in transmitted light with vital microscopy. A: Artery. avA: Arteriolar-venular anastomosis. pR: Polygonal ring. K: Capillary. V: Vein. ×80.

and 0.2–0.5 mm/s in venules. The corresponding rates for the marrow were lower, being 0.5 mm/s and 0.1–0.3 mm/s respectively. When the data from the rabbit tibia are compared with those from the rat incisor periodontal ligament recorded by Gängler and Merte (1979b), a marked difference can be discerned. A capillary flow rate in the periodontal ligament of only 0.02–0.04 mm/s was measured. The rate in the venules was 0.1 mm/s. Thus, the bone capillary flow rates are more than ten times greater than periodontal capillary rates. At the time of writing, it is difficult to evaluate whether such differences are real, are due to experimental difficulties (for example, in maintaining blood flows at normal rates), or represent species differences. Since the capillaries of the bone marrow have diameters of

8 μm (Brånemark, 1959) compared with the diameters of 5–7 μm for periodontal ligament capillaries (Gängler and Merte, 1979b), it is possible that there are more branches and anastomoses in the periodontal ligament than in the bone marrow. If this is so, a slower blood flow in the periodontal ligament is to be expected.

Blood flow as studied by indirect techniques

Because of the technical problems involved in measuring blood flow exclusively in a tissue having a thickness of only $\sim$0.2 mm, quantitative measurements of the blood flow in the periodontal ligament using

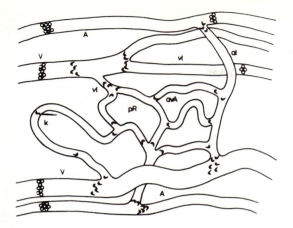

FIG. 8. Diagrammatic representation of the longitudinally arranged vascular bed in the periodontal ligament of the rat incisor. A: Artery. V: Vein. al: Arteriole. k: Capillary. vl: Venule. avA: Arteriolar—venular anastomosis. pR: Polygonal ring.

indirect techniques have not been made. In addition, that the periodontal ligament receives its blood supply via fine vessels from diverse sources indicates that its vascular bed is not an isolated functional unit.

One technique that has been employed to study blood flow in the oral tissues involves the use of radiolabelled microspheres. Using 15 ± 5 μm microspheres, Kaplan, Jeffcoat and Goldhaber (1978) estimated blood flow in the alveolar bone in dogs to be about 0.1 ml/min/g. Previously, Meyer (1970) and Path and Meyer (1977) reported higher flows — in the range of 0.1—0.5 ml/min/g. Comparisons between blood flow in mandibular alveolar bone and in gingiva were made by Kaplan, Davis and Goldhaber (1978) from studies using radiolabelled microspheres and a diffusible tracer (^{86}Rb). They reported significantly higher flow values in the gingiva (0.5 ml/min/g in gingiva and 0.1 ml/min/g in alveolar bone). To date, these techniques have not been applied to the study of the periodontal ligament vasculature.

Another indirect method to study local blood flow involves the measurement of the local clearance of a diffusible, inert, radioactive tracer injected directly into the tissue. This technique was devised by Kety (1949). Kety used radioactive sodium, but nowadays the inert lipid soluble gas ^{133}Xe or ^{125}I as iodide is more commonly used. These tracers

(especially Xe) pass so rapidly from the tissue to the blood that in most instances the rate of wash-out from the injection site is limited only by blood flow. If the tissue in which the injected depot is located is perfused uniformly and constantly with blood, the rate at which the tracer is washed out has a mono-exponential function. Thus, when tracer concentration is plotted against time on semilog paper, the wash-out curve forms a straight line. The slope of this curve is related to the rate of blood flow. For example, the curve becomes horizontal if blood flow is arrested suddenly. It must be emphasized that, since this technique reflects the rate of exchange of solutes between tissue and blood, the nutritive function of the blood flow is accentuated. Consequently, blood shunted away from capillaries via arterio-venous anastomoses will not be discerned by this technique. Edwall and Kindlová (1971) used tracer disappearance techniques to obtain some measure of blood flow in various oral tissues, including the periodontal ligament. Although the method did not allow quantitative calculations of blood flow, their results suggested that there were no significant differences between the rates of disappearance of tracers in periodontal ligament, gingiva, dental pulp and alveolar submucosa. Thus, blood flow seems to be of the same order of magnitude in these tissues. However, the techniques involved (i.e. injection of 10—20 μl of fluid into the periodontal space in the bifurcation area of a mandibular molar of the dog via a channel drilled from the pulp chamber) might have resulted in spread of the depot fluid into the adjacent alveolar bone. Therefore, their data for the periodontal ligament probably reflect a combined effect in both the ligament and the adjacent bone.

Linden (1975) has assessed the effects of stimulating the cervical sympathetic trunk on the periodontal ligament by monitoring temperature changes within the tissue. This technique offers another possibility for indirectly assessing changes in periodontal ligament blood flow, though precise data cannot be provided. His results will be discussed further in the section concerned with the control of the blood circulation (page 165).

Blood volume changes monitored by plethysmographic techniques

Plethysmography involves the measurement of volume changes in the tissue under study. If the venous outflow can be obstructed intermittently, the technique can measure total blood flow. Unfortunately, it is not possible to measure precisely volume changes in the periodontal ligament nor to control venous outflow. Thus, plethysmography can only hint at changes in blood flow within the periodontal ligament.

Packman, Shoher and Stein (1977) used photoelectric plethysmography to monitor changes in the microcirculation of the human periodontal ligament. The technique is based on the principle that, when a tissue is transilluminated, some of the light is absorbed by the vascular components of the tissue. Whilst certain non-vascular components of the tissue can also absorb light, their opacity remains essentially constant over short periods of time. Thus, any rapid variation of light absorption represents vascular changes. The main difficulty with this technique concerns the conversion of the light intensity data into changes in basic circulatory parameters (e.g. blood volume), because light absorption also depends on other factors (e.g. the local hematocrit). In the study of Packman et al. (1977), light was conducted to and from the periodontal tissues either via miniature fibre optics placed within the roots of endodontically treated teeth or by trans-illuminating the ligament from the gingiva. They monitored circulatory activity with the teeth at rest and under intrusive and horizontal loads. Pulsatile changes were recorded at rest which were synchronous with the heart beat. They reported that loading a tooth produced a decrease in blood volume in areas under compression. In an area under tension, however, an initial increase in blood volume was followed by a decrease as the magnitude of force rose. However, their results may not only reflect circulatory changes in the periodontal ligament but may also relate to changes in the alveolar bone and, in the case of transillumination, in the gingiva.

Another way to use the principle of plethysmography to investigate the periodontal vasculature involves monitoring changes in tooth position. A number of studies have reported that the ligament allows minute movements of the tooth which are synchronous with pulsatile changes in blood pressure (e.g. Hofmann and Diemer, 1963; Körber, 1963; Körber and Körber, 1965; Körber, 1970) (Figs. 9 and 10). The amplitude of movement is usually less than 0.5 μm (e.g. Hofmann and Diemer, 1963; Körber and Körber, 1965), the pulsatile movements axially being less than those labially. These tooth movements can only be interpreted in terms of pulsatile changes in local tissue and blood pressures. Using displacement transducers which are sensitive enough to allow continuous monitoring of tooth position, it has been possible to study tooth position in rabbit and rat incisors and ferret and cat canines (Matthews and Berkovitz, 1972; Lisney, Matthews and Sharp, 1972; Moxham, 1975, 1976, 1978, 1979 a, b; Aars, 1976, 1978; Myhre, Preus and Aars, 1978, 1979; Burn-Murdoch and Picton, 1978; Linden and Aars, 1979; Moxham and Berkovitz, in press). Many of these studies report clear-cut changes following experimental interference with the vascular system (e.g. see Fig. 11 and Chapter 10) and it seems that the resting position of the tooth is influenced by the arterial blood pressure via the periodontal vessels (the probable mechanism being an alteration in vascular volumes or tissue pressures in the periodontium). Such techniques also have been used to investigate the vasomotor control of the periodontal vasculature (see pages 165, 166) and to study the mechanisms of tooth support and eruption (see Chapters 11 and 10 respectively).

The measurement of interstitial pressures in the periodontal ligament

Few investigations have dealt with tissue pressure of the periodontal ligament. Schärer and Hayashi (1969) were the first to report on periodontal ligament tissue pressure, recording changes in pressure following force application. Subsequently, Lamb and Van Hassel (1972) and Palcanis (1973) studied the pressures during resting conditions and following traumatic occlusion, tissue damage and infiltration of Lidocaine with adrenaline (Fig. 12). The resting tissue pressure in the canine tooth of the dog was

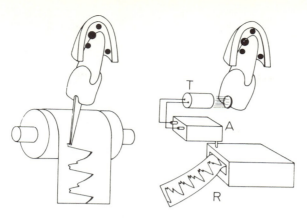

FIG. 9. Diagrams to show methods of recording periodontal pulsation. Right: system of electronic measurement without touching the tooth. T: Transducer. A: Amplifier. R: Recorder.

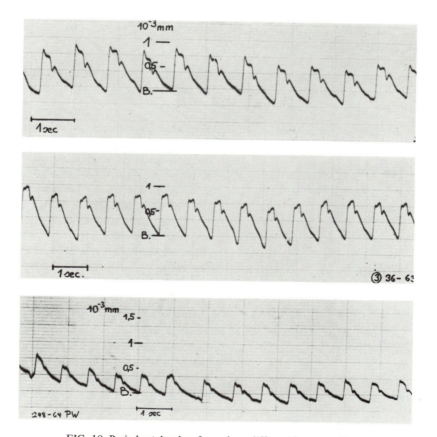

FIG. 10. Periodontal pulses from three different human subjects.

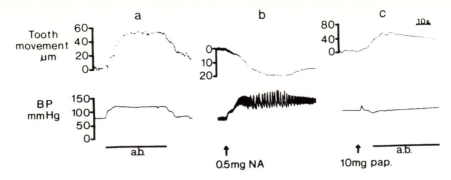

FIG. 11. Changes in position of rabbit incisor resulting from alteration of arterial blood pressure and injection of vasoactive drugs. Responses to: (a) inflation of a balloon in the descending aorta; (b) i.v. injection of noradrenaline; (c) i.v. injection of papaverine. Reduction in arterial pressure after injection of papaverine was avoided by inflation of the aortic balloon (a.b.).

seen to average 9–10 mm Hg above atmospheric pressure. Trauma was found to double the pressure. Infiltration of the vasoconstrictor agent reduced the periodontal ligament tissue pressure. More recently, however, Walker, Ng and Burke (1978) reported that the resting periodontal ligament pressure was about 2 mm Hg below atmospheric pressure. It is known from studies of pulpal interstitial pressure (e.g. Nähri, 1978) that marked pressure gradients

occur over a distance of only a few millimetres within the tissue. It is possible, therefore, that the tissue pressures recorded in the periodontal ligament reflect very localized pressures at the sites of measurement.

Control of the periodontal ligament vasculature

The vascular control in the periodontal ligament has only recently attracted attention. Using tracer disappearance techniques (see page 161), Edwall and Kindlová (1971) studied the effects of sympathetic nerve activation on the periodontal ligament vasculature in the dog. They reported that the wash-out rates were reduced following sympathetic activation and that there was a clear frequency-response relationship between the stimulation frequency and the reduction of nutritive blood flow. This study also involved monitoring blood flow in other tissues (i.e. pulp, gingiva, alveolar submucosa and gastrocnemius muscle). Sympathetic nerve stimulation induced reduction of up to 70% in tracer disappearance rate in all the oral tissues investigated with the exception of the periodontal ligament where the response was higher (about 90% reduction). This 90% reduction, however, concerns also the alveolar bone because of the possibility of spread of the depot and the route of drainage from the ligament. Sympathetic nerve stimulation produced responses in the oral

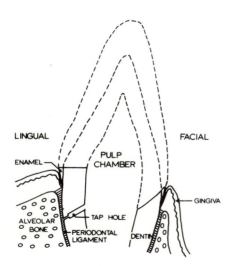

FIG. 12. Diagram explaining the method of preparing a canine tooth in the dog for recording interstitial pressure in the periodontal ligament. The portion of the tooth sketched by dotted lines was removed during preparation.

tissues of the same order of magnitude as those obtained in skeletal muscle (gastrocnemius) using a similar technique. A typical experiment protocol is illustrated in Fig. 13. Here, the effects of three sympathetic stimulations with different frequencies are shown on the semilog plot of the wash-out curve. Note that, in spite of pronounced elevation of systemic arterial pressure (third stimulation), the k-value (representing the fractional elimination of the depot per minute) is close to zero, indicating a pronounced reduction of nutritive blood flow. These effects were seen at stimulation frequencies of 0.1–6 Hz (frequencies which are within the physiological range of discharge in sympathetic nerves). In experiments on the pulp and submucosa, α-adrenoceptor blocking agents were able to block the reduction in k-value. It is not unreasonable to assume that the responses obtained in the periodontal ligament also were mediated by adrenoceptors of the α-type.

Moxham (1975, 1976, 1978) reported that stimulation of the peripheral cut end of the ipsilateral cervical sympathetic trunk produced intrusive movements of the rabbit mandibular incisor. Aars (1976) reported that sympathetic nerve activation induced abrupt intrusion of the rabbit maxillary incisor and that unilateral cutting of the sympathetic trunk resulted in 20–40 μm extrusion of the tooth.

Bilateral sectioning was seen to double the extrusion. Subsequent electrical stimulation of the sectioned nerves made the tooth move back into its socket, the position held prior to nerve section being obtained with stimuli between 0.5 and 1 Hz. About 90% of the maximal inward movement was seen following bilateral stimulation with 4 Hz. Aars (1978) found that the intrusion induced by sympathetic activation could be blocked by α-adrenoceptor agents. This observation supports the contention of Edwall and Kindlová (1971) that sympathetically innervated α-adrenoceptors mediate the vasoconstriction. Aars (1978) suggested that the precapillary resistance vessels were targets for the vasoconstrictor influence.

Linden (1975) investigated the effects of nerve stimulations and transections on periodontal ligament temperature. Stimulation of the cervical sympathetic trunk was associated with a fall in ligament temperature. Transection of the inferior alveolar nerve was found to prevent this fall in ligament temperature. Since similar results have been reported in studies on pulpal blood flow (Tønder and Naess, 1978; Gazelius and Olgart, 1980), this indicates that the sympathetic pathway to the mandibular teeth is contained in the inferior alveolar nerve (see also Chapter 8, page 192). When Linden (1975) stimulated the distal end of the transected inferior nerve, how-

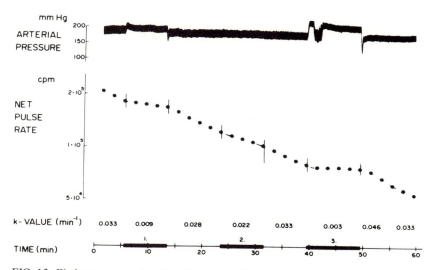

FIG. 13. Wash-out curve of radioactive xenon illustrating changes in nutritive blood flow in the periodontal ligament and adjacent alveolar bone of the dog. Signals on the abscissa show periods of sympathetic nerve stimulation. 1: Stimulation with 2.5 Hz. 2: Stimulation with 0.25 Hz. 3: Stimulation with 6 Hz.

ever, the full effect of sympathetic stimulation could not be reproduced. More recently, Gazelius and Olgart (1980) reported that stimulation of the transected inferior alveolar nerve antidromically induced a biphasic vascular response in the pulp which was converted to a clear-cut increase in pulp blood flow after α-adrenoceptor blockade. These observations indicate that the inferior alveolar nerve, apart from containing sympathetic nerve fibres, possesses fibres which have a vasodilator function. It has been suggested that this dilator effect is mediated by Substance P (Gazelius and Olgart, 1980) and it will be important to see whether this mechanism is also present in the periodontal ligament.

Aars (1978) reported that β-adrenoreceptor blockade produced by infusion of propranolol extruded the tooth while infusion of isoprenaline reversed or prevented this movement. This result indicates a double adrenergic control of the periodontal ligament vasculature: (i) sympathetically innervated α-adrenoceptors mediating constriction of precapillary vessels, and (ii) β-adrenoreceptors mediating dilation of post-capillary resistance vessels. The results reported by Aars (1976, 1978) also suggest that both the pre- and post-capillary resistance vessels were under the influence of a sympathetic tone (nervous and humoral) during the experiment; nerve transection or propranolol both induced extrusion. Since the experiments were performed under general anaesthesia, however, it cannot be stated to what extent such sympathetic tone is present in the conscious animal.

There seems to be little information about other types of nervous vasomotor control (e.g. cholinergic, peptidergic control). Aars (1978) noted that atropine had no effect on the resting position of the rabbit incisor. In the cat, however, Linden and Aars (1979) observed that activation of low-threshold fibres in the sympathetic nerve could induce extrusion, possibly mediated by cholinergic, vascular receptors.

Little is known about the extent to which humoral agents affect the periodontal ligament vessels. Aars (1978) suggested that the β-adrenergic vasodilatation in the post-capillary resistance vessels was due to circulating noradrenaline. Moxham (1977, 1978, 1979b) and Myhre, Preus and Aars (1978) found that noradrenaline infused intra-vascularly resulted in an intrusive movement of the rabbit incisor.

Since it is established that there is a sympathetic vasoconstrictor control of the periodontal vasculature, it seems appropriate to consider the neuroeffector arrangement. Generally, arterioles are densely innervated in most vascular beds, while relatively few adrenergic nerve fibres reach the precapillary 'sphincters'. Veins show a density of innervation which varies in different vasculatures. At present, no information is available about the location of the adrenergic nerve fibres and terminals which control the periodontal ligament blood flow. If few adrenergic fibres are in the ligament, then perhaps its blood flow is regulated by nerves located in the adjacent alveolar bone. A similar arrangement has been found in the rat incisor pulp. Here the tissue seems to lack adrenergic fibres (Pohto and Antila, 1968) despite having a sympathetic vasomotor control of remarkable efficiency (Scott Jr. et al., 1972). On the other hand, in the cat dental pulp there is a sympathetic vasomotor control of similar efficiency (Edwall, unpublished) but with an adrenergic innervation in the major part of the tissue (Pohto and Antila, 1968).

The nutritive role of the periodontal ligament vasculature for the tooth

Wasserman et al. (1941) demonstrated that pulpless teeth continue to take up phosphorus via the cementum of the root and that about 10% of the amount of phosphorus taken up by normal teeth during 24 hours enters via the periodontal ligament. Gilda, McCauley and Johansson (1943) performed similar experiments and reported that 25% of the phosphorus uptake during 36 hours had entered via the ligament vasculature. Stüben and Spreter von Kreudenstein (1960) reported similar results for penicillin. Thus, there is good evidence that substances pass from the vessels of the periodontal ligament into the hard tissues of the root.

AGE CHANGES IN THE PERIODONTAL LIGAMENT VASCULATURE

Bernick (1962) investigated the effects of age using the molar teeth of rats (ranging from 1 to 18 months).

In the older animals, cellular cementum was formed in the apical third of the root. This was associated with the presence of capillary terminals adjacent to the cellular cementum. With further ageing, a progressive decrease in the number of interstitial vessels and their perforating branches was seen. Severson *et al.* (1978) studied eighty periodontal ligaments from twenty-four human cadavers ranging in age from 20 to 90 years. In the young specimens, numerous periodontal fibres surrounded the small, vascularized, interstitial spaces. In older specimens, these vascularized spaces appeared larger and encroached upon areas formerly occupied by periodontal fibres and bone. It is not yet clear, however, whether this change was also associated with an increase in the density of vessels within the ligament. Severson *et al.* (1978) reported that the older specimens contained a larger number of blood vessels in the interdental and interradicular bone. However, it was not stated how this comparison was accomplished.

LYMPHATIC VESSELS OF THE PERIODONTAL LIGAMENT

The existence of lymphatic vessels in the dental tissues has been a matter of much debate for many years. The periodontal ligament also has been involved in this dispute ever since Schweitzer (1907) stated that it has a rich network of lymphatic capillaries. Levy and Bernick (1968) and Bernick and Grant (1978) reported that staining thin sections by the PAS-hematoxylin reaction and thick sections with iron hematoxylin allowed a differentiation between lymphatic vessels and blood vessels. They stated that the lymphatic capillary consists only of an endothelial cell lining with no basement membrane, while the blood capillary consists of a single layer of endothelial cells and a well-defined basement membrane. In their earlier paper they claimed that lymph capillaries originated as blind endings in the stroma of the periodontal ligament and emptied into collecting lymph vessels. These collecting vessels supposedly had three pathways in the ligament; either they passed over the alveolar crest to drain into submucosal regions of palate and gingiva; or they perforated the alveolar

bone to traverse the spongiosa, or they passed directly apically in the periodontal ligament. However, the reliability of the morphological criteria for differentiating lymphatic and blood vessels is questionable.

More direct and convincing evidence of the presence of lymphatic vessels in the periodontal ligament can be found in the study on dogs by Ruben *et al.* (1971). By means of retroauricular (subcutaneous and deep) injections of Patent blue violet, the deep cervical lymphatic channels were located, ligated, and slowly perfused in the retrograde direction with Carbon black suspension. In this way, lymphatic vessels could be demonstrated in histological sections of the periodontal ligament, periosteum, gingiva, alveolar bone and dental pulp. Numerous lymphatic channels were seen on the alveolar side of the periodontal ligament (Figs. 14 and 15). The main drainage appeared to be in an apical direction, although lymphatic communications also were seen between the ligament, the

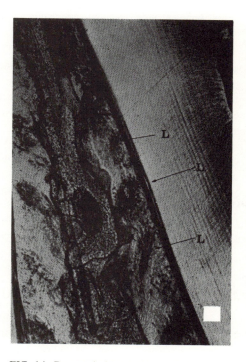

FIG. 14. Dog periodontal ligament after retrograde carbon perfusion of lymphatic vasculature. Carbon arranged in clusters. Lymph channels (L) found in the loose connective tissue between the fibre bundles.

FIG. 15. Same technique as previous figure. Tangentially cut area of periodontal ligament. Tooth is at left. Lymph vessels coursing between fibre bundles, with frequent intercommunications.

periosteum and the perivascular intraosseous channels. The authors emphasized that quantitatively the lymphatic system of the periodontal tissues appeared to be very small compared to its blood/vascular system.

Using intravital microscopy, Gängler and Merte (1979b) could not observe any lymphatic vessels. It is to be hoped that future studies using this technique in conjunction with retroauricular injection of Patent blue violet and retrograde lymphatic perfusion with carbon suspension will provide a means of visualizing periodontal ligament lymphatic vessels.

SUMMARY AND CONCLUDING REMARKS

1. The blood supply of the periodontal ligament is derived from arterial branches from the alveolar bone marrow, the periosteum and the gingiva. Communications with pulpal vessels also have been reported.

2. The blood vessels within the ligament are located between the principal collagen fibres near the alveolar bone in interstitial spaces which also contain loose connective tissue and nerves.

3. The veins from the ligament join larger veins in the septi of the alveolar bone and are connected to a rich venous network surrounding the apex of each alveolus.

4. The periodontal ligament and the adjacent bone marrow contain blood vessels (preferential channels and/or shunts) wider than the corresponding vessels in the gingiva and periosteum.

5. There have been many reports claiming that there are structures resembling renal glomeruli (possibly arterio-venous shunts) above the alveolar crest and sometimes in the periodontal ligament proper.

6. Vital microscopic studies suggest that blood flow may be slower in the periodontal ligament than in alveolar bone (perhaps due to a rich network of anastomosing vessels in the ligament). However, no short arterio-venous shunts have been seen with these techniques.

7. It has not yet been possible to obtain reliable values for blood flow in the periodontal ligament.

8. Changes in vascular volume or tissue pressure in the periodontal ligament influence the resting position of the tooth.

9. The resting tissue pressure in the periodontal ligament of the dog is about 10 mm Hg above atmospheric pressure; the pressure is increased by tissue damage and reduced by infiltration of a vasoconstrictor agent. However, one report states that the tissue pressures are subatmospheric.

10. Activation of sympathetic nerves to the jaws reduces the nutritive blood flow in the periodontal ligament, the effects being related to the frequency of stimulation, even within the physiological range of discharge in sympathetic nerves.

11. A double adrenergic vasomotor control of the periodontal ligament has been proposed: (i) α-adrenoceptors inducing constriction of precapillary resistance vessels and (ii) β-adrenoceptors mediating dilation of post-capillary resistance vessels.

12. A lymphatic system has been described in the periodontal ligament, though it is relatively minor compared to its blood/vascular system.

The periodontal ligament undoubtedly has unique functions among the connective tissues in the mammalian body. Its ability to tolerate high, intermittent pressures, combined with a sensory ability to detect small tactile stimuli as well as to discriminate between loads in the range up to 5 N (e.g. Anderson, Hannam and Matthews, 1970), is impressive. Therefore, it seems not unreasonable to expect that the vascular system in the periodontal ligament may also show characteristics not normally associated with connective tissues. However, such characteristics have not yet been reported (though one may be the high, supra-atmospheric, tissue pressure). One obvious reason for this is that few studies have been undertaken. Indeed, vital microscopy and studies on the vascular control of the periodontal ligament have only recently commenced. Among the basic information still lacking is: (i) the location and structural organization of the vasomotor innervation, (ii) the nervous and humoral vascular control (especially by adrenergic and peptidergic mechanisms and by biogenic agents involved in tissue damage), and (iii) the interaction between nutritional blood flow through exchange vessels and shunted blood flow through arterio-venous shunts. Techniques for analysis of these problems are becoming available and hopefully such work will be undertaken soon.

REFERENCES

AARS, H. (1976) Sympathetic nervous control of axial position of the rabbit incisor tooth. *Acta physiol. Scand.* Suppl. **440**, 131.

AARS, H. (1978) Adrenergic receptors in periodontal vessels. *Acta physiol. Scand.* **102**, 34–35A.

ANDERSON, D. J., HANNAM, A. G. & MATTHEWS, B. (1970) Sensory mechanisms in mammalian teeth and their supporting structures. *Physiol. Rev.* **50**, 171–195.

BERNICK, S. (1962) Age changes in the blood supply to molar teeth of rats. *Anat. Rec.* **144**, 265–274.

BERNICK, S. & GRANT, D. (1978) Lymphatic vessels of healthy and inflamed gingiva. *J. dent. Res.* **57**, 810–817.

BEVELANDER, G. & NAKAHARA, H. (1968) The fine structure of the human peridental ligament. *Anat. Rec.* **162**, 313–326.

BIRN, H. (1966) The vascular supply of the periodontal membrane. *J. periodont. Res.* **1**, 51–68.

BOYER, C. C. & NEPTUNE, C. M. (1962) Patterns of blood supply to teeth and adjacent tissues. *J. dent. Res.* **41**, 158–171.

BRÅNEMARK, P.-I. (1959) Vital microscopy of bone marrow in rabbit. *Scand. J. clin. Lab. Invest.* **11**, 38.

BRÅNEMARK, P., LUNDSKOG, J. & LUNDSTRÖM, J. (1968) Biomicroscopic evaluation of micro-angiographic methods. In: *Advances in Microcirculation.* H. HARDES (ed.), pp. 152–160. Basel, S. Karger.

BURN-MURDOCH, R. A. & PICTON, D. C. A. (1978) A technique for measuring eruption rates in rats of maxillary incisors under intrusive loads. *Archs. oral Biol.* **23**, 563–566.

CARRANZA, F. A., ITOIZ, M. E., CABRINI, R. L. & DOTTO, C. A. (1966) A study of periodontal vascularization in different laboratory animals. *J. periodont. Res.* **1**, 120–128.

CASTELLI, W. (1963) Vascular architecture of the human adult mandible. *J. dent. Res.* **42**, 786–792.

CASTELLI, W. A. & DEMPSTER, W. T. (1965) The periodontal vasculature and its responses to experimental pressure. *J. Amer. Dent. Assoc.* **70**, 890–905.

COHEN, L. (1959) The venous drainage of the mandible. *Oral Surg.* **12**, 1447–1449.

COHEN, L. (1960) Further studies into the vascular architecture of the mandible. *J. dent. Res.* **39**, 936–946.

CUTRIGHT, D. E. & HUNSUCK, E. E. (1970) Microcirculation of the perioral regions in the *Macaca rhesus.* Part II. *Oral Surg.* **29**, 926–934.

DRESEL, P., FOLKOW, B. & WALLENTIN, I. (1966) Rubidium[86] clearance during neurogenic redistribution of intestinal blood flow. *Acta physiol. Scand.* **67**, 173–184.

EDWALL, L. & KINDLOVÁ, M. (1971) The effect of sympathetic nerve stimulation on the rate of disappearance of tracers from various oral tissues. *Acta odont. Scand.* **29**, 387–400.

FOLKE, L. E. A. & STALLARD, R. E. (1967) Periodontal microcirculation as revealed by plastic microspheres. *J. periodont. Res.* **2**, 53–63.

FRANK, R. M., FELLINGER, E. & STEUER, P. (1976) Ultrastructure du ligament alvéolo-dentaire du rat. *J. Biol. Buccale* **4**, 295–313.

GÄNGLER, P. & MERTE, K. (1979a) Die vitalmikroskopische Untersuchung der periodontalen Blutzirkulation an Ratteninzisivus. *Zahn-, Mund- u. Kieferheilkd.* **67**, 129–136.

GÄNGLER, P. & MERTE, K. (1979b) Die System- und Mikrozirkulation des Periodontiums – vitalmikroskopische und histologische Untersuchungen an Ratteninzisivi. *Zahn-, Mund- u. Kieferheilkd.* **67**, 459–466.

GAZELIUS, B. & OLGART, L. (1980) Vasodilatation in dental pulp produced by electrical stimulation of the inferior alveolar nerve in the cat. *Acta. physiol. Scand.* **108**, 181–186.

GILDA, J. E., McCAULEY, M. C. & JOHANSSON, E. G. (1943) Effect of pulp extirpation on the metabolism of phosphorus in the teeth of a dog as indicated by radioactive phosphorus. *J. dent. Res.* **22**, 200.

GRIFFIN, C. J. & SPAIN, H. (1972) Organization and vasculature of human periodontal ligament mechanoreceptors. *Archs. oral Biol.* **17**, 913–921.

HARRIS, R. & GRIFFIN, C. J. (1974) Innervation of the human periodontium. Fine structure of the complex mechanoreceptors and free nerve endings. *Austral. dent. J.* 326–331.

HAYASHI, S. (1932) Untersuchungen über die arterielle Blutversorgung des Periodontiums. *Dtsch. Mschr. Zahnheilk.* **50,** 145–179.

HOFMANN, M. & DIEMER, R. (1963) Die Pulsation des Zahnes. *Dtsch. zahnärztl. Zschr.* **18,** 1268–1274.

ICHIKAWA, T., WATANABE, O. & YAMAMURA, T. (1977) Vascular architecture in oral tissues by vascular casts method for scanning electron microscopy. *9th Europ. Conf. Microcirc. Bibl. Anat.* No. **15,** 544–546.

ISHIMITSU, K. (1960) Beitrag zur Kenntnis der Morphologie und Entwicklungsgeschichte der Glomeruli Periodonti. *Yokohama Med. Bull.* **11,** 415–432.

KAPLAN, M. L., DAVIS, M. A. & GOLDHABER, P. (1978) Blood flow measurements in selected oral tissues in dog using radiolabelled microspheres and rubidium[86]. *Archs. oral Biol.* **23,** 281–284.

KAPLAN, M. L., JEFFCOAT, M. K. & GOLDHABER, P. (1978) Radiolabeled microsphere measurements of alveolar bone blood flow in dogs. *J. periodont. Res.* **13,** 304–308.

KENNEDY, J. (1969) Experimental ischemia in monkeys: II. Vascular response. *J. dent. Res.* **48,** 888–894.

KENNEDY, J. E. & ZANDER, H. A. (1969) Experimental ischemia in monkeys. I. Effect of ischemia on gingival epithelium. *J. dent. Res.* **48,** 696–701.

KETY, S. S. (1949) Measurement of regional circulation by the local clearance of radioactive sodium. *Amer. Heart J.* **38,** 321–328.

KHOUW, F. E. & GOLDHABER, P. (1970) Changes in vasculature of the periodontium associated with tooth movement in the rhesus monkey and the dog. *Archs. oral Biol.* **15,** 1125–1132.

KINDLOVA, M. (1965) The blood supply of the marginal periodontium in *Macaca rhesus. Archs. oral Biol.* **10,** 869–874.

KINDLOVÁ, M. & MATĚNA, V. (1959) Blood circulation in the rodent teeth of the rat. *Acta anat.* **37,** 163–192.

KINDLOVÁ, M. & MATĚNA, V. (1962) Blood vessels of the rat molar. *J. dent. Res.* **41,** 650–660.

KÖRBER, K. (1963) Oszillographie der Parodontaldurchblutung. *Dtsch. zahnärztl. Z.* **17,** 271–277.

KÖRBER, K. (1970) Periodontal pulsation. *J. Periodont.* **41,** 382–390.

KÖRBER, K. H. & KÖRBER, E. (1965) Patterns of physiological movement in tooth support. In: *Mechanisms of tooth support,* D. J. ANDERSON, J. E. EASTOE, A. H. MELCHER & D. C. A. PICTON (eds.). Bristol, Wright.

LAMB, R. E. & VAN HASSEL, H. J. (1972) Tissue pressure in the periodontal ligament. *J. dent. Res.* **51,** Special Issue of I.A.D.R. Abstracts, p. 240.

LENZ, P. (1968) Zur Gefässtruktur des Parodontiums. *Dtsch. zahnärztl. Z.* **23,** 357–361.

LENZ, P. (1974) Zur Gefässtruktur des marginalen Parodontiums rasterelektronenmikroskopisch Untersuchungen. *Dtsch. zahnärztl. Z.* **29,** 868–870.

LEVY, B. M. & BERNICK, S. (1968) Studies on the biology of the periodontium of marmosets: V. Lymphatic vessels of the periodontal ligament. *J. dent. Res.* **47,** 1166–1170.

LINDEN, R. W. A. (1975) Intraoral mechanoceptors: a study in man and animals. Ph.D. Thesis. Bristol University.

LINDEN, R. W. A. & AARS, H. (1979) Movements of the cat canine tooth in response to sympathetic nerve stimulation. *Acta physiol. Scand.* **105,** 42–43A.

LISNEY, S. J. W., MATTHEWS, B. & SHARP, S. E. (1972) Observations on eruption with use of a continuous recording technique. *J. dent. Res.* **51,** 1265.

MATĚNA, V. (1973) Periodontal ligament of rat incisor tooth. *J. Periodont.* **44,** 629–635.

MATTHEWS, B. & BERKOVITZ, B. K. B. (1972) Continuous recording of tooth eruption in the rabbit. *Archs. oral Biol.* **17,** 817–820.

MEYER, M. W. (1970) Distribution of cardiac output to oral tissues in dogs. *J. dent. Res.* **49,** 787–794.

MOXHAM, B. J. (1975) The use of a continuous recording technique for the assessment of the haemodynamic hypothesis of tooth eruption. *J. Physiol.* **245,** 43P.

MOXHAM, B. J. (1976) The effects of cervical sympathetic nerve section and stimulation on tooth eruption. *J. dent. Res.* **55,** 113.

MOXHAM, B. J. (1977) The effects of a variety of pharmacological agents with known vasoactive properties on tooth movements. *J. dent. Res.* **56,** Special Issue D, 131.

MOXHAM, B. J. (1978) An assessment of the vascular or tissue hydrostatic pressure hypotheses of eruption using a continuous recording technique for monitoring movements of the rabbit mandibular incisor. Ph.D. Thesis. Bristol University.

MOXHAM, B. J. (1979a) Recording the eruption of the rabbit mandibular incisor using a device for continuously monitoring tooth movements. *Archs. oral Biol.* **24,** 889–899.

MOXHAM, B. J. (1979b) The effects of some vaso-active drugs on the eruption of the rabbit mandibular incisor. *Archs. oral Biol.* **24,** 681–688.

MOXHAM, B. J. & BERKOVITZ, B. K. B. (in press) Some physiological comparisons between the periodontal tissues of teeth of continuous and limited growth. *J. dent. Res.*

MYHRE, L., PREUS, H. R. & AARS, H. (1978) Mechanisms controlling mobility and position of the rabbit's incisor tooth. *Acta physiol. Scand.* **102,** 34–35A.

MYHRE, L., PREUS, H. R. & AARS, H. (1979) Influences of axial load and blood pressure on the position of the rabbit's tooth. *Acta odont. Scand.* **37,** 153–159.

NÄHRI, M. (1978) Activation of dental pulp nerves of the cat and the dog with hydrostatic pressure. Thesis. *Proc. Finn. Dent. Soc.* **74,** Suppl. V, pp. 1–64.

NOYES, F. B. (1897) The structure of the peridental membrane. *Dent. Rev.* **11,** 448–458.

PACKMAN, H., SHOHER, I. & STEIN, R. S. (1977) Vascular responses in the human periodontal ligament and alveolar bone detected by photoelectric plethysmography. *J. Periodont.* **48,** 194–200.

PALCANIS, K. G. (1973) Effect of the occlusal trauma on interstitial pressure in the periodontal ligament. *J. dent. Res.* **52,** 903–910.

PATH, M. G. & MEYER, M. W. (1977) Quantification of pulpal blood flow in developing teeth in dogs. *J. dent. Res.* **56,** 1245–1254.

PERINT, J. (1949) Detailed roentgenologic examination of the blood supply in the jaws and teeth by applying radiopaque solutions. *Oral Surg.* **2,** 2–20.

POHTO, P. & ANTILA, R. (1968) Acetylcholinesterase and noradrenalin in the nerves of mammalian dental pulps. *Acta odont. Scand.* **26**, 641–656.

RUBEN, M. P., PRIETO-HERNANDEZ, J. R., GOTT, F. K., KRAMER, G. M. & BLOOM, A. A. (1971) Vizualization of lymphatic microcirculation of oral tissues. II. Vital retrograde lymphography. *J. Periodont.* **42**, 774–784.

SAUNDERS, R. L. DE C. H. & RÖCKERT, H. O. E. (1967) Vascular supply of dental tissues including lymphatics. In: *Structural and chemical organization of teeth*, Vol. 1, A. E. W. MILES (ed.), pp. 199–245. London, Academic Press.

SCHÄRER, P. & HAYASHI, Y. (1969) A qualitative study on intraperiodontal pressure. *Parodontologie* **23**, 3–10.

SCHWEITZER, G. (1907) Über die Lymphgefässe des Zahnfleisches und der Zähne beim Menschen und bei Säugetieren. *Arch. mikr. Anat.* **69**, 807–908.

SCOTT, D. Jr., SCHEININ, A., KARJALAINEN, S. & EDWALL, L. (1972) Influence of sympathetic nerve stimulation on flow velocity in pulpal vessels. *Acta odont. Scand.* **30**, 277–287.

SEVERSON, J. A., MOFFETT, B. C., KOKICH, V. & SELIPSKY, H. (1978) A histologic study of age changes in the adult human periodontal joint (ligament). *J. Periodont.* **49**, 189–200.

SICHER, H. (ed.) (1966) *Orban's oral histology and embryology*, 6th ed. Saint Louis, Mosby.

SIMS, M. R. (1975) Oxytalan–vascular relationships observed in histologic examination of the periodontal ligaments of man and mouse. *Archs. oral Biol.* **20**, 713–717.

SIMS, M. R. (1976) Reconstitution of the human oxytalan system during orthodontic tooth movement. *Amer. J. Orthod.* **70**, 38–58.

STEINHARDT, G. (1935) Die Gefässversorgung des gesunden, kranken und zahnlosen Kiefer. *Dtsch. Zahn-, Mund- u. Kieferheilkd.* **2**, 265–339.

STÜBEN, J. & SPRETER VON KREUDENSTEIN, T. (1960) Experimentelle Untersuchungen über die Beteiligung des Zahnmarks am Stoffaustausch zwischen Blut und Dentinliquor. *Dtsch. zahnärztl. Z.* **15**, 967–971.

TØNDER, K. J. H. & NAESS, G. (1978) Nervous control of blood flow in the dental pulp in dogs. *Acta physiol. Scand.* **104**, 13–23.

TURNER, H., RUBEN, M. P., FRANKL, S. N., SHEFF, M. & SILBERSTEIN, S. (1969) Visualization of the microcirculation of the periodontium. *J. Periodont.* **40**, 222–230.

VANDERSALL, D. C. & ZANDER, H. A. (1967) Experimental obstruction of the periodontal blood circulation. *Helv. odont. Acta* **11**, 74–79.

WAERHAUG, J. (1954) Over- og underkjevens karforsyning med saerlig henblikk pa gingiva, tenene og deres støtteve. *Norske Tannlaegeforen. tid.* **64**, 159–169.

WALKER, T. W., NG, G. C. & BURKE, P. S. (1978) Fluid pressures in the periodontal ligament of the mandibular canine tooth in dogs. *Archs. oral Biol.* **23**, 753–765.

WASSERMAN, F., BLAYNEY, J. R., GROETZINGER, G. & DE WITT, T. G. (1941) Studies on the different pathways of exchange of minerals in teeth with the aid of radioactive phosphorus. *J. dent. Res.* **30**, 389–398.

WAUGH, I. L. M. (1904) The alveolo-dental membrane: its minute structure from a practical standpoint. *Dent. Cosmos* **XVI**: 744–747.

WEDL, C. (1881) Über Gefässknäuel im Zahnperiost. *Virchows Arch.* **85**, 175–177.

ZWEIFACH, B. (1961) *Functional behaviour of the microcirculation*. Springfield, Thomas.

Chapter 8

THE INNERVATION OF THE PERIODONTAL LIGAMENT

A. G. Hannam

SENSORY INNERVATION

Introduction

The generation of interocclusal forces during function demands sophisticated neural control, reliant to a great extent upon afferent, sensory feedback. The periodontal innervation provides a major source of this kind of information. Yet, judged by most major reviews, our comprehension of its structural and functional relationships has remained incomplete (Anderson, Hannam and Matthews, 1970; Harris, 1975; Hannam, 1976; Dubner, Sessle and Storey, 1978). Perhaps we should not be unduly surprised.

It will be seen not only that there are species differences in the periodontal innervation, but that disproportionate numbers of various species have been employed in what are clearly unrelated anatomical and physiological studies. Findings from one discipline are consequently of lessened relevance to those from the other. Furthermore, while anatomists have not only described, but physically located, specific features of the innervation, physiologists,

however descriptive of function, generally have failed to pinpoint the position of the receptors under investigation (Hannam, 1976; Dubner et al., 1978). There are, in fairness, technical reasons for this, not the least being preservation of a viable preparation.

Another problem has been introduced by the bias of recording sites in physiological studies. For example, neural activity as a consequence of loading the teeth in cats has been recorded near the terminations of peripheral nerves, in the trigeminal ganglion, and in the mesencephalic nucleus of the trigeminal nerve (Anderson et al., 1970; Hannam, 1976; Dubner et al., 1978). Although each site represents collections of first-order neurones serving periodontal receptor endings, each has its own sampling bias; recordings made from peripheral nerves inevitably mean regional selection (Robinson, 1979), while data collected from one central site necessarily ignore neural contributions from the other (Linden, 1978).

The final major source of difficulty in correlating the results of morphological and physiological studies involves methods of classification and nomenclature. The plethora of terms used to describe putative nerve terminals observed by microscopy in the oral mucosa and periodontal ligament has been noted by others (Rapp, Kirstine and Avery, 1957; Dixon, 1961; Anderson *et al.*, 1970; Hannam, 1976; Kubota and Osanai, 1977; Byers and Holland, 1977; Everts, Beertsen and van den Hooff, 1977; Dubner *et al.*, 1978). Wholesale acceptance of all the categories proposed burdens us with a range of end-organs far in excess of that described for most other tissues, as well as the prospect of species differences of greater magnitude than one might expect. Differences in techniques and standards of preparation, as well as a natural enthusiasm for describing detail, undoubtedly contribute to this impressive array of descriptive terms, making comparisons ever difficult.

Morphology

THE CUTANEOUS INNERVATION

Our seemingly bleak chances of correlating structure and function in the periodontal innervation nevertheless can be offset by recourse elsewhere. It is a rewarding experience to review what is known of the cutaneous innervation before interpreting similar data about the periodontal tissues, and the reader herewith is encouraged to read the work of Munger (1971), Chambers *et al.* (1972), Andres and von Düring (1973), Burgess and Perl (1973), Munger (1975), Iggo (1976), Breathnach (1977), Munger (1977), Horch, Tuckett and Burgess (1977), Biemesderfer *et al.* (1978) and Dubner *et al.* (1978).

Peripheral, cutaneous, afferent nerves demonstrate a variety of endings, some of which are derived from branched terminal axons and some of which are not. Elaborate endings are associated universally with myelinated parent nerve fibres, and traditionally have been implicated in the sensations of touch, pressure, stretch and temperature. Simpler terminations associated with fine, myelinated and unmyelinated fibres are involved with mechanosensitive, thermosensitive and nociceptive sensations.

Fine terminations of nerves (neurites), whether derived from myelinated or unmyelinated fibres, may be associated with enveloping Schwann cells only (Fig. 1). In addition, free receptor axons, derived from myelinated fibres and encased by flattened Schwann cells, may arborize with frequent close contact between the receptive terminals and collagenous fibres. These are known as branched, lanceolate terminals (Fig. 2). Alternatively, neurites may be involved with a more specialized cell or organization of cells. The Merkel cells of the epithelial layer

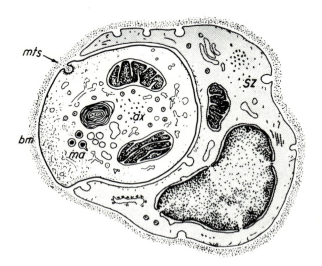

FIG. 1. Schematic cross-section of a free receptor terminal in the sinus hair of the rat, showing axoplasm (ax), basement membrane (bm), receptor matrix (ma), a coated pit (mts) and Schwann cell (sz).

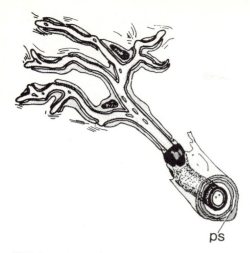

FIG. 2. Schematic representation of a free, branched, lanceolate terminal associated with a myelinated nerve fibre. The perineural sheath (ps) begins at the myelinated part of the axon. The terminal neurites may be incompletely encased by Schwann cells and may closely approximate collagen fibres in the connective tissue.

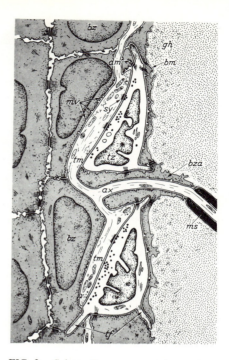

FIG. 3. Schematic representation of a Merkel cell–neurite complex from the external root sheath of a sinus hair. The myelinated axon loses its myelin and contacts the Merkel touch cells (tz). In the skin, the Merkel cells are on the opposite side of the neurite discs, nearer the basement membrane. The figure illustrates the sensory axon (ax), basement membrane (bm), basal cells (bz), desmosomes (dm), glassy membrane (gh), process of the touch cell (tf), Merkel discs (tm), and the contact zone of the Merkel cell (sy), myelin sheath (ms).

and the layers of differentiated, lamellar cells as in the Golgi–Mazzoni and Vater–Pacini corpuscle of the dermal tissues (Figs. 3 and 4) are both examples of specialized terminations. Even more elaborate endings are comprised of combinations of nerves and neurites with lamellar cells, collagen fibres, and a capsule which separates the conglomerate from dermal connective tissue. Examples of the latter include Ruffini and Meissner corpuscles (Figs. 5 and 6). Most mechanosensitive, cutaneous nerve endings fall into one or other of these general categories.

Sustained, mechanical stimulation of a mechano-receptor at innocuous intensities is only likely to evoke a sustained neural response if the threshold to stimulation is low enough, and if the receptor is coupled to the stimulus in a fairly direct fashion. Should a simple receptor (e.g. the free, penicillate or branched lanceolate endings of Fig. 2) lie among collagen fibres, the chances for such coupling are increased. However, the best opportunity for a sustained response occurs in more elaborate receptors, such as the Ruffini corpuscles (Fig. 5) where collagen fibres running within and through the capsule provide a direct mechanical link to the neurites (Andres and

von Düring, 1973; Iggo, 1976; Biemesderfer *et al.*, 1978).

In the opposite sense, simple endings distant from the site of stimulation and surrounded by a relatively viscous environment do not respond well to sustained stimulation. Elaborate receptors, notably those with a loose internal structure, or with a heavily lamellated capsule or corpuscle surrounding their neurites (for example, Meissner, Golgi–Mazzoni or Paciniform corpuscles) provide their own buffer against sustained deformation. Given an appropriate threshold for excitation, these receptors are good sensors of transient data, and are assumed to monitor the rapidly changing events associated

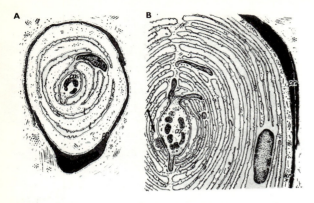

FIG. 4. Schematic representation of a simple type of lamellated sensory terminal from the foot-sole skin of Tupaia (A) and a Golgi–Mazzoni corpuscle from the hairy skin of the cat (B). The figures show axons (ax), Schwann cell lamellae (l), capsule spaces (kr), and perineural sheaths (pn). The arrow in B indicates a terminal of an unmyelinated axon lying on another axon terminal.

with mechanical stimulation (Andres and von Düring, 1973; Iggo, 1976).

The relationship between structure and function with regard to the pain experience is a complex one, and the reader is referred to Dubner *et al.* (1978) for current views on the subject. It is sufficient here to indicate that the receptors involved include morphologically simple, thermosensitive, high-threshold, mechanosensitive endings, as well as so-called polymodal endings which respond to more than one kind of stimulus.

THE INNERVATION OF THE PERIODONTIUM

Receptors responding to stimuli transmitted to the periodontal tissues may be found in three sites: the gingiva, the periodontal ligament and the periosteum of alveolar bone (Hannam, 1976; Dubner *et al.*, 1978). The gingival and periosteal innervations are relevant to this review because they share common morphological and physiological features with the periodontal innervation. Their territory is frequently continuous with that of the ligament, at least in a neurological context, and the respective contributions from all three sites are difficult, or impossible, to separate on functional grounds. The imbalance between structural and functional data for the periodontal region also encourages a critical appraisal

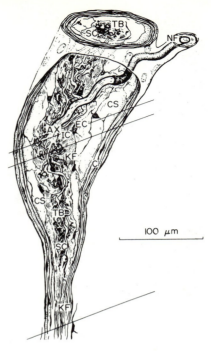

FIG. 5. Reconstruction of a Ruffini ending of the cat's skin from a series of semithin sections and from electron-microscope step-cuts. The picture shows two-thirds of the 0.5-mm-long Ruffini organ, and illustrates nerve fibres (NF), axon (AX), its terminal ramifications (TB), inner core of the corpuscle (IC), collagenous fibrils (KF), Schwann cells (SC), endoneural capsule space (CS), endoneural cell (EC), and perineural capsule (C).

of contiguous innervations for which some morphological data have been correlated with function. Accordingly, the three sources of innervation will be considered separately, and in turn.

The gingival innervation

Autoradiographic demonstrations of labelled nerve endings in cat (Weill, Bensadoun and de Tourniel, 1975) and rat (Byers and Holland, 1977; Pimenidis and Hinds, 1977), as well as light microscopy in a variety of animals, including man (Lewinsky and Stewart, 1938; Gairns and Aitchison, 1950; Dixon, 1961), indicate the presence of fine, free nerve endings in the epithelium of the gingival tissues.

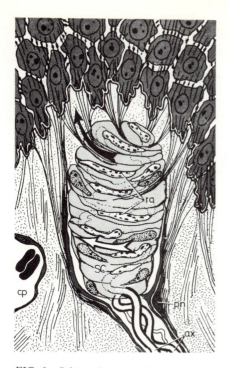

FIG. 6. Schematic representation of a Meissner corpuscle showing tonofibrils of the epithelial cells in continuity with collagen fibres of the corium, the capsule and the endoneural sheath. Differential movement in the manner indicated by the arrows may account for the rapidly adapting nature of this receptor. Coiled receptor axon, ra; Schwann cells, SC; perineural sheath, pn; myelinated axons, ax; capillary, cp.

(Quilliam, 1966; Andres and von Düring, 1973). They have an equally uncertain significance. Although prominent elsewhere in the oral epithelium (Munger, 1975), the presence of Merkel cell—neurite complexes in gingival tissue (though possible) is virtually unreported. These intra-epithelial neural complexes have been described by Andres and von Düring (1973), Munger (1975, 1977), Iggo (1976) and Dubner *et al.* (1978). An unusual epithelial cell, the Merkel cell, is usually found near the basal layers. It contains numerous secretory granules polarized towards the contiguous neurite which lacks a Schwann cell (Fig. 3). Whether or not these granules are associated with synaptic events is still uncertain. Clusters of such complexes may protrude into the stroma of the connective tissue, and Munger (1977) has described these as Merkel rete papillae.

The remainder of the gingival innervation is more conventional. Branched, free nerve endings abound in the subepithelial papillae (Dixon, 1961; Desjardins, Winkelmann and Gonzalez, 1971; Kubota and Osanai, 1977), while organized encapsulated endings have been reported in a variety of species. These endings include the clearly defined Meissner corpuscle (Kadanoff, 1928; Rapp *et al.*, 1957), the complex ultrastructural organization of which has been described by others (Andres and von Düring, 1973; Munger, 1975, 1977; Dubner *et al.*, 1978). It is sufficient to remind the reader of a capsulated, sensory nerve ending, characterized by a winding, terminal neurite, sandwiched between stacks of cytoplasmic lamellae which are derived from a core, lamellar cell (probably a specialized Schwann cell) (Fig. 6). Meissner corpuscles are common elsewhere in the oral mucosa (Munger, 1975).

Corpuscular, lamellated receptors (usually with a bulbous appearance) often have been observed in the gingival tissues (Rapp *et al.*, 1957; Dixon, 1961; Desjardins *et al.*, 1971; Martinez and Pekarthy, 1974). They vary in size, and apparently in form. Munger's (1975) description of glomerular corpuscles in the oral epithelium is a case in point, for here each tangled coiled neurite is surrounded by loose lamellae and connective tissue to form a corpuscular ending which Munger considers to be relatively non-specific, resembling a Krause end-bulb, genital end bulb or mucocutaneous end organ. Another example is the encapsulated gingival endings described by Martinez

Byers and Holland (1977) suggest that some of these endings can be quite large and arborized (Fig. 7), particularly in the crest of the free gingiva. The observations are significant because deeply penetrating, free, intra-epithelial, nerve endings seem to be relatively rare elsewhere in the body (including other regions of the oral mucosa) (Breathnach, 1977; Munger, 1977). Where they do occur, they usually retain their Schwann cells and are thought to have little functional significance (Breathnach, 1977). Specific cold thermoreceptors are also thought to present as fine, free terminals which penetrate a short distance into the epithelium (Hensel, 1973), but the gingival intra-epithelial endings that have been reported most resemble the intra-epithelial component of the Eimer's corpuscle of the mole

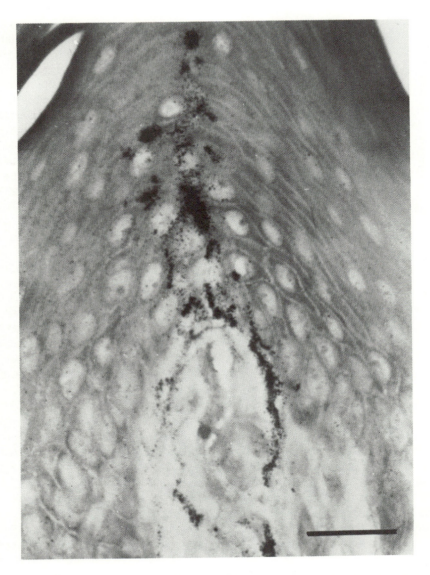

FIG. 7. Arborized intra-epithelial nerve endings and axons or endings in connective tissues, revealed by autoradiography. The section was through the right, buccal crestal epithelium adjacent to the third maxillary molar, in a rat injected 16 hours before fixation. Scale bar — 25 μm.

and Pekarthy (1974) which are illustrated in Fig. 8. These endings are found almost exclusively within the connective tissue papillae adjacent to the epithelium, often near blood vessels. The neurite endings (supplied here by single axons) are surrounded by a dense core of lamellar cells, devoid of interlaminar collagen. These in turn are surrounded by capsular cells which Martinez and Pekarthy consider resemble fibroblasts; it is conventionally held that such cells are derived from the perineurium (Munger, 1977). To complicate matters, the appearance of both terminals is not unlike Andres and von Düring's (1973) description of Golgi—Mazzoni endings. This forces one to question the functional significance of classifications based upon fine morphological distinctions.

Gingival nerve endings are probably not equally distributed around the teeth or even around the dental arch. Results from an autoradiographical study in the rat suggest that the junctional epithelium and the marginal side of the crestal epithelium are both well innervated, while the attached gingiva is not so well endowed (Byers and Holland, 1977). This is true at least for those endings supplied by neurones with cell bodies in the trigeminal ganglion. Desjardins *et al.* (1971) have reported the mean number of organized endings in man to be greatest in the incisor region and least in the molar region of the maxilla. Curiously, the opposite seems true for the mandible, where the number of endings found in the molar region is not only greater than that at the incisors, but greater than the number found in the molar region of the maxilla.

The periodontal ligament innervation

Earlier references to the vast array of terms used to describe nerve endings are most appropriate here. Factors contributing towards today's impressive lexicon of descriptive terms probably include the expressive flair of different observers, their difficulties in working with calcified tissues and in choosing meaningful planes of section through complex end organs (Bonnaud, Proust and Vignon, 1978), and real species differences in the periodontal innervation.

As for the gingiva, there is ample evidence of free nerve endings in the periodontal ligament (Lewinsky

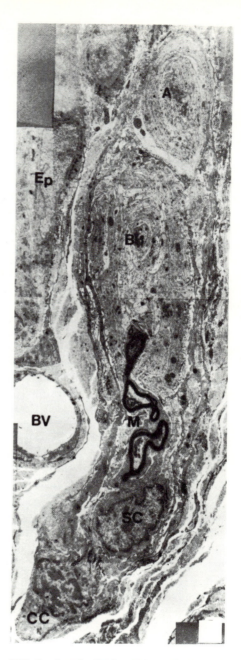

FIG. 8. Longitudinal section of gingival, encapsulated nerve ending lying adjacent to epithelium (Ep) and a blood vessel (BV) in the rat. The corpuscular ending consists of a Schwann cell (SC), a capsular cell (CC), a myelinated axon (M) and unmyelinated axons (A and B). ×3400.

and Stewart, 1937; Bernick, 1957; Rapp *et al.*, 1957; Hattyasy, 1959; Kizior, Cuozzo and Bowman, 1968; Griffin and Harris, 1968; Pimenidis and Hinds, 1977), but the exact nature of these endings is not entirely clear at the ultrastructural level.

In the skin, free terminals are derived from both unmyelinated and myelinated parent axons, and their ultrastructural appearance seems dependent upon which axon is involved. Unmyelinated axons tend to distribute in a plexiform fashion, forming penicillate endings with Schwann cell thickenings at the primary ramification. Branches exchange axons with other branches. Each penicillate ending contains few mitochondria and few other morphologically distinct components. On the other hand, myelinated axons may terminate in fine papillary endings, each consisting of several axon terminals containing mitochondria and pinocytotic vesicles, enclosed in a Schwann cell sheath (Cauna, 1976). Free endings in the periodontal ligament probably belong in both categories. The arborized, beaded appearance of fine endings so frequently reported may reflect Cauna's penicillate network, and there are sufficient descriptions of non-myelinated neurites rich in mitochondria and surrounded by Schwann cells (or Schwann-like cells) to mirror his papillary endings (Griffin, 1972; Everts *et al.*, 1977; Berkovitz and Shore, 1978; Bonnaud *et al.*, 1978). Difficulties in reconciling these observations should not be underestimated, however. Bonnaud *et al.* (1978) have highlighted the problem of deciding whether a terminal or subterminal region has been sectioned, and therefore whether one is looking at a collection of fine axons en route to the endings, or at components of an organized receptor, or at free endings.

There is also some uncertainty regarding the nature of the cells investing the neurites. In the mouse, Everts *et al.* (1977) refer to these as 'K' or 'kidney' cells (Fig. 9) and similar, investing cells observed by Berkovitz and Shore (1978) are considered by them to be atypical of Schwann cells. The vesicular components of these cells (which may also be present in Schwann cells) are reminiscent of those in the Merkel cell and have an equally unsubstantiated function.

Although free nerve endings appear to exist in the periodontal ligaments of all species, they appear to be the only source of periodontal innervation in the Japanese shrew-mole (Kubota and Osanai, 1977), thereby providing us with an example of a probable species difference.

Organized endings derived from myelinated fibres are frequent in most species and seem to be variable in appearance. Again, however, one must make allowances for a wide range of experimental approaches. Most of the variants centre upon apparent differences in the extent of branching and details of the precise method of termination. Observers have used terms such as arborizations, small rounded bodies (Lewinsky and Stewart, 1936), spindle-like structures (Lewinsky and Stewart, 1937; Bernick, 1957; Hattyasy, 1959), capsulated and ovoid with interweaving neurofibrils, and neural coils (Rapp *et al.*, 1957; Kizior *et al.*, 1968; Griffin, 1972) to describe organized nerve endings in the periodontal ligament.

The presence of lamellar, knob-like, neural terminations has been confirmed ultrastructurally in rat and mouse (Beertsen, Everts and van den Hooff, 1974; Everts *et al.*, 1977; Copron *et al.*, 1980). Here the terminal neurites, closely associated with kidney-shaped investing cells, are frequently surrounded by the fine, irregular, lamellar layers shown in Fig. 9. A more fully developed lamellar pattern has been reported by Bonnaud *et al.* (1978) for the cat. These endings apparently are characterized by their association with bundles of nerve fibres, lying within the cellular layer surrounding the nerve fibres. Their structure is thought by Bonnaud *et al.* to resemble that of Vater—Pacini corpuscles.

Even more elaborate lamellar endings have been described by Berkovitz and Sloan (1979) for the periodontal ligament of the Caiman. Considered by Berkovitz and Sloan to resemble avian Herbst corpuscles, they consist of unmyelinated nerve fibres, surrounded by closely arranged, fine cell processes that are separated by an amorphous ground substance with a few collagen fibrils (Fig. 10). The suggestion that the human periodontal ligament may be devoid of lamellar corpuscles, at least of the densely organized kind (Byers and Holland, 1977), as well as the uniqueness of the Herbst-like corpuscles in the Caiman (Berkovitz and Sloan, 1979) infer a species difference for this kind of end organ.

The morphology of organized endings in the

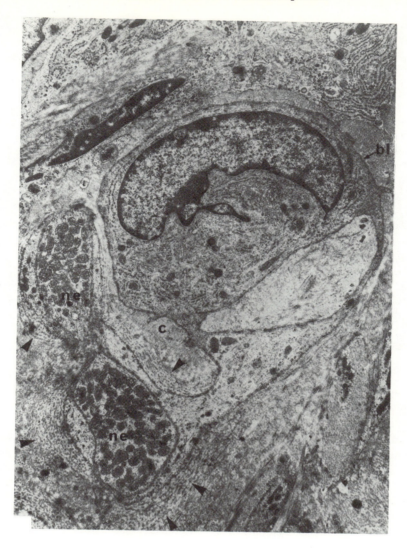

FIG. 9. Nerve endings in the periodontal ligament of a mouse. There is a K cell in close apposition to the nerve endings (ne) which contain numerous mitochondria. Where the cell extensions form a sheath around the neurite endings, layers of lamellar material can be seen (arrowheads). Also visible are the basal lamina (bl) and collagen (c). ×10,000.

human periodontal ligament depicted by Rapp *et al.* (1957) with the light microscope (Fig. 11) is consistent with Berkovitz and Shore's (1978) ultrastructural observations in the rat where single, myelinated nerve fibres are surrounded by bundles of small unmyelinated fibres, both separated from a discrete capsule of cells by fairly dense collagen (Fig. 12). This description is generally similar to those

reported by Bonnaud *et al.* (1978) in the cat, and by Griffin (1972), Griffin and Spain (1972), Griffin and Malor (1974) and Harris (1975) in man. Although in the rat it seems as though single, myelinated fibres give rise to the unmyelinated terminal arborizations within such structures, groups of myelinated fibres may be involved in some of the complexes seen in man (Harris, 1975). Despite the apparent

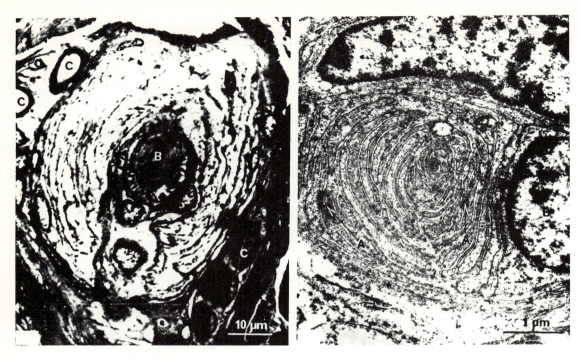

FIG. 10. Specialized, putative nerve endings in the Caiman periodontal ligament. On the left, a semi-thin section of a corpuscle shows outer circular membranes (A) surrounding an inner, central core (B). A number of myelinated nerves (C) are in close apposition. On the right, an electron micrograph of a corpuscle shows a number of lamellar, cell processes, attachment plaque (A) and nuclei (B).

collective tidiness of the data from these studies, technical and semantic differences continue to exist. Bonnaud *et al.* (1978) have warned against labelling sections such as that in Fig. 12 as terminal, as opposed to subterminal, structures. The question of whether the term 'nerve-ending' should be applied to an entire, capsulated end organ including any internally branched axons, or to the termination of one of its component neurites therefore becomes important when interpreting the results of a given study. Unfortunately, this distinction is made all too infrequently in the literature.

When considering gaps or inconsistencies in descriptions of periodontal receptor morphology, we should recall the structure of simple, lamellated corpuscles elsewhere in the body (particularly in Golgi—Mazzoni and Vater—Pacini corpuscles) and of terminal neural structures containing branching nerve fibres as well as collagenous elements (e.g. in simple, branched, lanceolate endings, and in the central regions of Ruffini corpuscles). The hint of common,

structural threads for many cutaneous and periodontal nerve terminations then becomes apparent, and later we shall find these useful in correlating periodontal receptor morphology with function.

Suggestions that nerve endings are not distributed equally within the periodontal ligament, but are most frequently seen around the root apices (Byers and Holland, 1977; Dubner *et al.*, 1978) are supported by a detailed analysis of innervation density provided for the mole by Kubota and Osanai (1977). In this mammal, the apical innervation is far denser than that in the intermediate zone. Furthermore, the ratio of these relative densities in the upper dentition (8 : 1) is greater than that found for the lower teeth (5 : 1). Large differences in these ratios for individual teeth imply functional correlations, but neither the innervation ratios nor any appropriate functional characteristics have been determined for other species.

Everts *et al.* (1977) have shown that neural elements within the periodontal ligament of the mouse incisor are found exclusively in the lateral, alveolar

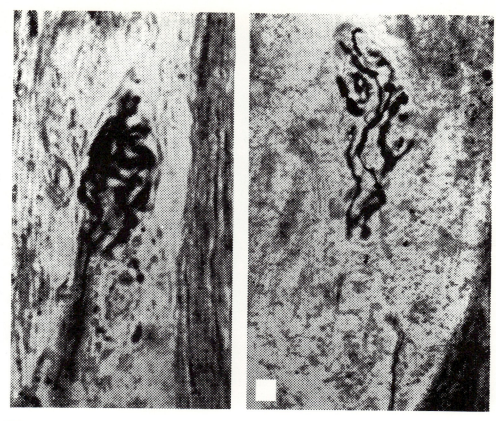

FIG. 11. Organized nerve endings in the human periodontal ligament. These two examples appear to be encapsulated and composed of branching and interwoven terminal fibres, both myelinated and unmyelinated. Light microscope, magnification unavailable.

compartment of the ligament around and between the vascular spaces. As the more central, avascular, tooth-related part of the ligament (that part which may move as the incisor erupts, e.g. Beertsen and Everts, 1977) does not contain neural endings, it may be that in the rodent incisor nerve endings remain relatively fixed *in situ*.

The periosteal innervation

Given the demonstration of a rich periosteal innervation in the facial bones and alveolar processes by Sakada (1971, 1974), and Picton's (1965) evidence for alveolar bone distortion when forces as low as 100 g (1 N) are applied to the teeth, it is likely that nerve endings in the alveolar periosteum provide sensory information which complements that furnished by endings in the gingival and periodontal tissues.

The periosteal innervation includes free endings, some of which may be arborized and unencapsulated (branched, lanceolate terminations), as well as organized corpuscular terminations similar to the lightly lamellated Golgi–Mazzoni ending (Sakada, 1971, 1974). The Golgi–Mazzoni endings appear to be frequent and are found most commonly in the medial facial structures, e.g. in the periapical region of the maxillary canine tooth and the mental region of the mandible. They occur singly or in groups within the inner and outer layers of the periosteum, sometimes in close association with nerve trunks (Sakada, 1971).

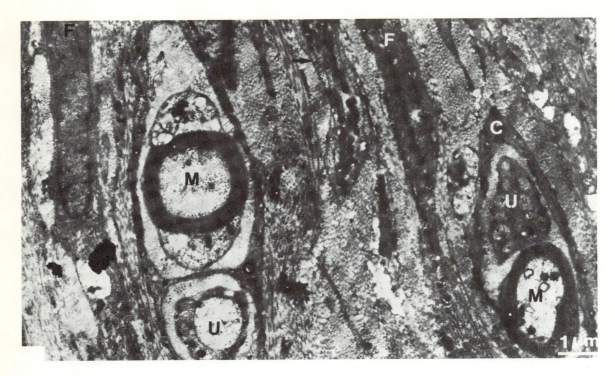

FIG. 12. Putative nerve terminals in the periodontal ligament of the rat incisor. Here are two examples of single, myelinated nerves (M) each with a bundle of unmyelinated nerve fibres (U) surrounded by a capsule of cells (C), from which they are separated by many collagen fibrils. The nerves are in cross-section. An unmyelinated, mitochondria-rich nerve fibre (arrowed) passes between the encapsulated nerves. Periodontal fibroblasts (F) are also evident.

THE PERIPHERAL AFFERENT NERVES

Nerve endings in the oral mucosa, gingivae and periosteal tissues are derived from extensive, plexiform networks of nerve fibres (Dixon, 1961, 1963; Desjardins et al., 1971; Sakada, 1971). Mucosal and gingival networks tend to be layered, appearing as deep, densely woven, submucous bundles of fibres which give rise to more superficial, finer, subepithelial arborizations (Dixon, 1963). In both tissues, interchanges of fibres between component nerve bundles are common. The densities of these neural nets are greatest in the dorsum of the tongue, the hard palate and the gingivae, especially in the anterior part of the mouth. Gingival plexuses seem to be more prominent anteriorly at least in the maxilla (Dixon, 1963; Desjardins et al., 1971), and are particularly dense in the region of the junctional epithelium (Kubota and Osanai, 1977; Byers and Holland, 1977). Sakada's

(1971) description of the periosteum suggests that the fairly even maxillary innervation is not found in the mandible where the buccal side shows a denser network than the lingual.

Nerve endings in the periodontal ligament are served by fibres from branches of coarse bundles ascending through the apical region, or from finer branches arriving via the lateral foramina of the alveolus (Bernick, 1957; Rapp et al., 1957; Anderson et al., 1970; Harris, 1975; Dubner et al., 1978). These are illustrated diagrammatically in Fig. 13.

The gingival, periosteal and periodontal networks associated with the sensory innervation described above are supplied by recognized branches of the major divisions of the trigeminal nerve and perhaps in some areas by fine branches of the cervical nerves. Whereas the general, regional distribution of such peripheral nerves is well known (and can be found in any standard anatomical text), the exact manner of

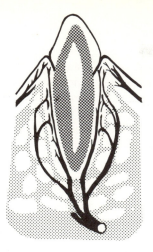

FIG. 13. Diagrammatic representation of peripheral nerves supplying the periodontal tissues. The supply is derived from a variety of conventionally recognized sensory branches depending upon whether the tooth concerned is maxillary or mandibular. Nerve endings in the periodontal ligament may be served by peripheral branches descending via an apical path, or leaving by a lateral route through the wall of the alveolus. Endings in the gingival tissues may be associated with nerves descending through the periodontal ligament, but more commonly with superficial submucous networks. Periosteal endings are also presumed to be served by the latter supply.

tance of combined anatomical and physiological approaches to correlate structure with function.

The diameters of the peripheral nerves supplying the periodontal tissues reflect the spectrum one might expect in other somatic afferents, but there may be variations depending upon the species studied and the region of the peripheral nerves sampled. Young (1977) has demonstrated that whereas unmyelinated fibres comprise about 65% of the total number of nerve fibres in the frog trigeminal sensory nerve root, they only represent 50% of the total in cat and man. The disproportionately large number of myelinated fibres in more evolutionarily advanced species possibly provides an example of the phylogenetic process of cephalization. Young's data (essentially the same for both cat and man) suggest a total fibre spectrum of 0.2–11 μm in the nerve root, most unmyelinated fibres having diameters in the region of 0.4–0.6 μm.

Other estimations, made more peripherally, include those of Brashear (1936) and Kizior *et al.* (1968) for the whole inferior dental nerve in the cat. Here myelinated fibres were reported to be from 2 to 16 μm in diameter, the unmyelinated fibre content (which was not measured) being estimated at between 14–22% of the total fibre count. The latter range is probably on the low side in view of Young's (1977) observations with the electron microscope. Similar whole-nerve ranges from myelinated fibres have been reported by others (de Lange, Hannam and Matthews, 1969 (1–16 μm); Sakada, 1974 (1–14 μm)), and assessments made on more terminal branches of the cat generally reflect the same spectrum. De Lange *et al.* (1969) found the majority to be from 5 to 6 μm in diameter in a monomodal distribution, whereas Mei, Hartmann and Aubert (1977) reported a bimodal distribution of 0–5 μm and 10–15 μm respectively. Griffin and Spain (1972) quoted a mean diameter for identified periodontal nerve plexuses of 4.5 μm, 20% of these fibres being over 5.5 μm in diameter, while Sakada (1971) has reported that the myelinated nerves supplying the Golgi–Mazzoni corpuscles of the periosteum have diameters in the range of 3–10 μm.

Given the technical problems in measuring such diameters, there is clearly a consensus between these studies. We can reasonably expect the periodontal tissues to be served by afferent nerve fibres

their terminal branching is far from clear. Robinson (1979) has shown in the cat that branches of the inferior dental nerve contain nerve fibres supplying two or more adjacent tissues (one branch serving, for example, periodontal ligament, pulp, mucous membrane and skin), and that the nerves supplying one tooth do not all travel in the same branch. Furthermore, Lisney and Matthews (1978) have provided physiological evidence that single nerve fibres may branch to supply both pulp and gingival tissues. Studies like these, unfortunately rare in other regions and in other species, emphasize the impor-

ranging from the fine, unmyelinated variety, about 0.5 μm in diameter (conceivably comprising almost a half of the total supply), to the myelinated kind, ranging from less than 5 μm to almost 16 μm in diameter. However, it is uncertain how many of the unmyelinated variety originate from the autonomic nervous system.

Peripheral afferent nerves can be viewed as long cellular extensions of cell-bodies located more centrally in the nervous system. It is now well established that the majority of cell-bodies belonging to first-order, trigeminal, sensory neurones are found in the trigeminal ganglion. Although one might expect peripheral nerve endings in the gingival, periodontal and periosteal tissues to conform to this general pattern, there are exceptions. Cell-bodies of neurones serving the periodontal tissues also can be found in the trigeminal mesencephalic nucleus (Anderson et al., 1970; Hannam, 1976; Dubner et al., 1978), and recent autoradiographic evidence provided by Byers and Holland (1977) in the rat suggests that the majority of periodontal neurones are served exclusively by cell-bodies in the mesencephalic site. The inference is that neurones of the gingival, and perhaps the periosteal, tissues are furbished by cell-bodies in the trigeminal ganglion. The functional correlates and implications of this dual representation are discussed later.

First-order neurones, wherever the location of their cell-bodies, necessarily relay to second-order neurones and beyond. While it is inappropriate here to review in detail the central neuronanatomy (the interested reader is referred to Dubner et al. (1978) for a complete description), we should note the projection of cell-bodies in the trigeminal ganglion to the trigeminal sensory complex of the brainstem for synaptic relay to the thalamus and cerebral cortex, and the uncertain fate of the projections from periodontal cell-bodies in the mesencephalic nucleus. In the latter instance, we should also remind ourselves of the strong projections of other cell-bodies in this nucleus, notably those associated with muscle afferents, to the motor nucleus of the fifth cranial nerve.

Physiology

Determining the response of a labelled nerve ending and pinpointing its physiological consequences is no simple task, and it is not surprising to find that directly correlative studies hardly exist. Most of our useful information has been gleaned from recordings of the activity in single nerve fibres or the cell-bodies of these fibres. Activity in the single neurone serving a nerve terminal or terminals usually is referred to as that from a single unit. Such units conventionally are identified and classified by physiological criteria, for example by their responsiveness to particular kinds of natural stimulation and by the characteristics of their response. The nature of the recording environment is such that the experimenter, having opted to sample the activity from a particular neural site, and having identified a unit which responds to stimulation of a given tooth, still has very little way of knowing whether the ending was actually located in the gingival, periodontal, or periosteal tissues around, or even near, the tooth stimulated. The tendency has been, therefore, for researchers to classify all such units as 'periodontal' or 'dental' units, and we must keep this in mind when considering the physiological data.

Although dental mechanosensitive units are not the sole kind found around the teeth, they are nevertheless the most studied. They have been found to conduct nerve impulses from 28 to 83 m/s, mostly about 50 m/s (Pfaffmann, 1939; Hannam, 1968; Linden, 1978), observations which correlate with measurements of fibre diameter discussed earlier.

Single units which respond to the stimulation of more than one adjacent tooth are not infrequent (Hannam, 1970; Sakada and Kamio, 1971). The phenomenon can be accounted for either by assuming that movement of one tooth can occasionally cause movement of its neighbour (or at least disturb the environment of its neighbour's receptor system), or that some peripheral afferent nerve fibres may branch (see page 185). The functional significance of such behaviour is unknown.

The qualities and characteristics of dental mechanosensitive units have been reviewed in detail elsewhere (Anderson et al., 1970; Hannam, 1976; Dubner et al., 1978). We can summarize them as follows:

SLOWLY ADAPTING MECHANOSENSITIVE UNITS

These units respond to small displacements (usually 2–10 μm) of the teeth (Yamada and Kumano, 1969), and they can be activated by forces as low as 1–2 g ($\sim$0.01–0.02 N) (Hannam, 1969a). There is a range of thresholds, however, and these may overlap to a considerable extent. Slowly adapting units respond to mechanical stimulation in different ways (see Fig. 14). Many fire trains of impulses for as long as the stimulus is applied (hence the descriptor, slowly adapting) with a frequency of discharge related to the amplitude of the stimulus. This kind of response is quite common in periodontal units of all species. It is seen usually in units with low thresholds to stimulation, relaying very precise information about the amplitude of the stimulus, and consequently any incremental changes in it (Hannam and Farnsworth, 1977; see Fig. 15). We must assume that this capacity is of value in the

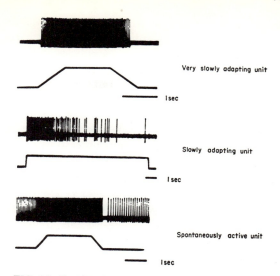

FIG. 14. Slowly adapting responses from periodontal mechanosensitive units. In each case, the upper trace represents the discharge of the unit and the lower trace a record of the force applied to the tooth concerned (100 g). The most common responses are the upper two.

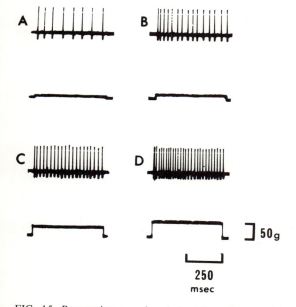

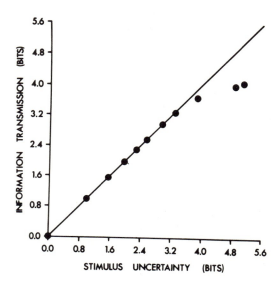

FIG. 15. Responsiveness of periodontal mechanosensitive units to small, incremental changes in stimulus strength. On the left, graded sequences of action potentials (upper traces) recorded from a single neuron are shown with corresponding increases in the force applied to the tooth (A–D). On the right, the ability of a periodontal unit to transmit information about stimulus amplitude (Information Transmission, expressed in binary integers) has been plotted against a measure of the number of stimulus categories used (Stimulus Uncertainty, also expressed in binary integers). The solid line represents perfect information transmission. This particular neurone's maximum information-carrying capacity was approximately 4.00 bits; it was therefore capable of discriminating sixteen different levels of force when thirty-two were applied to the tooth in the range 0–200 g.

sensory discrimination of force between the teeth. Although the sustained nature of the neural discharge also means that these units can indicate stimulus duration with some accuracy, not all of them have this ability. Figure 14 also illustrates a unit which, although adapting slowly to a sustained stimulus, nevertheless ceases to fire before the end of stimulation. Definition of a given slowly adapting unit therefore becomes a somewhat semantic process.

Individually, slowly adapting units are very sensitive to the direction in which the tooth is moved (Fig. 16). One unit, for example, may respond typically to several directions of stimulation, while exhibiting its maximum response in one (Hannam, 1970; Sakada and Kamio, 1971). The multiplicity of effective directions for exciting a given unit means that there is a considerable overlap for groups of units. Whether the periodontal innervation for the tooth as a whole imparts a marked directional sense to the central nervous system is unclear.

We can be reasonably certain that the slowly adapting responses recorded in experimental animals are also representative of those in man. The remarkable recordings of human mechanosensitive units activated by stimulation of the teeth by Johansson and Olsson (1976) confirm not only their presence, but also demonstrate their similar responsiveness

to small forces, to different magnitudes of sustained force, and to different directions of stimulation (Fig. 17).

There is the suggestion of a species difference, however, with regard to a particular kind of slowly adapting unit reported principally in the rabbit and dog (Ness, 1954; Wagers and Smith, 1960; Hannam, 1969b). Known as spontaneously discharging units and characterized by continuous activity even at rest, these seem to be rare or absent in the cat whether recordings are from peripheral nerves (personal observations), the trigeminal ganglion (Kerr and Lysak, 1964; Beaudreau and Jerge, 1968), or from the mesencephalic nucleus (Jerge, 1963; Linden, 1978).

We have no direct evidence as to the morphology of the slowly adapting mechanoreceptor. Pinpointing their location might assist us in choosing the likely morphological analogues, but even this can be difficult. Linden's (1978) work suggests that a significant number of slowly adapting units recorded in the mesencephalic nucleus may be associated with nerve terminals located in sutures (e.g. the palatomaxillary suture). Free fibre endings in the periosteal tissues are also capable of providing slowly adapting responses to mechanical deformation (Sakada, 1974); these undoubtedly are found in both the gingival and

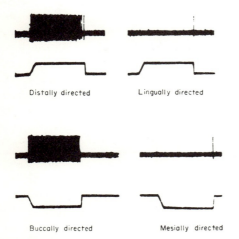

FIG. 16. Responses of a slowly adapting periodontal unit which is sensitive to forces applied to a tooth in more than one direction. In each case a force of 100 g lasting for 10 seconds was used, and is represented by the record beneath each response.

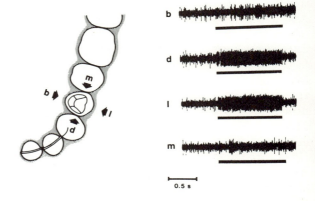

FIG. 17. Afferent signals recorded from a slowly adapting, periodontal mechanosensitive unit in man. The first premolar tooth of the left lower jaw was stimulated with a force of around 2 N applied in the buccal (b), distal (d), lingual (l) and mesial (m) directions. The responses were recorded from the inferior alveolar nerve.

periodontal tissues, and could produce similar response characteristics.

A better clue to structural and functional correlations can be provided by developing a composite picture of the behaviour of slowly adapting dental units, using features such as responses to sustained and dynamic stimuli, maintenance of tonic or resting discharges, directional characteristics, and neural conduction velocities to create it. When a picture like this is compared with those of mechanosensitive skin units, it is clear that dental units most resemble Type II skin units, as well as the Guard and Field units of hairy skin described by Chambers *et al.* (1972), Burgess and Perl (1973) and Horch *et al.* (1977). The morphology of Type II skin units is generally conceded to be that of the Ruffini terminal (Chambers *et al.,* 1972; Burgess and Perl, 1973). Ruffini terminals do not necessarily constitute a morphologically uniform group, even though they may be fundamentally similar (an example of a variant is the pilo-Ruffini complex described by Biemesderfer *et al.* (1978)). However, the feature of branched, terminal, neural ramifications in close approximation to collagenous fibrils emerging from the capsule to link the neurites with the connective tissue of the dermal corium seems to be a common element. In the pilo-Ruffini complex, extremely fine terminal branches lie in a matrix of densely packed collagen fibres.

Parallels between the above description and the situation in the periodontal ligament are obvious. Any terminal consisting of a loosely defined capsule but containing branched nerve terminals in close association with collagen fibres is likely to behave in a similar way to a Ruffini corpuscle (even if it lacks the latter's size). The special nature of the viscoelastic, collagenous investing environment of the periodontal ligament, when taken with the internal structure of the organized, periodontal end-organs described by Rapp *et al.* (1957), Griffin and Malor (1974), Harris (1975), Bonnaud *et al.* (1978) and Berkovitz and Shore (1978), almost guarantees the kinds of tonic response and directional characteristics that are observed in most slowly adapting dental units. When a tooth is stimulated mechanically, the degree of morphological complexity of a nerve ending, its location in the periodontal ligament relative to a given movement of the tooth, and its relationship

to the enveloping, collagenous elements of the periodontal ligament will together determine its threshold, its static and dynamic response characteristics, and its particular directional sensitivity.

The influence of the local environment upon slowly adapting receptors also may go beyond that of a constant, static one. Anderson and Linden (1977) have shown that prior stimulation of the cervical sympathetic trunk in the cat can reduce the response of these units to controlled, mechanical stimulation of the canine tooth. Altering the blood flow in the periodontal ligament may change the viscoelastic coupling without or within a given nerve terminal, thereby affecting the transduction process. Though it has been shown that sympathetic nerve stimulation also affects tooth position (Moxham, 1975), the possibility of interrupting a dynamic, central modulating influence upon peripheral receptor activity should be considered whenever experiments on peripheral nerves involve the commonly used technique of nerve section as part of the procedure.

Before leaving slowly adapting responses, we should remember our original proposition that Merkel cell—neurite complexes probably exist in the basal epithelial layers of the gingival tissues. In the skin, these terminals are known to be associated with Type I unit activity, the latter's principal features including high frequencies of discharge, relatively poor responses to sustained stimulation, greater dynamic sensitivity and frequently a more irregular discharge pattern (Horch *et al.,* 1977; Biemesderfer *et al.,* 1978). In peripheral nerve recordings of dental units such responses can be encountered but these have not been documented with care. We can reasonably speculate, in the absence of more direct evidence, that some of these responses represent activity recorded from Merkel cell—neurite complexes in the gingivae.

RAPIDLY ADAPTING MECHANOSENSITIVE UNITS

In the main, rapidly adapting dental units have high thresholds to mechanical stimulation of the teeth, better expressed perhaps in terms of tens of grammes instead of the few grammes more commonly seen in slowly adapting units (Hannam, 1969a; Anderson *et al.*, 1970). Their response is limited to the transient part of the stimulus, for example its on or off phases. As a result, these units can signal rates of change of stimulation (Fig. 18), but they are poor indicators of sustained tooth displacement. They have not received the attention of investigators to the same extent as slowly adapting dental units. Whether this reflects a true lower incidence and a consequent sampling bias, or more simply the inclination of the researchers themselves, is unknown.

Positive identification of the terminals associated with rapidly adapting units is at least partly possible. Sakada's (1971) direct comparison of receptor morphology with specific response characteristics in cat periosteal tissues makes it highly probable that, when rapidly adapting responses originate in the periosteal tissues, they are generated by Golgi—Mazzoni corpuscles. The high thresholds of many

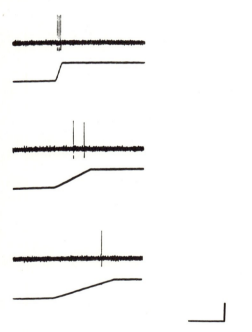

FIG. 18. The effect of changing the rate of application of force upon the response of a rapidly adapting periodontal mechanosensitive unit. The unit responded most vigorously when the rate of application was 2.5 kg/s (top) and less vigorously as it lowered to 400 g/s (centre) and then to 240 g/s (bottom). In each case, the force applied to the tooth is shown below the response. Vertical calibration bar 120 g, horizontal bar 0.25 second.

rapidly adapting dental units would be consistent with an hypothesis of periosteal involvement when transient mechanical stimulation of the teeth occurs. More uncertain, however, is the morphological basis of rapidly adapting, mechanosensitive responses of gingival or periodontal origin. Here we must rely upon the well-established links between lamellated endings and rapidly adapting responses in the skin (Burgess and Perl, 1973). Our candidates would include Meissner corpuscles, and the other corpuscular, lamellated receptors described by Rapp *et al.* (1957), Dixon (1961), Desjardins *et al.* (1971) and Martinez and Pekarthy (1974) in the gingival tissues, and organized lamellar endings of the kind described by Bonnaud *et al.* (1978) and Berkovitz and Sloan (1979) for the periodontal ligaments of the cat and Caiman respectively.

Finally, one should remember that a free terminal can respond in a rapidly adapting fashion if it is in a site which, though not providing a direct link for sustained transformation of a mechanical stimulus, acts as a viscous buffer. It can also exhibit a high threshold to stimulation if it is sufficiently remote from the point of stimulus application.

NOCICEPTIVE UNITS

Though factually obvious, the presence of units responding to painful or noxious stimulation of the periodontal tissues has only been shown recently by Mei, Hartmann and Aubert (1977). They recorded neural activity from units located in the periodontal ligament of the cat. These slowly conducting units (7 m/s) responded only to strong, noxious mechanical stimulation of the teeth, to warming, and to chemical stimulation with bradykinin, being insensitive to normal physiological stimuli. Their specific response pattern strongly suggests that the units are nociceptive. We can only speculate upon their relative distribution within the periodontal ligament, and upon their morphology. Most likely they are related to some of the finely myelinated and unmyelinated free terminals so common here and in gingival and periosteal tissues.

GENERAL COMMENTS

The functional implications of the dense collection

of endings distributed around the teeth have not escaped comparison with those of similar neural distributions elsewhere in the body. Burgess and Perl (1973) and Kubota and Osanai (1977) have observed similarities between the dental innervation and that of sturdy body hairs such as the vibrissae and sinus hairs. Burgess and Perl point out that there is minimal sustained activity when such structures are in their rest position. However, when the structure is moved in a given direction, particular receptors discharge in a graded fashion related to the degree of displacement. Return of the structure to its original position and displacement in the opposite direction evokes similar, progressive activity in another group of receptors. Terming this an 'opponent' system, they contrast it with an alternative one in which each receptor is capable of responding over the full range of directional movement. Although greater numbers of receptors are necessary in the 'opponent' system, it has the advantage of being relatively silent in the rest position of the structure concerned. This is conceivably a useful feature when peripheral information is to be processed centrally.

We have seen that the periodontal innervation is capable of signalling a wide variety of data when peripheral stimuli affect the tooth-supporting tissues. The speed, amplitude and duration of tooth displacement in response to applied occlusal forces are all coded with some accuracy. It is possible, though unproven, that information regarding direction may also be provided. Finally, should any stimuli reach noxious levels, we must assume that the appropriate signals are accordingly generated and relayed centrally.

FUNCTIONAL ROLE

Though a full consideration of the central, neurophysiological implications of periodontal input is beyond the scope of this chapter (the reader is referred elsewhere to reviews by Anderson et al. (1970), Sessle and Hannam (1976), Anderson and Matthews (1976), Perryman (1978), Dubner et al. (1978), Hannam (1979 a, b)), certain aspects are of particular relevance.

At the level of the brainstem, periodontal signals are processed so that alone (or in combination with inputs from other oro-facial sites) they may result in transient, reflex inhibition of activity in the jaw-closing muscles. The effect is mediated via the trigeminal sensory complex. If the peripheral stimuli are large enough, this inhibition can be profound. When combined with activation of the jaw-opening muscles, it can be manifested as a frank jaw-opening reflex. This reflex is viewed by some as an oral manifestation of the flexion-withdrawal, protective response seen in the limbs.

The implications of a periodontal projection via the mesencephalic nucleus of the trigeminal nerve are less clear. That this nucleus also happens to contain the cell bodies of afferent nerves supplying the muscle spindles of the jaw-closing muscles indicates a possible close relationship between activity in the muscle spindle afferents and periodontal afferents. Such a close interaction would have implications in the control of elevator muscle activity during function. However, whether periodontal influences via this route are excitatory, inhibitory, or both is unclear; certainly any reflex events appear to be very rapid and are not polysynaptic as they are elsewhere in the trigeminal sensory complex (Taylor et al., 1978).

Our understanding of the reasons for a dual periodontal representation in the brainstem can be improved if we view the issue from another perspective. Selachian fish do not contain muscle spindles in their jaw-closing muscles, but they do possess a very strong mesencephalic projection of peridental afferents from the tooth-attachment tissues (Taylor et al., 1978). Roberts and Witkowsky (1975) have shown this input to be excitatory to the jaw-closing muscles. Consequently, pressure on the teeth in these fish results in reflex snapping, jaw closure. Though perhaps a biological asset to the shark, such simple reflex behaviour may have proved less advantageous to species with demands for a more highly developed system for controlling jaw movement. Our present 'hybrid' periodontal projection in the brainstem may therefore merely signify stages in the evolutionary development of the masticatory apparatus.

Brainstem-mediated effects associated with periodontal stimulation are not limited to jaw-opening reflexes, or to brief, excitatory or inhibitory events in the jaw-closing muscles. Reflex, lateral jaw movements in response to dental stimuli have been reported by Lund, McLachlan and Dellow (1971). Furthermore, periodontal influences upon the brainstem 'pattern generator' responsible for the rhythmicity of jaw movements have been described (Lund, Smith and Lamarre, 1978; Hannam and Lund, in press). Obviously, the periodontal innervation plays an extensive role at the brainstem level, one which can be quite independent of any influence upon conscious perception or the sensorimotor events that accompany it.

As we ascend the neuraxis, correlations between the periodontal innervation and its behavioural influences become less distinct. Not only have the projections themselves been incompletely described (a task whose difficulty is compounded by the neuronal convergence and interactions which occur with greater frequency as the neuraxis is scaled), but the use of intact or near-intact preparations has introduced the usual complications that accompany all behavioural studies and their design. We may assume, however, that the periodontal innervation, via its thalamocortical projection, contributes to the conscious perception of interocclusal forces, and subsequently to their grading during voluntary effort. If mastication can be considered to be a learned skill (Welford, 1979), then periodontal feedback is likely to be used at a conscious level during its performance. It also seems as if periodontal afferents may be involved in the conscious perception of very small particles between the teeth (Hannam 1979a). How this occurs is obscure, however, because conventionally it is believed that thickness estimation (whatever the magnitude involved) is largely a function of input from joint and muscle (Dubner *et al.,* 1978; Hannam, 1979a).

It is hard to assess just how important feedback from the tooth-supporting structures is to the human subject. We must remember that there are many other receptor systems in and around the oral cavity which can provide sensory cues useful in controlling muscle activity and jaw movement, and that the human capacity for neuromuscular adaptation is considerable. Furthermore, man can clearly function tolerably well in the edentulous state, at least well enough to sustain his general health and well-being. However, dentate subjects have the ability to produce much higher interocclusal forces and to discriminate between fine particles with much greater accuracy. To a large extent these qualities depend upon an

intact periodontal innervation. If such qualities confer a biological advantage to their owners, we must assume that the sensory nerves supplying the periodontal tissues have equal significance.

AUTONOMIC INNERVATION

Compared with its common sensory innervation, the autonomic supply of the periodontal ligament has received scant attention. Furthermore, the few descriptions available are confined to the sympathetic division alone. There is no evidence for the existence of a parasympathetic component.

Even the routes by which sympathetic autonomic fibres travel to the periodontium are not properly understood. In man, it is commonly taught that post-ganglionic nerve fibres travel from the paravertebral superior cervical ganglion to the teeth via branches on the external carotid artery arising from the external carotid plexus. Yet, Matthews and Robinson (1979, 1980) have shown experimentally that sympathetic efferent fibres in the cat are present in the infraorbital and inferior alveolar nerves. These fibres apparently travel from the superior cervical ganglion with the internal carotid plexus; the majority then enter the middle cranial fossa through the foramen lacerum and are distributed thereafter with the mandibular division of the trigeminal nerve. Thus, the manner by which the post-ganglionic fibres reach the vessels may well be a dual one, involving vascular branches of the external carotid artery as well as the terminal branches of the superior and inferior dental nerves.

The sympathetic fibres are mostly unmyelinated (probably from 0.2 to 1 μm in diameter) and at best conduct nerve impulses no faster than 1.3 m/s (Matthews and Robinson, 1980). If they follow the general trend elsewhere in the body, the post-ganglionic axons become varicose on approaching their destinations and branch into long terminal fibres approximately 0.1 to 0.5 μm in diameter (Burnstock and Bell, 1974). Mingling before reaching effector cells, they ramify to form basket-like arrangements around the vessels. Throughout the periodontium, networks, arborizations and collections of free nerve terminals have been observed in close association with blood vessels and it is reasonable to assume that many of these originate from the autonomic nervous system (see Dubner *et al.,* 1978). Individual fibres probably innervate many effector cells, and display bead-like series of varicosities each from 0.5 to 2 μm in diameter and about 3–5 μm apart (Burnstock and Bell, 1974; Bhagat, Young and Biggerstaff, 1977). The varicosities are believed to contain the small, dense-core vesicles responsible for the synthesis, storage and release of noradrenaline. Fluorescence microscopy of human gingival material indicates that such catecholamine-containing endings are present near the outer border of the smooth muscle layer of the blood vessels (Frewin *et al.,* 1971), an observation in agreement with the distribution of adrenergic endings in muscular arteries and arterioles elsewhere. We can only assume that a similar arrangement exists in the periodontal ligament, and that the varicose, ramifying terminals here exert their effects upon alpha-adrenergic receptor sites in the underlying smooth muscle. This would be consistent with putative sympathetic nerve terminations in blood vessels of the pulp (Dubner *et al.,* 1978), alveolar submucosa (Edwall and Kindlová, 1971) and skin (Burnstock and Bell, 1974; Bhagat *et al.,* 1977).

The most profound physiological effect of sympathetic autonomic activity in the periodontal ligament is upon regional blood flow (Edwall and Kindlová, 1971; Edwall, 1972; Loginova and Khayutin, 1974; Dubner *et al.,* 1978); and vasoconstriction is the most plausible reason for the sympathetically induced changes in periodontal mechanoreceptor discharge described earlier (see page 189). A reduced blood supply or a reduced local tissue fluid pressure could alter the milieu of mechanoreceptors enough to produce the effects seen in the mesencephalic nucleus by Anderson and Linden (1977) and occasionally in afferent neurones of the trigeminal ganglion by Cash and Linden (1980). No influence of sympathetic stimulation upon the discharge of periodontal nociceptors has been reported. The functional significance of sympathetic modulation of mechanoreceptor input remains a problem. It is possible that vasodilation due to reduced sympathetic activity (or even to the release of endogenous chemical vasodilators) can also effect sensory input from the periodontal ligament. Whether this central modulation of peripheral responses is a useful means for preserving the coding of information despite fluctuations of pressure in the immediate receptor environment, or whether the changes in receptor responses are simply secondary to more significant events elsewhere, is unknown.

Other physiological implications of sympathetic activity in the vascular system of the periodontal ligament are dealt with specifically elsewhere (see Chapter 7), including its possible influence upon tooth position and eruption (see Chapter 10). For a detailed consideration of the general reflex behaviour of the autonomic nervous system as it applies to the oro-facial region, the reader is referred to Dubner *et al.* (1978).

REFERENCES

ANDERSON, D. J. & LINDEN, R. W. A. (1977) Sympathetic modulation of intraoral mechanoreceptor activity. *J. dent. Res.* **56**, D125.

ANDERSON, D. J. & MATTHEWS, B. (eds.) (1976) *Mastication.* Wright, Bristol.

ANDERSON, D. J., HANNAM, A. G. & MATTHEWS, B. (1970) Sensory mechanisms in mammalian teeth and their supporting structures. *Physiol. Rev.* **50**, 171–195.

ANDRES, K. H. & VON DÜRING, M. (1973) Morphology of cutaneous receptors. In: *Somatosensory system. Handbook of sensory physiology,* Vol. II, A. IGGO (ed.), pp. 3–28. Berlin, Springer-Verlag.

BEAUDREAU, D. E. & JERGE, C. R. (1968) Somatotopic representation in the Gasserian ganglion of tactile peripheral fields in the cat. *Archs. oral Biol.* **13**, 247–256.

BEERTSEN, W. and EVERTS, V. (1977) The site of remodelling of collagen in the periodontal ligament of the mouse incisor. *Anat. Rec.* **189**, 479–498.

BEERTSEN, W., EVERTS, V. & VAN DEN HOOFF, A. (1974) Fine structure and possible function of cells containing leptomeric organelles in the periodontal ligament of the rat incisor. *Archs. oral Biol.* **19**, 1099–1100.

BERKOVITZ, B. K. B. & SHORE, R. C. (1978) High mitochondrial density within peripheral nerve fibres of the periodontal ligament of the rat incisor. *Archs. oral Biol.* **23**, 207–213.

BERKOVITZ, B. K. B. & SLOAN, P. (1979) Attachment tissues of the teeth in Caiman sclerops (Crocodilia). *J. Zool. Lond.* **187**, 179–194.

BERNICK, S. (1957) Innervation of teeth and periodontium after enzymatic removal of collagenous elements. *Oral Surg. Oral Med. Oral Path.* **10**, 323–332.

BHAGAT, B. D., YOUNG, P. A. & BIGGERSTAFF, D. E. (1977) *Fundamentals of visceral innervation.* Springfield, Thomas.

BIEMESDERFER, D., MUNGER, B. L., BINCK, J. & DUBNER, R. (1978) The pilo—Ruffini complex: a non-sinus hair and associated slowly-adapting mechanoreceptor in primate facial skin. *Brain Res.* **142**, 197–222.

BONNAUD, A., PROUST, J. P. & VIGNON, C. (1978) Terminaisons nerveuses buccales chez le chat. *J. Biol. Buccale,* **6**, 111–120.

BRASHEAR, A. D. (1936) The innervation of the teeth. An analysis of nerve fibre components of the pulp and periodontal tissues and their probable significance. *J. Comp. Neurol.* **64**, 169–185.

BREATHNACH, A. S. (1977) Electron microscopy of cutaneous nerves and receptors. *J. Invest. Dermatol.* **69**, 8–26.

BURGESS, P. R. & PERL, E. R. (1973) Cutaneous mechanoreceptors and nociceptors. In: *Somatosensory system. Handbook of sensory physiology,* Vol. II, A. IGGO (ed.), pp. 29–78. Berlin, Springer-Verlag.

BURNSTOCK, G. and BELL, C. (1974) Peripheral autonomic transmission. In: *The peripheral nervous system,* J. I. HUBBARD (ed.), pp. 277–327. London, Plenum.

BYERS, M. R. & HOLLAND, G. R. (1977) Trigeminal nerve endings in gingiva, junctional epithelium and periodontal ligament of rat molars as demonstrated by autoradiography. *Anat. Rec.* **188**, 509–524.

CASH, R. M. & LINDEN, R. W. A. (1980) The effect of sympathetic stimulation on periodontal mechanoreceptor activity recorded in trigeminal ganglion of cat. *J. dent. Res.* **59**, Special Issue D, 1839.

CAUNA, N. (1976) Morphological basis of sensation in hairy skin. In: *Somatosensory and visceral receptor systems. Progress in brain research,* Vol. 43, A. IGGO & O. ILYINSKY (eds.), pp. 35–45. Amsterdam, Elsevier.

CHAMBERS, M. R., ANDRES, K. H., VON DUERING, M. & IGGO, A. (1972) The structure and function of the slowly adapting type II receptor in hairy skin. *Quart. J. expl. Physiol.* **57**, 417–445.

COPRON, R. E., AVERY, J. K., LEE, S. D. & MORAWA, A. P. (1980) Ultrastructure of a presumptive Golgi–Mazzoni receptor in the periodontal ligament in mice. *J. dent. Res.* **59**, 134.

DESJARDINS, R. P., WINKELMANN, R. K. & GONZALEZ, J. B. (1971) Comparison of nerve endings in normal gingiva with those in mucosa covering edentulous alveolar ridges. *J. dent. Res.* **50**, 867–879.

DIXON, A. D. (1961) Sensory nerve terminations in the oral mucosa. *Archs. oral Biol.* **5**, 105–114.

DIXON, A. D. (1963) Nerve plexuses in the oral mucosa. *Archs. oral Biol.* **8**, 435–447.

DUBNER, R., SESSLE, B. J. & STOREY, A. T. (1978) *The neural basis of oral and facial function.* New York, Plenum.

EDWALL, L. (1972) Nervous control of blood circulation in the dental pulp and periodontal tissues. In: *Oral physiology,* N. EMMELIN & Y. ZOTTERMAN (eds.). Oxford, Pergamon.

EDWALL, L. & KINDLOVÁ, M. (1971) The effect of sympathetic nerve stimulation on the rate of disappearance of tracers from various oral tissues. *Acta Odontol. Scand.* **29**, 387–400.

EVERTS, V., BEERTSEN, W. & VAN DEN HOOFF, A.

(1977) Fine structure of an end organ in the periodontal ligament of the mouse incisor. *Anat. Rec.* **189**, 73–90.

FREWIN, D. B., HUME, W. R., WATERSON, J. G. & WHELAN, R. F. (1971) The histochemical localization of sympathetic nerve endings in human gingival blood vessels. *Aust. J. exp. Biol. med. Sci.* **49**, 573–580.

GAIRNS, F. W. & AITCHISON, J. (1950) A preliminary study of the multiplicity of nerve endings in the human gum. *Dent. Rec.* **70**, 180–194.

GRIFFIN, C. J. (1972) The fine structure of end-rings in human periodontal ligament. *Archs. oral Biol.* **17**, 785–797.

GRIFFIN, C. J. & HARRIS, R. (1968) Unmyelinated nerve endings in the periodontal membrane of human teeth. *Archs. oral Biol.* **17**, 913–921.

GRIFFIN, C. J. & MALOR, R. (1974) An analysis of mandibular movement. In: *Physiology of mastication. Frontiers of oral physiology,* Vol. 1, Y. KAWAMURA (ed.), pp. 159–198. Basel, Karger.

GRIFFIN, C. J. & SPAIN, H. (1972) The organization and vasculature of human periodontal ligament mechanoreceptors. *Archs. oral Biol.* **17**, 913–922.

HANNAM, A. G. (1968) The conduction velocity of nerve impulses from dental mechanoreceptors in the dog. *Archs. oral Biol.* **13**, 1377–1383.

HANNAM, A. G. (1969a) The response of periodontal mechanoreceptors in the dog to controlled loading of the teeth. *Archs. oral Biol.* **14**, 781–791.

HANNAM, A. G. (1969b) Spontaneous activity in dental mechanosensitive units in the dog. *Archs. oral Biol.* **14**, 793–801.

HANNAM, A. G. (1970) Receptor fields of periodontal mechanosensitive units in the dog. *Archs. oral Biol.* **15**, 971–978.

HANNAM, A. G. (1976) Periodontal mechanoreceptors. In: *Mastication,* D. J. ANDERSON & B. MATTHEWS (eds.), pp. 42–49. Bristol, Wright.

HANNAM, A. G. (1979a) Neuromuscular control of overdentures. In: *Precision attachments in dentistry* (3rd ed.), H. W. PRIESKEL (ed.), pp. 156–161. London, Kimpton.

HANNAM, A. G. (1979b) Mastication in man. In: *Oral motor behaviour: Impact on oral conditions and dental treatment,* P. BRYANT, E. GALE and J. RUGH (eds.), pp. 87–118. Washington, Nat. Inst. Health Publication (79–1845).

HANNAM, A. G. & FARNSWORTH, T. J. (1977) Information transmission in trigeminal mechanosensitive afferents from teeth in the cat. *Archs. oral Biol.* **22**, 181–186.

HANNAM, A. G. & LUND, J. P. (in press) The effect of intraoral stimulation on the human masticatory cycle. *Archs. oral Biol.*

HARRIS, R. (1975) Innervation of the human periodontium. In: *The temporomandibular joint syndrome,* Monographs in Oral Science, Vol. 4, C. J. GRIFFIN & R. HARRIS (eds.), pp. 27–44. Basel, Karger.

HATTYASY, D. (1959) Zur Frage der Innervation der Zahnwurzelhaut. *Z. Mikr. Anat. Forsch.* **65**, 413–433.

HENSEL, H. (1973) Cutaneous thermoreceptors. In: *Somatosensory system. Handbook of sensory physiology,*

Vol. II, A. IGGO (ed.), pp. 79–110. Berlin, Springer-Verlag.

HORCH, K. W., TUCKETT, R. P. & BURGESS, P. R. (1977) A key to the classification of cutaneous mechanoreceptors. *J. Invest. Dermatol.* **69**, 75–82.

IGGO, A. (1976) Is the physiology of cutaneous receptors determined by morphology? In: *Somatosensory and visceral receptor systems. Progress in brain research,* Vol. 43, A. IGGO & O. ILYINSKY (eds.), pp. 15–31. Amsterdam, Elsevier.

JERGE, C. R. (1963) Organization and function of the trigeminal mesencephalic nucleus. *J. Neurophysiol.* **26**, 379–392.

JOHANSSON, R. S. & OLSSON, K. A. (1976) Microelectrode recordings from human oral mechanoreceptors. *Brain Res.* **118**, 307–311.

KADANOFF, D. (1928) Über die intraepithelialen Nerven und ihre Endigungen beim Menschen und bei Saugetieren. *Z. Zellforsch. mikr. Anat.* **7**, 553–576.

KERR, F. W. L. & LYSAK, W. R. (1964) Somatotopic organization of trigeminal ganglion neurones. *Arch. Neurol.* **11**, 593–602.

KIZIOR, J. E., CUOZZO, J. W. & BOWMAN, D. C. (1968) Functional and histologic assessment of the sensory innervation of the periodontal ligament of the cat. *J. dent. Res.* **47**, 59–64.

KUBOTA, K. & OSANAI, K. (1977) Periodontal sensory innervation of the dentition of the Japanese shrewmole. *J. dent. Res.* **56**, 531–537.

DE LANGE, A., HANNAM, A. G. & MATTHEWS, B. (1969) The diameters and conduction velocities of fibres in the terminal branches of the inferior dental nerve. *Archs. oral Biol.* **14**, 513–519.

LEWINSKY, W. & STEWART, D. (1936) The innervation of the periodontal membrane. *J. Anat.* **71**, 98–103.

LEWINSKY, W. & STEWART, D. (1937) The innervation of the periodontal membrane of the cat with some observations on the function of the end-organs found in that structure. *J. Anat.* **71**, 232–235.

LEWINSKY, W. & STEWART, D. (1938) The innervation of the human gum. *J. Anat.* **72**, 531–536.

LINDEN, R. W. A. (1978) Properties of intraoral mechanoreceptors represented in the mesencephalic nucleus of the fifth nerve in the cat. *J. Physiol. (Lond.)* **279**, 395–408.

LISNEY, S. J. W. & MATTHEWS, B. (1978) Branched afferent nerves supplying tooth pulp in the cat. *J. Physiol. (Lond.)* **279**, 509–517.

LOGINOVA, N. K. & KHAYUTIN, V. M. (1974) Quantitative characteristics of the effect of constrictor fibres of the cervical sympathetic nerve on resistive vessels of the mandible. *Stomatolog.* **53**, 3–6.

LUND, J. P., McLACHLAN, R. S. & DELLOW, P. G. (1971) A lateral jaw movement reflex. *Expl. Neurol.* **31**, 189–199.

LUND, J. P., SMITH, A. M. & LAMARRE, Y. (1978) Sensory control of mandibular movements and its modulation by set and circumstances. In: *Oral physiology and occlusion,* J. H. PERRYMAN (ed.), pp. 115–135. Oxford, Pergamon.

MARTINEZ, R. & PEKARTHY, J. M. (1974) Ultrastructure of encapsulated nerve endings in rat gingiva. *Amer. J. Anat.* **140**, 135–138.

MATTHEWS, B. & ROBINSON, P. P. (1979) The course of postganglionic sympathetic fibres to the face and jaws in the cat. *J. Physiol. (Lond.)* **293**, 46P.

MATTHEWS, B. & ROBINSON, P. P. (1980) The course of the postganglionic sympathetic fibres supplying the mandibular region in the cat. *J. dent. Res.* **59** (Special Issue D), 1840.

MEI, N., HARTMANN, F. & AUBERT, M. (1977) Periodontal mechanoreceptors involved in pain. In: *Pain in the trigeminal region,* D. J. ANDERSON & B. MATTHEWS (eds.), pp. 103–110. Amsterdam, Elsevier.

MOXHAM, B. J. (1975) The use of a continuous recording technique for the assessment of the haemodynamic hypothesis of tooth eruption. *J. Physiol. (Lond.)* **245**, 43P.

MUNGER, B. L. (1971) The comparative ultrastructure of slowly and rapidly adapting mechanoreceptors. In: *Oral-facial sensory and motor mechanisms,* R. DUBNER & Y. KAWAMURA (eds.), pp. 83–103. New York, Appleton-Century Crofts.

MUNGER, B. L. (1975) Cytology of mechanoreceptors in oral mucosa and facial skin of the rhesus monkey. In: *The basic neurosciences. The nervous system,* Vol. 1, D. TOWER (ed.), pp. 71–79. New York, Raven Press.

MUNGER, B. L. (1977) Neural–epithelial interactions in sensory receptors. *J. Invest. Dermatol.* **69**, 27–40.

NESS, A. R. (1954) The mechanoreceptors of the rabbit mandibular incisor. *J. Physiol. (Lond.)* **126**, 475–493.

PERRYMAN, J. H. (ed.) (1978) *Oral physiology and occlusion.* New York, Pergamon.

PFAFFMANN, C. (1939) Afferent impulses from the teeth due to pressure and noxious stimulation. *J. Physiol. (Lond.)* **97**, 207–219.

PICTON, D. C. A. (1965) On the part played by the socket in tooth support. *Archs. oral Biol.* **10**, 945–955.

PIMENIDIS, M. Z. & HINDS, J. W. (1977) An autoradiographic study of the teeth. II. Dental pulp and periodontium. *J. dent. Res.* **56**, 835–840.

QUILLIAM, T. A. (1966) Structure of receptor organs: unit design and array patterns in receptor organs. In: *Touch, heat and pain,* A. V. S. DE REUCK & J. KNIGHT (eds.), pp. 86–112. London, Churchill.

RAPP, R., KIRSTINE, W. D. & AVERY, J. K. (1957) A study of neural endings in the human gingiva and periodontal membrane. *J. Can. Dent. Ass.* **23**, 637–643.

ROBERTS, B. L. & WITKOWSKY, P. (1975) A functional analysis of the mesencephalic nucleus of the fifth nerve in the selachian brain. *Proc. Roy. Soc.* B **19**, 473–495.

ROBINSON, P. P. (1979) The course, relations and distribution of the inferior alveolar nerve and its branches in the cat. *Anat. Rec.* **195**, 265–272.

SAKADA, S. (1971) Response of Golgi–Mazzoni corpuscles in the cat periostea to mechanical stimuli. In: *Oral-facial sensory and motor mechanisms,* R. DUBNER & Y. KAWAMURA (eds.), pp. 105–122. New York, Appleton-Century Crofts.

SAKADA, S. (1974) Mechanoreceptors in fascia, periosteum and periodontal ligament. *Bull. Tokyo Med. Dent. Univ.* **21**, (Suppl), 11–13.

SAKADA, S. & KAMIO, E. (1971) Receptive fields and directional sensitivity of single sensory units innervating the periodontal ligaments of the cat mandibular teeth. *Bull. Tokyo Dent. Coll.* **12**, 25–43.

SESSLE, B. J. & HANNAM, A. G. (eds.) (1976) *Mastication and swallowing. Biological and clinical correlates.* Univ. Toronto Press, Toronto.

TAYLOR, A., STEPHENS, J. A., SOMJEN, G. & HARRISON, L. M. (1978) Muscle spindles and tooth mechano-receptors in the control of mastication. In: *Oral physiology and occlusion,* J. H. PERRYMAN (ed.), pp. 22–40. Oxford, Pergamon.

WAGERS, P. W. & SMITH, C. M. (1960) Responses in dental nerves of dogs to tooth stimulation, and the effects of systemically administered procaine, lidocaine and morphine. *J. Pharm. Expl Therap.* **130**, 89–105.

WEILL, R., BENSADOUN, R. & DE TOURNIEL, F. (1975) Démonstration autoradiographique de l'innervation de la dent et du parodonte. *C. R. Acad. Science Paris.* Series D, 647–650.

WELFORD, A. T. (1979) Principles of motor control and their application to dental problems. In: *Oral motor behaviour: impact on oral conditions and dental treatment,* P. BRYANT, E. GALE & J. RUGH (eds.), pp. 199–212. Washington, Nat. Inst. Health Publication (79–1845).

YAMADA, M. & KUMANO, T. (1969) Mobility and assessment of the tactile sensation of teeth. *Int. Dent. J.* **19**, 295–296.

YOUNG, R. F. (1977) Fiber spectrum of the trigeminal sensory root of frog, cat and man determined by electromicroscopy. In: *Pain in the trigeminal region,* D. J. ANDERSON and B. MATTHEWS (eds.), pp. 137–147. Holland, Elsevier.

Chapter 9

DEVELOPMENT OF THE PERIODONTAL LIGAMENT

S. Bernick and D. A. Grant

INTRODUCTION

The tissues of attachment of a tooth (cementum, periodontal ligament and the alveolar bone of the tooth socket) are derived from the dental follicle. The dental follicle is first recognized as a condensation of mesenchymal tissue surrounding the developing tooth anlage at the cap stage. By the bell stage, the mesenchymal tissue between the enamel organ and the wall of the alveolar crypt consists of three layers (Tonge, 1963). The inner layer is a vascular, fibrocellular condensation, three to four cells thick. The outer layer lining the developing alveolus is also comprised of a vascular mesenchyme. Between these two layers is a loose connective tissue which is relatively avascular. That there is some anatomical basis for separation between inner and outer layers of the follicle is indicated by the observation that tooth germs extracted from the jaw are surrounded by the inner, but not the outer, layer (Ten Cate, Mills and Solomon, 1971).

The term dental follicle has been used by different authors to mean different things and the problems associated with terminology have been reviewed by Tonge (1963) and Ten Cate (1969). Ten Cate (1969, 1972) is of the opinion that the term dental follicle should be reserved for the inner layer in contact with the tooth germ, believing that it alone gives rise to all the major components of the periodontium. He terms the remaining tissue perifollicular.

There has also been some debate about the precise origin of the cells comprising the dental follicle. Whilst traditionally it is held that the cells are derived from mesoderm near the site of the developing tooth, Ten Cate (1969) believes they originate, at least in part, from neural crest cells which have migrated to the region of the developing jaws.

The formation and organization of the periodontal ligament from the dental follicle has been studied primarily by histological and transplantation techniques. Autoradiographical studies have also provided some information relating to turnover and remodelling in the developing periodontal ligament.

HISTOLOGICAL STUDIES

The general sequence of events associated with root formation are well established. Root formation commences with the appearance of the epithelial root sheath. This is thought to induce the adjacent cells of the dental papilla to differentiate into odontoblasts and form root dentine. With root development, the epithelial cells lose their continuity, become separated from the surface of the forming root dentine, and later become the epithelial cells rests in the periodontal ligament. Mesenchymal cells of the dental follicle adjacent to root dentine differentiate into cementoblasts which commence cementogenesis. Following the onset of root formation, changes become apparent within the dental follicle associated with the development of the principal fibre groups of the periodontal ligament. However, at the growing root apex the dental follicle retains the layered appearance seen at the bell stage (Tonge, 1963; Ten Cate, 1969; Grant and Bernick, 1972).

Species differences in root formation do exist. Lester (1969) has noted that during root formation in molar teeth of rats, cells of the epithelial root sheath are embedded *en masse* between the forming cementum and dentine. Furthermore, he suggested the possibility that the epithelial cells may have a role to play in information transfer. Though it has been assumed generally that cementum is a product of cementoblasts, there is evidence in dogs (Owens, 1974), cats (Sloan and Benyon, in press) and man (Owens, 1974; Sloan and Benyon, in press) that the innermost layer of cementum is odontoblastic in origin.

Formation of the principal collagen fibre groups of the periodontal ligament

This has been described for the deciduous teeth of the marmoset (Levy and Bernick, 1968) and cat (Tonge, 1963), for the rodent molar (Sicher, 1923; Eccles, 1959; Bernick, 1960; Trott, 1962; Magnusson, 1968; Atkinson, 1972) and incisor (Eccles, 1964), for the permanent molars of the dog (Orban, 1927), marmoset (Grant *et al.*, 1972), macaque monkey (Magnusson, 1968) and man (Noyes, Schour and Noyes, 1943; Orban, 1957) and for the premolars of the squirrel monkey (Grant and Bernick, 1972) and of the marmoset (Grant *et al.*, 1972). The information which follows is based upon detailed studies of the sequential histogenesis of the periodontal ligament in squirrel monkey premolar teeth by Grant and Bernick (1972) and in marmoset premolar and molar teeth by Grant *et al.* (1972). This appears to agree with what is known about the situation in man.

FORMATION OF PREMOLAR PERIODONTAL LIGAMENT

(a) *Pre-emergence stage*

Prior to eruption into the oral cavity, the premolars are enclosed in a bony crypt. Periodontal ligament formation proceeds in a corono-apical sequence. When approximately one-third of the root has formed, the developing periodontal ligament appears to consist of loosely structured collagenous elements. Near the amelo-cemental junction (Fig. 1), fibres arising from

---

FIG. 1. The erupting permanent premolar is enclosed within a bony crypt. Predentogingival fibres are demonstrable, while more apically the periodontal ligament is composed of unorganized connective tissue elements. (Mallory's connective tissue stain, ×30.)

FIG. 2. At the cementoenamel junction of the tooth shown in Fig. 1, organized fibres can be observed emanating from cementum. These fibres course occlusally as they follow the outline of the crown. Intense osteoblastic activity is apparent at the bony margin. No fibres are seen emanating from bone. Apical to the cementoenamel junction, the periodontal ligament is occupied by loose, unorganized fibres. A, Cementoenamel junction. B, Alveolar bone. (Silver nitrate impregnation, ×115.)

FIG. 3. At the midroot region of the tooth shown in Fig. 1, brush-like fibres are seen emanating from cementum. The central zone is very wide and is occupied by loosely arranged collagenous elements. Osteoblasts line the bony margin which is almost devoid of fibre extrusions. A, Bone. B, Cementum. (Silver nitrate impregnation, ×200.)

FIG. 4. Apically, fibres arising from beneath the tooth course into the periodontal ligament. They are orientated parallel to the long axis of the tooth. (Silver nitrate impregnation, ×125.)

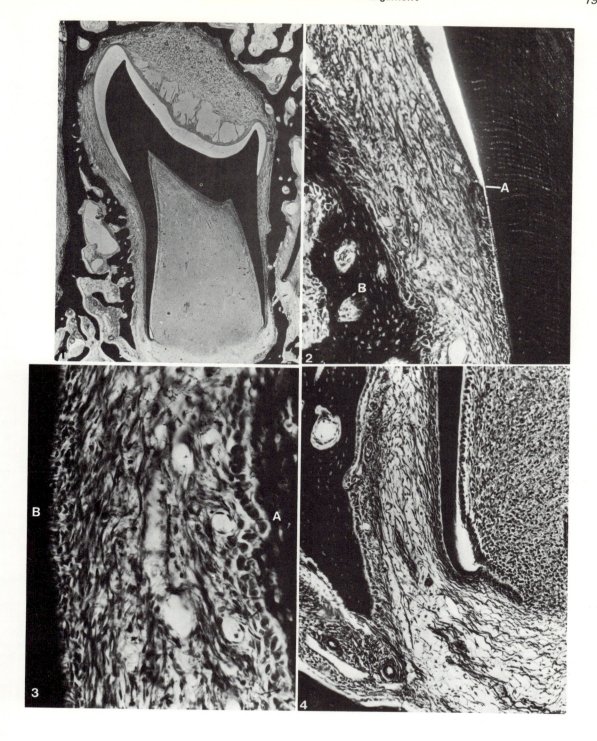

the cementum are demonstrable as an organized entity. They course coronally and follow the outline of the crown. In sections impregnated with silver nitrate (Fig. 2), fine argyrophilic fibres can be traced, originating from the cementum just below the amelo-cemental junction and coursing occlusally around the contour of the enamel surface. Although numerous osteoblasts line the margin of the adjacent crestal bone, no fibres can be seen emerging from the bone.

In the midroot region (Fig. 3), fine, short, closely spaced fibres can be seen emerging from cementum. In the middle three-quarters of the developing periodontal ligament there are loosely arranged fibres aligned parallel to the long axis of the root. Osteoblasts line the alveolar surface and only an occasional fibre can be seen emerging from bone.

In the periapical region (Fig. 4), fine collagenous fibres extend into the central third of the periodontal ligament and pass in an occlusal direction, parallel to the long axis of the root. Near the cementum, the fibres are densely packed and oriented in a superior-oblique direction from cementum toward the middle third of the ligament. Near the alveolar bone, fibre bundles emerging from the periapical zone course in a superior-oblique direction toward bone, in an alignment parallel to that of the fibres near cementum. They become packed more densely as they approach the osteoblast-lined bony margin, with the orientation changing to a coronal direction. The bundles finally become oriented in a superior-oblique direction from bone toward the broad central core of the developing ligament.

(b) *Emergence into the oral cavity*

The direction of the fibres during this period appears to be influenced by the precise stage of eruption of the emerging tooth and by its positional relationship to the adjacent teeth. Consider the situation where the third premolar of the squirrel monkey is emerging into the oral cavity (Fig. 5) (with the neighbouring first permanent molar in functional occlusion and the second premolar in a pre-eruptive stage of development).

With respect to the cervical region of the emerging third premolar, Figs. 5 and 6 show that organized fibre groups can be identified readily. Well-formed dento-gingival fibres can be seen emanating from the tooth. These course occlusally to terminate in the lamina propria of the interproximal gingiva. On the mesial surface, developing transseptal fibres appear beneath the dentogingival fibres to extend obliquely in an apical direction over the alveolar crest toward the amelo-cemental junction of the adjacent, unerupted premolar. On the distal surface, the developing trans-septal fibre group can be traced as it emanates from cementum to extend in a superior-oblique direction over the forming alveolar crest toward the first molar. Midway, an intermediate zone is present separating these fibres from the inferior obliquely oriented trans-septal fibres of the adjacent first molar (Fig. 7).

Further apically, the forming periodontal ligament is not so well organized into fibre bundles. In the region of the cervical third of the root of the emerging third premolar, fibres extend apically in an oblique direction from cementum toward the alveolar bone. In the middle third of the root (Fig. 8), organized fibre groups that are continuous from cementum to bone cannot be demonstrated. Widely spaced, argyrophilic fibres protrude from the surface of the alveolar bone and extend for a short distance toward the tooth. These are separated from the closely spaced, short, brush-like, cemental fibres by a wide zone of loosely

FIG. 5. Section showing the emergence into the oral cavity of the third premolar (P_3). As the tooth emerges, organized fibres are evident in the coronal and cervical areas. No principal fibres are demonstrable more apically in the periodontal ligament. Distally, the erupted first molar (M_1) shows a classically organized attachment apparatus. P_2 = second premolar. (Mallory's connective tissue stain, $\times 35$.)

FIG. 6. At higher magnification of the mesial surface of the emerging tooth (P_3), well-formed dentogingival fibres course occlusally to follow the outline of the enamel surface. Less distinct, obliquely orientated fibres course apically over the forming alveolar crest toward the cervical area of the unerupted second premolar (P_2). (Silver nitrate impregnation, $\times 90$.)

FIG. 7. On the distal surface of the erupting tooth (P_3), the developing transseptal fibres can be traced as they emanate from cementum to extend over the forming alveolar crest toward the first molar (M_1). More apically fibres from cementum are separated from those from bone by an ever-narrowing intermediate zone. (Silver nitrate impregnation, $\times 90$.)

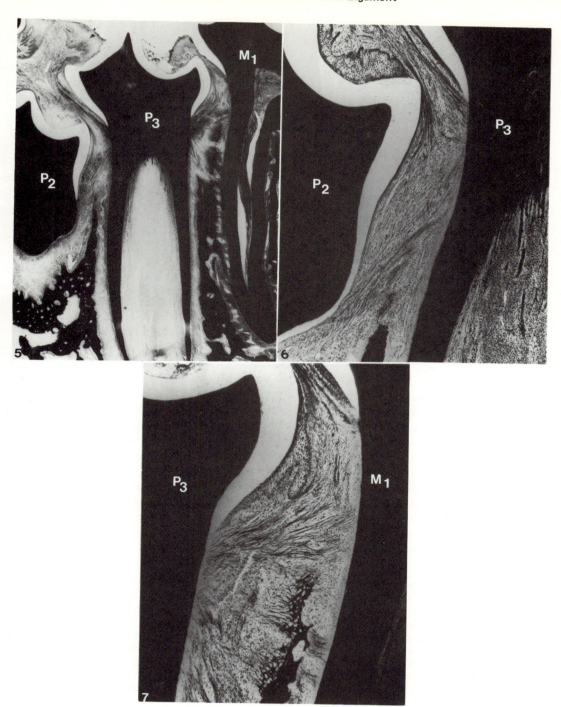

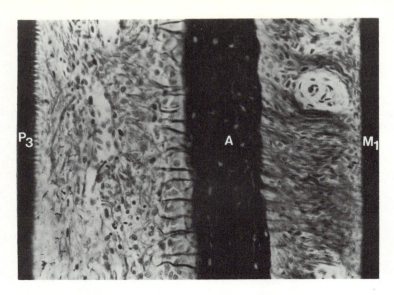

FIG. 8. At the midroot region of the teeth illustrated in Fig. 5, the classically organized and apparently continuous principal fibres of the functioning first molar (M_1) contrast with the still developing fibres of the third premolar (P_3). On the premolar, fine, short, brush-like fibres line the cemental surface and are separated from the longer, more widely spaced bony fibres by a broad zone of loosely structured collagenous elements. A, Interdental bone. (Silver nitrate impregnation, ×275.)

arranged connective tissue elements. Whilst this appearance is in accord with Sicher's observation in the guinea pig (Sicher, 1923), it is not supportive of Sicher's (1942b) and Orban's (1957) so-called 'intermediate plexus in man. In the region of the developing root apex of the third premolar, loosely organized collagenous elements like those seen in the pre-emergent premolar (Fig. 4) are evident. These fibres arise from the apical area of the tooth and course into the periodontal ligament space.

(c) First occlusal contacts

At this stage, fibre organization is further advanced. Figure 9 shows two premolars in closely successive stages of eruption from first occlusal contact to full

FIG. 9. Section showing two premolars in closely succeeding stages of eruption from first occlusal contact (tooth 'B') to full articulation (tooth 'A'). The dentogingival and transseptal fibre groups are well developed on tooth 'A'. On tooth 'B', obliquely orientated fibres course from cementum to bone at the cervical third of the root, while more apically the ligament becomes progressively less mature. (Mallory's connective tissue stain, ×40.)

FIG. 10. At higher magnification of tooth 'B' seen in Fig. 9, dense transseptal fibres extend from cementum over the alveolar crest. Apical to these, closely approximated fibres emerge from cementum to extend obliquely downward toward the alveolar bone. Near bone, these fibres appear to be joined with heavier, more widely spaced, Sharpey's fibres. Note the depth of penetration of the Sharpey's fibres into bone. A, Alveolar bone. (Silver nitrate impregnation, ×190.)

FIG. 11. A high-power view of Fig. 10 showing the joining of the cemental and osseous fibres. The heavier osseous fibres appear to 'unravel' as they splay out and apparently are joined with the more closely spaced, finer fibres that extend toward cementum. A, Alveolar bone. (Silver nitrate impregnation, ×400.)

FIG. 12. At midroot, the ligament of the emerging premolar (shown as tooth 'B' in Fig. 9) is poorly developed. Thick fibres project from bone and extend between osteoblasts into the periodontal ligament. These fibres splay outward, as if to unravel. The broad central zone of the ligament is occupied by loose collagenous elements. At the cemental surface, short, closely spaced fibres present a brush-like appearance. A, Alveolar bone. B, Cementum. (Silver nitrate impregnation, ×220.)

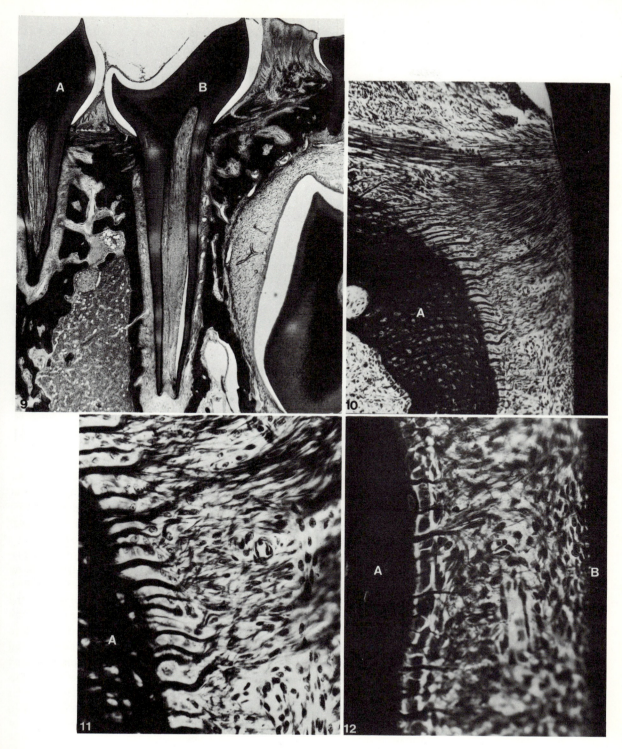

articulation. Between the premolars, the dentogingival and transseptal fibre groups are well developed and easily discerned. The alveolar crest and horizontal fibres can also be identified. However, they are less distinct than the more coronal fibre groups. More apically in the periodontal ligament, fibre development is less advanced in the tooth which has erupted less. At higher magnification in a section of this latter tooth impregnated with silver nitrate (Fig. 10), the features of the development of the periodontal ligament near the alveolar crest can be seen. A well-developed system of dense, intact, closely approximated, transseptal fibres is present. The alveolar crestal group of fibres passes from the cementum obliquely downward toward the alveolar bone. In the cervical third of the periodontal ligament proper, the cemental fibres appear to join with thicker, more widely spaced fibres that emerge from the alveolar bone. Figure 11 shows this area at higher magnification. Note the joining of the fibres from cementum with those from bone and the thick fibre bundles which emerge from the bone. Such fibres seem to 'unravel' as they arborize to join the less dense groups from cementum. In the midroot region of the premolar which has erupted less (Fig. 12), the fibres lose their continuity across the periodontal space. Extensions of Sharpey's fibres emerge from bone and project into the central zone. Separated from these fibres by the central zone, the diminutive cemental fibres are less perceptible as they emanate from the root into the developing periodontal ligament. By comparison, the periodontal fibres of the more erupted premolar show a more advanced stage of development in the midroot region (Fig. 13). Here, the fibres adjacent to alveolar bone are thicker and exhibit extensive branching as they appear to intertwine with the thinner fibres from cementum.

(d) *Full occlusal function*

Once the premolars become functional, all the classically described principal fibre groups become demonstrable (Fig. 14). A detailed description of fibres of the functional ligament is given in Chapter 3. At the functional stage, no central zone can be seen in the periodontal ligament, the fibre bundles forming a network passing directly from cementum to alveolar bone

(Figs. 14 and 15). Furthermore, with function the fibre bundles appear to thicken. This feature has also been reported in rat molars (Bernick, 1960; Trott, 1962) and incisors (Van Bladeren, 1971), though it was not confirmed by Atkinson (1972) for mouse molars.

The development of periodontal fibres for the monkey premolar is summarized diagrammatically in Figs. 16 and 17.

FORMATION OF PERMANENT MOLAR PERIODONTAL LIGAMENT

Periodontal ligament formation in teeth without primary predecessors (i.e. permanent molars) differs in several respects from that in secondary succedaneous teeth (Grant et al., 1972), and these are illustrated in Fig. 18. The main difference is the earlier appearance of the principal collagen fibres and the lack of an intermediate zone in the erupting molar teeth. In teeth without primary predecessors, periodontal ligament fibres are formed before eruption and are seen to emanate from bone and cementum (Fig. 19). Upon eruption, their obliquity appears lessened. Grant et al. (1972) showed the rapidity of principal fibre formation in two closely successive pre-eruptive stages in marmosets.

The differences between teeth with and without predecessors may be explained by a chronological variation in the sequence of deposition of alveolar bone. In permanent molars, deposition of alveolar bone is completed mainly before the crown emerges into the oral cavity. In contrast, the developing permanent premolars are completely enclosed by a bony crypt and erupt from a position lingual to the deciduous molars. During eruption, resorption of the bony roof and the lateral bony walls (as well as the overlying root) must await the subsequent deposition of alveolar bone which is deposited upon the residual cryptal bone. Thus, principal fibre formation must await the deposition of alveolar bone. The late appearance of the obliquely oriented group of dentoalveolar fibres in the succedaneous teeth is of relevance when considering the collagen-contraction hypothesis of tooth eruption (see Chapter 10).

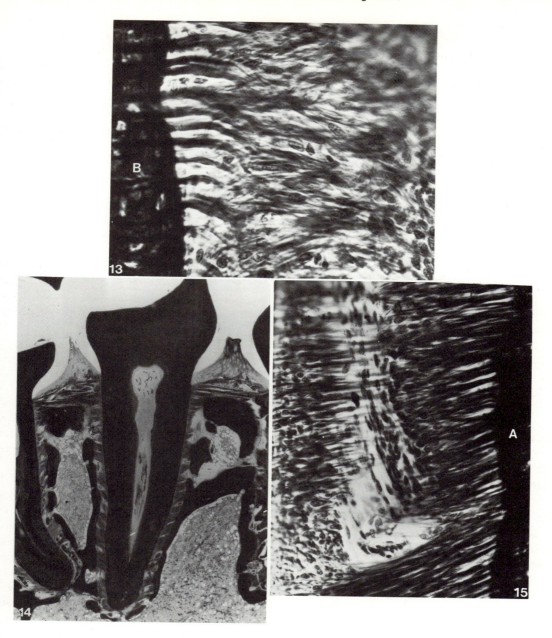

FIG. 13. In contrast with Fig. 12, fibres of the midroot periodontal ligament of the more functional premolar (tooth 'A' in Fig. 9) appear continuous from bone to cementum, as the branching Sharpey's fibres are intertwined with fibres from cementum. B, Alveolar bone. (Silver nitrate impregnation, ×190.)

FIG. 14. With function, the thick, classically oriented, principal fibres are demonstrable. (Mallory's connective tissue stain, ×30.)

FIG. 15. A higher magnification of the principal fibres of the functioning tooth shows thick fibres that appear to pass from bone to tooth. A, Alveolar bone. (Silver nitrate impregnation, ×250.)

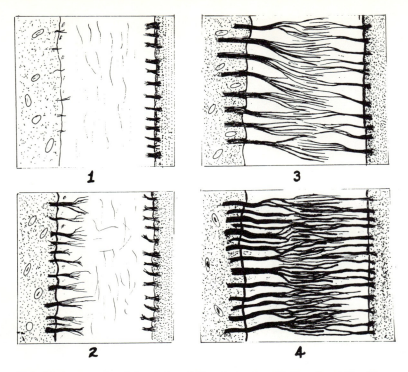

FIG. 16. A summary of alveolodental fibre formation. (1) Fine, brush-like fibres are first seen emanating from cementum. Only a few fibres project from the osteoblast-lined alveolar bone and extend into the non-organized, collagenous elements that occupy the broad central zone of the developing periodontal ligament. (2) Sharpey's fibres, thicker and more widely spaced than those from cementum, emerge from bone to extend toward the tooth and appear to unravel as they arborize at their ends. The closely spaced, cemental fibres are still short, giving the root a brush-like appearance. (3) The alveolar fibres extend further into the central zone to join the lengthening cemental fibres. (4) With occlusal function, the principal fibres become classically organized, thicker, and apparently continuous between bone and cementum.

Other features of the developing periodontal collagen fibres

Our observations of the fibre development in the periodontal ligaments of monkey permanent incisors and canines are in accord with the findings obtained for the premolars previously described.

With respect to the periodontal connective tissue directly beneath the root apex, particular attention has been focused on the so-called 'cushion hammock ligament'. This ligament was first described by Sicher (1942a) who, because of its supposed attachments to alveolar bone, considered that it provided a fixed, resistant base for the resolution of the forces produced by the growing root into an eruptive force. The ligament was said to be composed of a fibrous network with fluid-filled interstices. Though Sicher (1942b) was unable to observe a cushioned hammock ligament beneath multirooted teeth, its presence here was reported by Scott (1953). However, though subsequent authors (e.g. Hunt, 1959; Ness and Smale, 1959; Eccles, 1961; Ten Cate, 1969; Atkinson, 1972) have described the existence of a collagenous membrane beneath the developing root, it is not attached to the alveolar wall, but merges with fibres of the periodontal ligament more coronally (Fig. 4). For this reason, it is more satisfactorily termed the 'pulp-limiting membrane'. As for its function in eruption, root resection and tran-

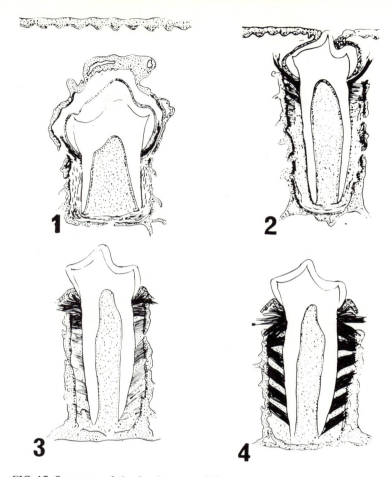

FIG. 17. Summary of the development of the principal collagen fibres of the periodontal ligament for the monkey premolar. (1) Pre-emergence. (2) Emergence into the oral cavity. (3) First occlusal contact. (4) Full occlusal function.

section studies in continuously growing incisors (e.g. Berkovitz and Thomas, 1969; Moxham and Berkovitz, 1974) show that root growth is not responsible for generating eruptive forces (see Chapter 10 for further details).

The intermediate plexus is a central zone in the periodontal ligament which separates the osseous and cemental fibres. It has attracted considerable attention and much controversy. The appearance and significance of the plexus in the functioning tooth is discussed in Chapter 3. In the developing tooth, it has been suggested that an intermediate plexus might permit eruptive and migratory tooth movements. Whilst we have not been able to observe an inter-

mediate plexus in the forming periodontal ligament of the monkey permanent molar (although Grant *et al.* (1972) observed a zone of loosely structured collagenous elements separating cemental and alveolar fibres in the early stage of the developing ligament near the root apex of the marmoset permanent molar), a central zone in the erupting monkey premolars is morphologically demonstrable at the light microscope level. However, suggestions that fibres of this zone become realigned to form or to contribute to principal fibre formation are not supported by our observations. On the other hand, the cells of the central zone, by their secretion of extracellular matrix, may participate in the lengthening and thickening of the principal fibres

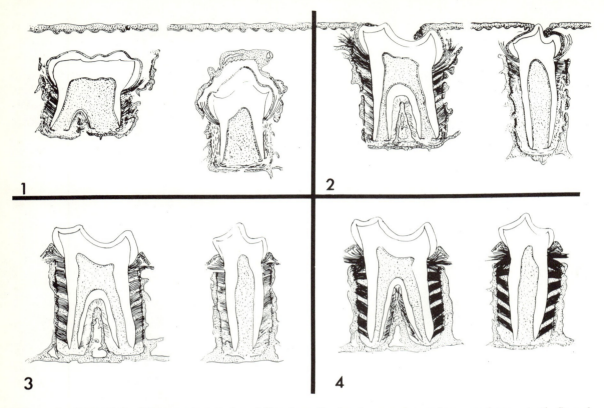

FIG. 18. A schema of the differences in periodontal fibre formation in primary and secondary succedaneous teeth. *Stage 1*. With root formation well advanced, the permanent molar (tooth without a predecessor) shows principal fibres extending from bone to cementum. The permanent premolar (tooth with a predecessor) shows only predentogingival fibres as an organized group. *Stage 2*. Upon emergence into the oral cavity, the permanent molar shows advanced fibre formation with apparently continuous principal fibres. The premolar shows organized fibres only at the alveolar crest. More apically, the periodontal ligament becomes progressively less organized. *Stage 3*. With occlusal function, the molar shows complete periodontal fibre apparatus. The premolar shows apparently continuous principal fibres, except near the apex where an intermediate zone is still demonstrable. *Stage 4*. With continued function, both molar and premolar show classically aligned, and apparently continuous, principal fibre groups.

(Baumhammers and Stallard, 1968). In this context, the study of suture development may be pertinent to the interpretations made during periodontal ligament histogenesis. Pritchard, Scott and Girgis (1956) studied the development of sutures between actively growing bones. They described middle layers bordered by cambial layers, somewhat similar to the intermediate plexus of the periodontal ligament. With maturation, collagen fibres directly united the bones across the width of the suture. This may be comparable to the imperceptibility of an intermediate plexus when tooth eruption has ceased. Trott (1962) and Atkinson (1972) both confirm the early appearance of obliquely oriented principal fibre bundles and the absence of a

loosely organized central zone during the development of the periodontal ligament of rat and mouse molars respectively. Magnusson (1968) found no evidence of an intermediate plexus during the development of permanent molars in *Macaca irus*. This may be due, however, to the absence of chronologically spaced specimens obtained within the short time interval during which fibre formation occurs in teeth without primary predecessors.

It has been reported that, as in marmoset molars, in the molars of the mouse (Atkinson, 1972), rat (Bernick, 1960; Thomas, 1965) and human (Thomas, 1965) periodontal fibres are present with an oblique orientation before the tooth has erupted. However,

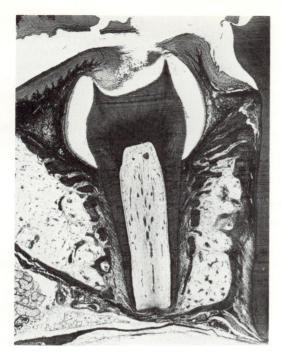

FIG. 19. The permanent second molar (a tooth without a predecessor) is just emerging into the oral cavity. The alveolar crest on both mesial and distal surfaces is at the midpoint of the crown. The periodontal ligament is composed of well-formed principal fibres that are oriented in a superior oblique direction from cementum to bone. (Mallory's connective tissue stain, ×15.)

ment of the collagen in the developing root. Owens (1979) has suggested that the basal lamina of the epithelial root sheath may play a role in orientating the first formed dentine collagen. The initial collagen fibres produced by cementoblasts are orientated at right angles to the root surface. The odontogenic and cementogenic fibres are then mineralized, the mineralization front proceeding outwards. This perpendicular arrangement of the collagen may play a role in orientating the developing principal fibre bundles. Subsequent development of cementum is controversial (for review see Formicola *et al.*, 1971) but involves entrapment of the principal fibres. Scanning electron-micrograph studies of developing periodontal attachment surfaces (Boyde and Jones, 1968; Jones and Boyde, 1974) showed that, as the fibres are entrapped, microcalcospherites form around them. The mineralization front of the Sharpey's fibre is concave and lags behind that of the surrounding collagen.

Though considerable data are available concerning turnover of extracellular protein for functioning teeth of both continuous and non-continuous growth (see Chapters 3, 4), few data are available for developing teeth. However, for developing rat and monkey molars the uptake of ^{3}H-proline and ^{35}S seems to be evenly distributed across the entire periodontal space (Magnusson, 1968; Kameyama, 1973).

Magnusson (1968) reported that a considerable portion of the root was formed before there was evidence of obliquely oriented fibres in the periodontal ligament of *Macaca irus* molars. Magnusson (1968) also noted that the inclination of the periodontal fibres decreased during eruption.

The mechanisms responsible for initiating and then maintaining the alignment of the different periodontal principal fibre groups are not known. However, it has been suggested that oblique fibre orientation is a reflection of lines of stress set up as a result of inward and upward growth of bone against the downward and usually inward root growth (Thomas, 1967). The oblique orientation of the fibroblasts, and hence the fibres, may be facilitated by their parallel alignment to the fibres of the pulp-limiting membrane (Atkinson, 1972). It is conceivable that the orientation of the developing principal fibre bundles relates to the arrange-

Development of oxytalan fibres

The development of these fibres has been described by Fullmer (1959, 1967) for human teeth. Oxytalan fibres are first demonstrable in connective tissues destined to become periodontal ligament when about 2 mm of dentine (measured in an apico-occlusal direction) has been produced in the developing root. Oxytalan fibres also form in the connective tissues of the oral mucosa superior to developing teeth. As the epithelial root sheath loses its continuity, oxytalan fibres are incorporated into cementum first at the cervical margin and gradually progress toward the root apex. With further development, and after functional demands are placed upon the teeth, oxytalan fibres undergo a rearrangement and increase in size. When oxytalan fibres are first seen, they are of a size approaching the limit of resolution of the light microscope (less than 0.5 μm in diameter). In the adult, oxytalan fibres are larger than when first formed and larger in the transseptal area than in any other area about the tooth. As the vascular system becomes established in the periodontium, some oxytalan fibres extend from the adventitia and become attached to the tooth.

As is evident from the above account, much more needs to be known about the development of oxytalan fibres.

Development of cells of the periodontal ligament

Particular attention has been paid to the changes occurring to the cells in the inner, investing layer of the dental follicle since they may be responsible for forming most of the periodontal tissues (see pages 211—212). From an ultrastructural study of the developing periodontal ligament of mouse first molars, Freeman and Ten Cate (1971) observed that prior to root formation the cells have the characteristics of undifferentiated or 'young' fibroblasts. Such cells were seen to contain few cytoplasmic organelles and dense accumulations of glycogen. At this time, the extracellular compartment is relatively structureless. With the onset of root formation, the cells show an increase in cytoplasmic organelles (particularly those associated with protein synthesis and secretion), a progressive sequence being seen such that the cells near the developing root apex have less organelles than those more coronally. Indeed, the evidence suggests that the cells are transformed into both cementoblasts and periodontal fibroblasts.

In developing roots of mouse molars, the transition from a loose connective tissue containing young fibroblasts and minimal extracellular collagen to a highly organized connective tissue consisting of actively functioning fibroblasts and dense extracellular bundles of collagen is abrupt (Freeman and Ten Cate, 1971). In addition to the investing layer of the dental follicle, Ten Cate (1972) has provided evidence that periodontal fibroblasts are derived by proliferation from perivascular cells located in the connective tissue immediately in advance of its organization into periodontal ligament.

Using tritiated proline as a marker for bone formation, Ten Cate (1975) has shown that osteoblasts lining the alveolar bone surface become organized and deposit new bone at the same time as organization of the periodontal ligament occurs. Our findings in sections impregnated with silver nitrate are in accord with this observation.

With regard to other types of connective tissue cells in the periodontal ligament (see Chapter 2), little information is available concerning their ontogeny.

Development of ground substance of the periodontal ligament

Little is known about changes in the ground substance during development. Using bovine periodontal ligament from molars at varying stages of development, Pearson et al. (1975) reported that the content of insoluble, non-collagenous glycoproteins and collagen hexoses was higher in developing than in mature ligament and that hyaluronic acid progressively decreased relative to chondroitin sulphate on eruption and maturation. The subject is considered further in Chapter 6, pages 136—137.

Development of innervation of the periodontal ligament

There is little information concerning the development of the nerve supply of the periodontal ligament. In the early bell stage of development of human teeth, there is a particularly rich innervation associated with small blood vessels in the inner, investing layer of the dental follicle (Fearnhead, 1967). Preliminary studies suggest that similar nerves in the mouse molar are adrenergic (Atkinson and Al-Takriti, 1980). Fearnhead (1967) also reported that the nerve fibres and the vessels associated with the external enamel epithelium disappeared when enamel formation neared completion. Prior to eruption, nerve fibres could be demonstrated in the pulp, but not in the periodontal ligament. With root formation and eruption, the nerves adjacent to the bone were seen to establish the periodontal innervation by growing into the developing ligament (most of them accompanying periodontal vessels). In the teeth of the marmoset (Levy and Bernick, 1968) and also in rat molars (Bernick, 1960), no sensory innervation was established until the ligament had become fully organized at the time of tooth eruption.

Development of vascular supply of the periodontal ligament

Few studies have been undertaken to investigate the vascular supply of the developing periodontal ligament.

Kindlová (1970) has described the development of the vasculature associated with the gingiva of rat molars. She noted that it was derived from vascular networks associated with the enamel organ and the alveolar mucosa. From this region, vessels spread apically to supply the developing periodontal ligament. Prior to eruption, the vascular bed of the periodontal ligament was found to be more uniform than in teeth subjected to masticatory loads, suggesting its pattern is influenced by function.

Cutright (1970) reported on the development of the vasculature of the periodontal ligament for permanent monkey teeth. The first indication of vascular development was the presence of a small, round, plexus of vessels derived from vessels in the adjacent alveolar bone, which had direct connections with the periodontal plexus of the overlying deciduous tooth. The encircling plexus gave rise to both pulp vessels and to the periodontal plexus. This latter plexus arose by 'a thinning and compression of the vessels of the encircling plexus, forming a dense network of flattened vessels within the periodontal membrane'. Direct vascular connections were noted between the periodontal plexuses of neighbouring teeth.

From our own observations on the developing rodent periodontal ligament, the vascular supply is derived from two sources. Blood vessels enter the periapical area of the ligament and pass occlusally to anastomose with perforating vessels that have coursed into, and through, the interseptal bone. As these vessels pass gingivally, their course is mainly in the alveolar-related part of the periodontal ligament. Terminal loops could not be demonstrated in the cemental part of the ligament in the rat. With eruption into functional occlusion, the vascular pathways through the periodontal ligament are not changed in the rat.

In the young adult spider monkey we observed vessels entering the periapical area of the ligament and also entering the interdental alveolar septum. The septal vessels arborized to enter and anastomose with ligament vessels. The vessels in the periodontal ligament formed two or more parallel ascending and descending channels with interconnecting loops (Grant, Stern and Everett, 1979). In the transseptal region, a rich anastomosing plexus is formed from branches from the mesial surface of one tooth, the distal surface of the adjacent tooth, and the crestal branches of the lingual and buccal gingival vessels. From this anastomosis, arborizations arise that proceed into the lamina propria of the gingiva to form terminal loops in the connective tissue papillae.

TRANSPLANTATION STUDIES

The important role played by the inner, investing layer of the dental follicle in the formation of the periodontal ligament has been shown by experiments in which developing tooth germs were transplanted from the jaw to other sites. Such tooth germs continued to develop in ectopic sites to produce a root, periodontal ligament and alveolar bone (Hoffman, 1960; Ten Cate et al., 1971). Following initial labelling of mitotic cells with tritiated thymidine to allow the transplanted cells to be recognized, Ten Cate et al. (1971) showed that the inner layer of the dental follicle gave origin to cementoblasts and fibroblasts of the periodontal ligament. The presence of lymphocytes around bone produced in the vicinity of subcutaneously transplanted tooth germs suggests that such 'alveolar' bone also arose from donor tissue (Ten Cate and Mills, 1972). Further evidence in support of this has been derived from studies in which developing first molar tooth germs from mice were implanted into holes prepared in the parietal bones of adult mice (Freeman, Ten Cate and Dickinson, 1975). It has been shown that a defect created in the rodent parietal bone is effected with fibrous tissue instead of new bone (Pritchard, 1946; Melcher, 1969). However, following implantation into the parietal defect, the tooth germs continued development with the formation of roots, periodontal ligament and new bone. This new bone fused with the old parietal bone and was presumably derived from cells of the investing layer associated with the original implant (Freeman et al., 1975).

The periodontal ligament of transplants shows organization of the principal collagen fibre groups, illustrating adaptation to later function (Atkinson and Lavelle, 1970; Ten Cate *et al.*, 1971).

Though the above experiments show that under certain conditions cells of the investing layer of the dental follicle give rise to all the supporting tissues, this does not preclude a contribution to the periodontal ligament from the outer layers of the dental follicle during normal development.

REFERENCES

ATKINSON, M. E. (1972) The development of the mouse molar periodontium. *J. periodont. Res.* **7**, 255–260.

ATKINSON, M. E. & AL-TAKRITI, S. (1980) A histochemical study of the innervation of developing teeth. *J. dent. Res.* **59**, Special Issue D, 1807.

ATKINSON, M. E. & LAVELLE, C. L. B. (1970) Experimental tooth transplantation in the mouse. *J. Anat.* **106**, 180.

BAUMHAMMERS, A. & STALLARD, R. E. (1968) ^{35}S–Sulfate utilization and turnover by the connective tissues of the periodontium. *J. periodont. Res.* **3**, 187–193.

BERKOVITZ, B. K. B. & THOMAS, N. R. (1969) Unimpeded eruption in the root-resected lower incisor of the rat with a preliminary note on root transection. *Archs. oral Biol.* **14**, 771–780.

BERNICK, S. (1960) The organization of the periodontal membrane fibres of the developing molars of rats. *Archs. oral Biol.* **2**, 57–63.

BOYDE, A. & JONES, S. J. (1968) Scanning electron microscopy of cementum and Sharpey fibre bone. *Z. Zellforsch.* **92**, 536–548.

CUTRIGHT, D. E. (1970) The morphogenesis of the vascular supply to the permanent teeth of *Macaca rhesus*. *Oral Surg.* **30**, 284–291.

ECCLES, J. D. (1959) The development of the periodontal membrane: the principal fibres of the molar teeth. *Dent. Practr. Dent. Rec.* **10**, 31–35.

ECCLES, J. D. (1961) Studies in the development of the periodontal membrane: The apical region of the erupting tooth. *Dent. Practr. Dent. Rec.* **11**, 153–157.

ECCLES, J. D. (1964) The development of the periodontal membrane in the rat incisor. *Archs. oral Biol.* **9**, 127–133.

FEARNHEAD, R. W. (1967) Innervation of dental tissues. In: *Structural and chemical organization of teeth*, Vol. 1, A. E. W. MILES (ed.), pp. 247–281. London, Academic Press.

FORMICOLA, A. J., KRAMPF, J. I. & WITTE, E. G. (1971) Cementogenesis in developing rat molars. *J. Periodont.* **42**, 766–773.

FREEMAN, E. & TEN CATE, A. R. (1971) Development of the periodontium: an electron microscope study. *J. Periodont.* **42**, 387–395.

FREEMAN, E., TEN CATE, A. R. & DICKINSON, J. (1975) Development of a gomphosis by tooth germ implants in the parietal bone of the mouse. *Archs. oral Biol.* **20**, 139–140.

FULLMER, H. M. (1959) Observations on the development of oxytalan fibres in the periodontium of man. *J. dent. Res.* **38**, 510–518.

FULLMER, H. M. (1967) The development of oxytalan fibres. In: *The mechanism of tooth support*, D. J. ANDERSON, J. E. EASTOE, A. H. MELCHER & D. C. A. PICTON (eds.), pp. 72–75. Bristol, Wright.

GRANT, D. & BERNICK, S. (1972) The formation of the periodontal ligament. *J. Periodont.* **43**, 17–25.

GRANT, D., BERNICK, S., LEVY, B. M. & DREIZIN, S. (1972) A comparative study of periodontal ligament development in teeth with and without predecessors in marmosets. *J. Periodont.* **43**, 162–169.

GRANT, D., STERN, I. & EVERETT, F. (1979) *Periodontics*, p. 84. St. Louis, C. V. Mosby & Co.

HOFFMAN, R. L. (1960) Formation of periodontal tissues around subcutaneously transplanted hamster molars. *J. dent. Res.* **39**, 781–798.

HUNT, A. M. (1959) A description of the molar teeth and investing tissues of normal guinea-pigs. *J. dent. Res.* **38**, 216–231.

JONES, S. J. & BOYDE, A. (1974) The organization and gross mineralization patterns of the collagen fibres in Sharpey fibre bone. *Cell Tiss. Res.* **148**, 83–96.

KAMEYAMA, U. (1973) An autoradiographic investigation of the developing rat periodontal membrane. *Archs. oral Biol.* **18**, 473–480.

KINDLOVÁ, M. (1970) The development of the vascular bed of the marginal periodontium. *J. periodont. Res.* **5**, 135–140.

LESTER, K. S. (1969) The unusual nature of root formation in molar teeth of the laboratory rat. *J. Ultrastruct. Res.* **28**, 481–506.

LEVY, B. M. & BERNICK, S. (1968) Development of organization of the periodontal ligament of deciduous teeth in marmosets (*Callithrix jacchus*). *J. dent. Res.* **47**, 27–33.

MAGNUSSON, B. (1968) Tissue changes during molar tooth eruption. *Trans. R. Schs Dent. Stockh. Umeå.* No. 13, 1–122.

MELCHER, A. H. (1969) Role of the periosteum in repair of wounds of the parietal bone of the rat. *Archs. oral Biol.* **14**, 1101–1109.

MOXHAM, B. J. & BERKOVITZ, B. K. B. (1974) The effects of root transection on the unimpeded eruption rate of the rabbit mandibular incisor. *Archs. oral Biol.* **19**, 903–909.

NESS, A. R. & SMALE, D. E. (1959) The distribution of mitoses and cells in the tissues bounded by the socket wall of the rabbit mandibular incisor. *Proc. R. Soc. B.* **151**, 106–128.

NOYES, F. B., SCHOUR, I. & NOYES, H. J. (1943) In: *Oral histology and embryology*, p. 170. Philadelphia, Lea & Febiger.

ORBAN, B. J. (1927) *Embryology and histogenesis. Fortschritte der Zahnheilkunde*, J. MISCHE (ed.), **3**, 749. Cited in ORBAN, B. J. (1944) *Oral histology and embryology*, 1st ed. St. Louis, C. V. Mosby & Co.

ORBAN, B. J. (1957) *Oral histology and embryology*, 4th ed., p. 185. St. Louis, C. V. Mosby & Co.

OWENS, P. D. A. (1974) A light microscopic study of the development of the roots of premolar teeth in dog. *Archs. oral Biol.* **19**, 528–538.

OWENS, P. D. A. (1979) A light and electron microscopic study of the early stages of root surface formation in molar teeth in the rat. *Archs. oral Biol.* **24**, 901–907.

PEARSON, C. H., WOHLLEBE, M., CARMICHAEL, D. J. & CHOVELON, A. (1975) Bovine periodontal ligament. An investigation of the collagen, glycosaminoglycan and insoluble glycoprotein components at different stages of tissue development. *Connect. Tiss. Res.* **3**, 195–206.

PRITCHARD, J. J. (1946) Repair of fractures of the parietal bone in rats. *J. Anat.* **80**, 55–60.

PRITCHARD, J. J., SCOTT, J. H. & GIRGIS, F. G. (1956) The structure and development of the facial sutures. *J. Anat.* **90**, 73–86.

SCOTT, J. H. (1953) How teeth erupt. *Dent. Practnr. Dent. Rec.* **3**, 345–350.

SICHER, H. (1923) Bau und Funktion des Fixationsapparates der Meerschweinenmolaren. *Z. Stomat.* **21**, 580. Cited in ORBAN, B. J. (1944) *Oral histology and embryology*, 1st ed. St. Louis, C. V. Mosby & Co.

SICHER, H. (1942a) Tooth eruption: the axial movement of continuously growing teeth. *J. dent. Res.* **21**, 201–210.

SICHER, H. (1942b) Tooth eruption: axial movement of teeth of limited growth. *J. dent. Res.* **21**, 395–402.

SLOAN, P. & BENYON, A. D. (in press) Development and structure of the cementum–dentine junction in man and cat. *J. dent. Res.*

TEN CATE, A. R. (1969) The development of the periodontium. In: *Biology of the periodontium*, A. H. MELCHER & W. H. BOWEN (eds.), pp. 53–89. London, Academic Press.

TEN CATE, A. R. (1972) Developmental aspects of the periodontium. In: *Developmental aspects of oral biology*, H. C. SLAVKIN & L. A. BAVETTA (eds.), pp. 309–324. London, Academic Press.

TEN CATE, A. R. (1975) Formation of supporting bone in association with periodontal ligament organization in the mouse. *Archs. oral Biol.* **20**, 137–138.

TEN CATE, A. R. & MILLS, C. (1972) The development of the periodontium. The origin of the alveolar bone. *Anat. Rec.* **173**, 69–78.

TEN CATE, A. R., MILLS, C. & SOLOMON, G. (1971) The development of the periodontium. An autoradiographic and transplantation study. *Anat. Rec.* **170**, 365–380.

THOMAS, N. R. (1965) The process and mechanism of tooth eruption. Ph.D. Thesis, Bristol University.

THOMAS, N. R. (1967) The properties of collagen in the periodontium of an erupting tooth. In: *The mechanism of tooth support*, D. J. ANDERSON, J. E. EASTOE, A. H. MELCHER & D. C. A. PICTON (eds.), pp. 102–106. Bristol, Wright.

TONGE, C. G. (1963) The development and arrangement of the dental follicle. *Trans. Eur. Orthod. Soc.* 118–126.

TROTT, J. R. (1962) The development of the periodontal attachment in the rat. *Acta Anat.* **51**, 313–328.

VAN BLADEREN, T. P. M. (1971) Tooth eruption and the development of the periodontal fibres. *Trans. Eur. Orthod. Soc.* 427–437.

Chapter 10

THE PERIODONTAL LIGAMENT AND PHYSIOLOGICAL TOOTH MOVEMENTS
B. J. Moxham and B. K. B. Berkovitz

INTRODUCTION

Physiological tooth movements are those a tooth makes to attain and maintain its functional position. Such movements include axial and non-axial movements during both the developmental stages of a tooth within the jaw and the functional stages within the oral cavity. They are associated with the processes of tooth growth, eruption and drift and with movements produced by (and following) the application of physiological external forces to the tooth. As will be shown, the periodontal tissues are involved in the generation of, or resistance to, many of these movements. This chapter is concerned primarily with eruption and drift. Chapters 11 and 12 deal with the effects on the periodontal tissues of external forces.

It is usual to describe eruption and drifting in relation to three phases in the development of a tooth: the pre-eruptive, prefunctional and functional phases (Sicher and Bhaskar, 1972). The pre-eruptive phase commences with the formation of the tooth bud and ends with the initiation of root formation. The prefunctional phase follows, terminating when the tooth reaches the occlusal plane. The functional phase refers to the situation after the tooth has reached the occlusal plane. This schema, like some others in developmental biology, can be criticized on the basis that it tends to oversimplify a complex series of events in a continuous process. Furthermore, although not based upon physiological characteristics, it has led to the view that different mechanisms might be operating during the different phases to produce similar tooth movements. Whilst this view is not unreasonable, little evidence is available to assess it. Despite these criticisms, such a schema does provide a convenient method for describing the various patterns of movement. We suggest a modification, however, to avoid the difficulty of deciding when a tooth becomes functional. We believe the terms 'prefunctional' and 'functional' are badly chosen and propose to subdivide the development of a tooth into pre-eruptive, eruptive and intra-oral phases. The pre-eruptive phase is as before. The eruptive phase begins with the onset of root development and ends when the crown penetrates the mucosa to appear in the oral cavity. Subsequently, the tooth is in its intra-oral phase.

Pre-eruptive phase

Throughout this phase the tooth remains in its developmental intra-osseous location. It is claimed that the pre-eruptive phase is characterized by concentric growth of the tooth within its follicle, any convergence of the occlusal surface of the developing tooth and the occlusal plane being attributed not to active bodily movement of the tooth but passively to growth of the tooth germ (Thomas, 1965; Darling and Levers, 1975, 1976). Figure 1 shows the distance from the mandibular canal to the centre of the follicle for three types of human teeth during their pre-eruptive and early eruptive phases (Darling and Levers, 1976). From this it was concluded that the centre of the follicle moves very little prior to the completion of the crown of the tooth. An alternative interpretation — that the mandibular canal and the centre of the follicle move in

unison over a period of several years — seemed unlikely. However, the graphs for the permanent mandibular second premolar and for the permanent mandibular second molar suggest that some axial movement towards the occlusal plane does take place during the pre-eruptive phase. Similar conclusions have been drawn from studies of the development of rat molar teeth (O'Brien, Bhaskar and Brodie, 1958; Thomas 1965). The studies of Darling and Levers (1975, 1976) are based primarily upon 'pseudo-longitudinal' surveys of radiographs from groups of children at different ages. Little information is available from true longitudinal surveys using standardized radiological techniques. Their use of the mandibular canal as a 'fixed' reference feature for recording relatively large eruptive movements may be acceptable. However, it may not be reliable enough to record smaller axial movements occurring during the pre-eruptive phase.

Studies of bone activity on the walls of the alveolar crypts containing the developing teeth suggest that there is drifting and tilting of the teeth during the pre-eruptive stage. For cat molars, bone deposition on the lingual walls and resorption on the buccal walls of the dental crypts is associated with a backward relocation of the teeth (Manson, 1968). Distolingual deposition of bone within the crypts of monkey mandibular permanent incisors is associated with a forward and outward relocation (Baume, 1953). Madder-feeding experiments using the pig indicate a considerable range of drifting movements during the pre-eruptive phase (Brash, 1928). Whether the bone activity observed in the above studies caused the tooth movements or was the response to movement produced by another agency has not been established. Drifting and tilting of human teeth prior to their eruption have also been observed. For example, changes in orientation and position of developing teeth occur with growth of the jaws and are particularly noticeable for a permanent tooth 'moving' with respect to its deciduous predecessor. As yet, the details of such movements have not been properly documented.

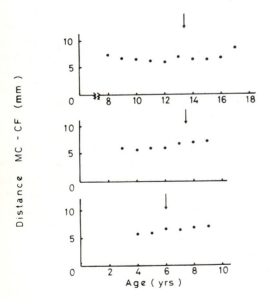

FIG. 1. Mean distance from the mandibular canal to the centre point of the dental follicle with age. The upper graph is for the mandibular third molar, the middle graph for the mandibular second molar, the lower graph for the mandibular second premolar. Arrows indicate age at crown completion.

Eruptive phase

This phase is characterized by axial migration of the tooth which involves its active bodily movement

(Carlson, 1944; Thomas, 1965; Björk and Skieller, 1972; Darling and Levers, 1975).

It is usually claimed that as the forming root grows towards the floor of the crypt there is resorption of bone in this location. With the onset of eruption, space is created for the forming root and resorption is no longer seen. Where the distance moved by the tooth is greater than the amount of root formed, bone is deposited on the crypt floor (Ten Cate, 1976). However, such claims have not been confirmed by study of the post-natal growth of the mandible in the rat, guinea pig and cat (Manson, 1968). Bone resorption was seen to predominate in the floors of the molar crypts throughout the period of root formation. Where bone deposition was seen, this was thought to be related to relocation of the crypt within the growing mandible rather than to eruption.

Darling and Levers (1976) have measured the axial movement of some types of human mandibular teeth during the eruptive phase using the mandibular canal as a reference feature (Fig. 2). They noted that eruption through the jaw commenced once the roots began to form. The calculated rates of eruption showed

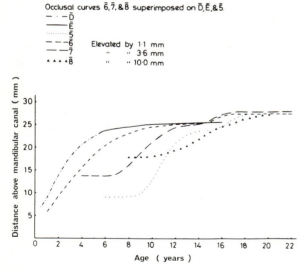

Occlusal curves 6̄, 7̄, & 8̄ superimposed on D̄, Ē, & 5̄.

FIG. 2. Composite graph showing mean distance from mandibular canal to occlusal surface with age. The curves show tooth movements during both the eruptive and intra-oral phases. Note that for some teeth, a second phase of axial movement occurs at about 16 years, after the tooth has reached the occlusal plane. The curves for the permanent molars have been elevated to make allowance for the curvature of the mandibular canal.

much variation, ranging from 1.2 mm/year for the permanent mandibular third molar to 3.5 mm/year for the permanent mandibular second premolar. The evidence in support of the view that the mandibular canal is a suitable reference feature for such studies is derived from the work of Björk (1963), Thomas (1965), Manson (1968) and Darling and Levers (1976). Using amalgam implants placed in human mandibles, Björk (1963) has shown that the mandibular canal remains in a relatively stable position. From observations of the pattern of bone deposition and resorption around the mandibular canal in experimental animals, Thomas (1965) and Manson (1968) came to similar conclusions. Darling and Levers (1976) found that the shape of the curve describing the eruption of a tooth using the mandibular canal for reference purposes was similar to the curve obtained using the occlusal surface of a submerging ankylosed tooth. Even if the mandibular canal maintains a stable position, care must be taken to ensure that errors in measuring eruptive distances do not arise from failure to take account of drifting of the teeth.

The development of the periodontal tissues during the eruptive phase is described in Chapter 9.

Significant changes occur within the tissues that cover a tooth during eruption. It has been suggested that the gubernacular tissue may play a role in the movements of the developing permanent teeth through the jaws (Scott, 1948, 1953, 1967; Thomas, 1965). During eruption, the gubernacular cords increase in thickness but become less dense (Scott and Symons, 1977) and the size of the gubernacular canal is increased to accommodate the crown of the erupting tooth (Cahill, 1974). Whether the gubernaculum provides a path of least resistance or whether the gubernacular tissue is actively engaged in moving the tooth has not been established. It cannot be implicated in the process of eruption once the tooth has breached the mucosa, nor can it be involved in the eruption of a deciduous tooth since it lacks a gubernaculum.

It is generally assumed that the formation of a pathway through the jaw for an erupting tooth results from continuous pressure exerted by the tooth. However, Cahill (1969) observed that apparently normal pathways formed where developing teeth were immobilized so that they could not exert pressure against the overlying bone.

As the tooth erupts, there is a reduction in density

of the connective tissue between the tooth and oral epithelium (McHugh, 1961). It has been suggested that the cells of the reduced enamel epithelium secrete enzymes which degrade collagen (Toto and Sicher, 1966; Melcher, 1967). Depolymerization of muco-polysaccharides has been detected in the connective tissue overlying erupting teeth in rats and humans (Engel, 1951). Electron-microscopic studies indicate that 'fibrocytes' in this connective tissue stop fibrillo-genesis, actively take up extracellular material and synthesize acid hydrolases (Ten Cate, 1971). These changes are followed by the degeneration of the cell. Ten Cate (1971) has suggested that reduced enamel epithelial cells are concerned with the removal of breakdown products. A relationship between degeneration of connective tissue and pressure exerted by the erupting tooth has not been established, though ischaemia has been mentioned as a contributory factor (Schour, 1960). However, pressure alone is unlikely to account for collagen degradation since the connective tissue above the erupting tooth always exhibits evidence of collagen formation (Fullmer, 1961). The changes in the connective tissue may allow a tooth to erupt along a path of least resistance. Abnormal changes within the tissue may increase the resistance to eruption. That human permanent maxillary incisors and canines with delayed eruption will erupt subsequent to the surgical removal of the overlying connective tissue (Duckworth, 1962; Howard, 1966; Johnston, 1969; Di Biase, 1971) supports this view. Histological and radiographical studies of the tissues overlying human maxillary incisors reveal that an enlarged dental follicle is often associated with retarded eruption (Di Biase, 1969).

Little is known about tilting and drifting movements of teeth during the eruptive phase. From a cephalometric appraisal of the eruption of human permanent maxillary incisors, evidence has been obtained to show that they erupt along a path of least resistance (Fletcher, 1963). Fletcher suggested that three elements offered resistance: the cortical bone of the outer and inner plates of the alveolus, neighbouring developing permanent teeth, and deciduous predecessors (or fragments of such teeth). Teeth were seen to be deflected in their eruptive path by such structures, showing tilting movements. Figure 3 summarizes the typical eruptive behaviour of the human permanent maxillary incisor. Di Biase (1976) has

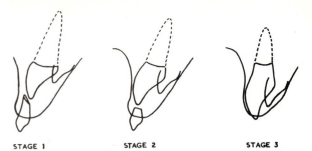

STAGE 1   STAGE 2   STAGE 3

FIG. 3. Diagram illustrating tilting movements of the crown of the maxillary central incisor during its eruptive phase. The crowns of the deciduous central and permanent lateral incisors are also shown. *Stage 1.* The permanent central incisor lies within its crypt with the permanent lateral incisor being situated distally. The teeth erupt buccally, perhaps in relation to the slope of the alveolar bone surface. *Stage 2.* As the labial surface of the permanent central incisor crown approaches the buccal surface of the alveolus, it uprights most rapidly, the fulcrum being supplied at a variable point of contact on the mesial surface of the lateral incisor. *Stage 3.* This shows the position of the permanent maxillary incisor at the time of its eruption into the oral cavity.

conducted surveys to study delayed eruption of human permanent maxillary incisors associated with supernumerary teeth. Following removal of the supernumerary he observed that, where there was space in the dental arch greater than the width of the crown of the permanent incisor, significant changes in the inclination of the incisor often occurred during its subsequent eruption. He also claimed that, whilst the eruptive path of the incisor through the bone was straight if it was upright in the alveolus, its path was curved where initially it was inclined mesially or distally.

Intra-oral phase

During this phase the tooth, having emerged into the oral cavity, continues to erupt to attain its functional position. However, the emergence may be facilitated by recession of the mucosa around the erupting tooth. The reader is referred to a review by Schroeder and Listgarten (1971) for information on the changes in the epithelial tissues of the oral mucosa and the reduced enamel epithelium during eruption.

Measurements of the rates of emergence of human teeth into the oral cavity before they reach the occlusal plane have been made by Burke and Newell (1958), Burke (1963), Berkovitz and Bass (1976) and Smith (1978). Burke and Newell (1958) reported that the rates of eruption of the permanent maxillary central incisors of one of their patients were greatest at the time of crown emergence, decreasing thereafter. During the first month of their emergence the teeth were seen to erupt by approximately 1 mm. Burke (1963) recorded the eruption of a large number of human permanent maxillary central incisors whose eruption was delayed. After surgical exposure, their initial rates of eruption were about 2 mm per month. Smith (1978) has measured eruption of human canine and premolar teeth. He found that the most rapid rate of movement was for a mandibular second premolar (4.5 mm in 14 weeks). Smith also recorded the changing depths of the gingival crevice during eruption. The crevices of teeth which had just penetrated the mucosa were found to exceed 7 mm in depth, but became more shallow as eruption continued. This reduction, he claimed, was associated partly with the eruptive movements and partly with gingival 'recoil'. The patterns of eruption and of gingival 'recoil' were characterized by rapid changes initially followed by slower ones (though considerable variations were found). The studies of Burke and Newell (1958), Burke (1963) and Smith (1978) used the occlusal plane as a datum for measurements. Because of the young age of the participants in these studies, however, the occlusal plane may not be stable. Berkovitz and Bass (1976) have determined the rates of emergence of human permanent maxillary third molars for a group of students with an average age of 19 years. They also employed the occlusal plane for measurements, believing that it was more stable for the older age group (see Darling and Levers, 1976). Where space was available, the maximum rate of eruption was found to be about 1 mm/3 months. In crowded dentitions, the rate was less than 1 mm/6 months. This study also indicated that exposure of the crown was the result of gingival recession as well as eruption of the tooth.

Burke and Newell (1958), Berkovitz and Bass (1976) and Smith (1978) report a decrease in eruption as the tooth approaches the occlusal plane. A similar observation has been made by Darling and Levers (personal communication). It has not been established whether this results from a fundamental change in the eruptive mechanism, is due to the retarding action of occlusal forces, and/or is the consequence of structural or biomechanical changes within the periodontium.

That axial, eruption-like movements are possible following the establishment of a tooth's functional position in the dental arch is well known. It is not uncommon for an unopposed tooth to overerupt (Boyle, 1955; Cohn, 1966; Moss and Picton, 1967; Pihlstrom and Ramfjord, 1971). Though an increase in dental cement formation around the root apex has been observed in these situations (Boyle, 1955; Pihlstrom and Ramfjord, 1971), the small amount of movement involved and the difficulty of distinguishing cause from effect have prevented identification of the mechanisms responsible. Cohn (1966) has studied the behaviour of molar teeth in mice following the extraction of varying combinations of opposing teeth. He concluded that the degree of overeruption depended upon: the position of the tooth with respect to the missing opposing molars, the degree of non-function to which the tooth was subjected, and the length of time the tooth remained out of function. In a study using *Macaca irus* monkeys, Moss and Picton (1967) observed that the mandibular cheek teeth of adult animals overerupted at a rate of approximately 75 μm/week following the extraction of opposing teeth.

Even in the presence of opposing teeth, eruption-like movements may be observed. Darling and Levers (1976) report that, though eruption stops once a tooth reaches occlusion, a second phase of axial movement in an occlusal direction may be observed at about 14—16 years of age (Fig. 2). They suggest that such movements occur as a response to condylar growth which effectively separates the jaws, producing disturbance of the occlusal 'equilibrium' and 'release' of the eruptive forces. Siersbaek-Nielsen (1971) has obtained similar results from studies using the analysis of jaw growth and tooth eruption with respect to metallic implants (Fig. 4). The findings suggest that incisor eruption rate shows a distinct spurt coincident with spurts of growth at puberty. It is often stated that eruption-like movements may also be seen in the adult to compensate for occlusal wear of the teeth and to prevent excessive loss of facial height (e.g. Murphy, 1959). However, Ainamo and Talari (1976) suggest that vertical growth within the alveolar pro-

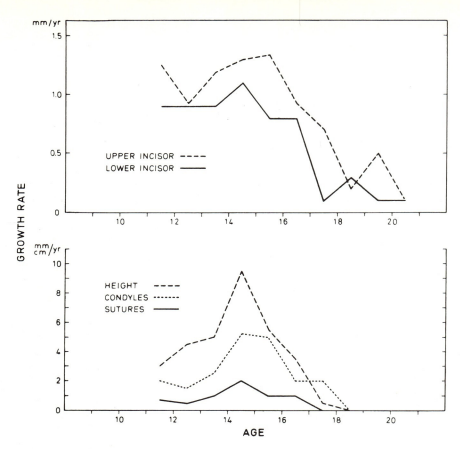

FIG. 4. Eruption rates of maxillary and mandibular central incisors versus growth rates for upper-face sutures, mandibular condyles and body height.

cesses occurs independently of both attrition and masticatory function. This claim is supported by the finding that, where the food is mainly non-abrasive, the lower facial height for adults may increase by 0.4 mm per year (Thompson and Kendrick, 1964). Furthermore, with a highly abrasive diet the amount of compensatory alveolar growth and eruption may be insufficient, leading to a reduction of the lower facial height (Murphy, 1959).

In addition to axial movements during the intra-oral phase, there may be movements of a tooth in the horizontal plane — approximal (mesial and distal) and lateral drift. Mesial drift has been the phenomenon to which most attention has been paid. It is assumed that mesial drift occurs as a response to approximal wear. As a consequence, mutual support of the teeth

under masticatory loads is said to be enhanced and the interdental tissues protected from trauma. From studies on Australian aboriginal skulls, Begg (1954) and Murphy (1959) have reported that contact with neighbouring teeth was maintained in both the deciduous and permanent dentitions despite progressive loss of approximal enamel and dentine. The existence of mesial drift in humans has been confirmed by studies reporting reduction in dental arch length with age (Goldstein and Stanton, 1935; Black, 1936; Cohen, 1940; Brown and Daugaard-Jensen, 1950; Speck, 1950; Barrow and White, 1952; Begg, 1954; Sved, 1955; Lysell, 1958; Moorrees, 1959; Knott, 1961; Vego, 1962; Sillman, 1964; Lammie and Posselt, 1965; Lundström, 1969; Yilmaz, 1973, 1976). However, Baume (1950), Clinch (1951), Sillman (1951) and Henriques (1953) failed to show any reduction. Using plaster casts with the palatal rugae as reference landmarks, Lebret (1967) has shown mesial drifting of the permanent maxillary first molar and canine from the time of their emergence into the oral cavity.

Considerable variations in rates of mesial drift in man have been reported. From the studies involving measurement of dental arch length in modern man, the rates range from about 0.05 mm/annum (Lammie and Posselt, 1965) to 0.7 mm/annum (Moorrees, 1959). It is conceivable that the variation in rates relates to such factors as age, diet, dimensions of the various types of teeth studied and methods of measurement. The data also suggest that the rates for mandibular teeth are greater than for maxillary teeth.

Mesial drift has been observed not only in man but also in monkeys (Baume and Becks, 1950; Latham and Scott, 1960; Moss and Picton, 1967), pigs (Brash, 1927; Yilmaz, 1976) and the elephant, manatee and dugong (Brash, 1927). However, Sicher and Weinmann (1944), Myers and Wyatt (1961) and Kronman (1971) have shown that approximal migration of rat and hamster molars occurs in a distal direction.

Lateral drift is associated usually with changes in the dimensions of the dental arch of the growing child. Study of plaster casts suggests that the well-documented labial drifting of the erupting permanent incisors as the deciduous teeth become exfoliated is a change in angulation rather than whole bodily drift (Picton, 1976). Many studies have been undertaken to determine the rates and timing of lateral expansion of the dental arches (e.g. Friel, 1945; Moorrees, 1964; Sillman, 1964). It seems that little increase in arch dimension occurs after the eruption of the permanent teeth. The final arch width in the canine, premolar and molar regions is achieved by 12—13 years, although growth of other oral tissues continues for several years. However, labiolingual changes are said to occur in the heavily worn dentition. Begg (1954) described a progressive trend to an edge-to-edge occlusion of the incisors in Australian aborigines. Little information is available concerning lateral drift in animals.

A final word of caution needs to be given about interpreting tooth movements. This relates to the work of Björk and Skieller (1972) who, using amalgam implants to provide reference features for studying movements of human permanent teeth, found that developmental rotation of the facial skeleton was associated with compensatory movements of the teeth. Thus, the growth of the jaws may be responsible for tooth movements which, to the unwary, might be attributed to another cause.

THE MECHANISMS OF TOOTH ERUPTION

Investigations into the eruptive mechanism have used mainly the continuously growing incisors of rodents and lagomorphs. Before reviewing these investigations, it is appropriate to describe the pattern and measurement of eruption of the continuously growing incisor and its relevance as a model for the study of the eruptive mechanism of a tooth of limited growth. The reader is referred to reviews by Schour and Massler (1942) and Ness (1964) for accounts of the structure of the continuously growing incisor.

Much early research involved determining eruption rates of continuously growing incisors in occlusion (i.e. impeded eruption rates). Since there appears to be some relationship between eruption and attrition (Ness, 1964), impeded eruption rates cannot always be considered a proper expression of eruption. Indeed, experimentally induced changes in impeded eruption rates may be more a reflection of changes in biting behaviour than of changes in the eruptive mechanism. To obviate variables associated with attrition, most recent research has involved monitoring eruption rates of incisors which have been cut out of occlusion (i.e. unimpeded eruption rates). Unimpeded eruption rates are consistently greater than impeded eruption rates (Ness, 1964): for the rat the unimpeded eruption rate is about 1 mm/day, the impeded eruption rate is approximately 0.4 mm/day. Although unimpeded eruption rates are generally considered to be a full expression of the eruptive potential which is 'released' with the removal of occlusal stresses, an unimpeded tooth may still have to bear some, if not considerable, loads. There is also evidence suggesting that normal unimpeded eruption rates are not realized immediately. Chiba, Tsuruta and Eto (1973) found that the unimpeded eruption rates of rat mandibular incisors were not fully reached until 12—16 hours after the teeth were removed from the bite. Using a technique for the continuous recording of eruption of the rabbit mandibular incisor, Moxham (1979a) calculated that

3 hours after the teeth became unimpeded the eruption rates were only equivalent to $\sim 700\,\mu m/day$. Five days after becoming unimpeded, however, the rates were equivalent to $\sim 1200\,\mu m/day$. A factor which needs to be considered when studying the unimpeded tooth concerns the possibility of fundamental changes in the periodontal tissues which may affect eruption. Beertsen and Everts (1977) have not observed any marked structural differences between the periodontal ligaments of impeded and unimpeded teeth at the ultrastructural level. However, some information is available suggesting the possibility of biomechanical changes. Details of this are given in Chapter 11, pages 264–265.

Two approaches have been adopted to study the behaviour of a tooth during its eruption. The most favoured approach relies upon the determination of eruption rates from measurements of changes in tooth position. Alternatively, the forces of eruption are measured.

Tooth movements may be determined from periodic measurements of tooth position or may be recorded continuously. Various techniques have been used for detecting periodic changes in the eruption of a continuously growing incisor (Schour and Van Dyke, 1932; Ness, 1954, 1956, 1965; Bryer, 1957; Adams and Main, 1962; Main and Adams, 1965; Michaeli and Weinreb, 1968; Chiba et al., 1973; Robins, 1979). These have relied upon measurements made by direct vision, using calipers, using a dissecting microscope incorporating a calibrated eyepiece or from standardized radiographs or photographs. Various anatomical features are used as reference points (e.g. the occlusal plane, alveolar crest and gingival margin) in association with marks on the teeth. Only the methods of Michaeli and Weinreb (1968) and Chiba et al. (1973) have been used to determine eruption rates at intervals of less than 24 hours. Details of a technique which is sensitive enough to allow the continuous recording of eruption of rabbit incisors have been published by Matthews and Berkovitz (1972) and Moxham (1979a). Briefly, this technique makes use of a variable capacitance displacement transducer consisting of two aluminium plates, one mounted on the incisor, the other fixed firmly to adjacent bone (Fig. 5). The plates are aligned parallel and behave as a capacitor when current is fed across them. They are part of a circuit whose output is proportional to the capacitance of the trans-

ducer. The sensitivity of the system is such that a change of 1 μm between the plates can produce a movement of 10 mm on a pen recorder. Figure 6 shows a typical trace of eruption of a rabbit mandibular incisor recorded using this transducer. Because of its sensitivity, the continuously recording technique has the advantage of being able to assess the immediate and short-term effects of experimental interference with eruption. Using this technique Moxham (1979a) has shown that eruption of a rabbit mandibular incisor is continuous, though there is considerable variation in the rates (even from minute to minute) for any given rabbit and also between rabbits (Fig. 7). Burn-Murdoch and Picton (1978) have described a technique for continuously monitoring eruption of a rat maxillary incisor and also reported variation in eruption rates. In addition, it is conceivable that the ultrasonic transit-time technique described by Aars (1976) and Myhre, Preus and Aars (1979) to record axial position of rabbit maxillary incisors may one day be used to monitor eruption.

Measurement of forces exerted by erupting teeth has been undertaken by Taylor and Butcher (1951), Miura and Ito (1968) and Thomas (1976). Taylor and Butcher (1951) and Miura and Ito (1968) used similar techniques of elastic traction to oppose the eruption of continuously growing incisors over periods of up to 3 weeks. Taylor and Butcher (1951) reported that a force equivalent to 5 g (~ 0.05 N) was sufficient to stop the eruption of rat mandibular incisors. Miura and Ito (1968) found that 7 g (~ 0.07 N) was required to prevent eruption of rabbit maxillary incisors. In both studies it was reported that the teeth were intruded into their sockets should the tension exceed that required to arrest eruption. The extent to which the continuous application of forces to the teeth over long periods might unduly disturb the periodontal tissues and their functioning was not assessed, and it remains a matter of conjecture whether physiological values for the forces that an erupting tooth can exert can be derived from techniques which physically prevent the tooth from erupting. Thomas (1976) has described briefly a technique for continuously monitoring forces exerted by erupting dog canines and rat incisors, recording 'eruptive forces' between 0.5 g (~ 0.005 N) and 2.5 g (~ 0.025 N) under a variety of experimental conditions. Whilst continuous recording of forces under normal and experimentally

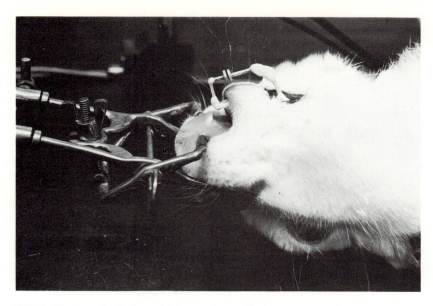

FIG. 5. Photograph of the variable capacitance displacement transducer mounted on the incisor and adjacent mandibular bone.

altered situations is potentially of great significance to the study of eruption, it is not yet possible to assess fully Thomas' experiments since there is insufficient information concerning the experimental protocol.

There is debate concerning the validity of extrapolating results from the study of the eruption of the continuously growing incisor to the mechanisms responsible for the eruption of teeth of limited growth. Since only teeth of limited growth are found in the earliest mammals, teeth of continuous growth have evolved from teeth of limited growth. It can be argued, therefore, that continuous eruption is based upon the exploitation of mechanisms already present in teeth of limited growth (Ness, 1956). This line of argument may be supported by the finding that continuous eruption has appeared in the teeth of mammals in widely divergent orders, and that both continuously and non-continuously erupting teeth may be found in the same dentition. As yet, however, there is little experimental evidence to show that the

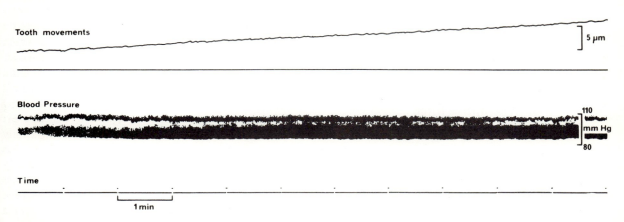

FIG. 6. A typical pen recorder trace of movements of a rabbit mandibular incisor obtained using the variable capacitance displacement transducer. The movement shown is in a direction favouring eruption.

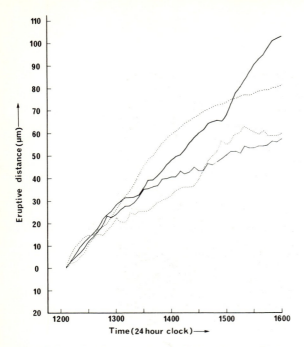

FIG. 7. Eruptive distances travelled by the right mandibular incisors of four rabbits over a 4-hour recording period determined using the variable capacitance displacement transducer.

eruptive mechanism in teeth of continuous growth is similar to that in teeth of limited growth. Some evidence to support the view that similar processes underlie eruption of both types of teeth can be derived from the finding that propylthiouracil retards the appearance in the oral cavity of molars in newborn rats (Paynter, 1954) and reduces the impeded eruption rates of adult rat incisors (Garren and Greep, 1955).

The role of the periodontal ligament in the generation of the eruptive force

Eruption has been attributed to a variety of causative agents. These may be broadly classified into those which are associated with the periodontal connective tissues and those which are not. In the first category are hypotheses related to contraction of periodontal collagen, migration or contraction of periodontal fibroblasts and to pressure exerted by vascular or fluid elements around or beneath the tooth. In the second category are hypotheses associated with alveolar bone growth, root growth and pulp cell proliferation.

Despite considerable research, there is conflicting evidence for and against all these hypotheses. However, experiments which involve surgically removing the odontogenic regions of teeth of continuous growth (resection) or the transverse bisection of such teeth (transection) have focused attention on the role of the periodontal tissues in the mechanism of eruption. Bryer (1957), Kostlán, Thořová and Škach (1960) and Pitaru et al. (1976) have shown that resected teeth continue to erupt (Fig. 8). Berkovitz and Thomas (1969) reported that the eruption rates of unimpeded resected teeth reached control values a few days after resection and were maintained until the tooth was about to drop out of its socket. Since a variety of agents (hydrocortisone, thyroxine, demecolcine, triethanomelamine and aminoacetonitrile) have the same effects upon the eruption of the normal and resected tooth (Berkovitz, 1969, 1972; Day, 1969; Berkovitz, Migdalski and Solomon, 1972), the mechanism of eruption of the resected tooth is considered to be similar to that of a normal tooth. Following transection of the continuously growing incisor, the segment distal to the site of surgery erupts without any contribution from the proximal segment (Fig. 8) (Massler and Schour, 1941; Bryer, 1957; Berkovitz and Thomas, 1969; Berkovitz, 1971; Moxham and Berkovitz, 1974). Berkovitz (1971) reported that the unimpeded eruption rates of the distal segments attained control values. Since alveolar bone growth, root growth and pulp cell proliferation are not essential to the eruption of the resected and transected tooth, and since eruption rates are the same in the resected and non-resected tooth under normal and experimentally altered conditions, it can be concluded that the periodontal ligament is the source of the eruptive mechanism.

The various hypotheses of eruption which are associated with the periodontal ligament will now be assessed in relation to the following criteria:

1. Any system proposed as the eruptive mechanism requires characteristics which enable it to sustain eruption.
2. The system must be capable of producing a force which is sufficient to move a tooth in a direction favouring eruption under physiological condi-

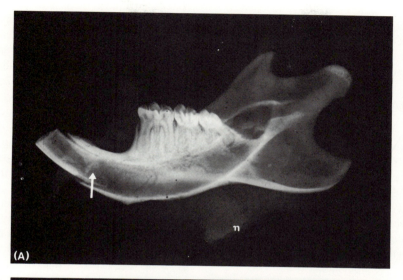

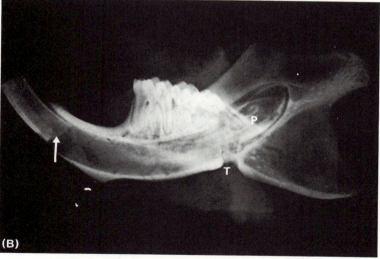

FIG. 8. Radiographs of rat mandibles to show the effects on the incisors of root resection (A) and root transection (B). Note that in both instances eruption of the remaining tooth segment has continued despite the surgical disturbance. For (A), the arrow indicates the base of the resected tooth. Note the absence of any dental tissues in the remainder of the socket. For (B) the arrow indicates the base of the distal segment of the transected tooth. Note the retained proximal segment (P). T = site of root transection.

tions, whilst experimentally induced changes in the system should cause predictable changes in tooth movements (without unduly influencing processes other than the eruptive mechanism). Though these criteria are not profound, guidelines of this kind have not been used previously to evaluate the relative significance of experiments conducted to investigate the eruptive mechanism.

THE PERIODONTAL COLLAGEN CONTRACTION HYPOTHESIS

This idea, originally conceived by Shrimpton (1960), was developed by Thomas (1965, 1976). Thomas has suggested a variety of biochemical mechanisms for the contraction of collagen including:

  (i) Decrease in entropy during electrostatic attraction of disordered tropocollagen macromolecules and alignment along lines of stress.
 (ii) Linear polymerization producing a decrease in length of macromolecules.
(iii) Shrinkage associated with dehydration.
 (iv) A system analogous to the sliding of actomyosin filaments.
  (v) Interfibrillar repulsion produced by the interaction of adjacent electrical double layers.
 (vi) Formation of intermolecular crosslinks.

According to our first criterion, the collagen contraction hypothesis requires a continuous, high rate of turnover of collagen in the periodontal ligament to sustain eruption since contraction would occur only during the maturation of the collagen. Autoradiographic studies using tritiated proline or glycine have shown high rates of turnover of protein in the periodontal ligament (see Chapter 3, pages 60–62). However, the rapid turnover might not be concerned with providing the motive force for eruption but could be a response to tooth movement produced by some other agency. Sodek (1978) has reported that the turnover times for collagen in the periodontal ligaments of rat molars are faster than in the continuously growing incisors. This suggests that the rate of movement of a tooth is not the sole factor which governs turnover time of components within the periodontal ligament.

In order to satisfy our first criterion there also needs to be a specialized system for remodelling of collagen in the periodontal ligament which allows new tooth positions gained during eruption to be maintained. The existence of an intermediate plexus within the periodontal ligament would provide such a system. Although there is little histological evidence for the presence of an intermediate plexus as originally described by Sicher (1942), there is evidence for a zone of shear between cemental and alveolar fibres which might allow remodelling of the ligament during eruption (Melcher, 1967; Beersten, 1973; Beertsen and Everts, 1977). (For further discussion see pages 58–62.) Whether such remodelling is associated with the production of eruptive forces or is an effect of them awaits further investigation.

With regard to our second criterion, it has yet to be shown that collagen can contract under physiological conditions. Furthermore, all mechanisms so far proposed to explain collagen contraction seem to be biochemically untenable (Bailey, 1968, 1976). Collagen can be made to contract *in vitro* by heating, or by its suspension in 6 M lithium bromide, guanidine or urea, but these are extreme conditions which cannot be regarded as physiological. Thomas' suggestion that it is the crosslinking between fibres that generates the tension necessary to pull a tooth out of its socket has been criticized by Bailey (1976) on the basis that, for crosslinking between fibres to cause a contraction, a highly organized fibre alignment and crosslink location would be required. However, there is no evidence of a collagen-type crosslink between fibres and, if there were, there would be no flexibility in the tissue (Bailey, 1976).

Despite the lack of evidence to show contraction of collagen, experiments have been designed to assess the collagen contraction hypothesis using vitamin-C-deficient diets, hydrocortisone, agents promoting cross linkages, and lathyrogens.

Gould (1968) and Barnes and Kodicek (1972) have shown that ascorbic acid plays an important role in the formation of collagen, at the step involving the hydroxylation of proline to hydroxyproline or of an unhydroxylated precursor to the hydroxylated compound. In scorbutic animals the synthesis of collagen is depressed (e.g. Ten Cate, Deporter and Freeman, 1976), as is collagen degradation (Prockop and Kivirikko, 1968). There is little or no new collagen formation in wounds and this deficiency may account for a loss of tensile strength (Harkness, 1968). It has been shown that both impeded (Dalldorf and Zall, 1930;

Berkovitz, 1974) and unimpeded (Berkovitz, 1974) eruption rates are retarded in scorbutic guinea pigs. Though these findings may be regarded as evidence for the contraction of collagen hypothesis, care must be taken in interpreting the results since other systems (such as the vascular system) will also be affected in the scorbutic animal (Chattergee, 1967; Kutsky, 1973).

Cortisone is known to inhibit cell division and growth in mesenchymal tissues (Palmer, Katonah and Angrist, 1951; Glickman and Shklar, 1954). It also inhibits the synthesis of collagen and promotes its catabolism (Baker and Whitaker, 1950; Castor and Baker, 1950; Smith and Allison, 1965; Berliner *et al.*, 1967; Kutsky, 1973; Liddle and Melmon, 1974; Russell, Russell and Trupin, 1978). On this basis, studies of the effects of cortisones on eruption may be considered pertinent to the assessment of the role of collagen in eruption. Accordingly, the administration of cortisone might be expected to decrease the eruption rate. Domm and Wellband (1960) and Garren and Greep (1960) found that daily doses of cortisone resulted in a significant increase in the eruption of rat incisors. Ball (1977) noted that maintaining mature rats in a hyperglucocorticoid state (using weekly, subcutaneous injections of methylprednisolone acetate) produced a significant increase in the eruption rates of the mandibular incisors. In all these studies the eruption rates were impeded eruption rates. It has been shown, however, that hydrocortisone also increases unimpeded rates in normal (Kay, 1969; Moxham and Berkovitz, 1980) and root-resected teeth (Berkovitz, 1969; Kay, 1969). Like the vitamin-C-deficiency experiments, however, interpretation of the results is complicated by the wide range of activities of the cortisone hormone (Liddle and Melmon, 1974).

Thomas (1976) and Tyler and Burn-Murdoch (1976) have attempted to evaluate the role of crosslinking of collagen in eruption by experiments involving the measurement of the forces that an erupting tooth can exert. Thomas (1976) reported that the 'eruptive force' of the rat incisor and dog canine was reduced following intra-arterial perfusion of 5OH tryptamine and noradrenaline. On the other hand, tolazoline (a smooth muscle relaxant) was said to raise the 'eruptive force'. Thomas admits that these changes might be produced by altering perfusion pressure consequent upon changes in arterial smooth-muscle activity. However, he claims that the same effects were observed

in vitro when the agents were added to a waterbath of physiological saline in which lay an isolated, dissected rat jaw. He states that these effects must be mediated, therefore, via the collagen of the periodontal ligament. On administration of glutaraldehyde (an agent which promotes crosslinking (Veis, 1967)), the 'eruptive forces' were said to be increased both *in vivo* and *in vitro* (Thomas, 1976). However, Tyler and Burn-Murdoch (1976) reported that, when glutaraldehyde was 'perfused' into the periodontia of rat or rabbit incisors in dissected mandibles from freshly killed animals, no changes in tooth movements were produced. Jackson (1976) and Bailey (1976) have criticized the use of glutaraldehyde in such experiments on the basis that the crosslinking introduced by glutaraldehyde is artificial and that the agent is not a physiological one. Furthermore, the extent to which the *in vitro* techniques described by Thomas (1976) and Tyler and Burn-Murdoch (1976) are of value to the study of the biochemical and biophysical properties of the periodontal ligament collagen *in vivo* is not known.

Much has been made of the finding that daily impeded and unimpeded eruption rates of rat mandibular incisors are markedly retarded when collagen maturation is interfered with following the administration in the diet of the lathyritic agent aminoacetonitrile (AAN) (Thomas, 1965, 1967). AAN acts by specifically inhibiting crosslinking in collagen (Tanzer, 1965; Ross, 1968; Shoshan and Finkelstein, 1968; Levene, 1973). Although Thomas (1965) did not evaluate his results statistically, he states that after about 3 days of administrating AAN to the drinking water the eruption rates decreased, approaching zero. Sarnat and Sciaky (1965) also reported a significant retardation in impeded eruption rates following the administration of AAN, though unimpeded eruption rates were not affected. It can be argued that the effects of AAN on impeded eruption rates may not be related to the eruptive mechanism but may be the result of occlusal stress acting upon a structurally weakened periodontal ligament. Since the studies of Thomas and Sarnat and Sciaky gave conflicting results for the effects on unimpeded eruption rates, Berkovitz, Migdalski and Solomon (1972) repeated the experiment, studying the effects of AAN on the unimpeded eruption of normal and root resected rat mandibular incisors. The root resection study was included to assess the contribution of the proliferative basal tissues to the eruption of the incisors of lathyrogen-treated animals. Whether normal or root resected, they reported that unimpeded eruption rates in the lathyrogen-treated animals were not significantly different from those in control animals. The disruption of the collagen of the periodontal ligament was evidenced by the ease with which the incisors of the lathyritic animals could be extracted with forceps. Subsequently, other studies confirmed that unimpeded, lathyritically affected teeth continue to erupt at high rates (Tsuruta, Eto and Chiba, 1974; Michaeli *et al.*, 1975; Thomas, 1976).

Further evidence against the collagen contraction hypothesis derives from the work of Magnusson (1968) and Grant *et al.* (1972). Magnusson (1968) has shown that the periodontal fibres at the time of the earliest eruptive movements of the molars of rats or monkeys are disorientated so that an effective eruptive force is unlikely to be produced. Grant *et al.* (1972) studied the development of the periodontal tissues in the permanent teeth of marmosets with and without deciduous predecessors. They demonstrated that in the periodontal ligaments of teeth which have predecessors only dentogingival, alveolar crest and horizontal principal collagen fibres at the alveolar crest are discernible upon emergence into the oral cavity. The remaining fibres in the periodontal space appear once the tooth becomes functional. It may be concluded, therefore, that the succedaneous teeth of marmosets do not require organized oblique principal fibres in the periodontal ligaments for their eruption.

In conclusion, there is little evidence for, and much evidence against, the concept that the eruptive forces are generated by the contraction of collagen fibres in the periodontal ligament. Nevertheless, the collagen may play some role in the eruptive process, if only by resisting the forces of eruption or, by its remodelling, allowing eruptive movements produced by some other system(s) to be maintained.

THE PERIODONTAL FIBROBLAST MOTILITY HYPOTHESIS

The possibility that fibroblasts within the periodontal ligament are responsible for generating the eruptive force was first suggested by Ness (1967). This sugges-

tion was made not from experimental observations, but from an appreciation that wound contraction may be mediated by fibroblasts in granulation tissue (James, 1964) and from an attempt to explain the rotation which occurs during the eruption of the tusk of a narwhal (*Monodon*). At that time, Ness was of the opinion that forces were generated by contraction of the fibroblasts. It has been shown that fibroblasts in culture are capable of generating a force (James and Taylor, 1969). Majno *et al.* (1971) have shown that wound granulation tissue, like smooth muscle, contracts with 5OH tryptamine, adrenaline, bradykinin and angiotensin, the contraction being mediated through fibroblasts. It has also been shown that fibroblasts from granulation tissue resemble smooth-muscle cells morphologically (Gabbiani, Ryan and Majno, 1971) and antigenically (Hirschel *et al.*, 1971). There is no evidence, however, that fibroblasts in the periodontal ligament have such characteristics and van den Brenk and Stone (1974) were unable to demonstrate any effect of smooth-muscle agents on uninjured connective tissue. Azuma *et al.* (1975) claim to be able to distinguish a sub-population of fibroblasts in the periodontal ligament which resemble smooth-muscle cells, the so-called myofibroblasts. Such findings, however, have not been confirmed by other workers (e.g. Ten Cate, 1972; Beertsen, Everts and van den Hooff, 1974; Garant, 1976; Shore and Berkovitz, 1979).

It has been proposed that the migration of fibroblasts through the periodontal ligament provides a tractional force which is capable of producing eruption (Ness, 1970; Beertsen *et al.*, 1974). Beertsen *et al.* (1974) have suggested that the oxytalan fibre system has a guiding or supporting role in the dynamics of the ligament. They have postulated that the fibroblasts are directed by the oxytalan fibres in their migration up the ligament, in so doing, effecting eruptive movements by their connections with the collagen fibres inserted into the cementum of the tooth.

According to our first criterion, the fibroblast motility hypothesis requires continuous production and movement of fibroblasts in the periodontal ligament from the base of the ligament to its gingival part, the rate of movement reflecting the rate of eruption. Studies by Melcher (1967), Chiba (1968), Robins (1972) and Beertsen (1973, 1976) suggest that fibroblasts migrate in an occlusal direction in the perio-

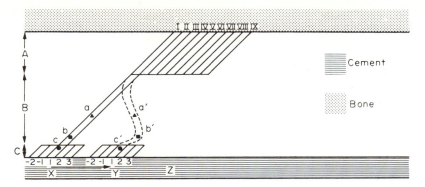

FIG. 9. Diagrammatic representation of the periodontal ligament showing three fibro-blasts (a, b, c) positioned along an obliquely orientated collagen fibre (1, I). As the tooth moves occlusally (from position X to Y), the fibre is now longer than the distance 1—I. The fibre could be envisaged to deform as shown, the fibroblasts being carried to new positions (a¹, b¹, c¹), thus giving the appearance of a differential rate of migration.

dontal ligaments of rodent incisors. Ness (1970) claims that fibroblasts are 'born' near the root apex of the tooth, whence they move upwards with the erupting tooth towards the gingival part of the ligament where they eventually die. Beertsen (1973) showed that migrating periodontal fibroblasts were located in the tooth-related part of the ligament. Nearer the alveolar bone, the periodontal fibroblasts did not appear to move. Beertsen (1976) reported that, in the perio-dontal tissues of the mouse incisor, the rate of movement of the fibroblasts in the tooth-related part of the ligament equalled the rate of eruption of the tooth, whether impeded or unimpeded. However, it is questionable whether the fibroblast movements are causing eruption or are an effect of it. In other words, are they actively moving or are they being carried passively with the tooth-related part of the ligament, the eruptive force being generated by another system? Evidence supporting the concept of active fibroblast migration may be obtained from the findings of Zajicek (1974). He found differential rates of fibro-blast migration in various zones across the ligament in the mouse incisor: fibroblasts 20—30 μm from the tooth moved occlusally 3 times faster than the rate of tooth eruption, whilst fibroblasts closer to the cement surface moved at the same rate as tooth eruption. Zajicek was unable to explain these findings on the basis of passive movements of the fibroblasts in associa-tion with adjacent collagen. However, Shore and

Berkovitz (1978) have described a model, based upon the deformation of collagen fibres in the periodontal ligament as a result of eruptive movements, which can explain differential rates of fibroblast migration within the ligament without recourse to active fibroblast movement. The principle of this interpretation is seen in Fig. 9. In addition, if periodontal fibroblasts gener-ated at the base of the tooth were to migrate at a rate 3 times that of eruption then, following removal of the proliferative basal tissues by root resection, it might be expected that the resected tooth should stop erupting when about one-third of the way along the socket. However, such surgically treated teeth erupt the complete length of the socket (Berkovitz, 1971).

If periodontal fibroblasts are moving actively with directional specificity, it might be expected that they should exhibit some of the specialized features asso-ciated with cell motility. Beertsen, Everts and van den Hooff (1974) claim that the fibroblasts have a well-developed system of microfilaments and microtubules, organelles implicated in active cell movement. How-ever, many non-motile cells also have microfilaments and microtubules (Gomez-Acebo and Garcia Hermida, 1973; Weiss, 1973). Also, it has been shown that microfilaments are associated with exocytosis and endocytosis (Allison, 1973), processes occurring in periodontal fibroblasts. Fibroblasts migrating in tissue culture show marked polarity of shape and the possession of polarized arrays of microfilament bundles and microtubules, particularly in the tail region (Wessels, Spooner and Ludvena, 1973; Goldman, Schloss and Starger, 1976; Vasiliev and Gelfand, 1976). Though fibroblasts appear polarized in longitudinal sections of the periodontal ligament of the rat incisor, it is necessary to view the cells in other planes to determine their overall morphology. When this is carried out, the fibroblast appears as an irregular flattened disc, lacking polarity in both morphology and in the distribution of its intracytoplasmic organelles. When present, microfilament bundles lack any preferential orientation (Shore and Berkovitz, 1979). In a further attempt to determine whether periodontal fibroblasts show any morphological evidence of directionally specific motility, Berkovitz and Shore (1978) have compared fibroblasts within the rat incisor ligament with fibroblasts adjacent to the enamel organ of the same tooth. These latter cells have never been implicated in the generation of an eruptive force. It was reported that the general morphology of the fibroblasts was similar.

There is, therefore, little evidence showing that periodontal fibroblasts are migrating actively. Furthermore, it has yet to be shown that migrating fibroblasts in the periodontal ligament can produce a force significant enough to cause tooth movement. Also, no experiments have yet been undertaken to show that experimentally induced changes in the movement of the fibroblasts produce predictable changes in tooth movement. Consequently, the evidence so far presented for the periodontal fibroblast motility hypothesis remains poor. However, it is possible that the effect of demecolcine in retarding eruption (Chiba, Narraway and Ness, 1968; Berkovitz, 1972) may be linked with an effect on fibroblast motility. Gail and Boone (1971) have shown that *in vitro* this drug significantly reduces fibroblast motility. However, colchicine also affects all proliferating cells in the body, increases viscosity of hyaluronic acid *in vitro* (Castor and Prince, 1964), reduces collagen synthesis (Bornstein, 1974), affects the contractility of granulation tissue (van den Brenk and Stone, 1974) and raises blood pressure by causing arterial constriction (Fergusson, 1952). Results of an electron-microscopic study of periodontal fibroblasts following administration of colchicine suggest that the drug inhibits the secretion of newly synthesized tropocollagen into the extracellular compartment with a subsequent increase

in the number of intracellular collagen profiles (Cho and Garant, 1978). These findings implicate the microtubule system in protein secretion and could, therefore, provide an alternative explanation for the decrease in eruption rate with colchicine in terms of collagen remodelling.

Finally, Beertsen, Everts and van den Hooff (1974) have suggested that the fibroblasts pull the tooth by means of the network of collagen fibres in the periodontal ligament. That the fibre system in the ligament is weakened by lathyrogen, without stopping eruption, seems to argue against this idea.

THE VASCULAR AND PERIODONTAL TISSUE HYDROSTATIC PRESSURE HYPOTHESES

Constant (1900) first suggested that the eruptive force was related to blood pressures. Ness and Smale (1959) developed this idea, in effect in terms of the Starling hypothesis (1909), the eruptive force being deemed to be derived from the hydrostatic pressure of the dental connective tissues (and therefore only indirectly from vascular pressures). The knowledge that ground substance is a major water-binding component of connective tissues (e.g. Schubert and Hamerman, 1968; Bentley, 1970; Melcher and Walker, 1976) might necessitate a further modification of this hypothesis. Guyton (1972) has shown that ground substance removed from a tissue and placed in an electrolyte medium will swell by 30–50% and will exert considerable pressure against any barrier that attempts to prevent its swelling. If the periodontal ligament is similar, tissue fluid may provide pressure in the ground substance sufficient to produce tooth movements. Tyler and Burn-Murdoch (1976) reported that incisor teeth in isolated (dissected) rat mandibles showed extrusive movements during periodontal infusion of distilled water and intrusive movements during infusion of saline. They thus claimed that changes in electrolyte balance can affect the periodontal tissues to produce changes in tooth movements. As shown in Chapter 6, however, too little is known about the periodontal ground substance to formulate views about its role in tooth eruption without being too speculative. Nevertheless, information about changes in the constituents of the ground substance during eruption is beginning to emerge (see Chapter 6, pages 136–137).

According to our first criterion, the tissue pressure hypothesis requires a high-pressure system within and around the tooth with either free mobility of fluid and/or differential pressures between the basal and coronal parts of the erupting tooth.

In the main, the tissue pressures recorded in and around the tooth have been high considering the low, and sometimes even negative, values (in relation to atmospheric pressure) which have been recorded from other connective tissues (e.g. Guyton, 1963, 1976). Pressures in the dental pulp of about 20 mm Hg (and up to 60 mm Hg) above atmospheric pressure have been reported (Wynn *et al.*, 1963; Beveridge *et al.*, 1964; Brown and Yankowitz, 1964; Brown and Beveridge, 1966; Brown, 1968; Brown *et al.*, 1969; Van Hassel and Brown, 1969; Van Hassel, 1971; Stenvik, Iversen and Mjör, 1972; Van Hassel and McMinn, 1972). Within the periodontal ligaments of dog canines, pressures of about 10 mm Hg above atmospheric pressure have been recorded (Lamb and Van Hassel, 1972; Palcanis, 1973), though Walker, Ng and Burke (1978) claim that the pressures are about 2 mm Hg below atmospheric pressure.

It has been argued that, if pressure in and/or around the tooth is to produce eruptive movements, there must be a pressure gradient, the direction of which favours axial movement of the tooth out of its socket. Ness (1964) suggested that this pressure acts in, and is restricted to, the basal region of the root, where 'the tooth forms one wall of a chamber containing fluid at a pressure sufficient to overcome forces holding the tooth in position but insufficient to move the other wall of the chamber'. Ness defined the walls as: 'the bone of the socket base and the periodontal ligament connective tissue whose density is considerable everywhere coronal from about 1 mm from the basal plane'. He assumed that these walls prevent the dissipation of the pressure head by providing a relatively high resistance to flow. With the exception of periapical effusions said to be of vascular origin described by Magnusson (1968), there is little evidence to support the ideas of Ness. Thomas (1976) is of the opinion that the results of resection and transection experiments argue against the tissue fluid hypothesis. It is his belief that the surgical treatment prevents the build up of pressure by 'opening the system'. However, it has been reported that fluid fills the space beneath the erupting resected tooth (Berkovitz, 1971).

The possibility that this fluid can attain a pressure which is sufficiently great to be responsible for the eruption of the resected tooth cannot be dismissed until it has been measured.

Thomas (1965, 1976), assuming that the tissue hydrostatic pressure is constant throughout the periodontal ligament, has argued that, because the basal diameter of the continuously growing incisor is greater than its coronal diameter, the resultant vector of pressure around the tooth would only serve to push the tooth back into its socket. At present, however, we know too little about the fluid dynamics within the periodontal ligament to make such predictions. Brown (1968) reported that tissue pressures recorded simultaneously at two sites within the same pulp chamber have similar values. If injection of fluid is made at one site, however, a pressure rise is only sometimes observed at the other site. He also noted that, if the tooth crown is ground down, the pulp pressure remains normal until the pulp exposure progresses to within a few millimetres of the recording site. These results may indicate a compartmentalization of pressures within the pulp. As yet, it is not known whether similar phenomena exist within the periodontal tissues. That there is a differential between the pressures in the tissues above and below an erupting tooth has been demonstrated by Van Hassel and McMinn (1972) (Fig. 10). They showed that the average tissue pressure above erupting teeth in young dogs was 10 ± 5 mm Hg above atmospheric pressure. The average pressure within the pulps of the erupting teeth was 23 ± 6 mm Hg above atmospheric pressure. In every case the pressure differential favoured eruptive movements, the mean differential being 13 ± 4 mm Hg. Assuming the tissue pressure at the base of the tooth to be the same as that for the coronal pulp tissue from which pressure recordings were monitored, the authors calculated that an average force of 15 g (~ 0.15 N) could be generated by the tissue fluid at the base of the tooth. It has yet to be determined, however, whether a force of 15 g (~ 0.15 N) is sufficient to cause a tooth to erupt since the nature and magnitude of the forces resisting eruption are unknown. The mechanism responsible for maintaining these pressure gradients is not known.

With regard to our second criterion, since teeth at rest show small pulsatile movements which are synchronous with the arterial pulse (e.g. Körber, 1970)

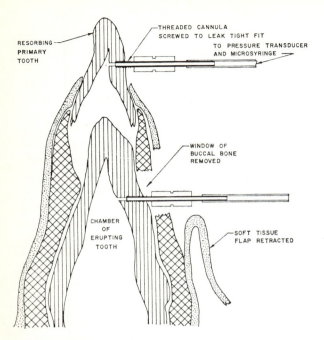

FIG. 10. Diagram of a buccal-lingual section through a dog mandible in the region of a posterior tooth to show sites of surgical access and cannulae placement in order to simultaneously record pressures in the pulps of an erupting tooth and its overlying deciduous predecessor.

vascular pressures can produce a force sufficient to move a tooth under physiological conditions. Using a variable capacitance displacement transducer to continuously record tooth movements, Moxham (1979a) has suggested that eruption is sensitive to changes in blood pressure. He reported that, whilst variations in the rate of eruption of the mandibular incisor of the rabbit occurred without comparable variation in arterial blood pressure (measured from the femoral artery), eruption ceased if the mean blood pressure fell to a level consistently below 70 mm Hg. Furthermore, for one rabbit he observed that significant changes in tooth position occurred associated with marked drops in arterial blood pressure (Fig. 11). After the animals were killed, eruption ceased with the sudden drop in arterial blood pressure and the cessation of the heart beat, the teeth gradually intruding once the arterial blood pressure dropped to zero (Fig. 12). Myhre, Preus and Aars (1979) have reported similar findings. Using an ultrasonic technique to monitor the axial position of a rabbit maxillary incisor,

they observed that the position was influenced greatly by arterial blood pressure. Following the death of the rabbits, tooth movements were seen similar to those described by Moxham (1979a).

Experimental investigations into the vascular and tissue hydrostatic pressure hypotheses have been based either upon a visual assessment of 'vascularity' (which required the evaluation of the area occupied by blood vessels in histological sections) or upon attempts to alter eruptive behaviour by changing indirectly blood flow and pressures within the vessels of the periodontal ligament.

Bryer (1957) studied the effects of nutritional disturbance and surgical interference on the eruption of the rodent incisor, relating the resulting changes in vascularity of the dental tissues to eruption rate. He reported that a reduction in eruption rates observed in vitamin A deficiency, rickets, vitamin D toxicity, cobalt administration, and various surgical interferences with the tissues and blood supply to the teeth was associated with a reduced vascularity. Increases in eruption during semistarvation and after localized sympathectomy were said to be associated with increased vascularity. Bryer concluded that 'the eruptive force of the rat's incisor is derived predominantly from the tissue tension within the pulp and periodontal tissues and that this tension is dependent upon the dynamics of the blood circulation'. The validity of this conclusion must be questioned on the basis that histological assessment of vascularity is not the same as a physiological assessment of vascular behaviour. Furthermore, vitamin C deficiency reduces eruption rates (Dalldorf and Zall, 1930; Berkovitz, 1974) but with hyperaemia and oedema of the pulp (Höjer and Westin, 1925; Key and Elphick, 1931; McLean, Sheppard and McHenry, 1939).

Experiments directed towards altering blood flow and pressures in the vessels of the tooth (and thereby, it was assumed, the tissue fluid pressure) have relied upon section of the vasomotor nerve supply or the administration of drugs with vaso-active properties.

Studies on the effect of sympathectomy using techniques for measuring eruption at discrete intervals of more than 24 hours are inconclusive. Increased impeded eruption rates have been recorded following sympathectomy for the incisors of rats (Breitner and Leist, 1927), guinea pigs (Leist, 1927) and rabbits (King, 1937). Unimpeded eruption rates of rat incisors

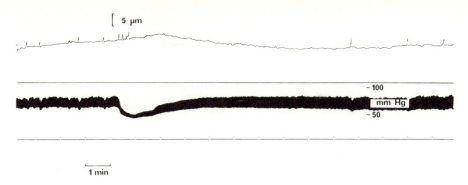

FIG. 11. Record of the movements of a rabbit's mandibular incisor monitored with a variable capacitance displacement transducer during a period when there was a spontaneous drop in arterial blood pressure lasting 2–3 minutes. Note the intrusive movement of the tooth as the arterial blood pressure returns to normal.

were reported to increase following sympathectomy (Bryer, 1957). However, similar experiments using rat incisors produced no effects on impeded eruption rates (Taylor and Butcher, 1951; Miller, 1957; Moss and Crikelair, 1960). Thus, the failure to establish any consistent change in eruption following sympathectomy may argue against the periodontal tissue hydrostatic pressure hypothesis. However, there is no certainty that nerve section caused the change in tissue hydrostatic pressure that one might have expected. Firstly, since sympathetic section will not only reduce arteriolar tone but can also reduce venomotor tone, it may not cause a rise in filtration pressure. Secondly, even though capillary filtration is increased, the tissue pressure may not rise because of tissue compliance. In the dog leg, Guyton, Granger and Taylor (1971) have shown that the volume of fluid can rise by nearly 100% with only a small change in tissue hydrostatic pressure. However, since the tooth and its supporting tissues are housed in a bony socket, it seems unlikely that there is such compliance. Thirdly, although there is evidence to suggest that the periodontal ligaments of the cat and dog have functional sympathetic innerva-

tions (Miura and Kondo, 1969; Edwall, 1971, 1972; Edwall and Kindlová, 1971), such evidence seems to be lacking for rodents. Fourthly, there is the possibility of the blood vessels re-establishing their calibre soon after sympathectomy (Barcroft and Swan, 1953). More recently, however, Moxham (1976, 1978), using a technique sufficiently sensitive to continuously record eruption of the rabbit incisor, has shown that section of the cervical sympathetic trunk was associated with an increase in the eruption rates of the ipsilateral incisor during the first 1½ hours after sympathectomy (Fig. 13). Stimulation of the peripheral cut end of the sympathetic trunk was associated with intrusive movements of the incisor (Fig. 14). Similar findings have been described in a preliminary report by Aars (1976) (see also page 165).

With regard to experiments using drugs with vasoactive properties, Main and Adams (1966) reported that daily intramuscular doses of the hypotensive agents guanethidine and hydrallazine to normotensive rats over a period of 8 days did not affect the rates of unimpeded eruption of their incisors. Litvin and de Marco (1973) have reported that twice-daily intra-

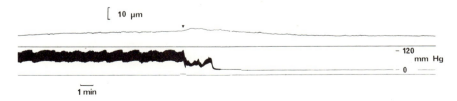

FIG. 12. Movements of a rabbit mandibular incisor recorded following death. At the marker arrow a lethal dose of urethane was injected intravenously.

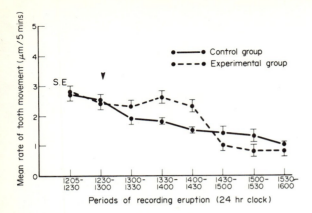

FIG. 13. Graphs showing group mean rates of movement (in μm/5 min) of erupting rabbit mandibular incisors for a control group of animals and an experimental group where the ipsilateral cervical sympathetic trunk was sectioned. These data were obtained using a variable capacitance displacement transducer measuring eruption over a 4-hour period (1200–1600 hours). The marker arrow indicates that sympathectomy was undertaken in each animal of the experimental group at 1300 hours.

muscular injections of the diuretic Lasix (furosemide) to female white rabbits over an 8-day period did not affect the unimpeded eruption of the maxillary and mandibular incisors. However, they reported that twice-daily intramuscular injections of the antidiuretic pitressin (vasopressin) to female white rabbits over an

8-day period increased the unimpeded eruption rate of the incisors from a group mean of 1.81 mm/4 days to 2.18 mm/4 days. Main and Adams (1966) and Litvin and de Marco (1973) used techniques for determining eruption rates which required an assessment of changes in tooth position at intervals of 2 and 4 days respectively. Since changes in the vasculature may only be short term, their techniques may not be sufficiently sensitive to monitor changes in eruptive behaviour. The increase in eruption rate following the administration of pitressin reported by Litvin and de Marco (1973) may not be reliable since their method of measurement (with calipers from the interdental papilla) is crude. Recently, the immediate and short-term effects of a variety of drugs with vaso-active properties have been studied using a technique to continuously monitor eruption of the rabbit mandibular incisor (Moxham, 1979b). Intravenous injections of the hypotensive agents hexamethonium, guanethidine and hydrallazine were found to produce significant (though relatively short term) increases in rates compared with those for control animals (Fig. 15). It might be thought that hypotensive agents should produce a decrease in eruption rates to be consistent with the vascular hypothesis. However, though main arterial blood pressure falls, for the microcirculation there is likely to be an increase in vascular pressures

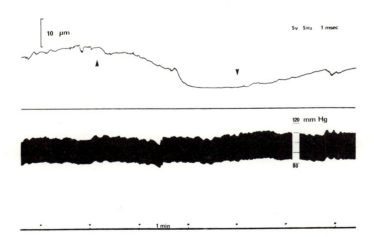

FIG. 14. Movements of a rabbit's mandibular incisor recorded using a variable capacitance displacement transducer when the peripheral cut end of the ipsilateral cervical sympathetic trunk was stimulated. In this instance the stimulus strength was 5 V, the frequency of the impulses was 5 Hz and the duration of each impulse was 1 ms. The period of stimulation was 3 minutes as indicated by the marker arrows.

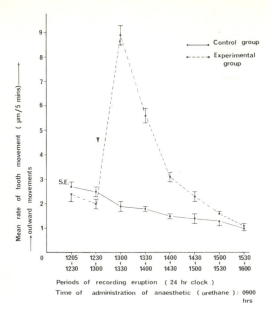

FIG. 15. Graphs showing group mean rates of movements (in μm/5 min) of erupting rabbit mandibular incisors for a control group of animals and an experimental group where a single dose of hexamethonium (10 mg/kg) was administered intravenously at 1300 hours (arrow) to each animal.

which, arguing from Starling's hypothesis, should result in an increase in tissue fluid pressures and hence an increase in eruption. Infusions of noradrenaline or acetylcholine into the subclavian artery were also found to have significant effects on tooth movements (Figs. 16 and 17). Myhre *et al.* (1979) also have observed intrusive movements of the rabbit maxillary incisor with i.v. noradrenaline and have reported extrusive movements with i.v. papaverine.

In summary, although the experiments based upon section of the vasomotor nerve supply to the teeth or the administration of drugs with vaso-active properties which used techniques of measuring eruption at intervals of 24 hours or more are inconclusive, similar experiments using techniques for continuously recording eruption (Aars, 1976; Moxham, 1978, 1979b; Myhre *et al.,* 1979) produced results which are consistent with the vascular or tissue hydrostatic pressure hypothesis of eruption. Further appreciation of the mechanisms underlying such findings may be achieved by investigations involving study of vascular physio-

logy, tissue pressures and metabolic activity in the dental tissues.

Several conclusions may be drawn from this section of the review:

1. The evidence suggests that all the systems in the periodontal ligament which have been implicated in the eruptive mechanism have characteristics which, if they generated the eruptive force, would allow such a force to be sustained. However, there is a problem of distinguishing between cause and effect. Consequently, it is not known to what extent the high turnover of collagen, the migration of fibroblasts and the tissue pressures are responses to eruptive movements.

2. There is little evidence to show that collagen contraction or fibroblast activity within the periodontal ligament can generate a force under physiological conditions which is sufficient to move a tooth in a direction favouring eruption. Furthermore, it has yet to be shown that experimental alteration of these systems produces significant and predictable changes in eruption.

3. There is evidence to show that teeth move under physiological conditions in synchrony with the arterial pulse and that experimental procedures expected to change vascular behaviour in and around a tooth produce changes in tooth movements which are consistent with the vascular hypotheses.

Some further considerations concerning the eruptive process

A major problem which needs to be resolved in order to understand the process of tooth eruption concerns the possibility that experimentally induced alterations in the eruption rates may be the result not of changes in the mechanisms generating the eruptive forces but of changes in the resistance of the tissues to such forces. To date, there have been few attempts to interpret the findings of experiments on eruption on this basis. Indeed, the manner (and extent) whereby the tissues surrounding a tooth resist extrusive loads has hardly been investigated. Such information is fundamental for the interpretation of data obtained from experiments on eruption. Preliminary studies towards this have been undertaken by Moxham and

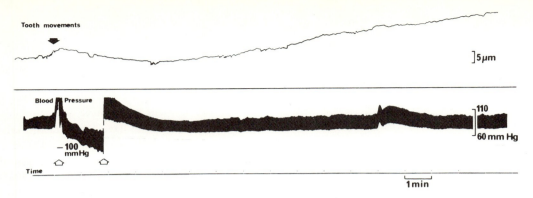

FIG. 16. Record of the movements of a rabbit's mandibular incisor showing the immediate effects of a close arterial injection of noradrenaline (0.003 mg/kg) (arrow). Note that eruption-like movements ceased on inject-ing the noradrenaline, the incisor intruding into its socket (by about 8 μm) for a period of approximately 5 minutes. Thereafter, eruption-like movements recommenced. The marker arrows on the blood-pressure trace indicate the use of an offsetting device.

Berkovitz (1979) and are described in Chapter 11 (pages 262—265).

In view of the controversies surrounding tooth eruption, many have been tempted to postulate that eruption is not the result of a prime mover but is multifactorial. Since a variety of agents are known to have significant and different effects upon erup-tion rates of continuously growing incisors then, if eruption is a multifactorial process, it is possible that different agents affect different factors. Based upon this premise, Moxham and Berkovitz (1980) assessed whether eruption is multifactorial by experiments involving the administration of combinations of drugs (namely hydrocortisone, thyroxine and cyclophospha-

mide). They observed that thyroxine and hydro-cortisone alone increased unimpeded eruption rates of rat incisors whilst cyclophosphamide alone decreased them. The combination of cyclophosphamide and hydrocortisone did not produce effects significantly different from those observed with cyclophosphamide alone. The enhanced increases in unimpeded eruption rates associated with the combination of thyroxine and hydrocortisone were consistent with the idea that the process of eruption is multifactorial. However, additional information regarding the effects of these drugs on the periodontal tissues is required to allow a fuller interpretation of these findings. Furthermore, the results do not necessarily imply that the mecha-

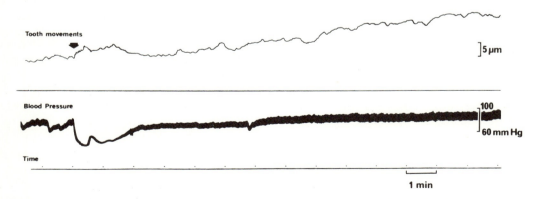

FIG. 17. The immediate effects of close arterial injection of acetylcholine (0.01 mg/kg) (arrow) on move-ments of a rabbit's mandibular incisor. In this instance, outward tooth movements resembling eruption were not recorded prior to the injection of acetylcholine. Immediately following the injection of acetylcholine, however, outward tooth movements were recorded at rates of approximately 7 μm/5 min.

nism generating the force of eruption is multifactorial. That eruption is multifactorial is not surprising since, though the eruptive force may be generated by one system within the periodontal ligament, its translation into sustained outward movement may depend upon other systems within the ligament (such as those related to turnover and remodelling). In addition, one or more of the drugs used in their experiments may have affected the resistance of the periodontal tissues to eruption.

THE MECHANISMS OF MESIAL DRIFT

Although approximal drift in both mesial and distal directions has been reported (pages 220–221), most attention has been paid to mesial drift since this is the main direction for human teeth. Consequently, this review is concerned primarily with mechanisms of mesial drift. It is possible, however, that similar kinds of mechanisms are responsible for distal drift.

Many hypotheses have been proposed to explain the mechanisms whereby the forces producing drift are generated. These can be classified broadly into those which relate to external loads placed upon the teeth and those which claim that drift is the result of forces generated in the periodontium. In the first category are factors related to the anterior component of occlusal force, to oral soft-tissue pressures and to erupting molars. In the second category are hypotheses relating to the deposition and resorption of alveolar bone and to contraction of the transseptal fibre system.

The anterior component of occlusal force

According to this hypothesis, when the teeth occlude part of the force is transmitted in a forward direction because the teeth are inclined mesially. That the long axes of most human teeth are inclined mesially is well known (e.g. Dewel, 1949). Stallard (1923), Osborn (1961) and Picton (1962) have demonstrated the reality of the anterior component of force in humans. Stallard (1923) showed that ivory blocks mounted in soft wax on denture bases moved mesially on clenching the jaws. Furthermore, a wire arm projecting at right angles from a maxillary canine of a patient was seen to move

anteriorly when the teeth were clenched. Osborn (1961) showed that more force was required to remove a steel strip placed between adjacent teeth when the teeth were clenched than when they were not. Mesial tilting of maxillary and mandibular cheek teeth and of maxillary central incisors was demonstrated using wire resistance strain gauges when axial loads of 2–5 kg ($\sim$ 20–50 N) were applied to the occlusal surfaces of the teeth (Picton, 1962). Further evidence that biting loads produce a forward force on the cheek teeth in man stems from the observation that interproximal contact points are often worn. However, whether the anterior component of occlusal force can be translated into the forward migration of mesial drift has not been clarified. In relation to this point, we do not yet know the magnitude and nature of the forces required to produce mesial drift (or to resist it). For example, has the force to be continuous or need it only be intermittent? That bone behaves differently to intermittent or continuous forces (Heřt, Lišková and Landrgot, 1969; Lišková and Heřt, 1971) indicates that this might be a significant consideration.

A variety of experiments have been conducted to test the anterior component of occlusal force hypothesis. Moss and Picton (1967) measured the approximal drift of the cheek teeth of *Macaca irus* monkeys by means of clinical, radiographic and histological methods for periods of between 10 and 32 weeks. The teeth were disced interproximally to encourage movement. It was reported that teeth with and without their antagonists in the opposing jaw drifted approximally. According to the anterior component of occlusal force hypothesis, no movement of the unopposed teeth should have occurred. Moss and Picton (1967) claim, therefore, that this hypothesis is disproved. However, overeruption of the unopposed teeth did occur and the direction of overeruption may have contributed towards the drift. The molars, being inclined mesially, drifted mesially; the premolars, being inclined distally, drifted distally. Thus, it might also be concluded that teeth tend to drift in the direction in which they are aligned. In another study, however, Picton and Moss (1974) reported no significant correlation between the angulation of the roots of the cheek teeth of *Macaca irus* monkeys and the direction or distance of approximal drift of these teeth. They concluded that the inclination of the roots was not an important factor contributing to drift. In their

1967 experiment, Moss and Picton reported increased rates of drift for those teeth without antagonists compared with those teeth with antagonists. In an attempt to explain this, Picton and Moss (1978) examined the effects of reducing cusp height on the rate of drift. They found that drift was significantly more rapid on the side with reduced cusps during the first 2 or 3 weeks and concluded that interdigitation of cusps during normal function retards drift.

Findings on approximal drift in *Macaca irus* monkeys which appear to conflict with those of Moss and Picton (1967) and Picton and Moss (1978) have been described by van Beek and Fidler (1977). They observed that the interdental spaces between the cheek teeth closed faster when the opposing teeth were in occlusion. In their experiments, they disced the interproximal surfaces of both the mandibular and the opposing maxillary cheek teeth so that, in occlusion, the molars could still move in pairs. They concluded that functional occlusion plays an important role in the mechanism of mesial tooth migration. In response to this, a study has been conducted by Picton and Moss (1979) in which the occlusal surfaces of cheek teeth of *Macaca irus* monkeys were sloped to gingival levels. On one side of the jaw PM_1, PM_2, and M_1 were sloped mesially while M_2 and M_3 were sloped distally. This pattern was thought to favour approximal drift. On the other side of the jaw, the teeth were sloped in the reverse direction so that the biting force tended to cause separation of teeth. The opposing teeth were undisturbed. After interdental spaces had been created by discing the teeth, approximal drift was noted in all test segments, the rates being similar for both patterns of occlusion. It appears, therefore, that an adverse component of force does not prevent drift. One problem concerning this interpretation relates to the possibility that the experimental occlusion may have interfered with mastication. Picton and Moss (1980) have carried out another study using the same animals from the earlier (1979) experiment. They fitted silver splints to the teeth in the test segments to restore the horizontal occlusal surfaces and disced the opposing teeth to create the steeply sloping occlusal surfaces which either encouraged or discouraged approximal drift. Following interproximal discing of the teeth with sloping occlusal surfaces, it was again seen that approximal drift occurred regardless of whether the slopes favoured or hindered the development of a horizontal component of biting force. That the silver splints showed brightly abraded surfaces demonstrated that tooth contacts were occurring during biting. This, together with lack of any reported abnormality in feeding behaviour, goes some way to showing that masticatory behaviour is not unduly affected by the experimental procedures adopted.

Soft-tissue pressures

That drift might be produced by forces exerted by the cheeks and the tongue was first suggested by Wallace (1904). Winders (1962), Gould and Picton (1964) and Lear *et al.* (1965) have demonstrated the reality of such forces on buccal and lingual surfaces of human teeth. Weinstein (1967) showed that if the morphology of buccal or lingual surfaces of teeth was altered by inlays, the balance of soft-tissue pressures was disturbed and teeth drifted.

Moss and Picton (1970) conducted experiments using *Macaca irus* monkeys to determine whether approximal drift occurs when forces from the cheeks and tongue are eliminated. This was achieved by placing an acrylic dome over the cheek teeth on one side of the arch. The cheek teeth on the other side of the arch served as controls, being left uncovered. Both the experimental and control cheek teeth were disced interproximally to encourage drift and the opposing cheek teeth on both sides extracted. After periods varying from 6 to 17 weeks the molars covered by the dome had drifted towards each other at approximately the same rate as the control teeth. This suggests that forces from the cheeks and tongue do not play a significant part in producing drift.

The eruptive force of molars

It has been suggested that erupting molars exert a force against the distal aspect of the teeth immediately anterior. This force is thought to produce mesial migration (Trauner, 1912; Korkhaus, 1938). Some clinical evidence in support of this view stems from the observation that space produced by extraction of premolars for orthodontic purposes is closed by drift of molars more rapidly in patients possessing third molars than in patients where third molars had been previously extracted (Schwarze, 1972, 1973). Further support for this view has been forwarded by van Beek (1979). He showed that mesial drifting of maxillary and mandibular first molars was reduced in *Macaca irus* if the interproximal contacts between first and second molars were disced. However, that forces from erupting molars are not essential for mesial drift is evident from observations that drift occurs (i) after the dentition has fully developed (e.g. Begg, 1954; Moss and Picton, 1967, 1970), (ii) in front of ankylosed teeth (Yilmaz, 1973) and (iii) in teeth where there are no contacts with adjacent teeth (Moss and Picton, 1967, 1970).

The deposition and resorption of alveolar bone

Mesial drifting of teeth has been attributed to bone deposition distal to the tooth with resorption mesially (Sicher and Weinmann, 1944). Although such histological changes are well documented (e.g. Moss and Picton, 1967), these may be the result rather than the cause of the migration. Furthermore, it is difficult to separate bone activity related to tooth movements from that related to jaw growth (e.g. Manson, 1968).

Contraction of the transseptal fibre system

Scott (1967) suggested that transseptal fibres might maintain contact between the teeth. Thompson *et al.* (1958), Boese (1969), Edwards (1970), Strahan and Mills (1970) and Pinson and Strahan (1974) have reported that the relapse of teeth moved orthodontically could be reduced when gingivectomy was undertaken. Murphey (1970) reported that, following extraction of the mandibular first molars in a young adult monkey, the adjacent premolars migrated distally once transseptal fibres developed across the healing socket. Such findings indicate that the gingival fibres may play a role in stabilizing tooth position and in restoring the position of displaced teeth.

On the basis of their early work, Moss and Picton (1967, 1970) concluded that, since approximal drift could occur in the absence of forces from the tongue,

cheeks and opposing teeth, the principal cause of drift lies in or around the roots of the teeth. They implicated contraction of the transseptal fibre system and conducted two experiments to assess this.

The first experiment (Picton and Moss, 1973) involved measuring the migration of the cheek teeth in macaque monkeys after the interdental soft tissues were scraped away or cut vertically to interrupt the continuity of the transseptal fibre system. They reported that, following interproximal discing, there was a significant reduction in the migration of these teeth when compared with teeth with non-traumatized gingivae in the same animal. However, the surgically treated teeth still drifted approximately 20 μm/week (compared with 55 μm/week for control teeth). This finding has not been adequately explained. It may be that some system in addition to the transseptal fibre system is involved in producing drift. Alternatively, the reduction could be the result of changes in resistance of the tissues to drifting. Histologically, the sites of trauma did not show transseptal fibres, though granulation tissue was seen. It is possible that the inflammatory changes influenced the results, perhaps by increasing the resistance to drift. In two animals where there was repeated surgical removal of interdental papillae without apparent effects on the deeper transseptal fibres, the rates of drift were not reduced. Moss and Picton concluded that, since papillectomy produced inflammatory changes similar to those seen when the transseptal fibres were damaged, inflammation was not a significant factor in retarding drift.

The second experiment (Moss and Picton, 1974) involved dividing first and second mandibular molars of macaque monkeys into mesial and distal fragments. Where the interdental tissues were not damaged, the mesial and distal fragments of a tooth moved apart. Where the interdental tissues were scraped away, mesial and distal fragments initially remained stationary but later moved together. The authors stated that 'The impression gained from the graphic records of all the animals was as though elastic bands joined the adjacent surfaces of neighbouring teeth prior to the experiment and at that time these elastics were under tension. When spaces were created between the teeth and then the roots of the first and second molars were divided, the elastic contracted, so drawing the fragments of the divided teeth away from each other. Such displacement did not occur on the side where the interdental soft tissues had been scraped away. The presence of intact bands of connective tissue extending from one tooth to the adjacent tooth, as revealed in the histological sections, provides a structural element in the right situation.' However, whether the transseptal fibres do indeed have these properties is not known. It may seem surprising that, where the interdental soft tissues were scraped away, the mesial and distal fragments came together. To explain this, Moss and Picton suggested that a fibre system capable of contraction may have developed within the granulation tissue between the fragments. To counter the possibility that the cusps of the opposing teeth had influenced the migration of the tooth fragments by driving between them, it was reported that the separation of tooth fragments still occurred for two animals where the occlusal surfaces of opposing teeth were flattened.

In summary, the evidence shows that drifting of teeth occurs without the application of external loads on the teeth and suggests that some factor(s) in the periodontium may be responsible. That most experiments on drift require discing the interproximal surfaces of teeth to create space raises the question – do the mechanisms operating during experimental drifting operate during physiological drifting with tooth contacts? This question is similar to one asked for the eruptive mechanism – in what way does unimpeded eruption resemble impeded eruption? We can assess the hypotheses proposed to explain drifting by adopting criteria similar to those used to assess the hypotheses relating to the eruptive mechanism (see pages 224–226). Any system proposed as the mechanism responsible for approximal drift must be shown capable of producing a force under physiological conditions which can move a tooth approximally. Experimentally induced changes in the system should cause predictable changes in drift.

Of the various hypotheses proposed, only the anterior component of occlusal force and oral soft-tissue pressures have been shown to produce forces under physiological conditions capable of moving teeth. However, experiments aimed at eliminating such forces produced results which are inconsistent with the anterior component of occlusal force and soft-tissue pressure hypotheses. Although the findings from the experiments of Picton and Moss (1973) and Moss and Picton (1974) suggested the involvement of the transseptal fibre system in drift, as yet the precise mechanisms responsible are not known. Initially, they postulated contraction of the collagen fibres. However, contraction of collagen has not been demonstrated under physiological conditions. More recently, Moss (1976) has suggested that the contractility might be associated with fibroblasts. However, there is also little evidence to support this. Experiments have yet to be conducted to see whether experimentally induced changes in collagen or fibroblast activity within the transseptal fibre system produce changes in drift.

Finally, to date we have insufficient information concerning the process of approximal drift to enable us to define the characteristics of the system necessary to produce it. For example, is it a continuous or intermittent process? What is the magnitude of the forces which produce (and resist) drift? If the transseptal fibre system is implicated, does it have the turnover and remodelling characteristics necessary to ensure that changes in tooth position are maintained?

ACKNOWLEDGEMENTS

The authors gratefully acknowledge the financial assistance obtained from the Medical Research Council.

REFERENCES

AARS, H. (1976) Sympathetic nervous control of axial position of the rabbit incisor tooth. *Acta Phys. Scand.* Suppl. **440**, 131.

ADAMS, D. & MAIN, J. H. P. (1962) A radiographic method of measuring unimpeded eruption rates in the rat incisor. *J. Physiol.* **160**, 1–2.

AINAMO, J. & TALARI, A. (1976) Eruptive movements of teeth in human adults. In: *The eruption and occlusion of teeth*, D. F. G. POOLE & M. V. STACK (eds.), pp. 97–107. London, Butterworths.

ALLISON, A. C. (1973) The role of microfilaments and microtubules in cell movement, endocytosis and exocytosis. In: *Locomotion of tissue cells* (CIBA Symposium 14), pp. 110–143. Amsterdam, Elsevier.

AZUMA, M., ENLOW, D. H., FREDRICKSON, R. G. & GASTON, L. F. (1975) A myofibroblastic basis for the physical forces that produce tooth drift and eruption, skeletal displacement of sutures, and periosteal migration. In: *Determinants of mandibular form and growth*, J. A. McNAMARA (ed.), pp. 179–207. University of Michigan.

BAILEY, A. J. (1968) The nature of collagen. *Comp. Biochem.* **26**, 297–423.

BAILEY, A. J. (1976) In: *The eruption and occlusion of teeth,* D. F. G. POOLE & M. V. STACK (eds.), pp. 306–307. London, Butterworths.

BAKER, B. L. & WHITAKER, W. L. (1950) Interference with wound healing by the action of adrenocortical steroids. *Endocrinology* 46, 544–551.

BALL, P. C. (1977) The effect of adrenal glucocorticoid administration on eruption rates and tissue dimensions in rat mandibular incisors. *J. Anat. Lond.* 124, 157–163.

BARCROFT, H. & SWAN, H. J. C. (1953) Sympathetic control of human blood vessels. *Monographs of the Physiological Soc.* No. 1.

BARNES, M. J. & KODICEK, E. (1972) Biological hydroxylations and ascorbic acid with special regard to collagen metabolism. *Vitam. Horm.* 30, 1–43.

BARROW, C. G. & WHITE, J. R. (1952) Developmental changes of the maxillary and mandibular dental arches. *Angle Orthodont.* 22, 41–46.

BAUME, L. J. (1950) Physiologic tooth migration and its significance for the development of occlusion. *J. dent. Res.* 29, 331–337.

BAUME, L. J. (1953) The development of the lower permanent incisors and their supporting bone. *Amer. J. Orthod.* 39, 526–544.

BAUME, L. J. & BECKS, H. (1950) Development of the dentition of *Macaca mulatta. Amer. J. Orthod.* 36, 723–748.

BEERTSEN, W. (1973) Tissue dynamics in the periodontal ligament of the mandibular incisor of the mouse: A preliminary report. *Archs. oral Biol.* 18, 61–66.

BEERTSEN, W. (1976) Cell movement in the periodontal ligament. In: *The eruption and occlusion of teeth,* D. F. G. POOLE & M. V. STACK (eds.), pp. 215–216. London, Butterworths.

BEERTSEN, W. & EVERTS, V. (1977) The site of remodelling of collagen in the periodontal ligament of the mouse incisor. *Anat. Rec.* 189, 479–498.

BEERTSEN, W., EVERTS, V. & VAN DEN HOOFF, A. (1974) Fine structure of fibroblasts in the periodontal ligament of the rat incisor and their possible role in tooth eruption. *Archs. oral Biol.* 19, 1087–1098.

BEGG, P. R. (1954) Stone Age man's dentition: with reference to anatomically correct occlusion, the etiology of malocclusion, and a technique for its treatment. *Amer. J. Orthod.* 40, 298–312, 373–383, 462–475, 517–531.

BENTLEY, J. P. (1970) The biological role of the ground substance mucopolysaccharides. *Adv. Biol. Skin* 10, 103–121.

BERKOVITZ, B. K. B. (1969) An experimental study into the mechanism of tooth eruption. Ph.D. Thesis. London University.

BERKOVITZ, B. K. B. (1971) The effect of root transection and partial root resection on the unimpeded eruption rate of the rat incisor. *Archs. oral Biol.* 16, 1033–1043.

BERKOVITZ, B. K. B. (1972) The effect of demecolcine and triethanomelamine on the unimpeded eruption rate of normal and root resected incisor teeth in rats. *Archs. oral Biol.* 17, 937–947.

BERKOVITZ, B. K. B. (1974) The effect of vitamin C deficient diet on eruption rates for the guinea pig lower incisor. *Archs. oral Biol.* 19, 807–811.

BERKOVITZ, B. K. B. & BASS, T. B. (1976) Eruption rates of human upper third molars. *J. dent. Res.* 55, 460–464.

BERKOVITZ, B. K. B., MIGDALSKI, A. & SOLOMON, M. (1972) The effect of the lathyritic agent aminoacetonitrile on the unimpeded eruption rate in normal and root-resected rat lower incisors. *Archs. oral Biol.* 17, 1755–1763.

BERKOVITZ, B. K. B. & SHORE, R. C. (1978) The ultrastructure of the enamel aspect of the rat incisor periodontium in normal and root-resected teeth. *Archs. oral Biol.* 23, 681–689.

BERKOVITZ, B. K. B. & THOMAS, N. R. (1969) Unimpeded eruption in the root-resected lower incisor of the rat with a preliminary note on root transection. *Archs. oral Biol.* 14, 771–780.

BERLINER, D. L., WILLIAMS, R. J., TAYLOR, G. N. & NABORS, C. J. (1967) Decreased scar formation with topical corticosteroid treatment. *Surgery* 61, 619–625.

BEVERIDGE, E., GROSS, R., YANKOWITZ, D. & BROWN, A. C. (1964) The relation between dental pulp tissue pressure and systemic arterial blood pressure. *J. dent. Res.* 43, 805.

BJÖRK, A. (1963) Variations in growth pattern of the human mandible. Longitudinal, radiographic study by the implant method. *J. dent. Res.* 42, 400–411.

BJÖRK, A. & SKIELLER, V. (1972) Facial development and tooth eruption. An implant study at the age of puberty. *Amer. J. Orthod.* 62, 339–383.

BLACK, G. V. (1936) *Operative dentistry,* Vol. 1. Chicago, Medico-Dental Pub. Co.

BOESE, L. R. (1969) Increased stability of orthodontically rotated teeth following gingivectomy in *Macaca nemestrina. Amer. J. Orthod.* 56, 273–290.

BORNSTEIN, P. (1974) The biosynthesis of collagen. *Ann. Rev. Biochem.* 43, 567–603.

BOYLE, P. E. (1955) *Kronfeld's histopathology of the teeth and their surrounding structures,* 4th ed. London, Kimpton.

BRASH, J. C. (1927) The growth of the alveolar bone and its relation to the movement of teeth, including eruption. Part II. *Dent. Rec.* 27, 1–27.

BRASH, J. C. (1928) The growth of the alveolar bone and its relation to the movements of the teeth including eruption. *Int. J. Orthod.* 14, 196–223, 283–293, 398–405, 487–494, 494–504.

BREITNER, C. & LEIST, M. (1927) Über den Einfluss des vegetativum Nervensystems auf die Zähne. *Z. Stomat.* 25, 772–776.

BROWN, A. C. (1968) Pulp tissue pressure and blood flow. In: *Biology of the dental pulp organ,* S. B. FINN (ed.), pp. 381–395. Alabama, University of Alabama Press.

BROWN, A. C., BARROW, B. L., GADD, G. N. & VAN HASSEL, H. J. (1969) Tooth pulp transcapillary osmotic pressure in the dog. *Archs. oral Biol.* 14, 491–502.

BROWN, A. C. & BEVERIDGE, E. E. (1966) The relation between tooth pulp pressure and systemic arterial pressure. *Archs. oral Biol.* 11, 1181–1193.

BROWN, A. C. & YANKOWITZ, D. (1964) Tooth pulp tissue pressure and hydraulic permeability. *Circ. Res.* 15, 42–50.

BROWN, V. P. & DAUGAARD-JENSEN, I. (1950) Changes in the dentition from the early teens to the early twenties. *Acta Odont. Scand.* 9, 177–192.

BRYER, L. W. (1957) An experimental evaluation of the physiology of tooth eruption. *Int. dent. J.* 7, 432–478.

BURKE, P. H. (1963) Eruptive movements of permanent maxillary central incisor teeth in the human. *Proc. R. Soc. Med.* 56, 513–515.

BURKE, P. H. & NEWELL, D. J. (1958) A photographic method of measuring eruption of certain human teeth. *Amer. J. Orthod.* 44, 590–602.

BURN-MURDOCH, R. A. & PICTON, D. C. A. (1978) A technique for measuring eruption rates in rats of maxillary incisors under intrusive forces. *Archs. oral Biol.* 23, 563–566.

CAHILL, D. R. (1969) Eruption pathway formation in the presence of experimental tooth impaction in puppies. *Anat. Rec.* 164, 67–78.

CAHILL, D. R. (1974) Histological changes in the bony crypt and gubernacular canal of erupting permanent premolars during deciduous premolar exfoliation in beagles. *J. dent. Res.* 53, 786–791.

CARLSON, H. (1944) Studies on the rate and amount of eruption of certain human teeth. *Amer. J. Orthod.* 30, 575–588.

CASTOR, C. W. & BAKER, B. L. (1950) Local action of adrenocortical steroids on epidermis and connective tissue of skin. *Endocrinology* 47, 234–241.

CASTOR, C. W. & PRINCE, R. K. (1964) Modulation of the intrinsic viscosity of hyaluronic acid formed by human fibroblasts *in vitro:* the effects of hydrocortisone and colchicine. *Biochim. Biophys. Acta* 83, 165–177.

CHATTERGEE, G. C. (1967) Effects of ascorbic acid deficiency in animals. In: *The vitamins,* Vol. 1 (2nd ed.), W. H. SEBRELL & R. S. HARRIS (eds.), pp. 407–457. London, Academic Press.

CHIBA, M. (1968) Movement during unimpeded eruption of the position of cells and of material incorporating tritiated proline, in the lingual periodontal membrane of the mandibular incisors of adult male mice. *J. dent. Res.* 47, 986.

CHIBA, M., NARRAWAY, J. M. & NESS, A. R. (1968) Impeded and unimpeded eruption of the mandibular incisor of the adult male rat and its stoppage by demecolcine. *J. dent. Res.* 47, 986.

CHIBA, M., TSURUTA, M. & ETO, K. (1973) A photographic method of measuring eruption rates of rat mandibular incisors. *Archs. oral Biol.* 18, 1003–1010.

CHO, M. & GARANT, P. R. (1978) Effects of colchicine on periodontal ligament fibroblasts of the mouse: 1. Cytoplasmic changes. *J. dent. Res.* 57, Special issue A, 139.

CLINCH, L. (1951) An analysis of serial models between three and eight years of age. *Dent. Rec.* 71, 61–72.

COHEN, J. T. (1940) Growth and development of the dental arches in children. *J. Amer. Dent. Ass.* 27, 1250–1260.

COHN, S. A. (1966) Disuse atrophy of the periodontium in mice following partial loss of function. *Archs. oral Biol.* 11, 95–105.

CONSTANT, T. E. (1900) The eruption of the teeth. *Int. dent. Congr.* 2, 180–192.

DALLDORF, G. & ZALL, C. (1930) Tooth growth in experimental scurvy. *J. Exp. Med.* 52, 57–63.

DARLING, A. I. & LEVERS, B. G. H. (1975) The pattern of eruption of some human teeth. *Archs. oral Biol.* 20, 89–96.

DARLING, A. I. & LEVERS, B. G. H. (1976) The pattern of

eruption. In: *The eruption and occlusion of teeth,* D. F. G. POOLE & M. V. STACK (eds.), pp. 80–96. London, Butterworths.

DAY, B. A. (1969) An investigation into the action of L-Na Thyroxine on the unimpeded eruption rate of the normal and root resected rat incisor. B.Sc. Thesis, University of Bristol.

DEWEL, B. F. (1949) Clinical observations on the axial inclination of teeth. *Amer. J. Orthod.* 35, 98–115.

DI BIASE, D. D. (1969) Mucous membrane and delayed eruption. *Trans. Br. Soc. Study Orthod.* 149–158.

DI BIASE, D. D. (1971) The effects of variations in tooth morphology and position on eruption. *Dent. Practnr dent. Rec.* 22, 95–108.

DI BIASE, D. D. (1976) Dental abnormalities affecting eruption. In: *The eruption and occlusion of teeth,* D. F. G. POOLE & M. V. STACK (eds.), pp. 156–168. London, Butterworths.

DOMM, L. V. & WELLBAND, W. A. (1960) Effects of adrenalectomy and cortisone on eruption rate of incisors in young female albino rats. *Proc. Soc. exp. Biol. Med.* 104, 582–584.

DUCKWORTH, R. (1962) Abnormal attachment of labial mucosa in maleruption of teeth. *Br. dent. J.* 113, 312–314.

EDWALL, L. (1971) Some effects of sympathetic nerve activation in oral tissues as studied by tracer disappearance. Ph.D. Thesis. Stockholm.

EDWALL, L. (1972) Nervous control of blood circulation in the dental pulp and the periodontal tissues. In: *Oral physiology,* N. EMMELIN & Y. ZOTTERMAN (eds.), pp. 139–149. Oxford, Pergamon.

EDWALL, L. & KINDLOVA, M. (1971) The effect of sympathetic nerve stimulation on the rate of disappearance of tracers from various oral tissues. *Acta Odont. Scand.* 29, 387–400.

EDWARDS, J. G. (1970) A surgical procedure to eliminate rotational relapse. *Amer. J. Orthod.* 57, 35–46.

ENGEL, M. B. (1951) Some changes in the connective tissue ground substance associated with the eruption of the teeth. *J. dent. Res.* 30, 322–330.

FERGUSSON, F. C. Jr. (1952) Colchicine. 1. General pharmacology. *J. Pharmacol. exp. Therap.* 106, 261–270.

FLETCHER, G. G. T. (1963) A cephalometric appraisal of the development of malocclusion. *Trans. Br. Soc. Study Orthod.* 124–154.

FRIEL, S. (1945) Migrations of teeth following extractions. *Proc. R. Soc. Med.* 38, 456–462.

FULLMER, H. M. (1961) A histochemical study of periodontal disease in the maxillary alveolar process of 135 autopsies. *J. Periodont.* 32, 206–218.

GABBIANI, G., RYAN, G. B. & MAJNO, G. (1971) Presence of modified fibroblasts in granulation tissue and their possible role in wound contraction. *Experientia* 27, 549–550.

GAIL, M. H. & BOONE, C. W. (1971) Cytochalasin effects on BALB-3T3 fibroblasts: dose dependent, reversible alterations of motility and cytoplasmic cleavage. *Exp. Cell Res.* 68, 226–228.

GARANT, P. R. (1976) Collagen resorption by fibroblasts. *J. Periodont.* 47, 380–390.

GARREN, L. & GREEP, R. O. (1955) Effects of thyroid hormone and propylthiouracil on eruption rate of upper incisor teeth in rats. *Proc. Soc. exp. Biol. Med.* **90**, 652–655.

GARREN, L. & GREEP, R. O. (1960) Effect of adrenal cortical hormones on eruption rate of incisor teeth in the rat. *Endocrinology* **66**, 625–628.

GLICKMAN, I. & SHKLAR, G. (1954) The effect of systemic disturbances on the pulp of experimental animals. *Oral Surg.* **7**, 550–558.

GOLDMAN, R. D., SCHLOSS, J. A. & STARGER, J. M. (1976) Organizational changes of action-like microfilaments during animal cell movements. In: *Cell motility Book A*, R. GOLDMAN, T. POLLARD & J. ROSENBAUM (eds.), pp. 217–245. Cold Spring Harbor Laboratory.

GOLDSTEIN, M. S. & STANTON, F. L. (1935) Changes in dimension and form of the dental arches with age. *Int. J. Orthod.* **21**, 357–380.

GOMEZ-ACEBO, J. & GARCIA HERMIDA, O. (1973) Morphological relations between rat β-secretory granules and the microtubular-microfilament system during sustained insulin release *in vitro. J. Anat. Lond.* **114**, 421–437.

GOULD, B. S. (1968) The role of certain vitamins in collagen formation. In: *Treatise on collagen,* Vol. 2, *Biology of collagen,* B. S. GOULD (ed.), pp. 323–365. London, Academic Press.

GOULD, M. S. E. & PICTON, D. C. A. (1964) A study of pressures exerted by the lips and cheeks on the teeth of subjects with normal occlusion. *Archs. oral Biol.* **9**, 469–478.

GRANT, D. A., BERNICK, S., LEVY, B. M. & DREIZEN, S. (1972) A comparative study of periodontal ligament development in teeth with and without predecessors in marmosets. *J. Periodont.* **43**, 162–169.

GUYTON, A. C. (1963) A concept of negative interstitial pressure based on pressures in implanted capsules. *Circ. Res.* **12**, 399–414.

GUYTON, A. C. (1972) Compliance of the interstitial space and the measurement of tissue pressure. *Pflugers Arch.* **336** (Suppl.), S1–S20.

GUYTON, A. C. (1976) In: *Textbook of medical physiology,* 5th ed. Philadelphia, Saunders.

GUYTON, A. C., GRANGER, H. J. & TAYLOR, A. E. (1971) Interstitial fluid pressure. *Physiol. Rev.* **51**, 527–563.

HARKNESS, R. D. (1968) Mechanical properties of collagenous tissues. In: *Treatise on collagen,* Vol. 2, *Biology of collagen,* B. S. GOULD (ed.), pp. 248–310. London, Academic Press.

HENRIQUES, A. C. (1953) The growth of the palate and the growth of the face during the period of the changing dentition. *Amer. J. Orthod.* **39**, 836–858.

HEŘT, J., LIŠKOVÁ, M. & LANDRGOT, B. (1969) Influence of the long term, continuous bending on the bone. *Folia morph. (Prague),* **17**, 389–399.

HIRSCHEL, B. J., GABBIANI, G., RYAN, G. B. & MAJNO, G. (1971) Fibroblasts of granulation tissue: immunofluorescent staining with antismooth muscle serum. *Proc. Soc. exp. Biol. Med.* **138**, 466–469.

HÖJER, A. & WESTIN, G. (1925) Jaws and teeth in scorbutic guinea pigs. *Dental Cosmos.* **67**, 1–24.

HOWARD, R. D. (1966) The unerupted incisor. *Trans. Br. Soc. Study Orthod.* 30–40.

JACKSON, D. S. (1976) In: *The eruption and occlusion of teeth,* D. F. G. POOLE & M. V. STACK (eds.), p. 306. London, Butterworths.

JAMES, D. W. (1964) Wound contraction – a synthesis. In: *Advances in biology of skin,* Vol. 5, W. MONTAGNA & R. E. BILLINGHAM (eds.), pp. 216–230. Oxford, Pergamon.

JAMES, D. W. & TAYLOR, J. F. (1969) The stress developed by sheets of chick fibroblasts *in vitro. Expl. Cell Res.* **54**, 107–110.

JOHNSTON, W. D. (1969) Treatment of palatally impacted canine teeth. *Amer. J. Orthod.* **56**, 589–596.

KAY, T. E. (1969) The effects of corticosteroids on the unimpeded eruption rate of the normal and root resected lower incisor of the rat. B.Sc. Thesis, University of Bristol.

KEY, K. M. & ELPHICK, G. K. (1931) A quantitative method for the determination of vitamin C. *Biochem. J.* **25**, 888–897.

KING, J. D. (1937) Dietary deficiency, nerve lesions and the dental tissues. *J. Physiol.* **88**, 62–77.

KNOTT, V. B. (1961) Size and form of the dental arches in children with good occlusion studied longitudinally from age 9 years to late adolescence. *Amer. J. Phys. Anthropol.* **19**, 263–284.

KÖRBER, K. H. (1970) Periodontal pulsation. *J. Periodont.* **41**, 686–708.

KORKHAUS, G. (1938) Clinical studies of the ontogenetic development of the dentition. *Dent. Rec.* **58**, 641–654.

KOSTLÁN, J., THOŘOVÁ, J. & ŠKACH, M. (1960) Erupce llodavého zubu po resekci jeho růstové zóny. *Čslká Stomat.* **6**, 401–410.

KRONMAN, J. H. (1971) Tissue reaction and recovery following experimental tooth movement. *Angle Orthod.* **41**, 125–132.

KUTSKY, R. J. (1973) In: *Handbook of vitamins and hormones.* New York, Van Nostrand Reinhold Company.

LAMB, R. E. & VAN HASSEL, H. J. (1972) Tissue pressure in the periodontal ligament. *J. dent. Res.* **51**, Special issue of IADR abstracts, p. 240.

LAMMIE, G. A. & POSSELT, U. (1965) Progressive changes in the dentition of adults. *J. Periodont.* **36**, 443–454.

LATHAM, R. A. & SCOTT, J. H. (1960) Mesial movement of the teeth in the Rhesus monkey. *Eur. Orthod. Soc.* 199–203.

LEAR, C. S. G., CATZ, J., GROSSMAN, R. C., FLANAGAN, J. B. & MOORREES, C. F. A. (1965) Measurement of lateral muscle forces on the dental arches. *Archs. oral Biol.* **10**, 669–689.

LEBRET, L. M. L. (1967) Tooth migration. In: *The mechanisms of tooth support,* D. J. ANDERSON, J. E. EASTOE, A. H. MELCHER & D. C. A. PICTON (eds.), pp. 120–125. Bristol, Wright.

LEIST, M. (1927) Über den Einfluss des vegetativum Nervensystems auf die Zähne. *Z. Stomat.* **25**, 765–771.

LEVENE, C. I. (1973) Lathyrism. In: *Molecular pathology of connective tissues,* R. PÉREZ-TAMAYO & M. ROJKIND (eds.). New York, Dekker.

LIDDLE, G. W. & MELMON, K. L. (1974) The adrenals. In: *Textbook of endocrinology,* 5th ed., R. H. WILLIAMS (ed.), pp. 233–322. Philadelphia, Saunders.

LIŠKOVÁ, M. & HEŘT, J. (1971) Reaction of bone to mechanical stimuli. Part 2. Periosteal and endosteal reaction of tibial diaphysis in rabbit to intermittent loading. *Folia morph. (Prague)* **19**, 301–317.

LITVIN, P. E. & DE MARCO, T. J. (1973) The effect of a diuretic and antidiuretic on tooth eruption. *Oral Surg.* **35**, 294–298.

LUNDSTRÖM, A. (1969) Changes in crowding and spacing of the teeth with age. *Dent. Practnr dent. Rec.* **19**, 218–223.

LYSELL, L. (1958) Qualitative and quantitative determination of attrition and the ensuing tooth migration. *Acta Odont. Scand.* **16**, 267–292.

MAGNUSSON, B. (1968) Tissue changes during molar tooth eruption. *Trans. R. Schs. Dent. Stochk. Umeå.* No. 13, 1–122.

MAIN, J. H. P. & ADAMS, D. (1965) Measurement of the rate of eruption of the rat incisor. *Archs. oral Biol.* **10**, 999–1008.

MAIN, J. H. P. & ADAMS, D. (1966) Experiments on the rat incisor into the cellular proliferation and blood pressure theories of tooth eruption. *Archs. oral Biol.* **11**, 163–179.

MAJNO, G., GABBIANI, G., HIRSCHEL, B. J., RYAN, G. B. & STATKOV, P. R. (1971) Contraction of granulation tissue *in vitro*: similarity to smooth muscle. *Science* **173**, 548–550.

MANSON, J. D. (1968) *A comparative study of the postnatal growth of the mandible.* London, Kimpton.

MASSLER, M. & SCHOUR, I. (1941) Studies on tooth development. Theories of eruption. *Amer. J. Orthod.* **27**, 552–576.

MATTHEWS, B. & BERKOVITZ, B. K. B. (1972) Continuous recording of tooth eruption in the rabbit. *Archs. oral Biol.* **17**, 817–820.

McHUGH, W. D. (1961) The development of the gingival epithelium in the monkey. *Dent. Practnr dent. Rec.* **11**, 314–324.

McLEAN, D. L., SHEPPARD, M. & McHENRY, E. W. (1939) Tissue changes in ascorbic acid deficient guinea pigs. *Br. J. Exptl. Pathol.* **20**, 451–457.

MELCHER, A. H. (1967) Remodelling of the periodontal ligament during eruption of the rat incisor. *Archs. oral Biol.* **12**, 1649–1652.

MELCHER, A. H. & WALKER, T. W. (1976) The periodontal ligament in attachment and as a shock absorber. In: *The eruption and occlusion of teeth*, D. F. G. POOLE & M. V. STACK (eds.), pp. 183–192. London, Butterworths.

MICHAELI, Y., PITARU, S., ZAJICEK, G. & WEINREB, M. M. (1975) Role of attrition and occlusal contact in the physiology of the rat incisor: IX. Impeded and unimpeded eruption in lathyritic rats. *J. dent. Res.* **54**, 891–898.

MICHAELI, Y. & WEINREB, M. M. (1968) Role of attrition and occlusal contact in the physiology of the rat incisor: II. Diurnal rhythm in eruption and attrition. *J. dent. Res.* **47**, 486–491.

MILLER, B. G. (1957) Investigations of the influence of vascularity and innervation on tooth resorption and eruption. *J. dent. Res.* **36**, 669–676.

MIURA, F. & ITO, G. (1968) Eruptive force of rabbits' upper incisors. *Trans. Eur. orthod. Soc.* 121–126.

MIURA, F. & KONDO, K. (1969) A study of blood circulation in the periodontal membrane by electrical impedance plethysmography. *J. Jap. Stomat. Soc.* **36**, 20–42.

MOORREES, C. F. A. (1959) *The dentition of the growing child.* Harvard University Press.

MOORREES, C. F. A. (1964) Dental development – a growth study based on tooth eruption as a measure of physiologic age. *Trans. Eur. orthod. Soc.* 92–105.

MOSS, J. P. (1976) A review of the theories of approximal migration of teeth. In: *The eruption and occlusion of teeth*, D. F. G. POOLE & M. V. STACK (eds.), pp. 205–212. London, Butterworths.

MOSS, J. P. & PICTON, D. C. A. (1967) Experimental mesial drift in adult monkeys (*Macaca irus*). *Archs. oral Biol.* **12**, 1313–1320.

MOSS, J. P. & PICTON, D. C. A. (1970) Mesial drift of teeth in adult monkeys (*Macaca irus*) when forces from the cheeks and tongue have been eliminated. *Archs. oral Biol.* **15**, 979–986.

MOSS, J. P. & PICTON, D. C. A. (1974) The effect on approximal drift of cheek teeth of dividing mandibular molars of adult monkey (*Macaca irus*). *Archs. oral Biol.* **19**, 1211–1214.

MOSS, M. L. & CRIKELAIR, G. F. (1960) Progressive facial hemiatrophy following cervical sympathectomy in the rat. *Archs. oral Biol.* **1**, 254–258.

MOXHAM, B. J. (1976) The effects of cervical sympathetic nerve section and stimulation on tooth eruption. *J. dent. Res.* **55**, 113.

MOXHAM, B. J. (1978) An assessment of the vascular or tissue hydrostatic pressure hypotheses of eruption using a continuous recording technique for monitoring movements of the rabbit mandibular incisor. Ph.D. Thesis, University of Bristol.

MOXHAM, B. J. (1979a) Recording the eruption of the rabbit mandibular incisor using a device for continuously monitoring tooth movements. *Archs. oral Biol.* **24**, 889–899.

MOXHAM, B. J. (1979b) The effects of some vaso-active drugs on the eruption of the rabbit mandibular incisor. *Archs. oral Biol.* **24**, 681–688.

MOXHAM, B. J. & BERKOVITZ, B. K. B. (1974) The effects of root transection on the unimpeded eruption rate of the rabbit mandibular incisor. *Archs. oral Biol.* **19**, 903–909.

MOXHAM, B. J. & BERKOVITZ, B. K. B. (1979) The effects of axially-directed extrusive loads on movements of the mandibular incisor of the rabbit. *Archs. oral Biol.* **24**, 759–763.

MOXHAM, B. J. & BERKOVITZ, B. K. B. (1980) An approach to the investigation of a multifactorial basis for the mechanism of tooth eruption. *J. dent. Res.* **59**, Special Issue D, 1840.

MURPHEY, W. H. (1970) Oxytetracycline microfluorescent comparison of orthodontic retraction into recent and healed extraction sites. *Amer. J. Orthod.* **58**, 215–239.

MURPHY, T. (1959) Compensatory mechanisms in facial height adjustment to functional tooth attrition. *Aust. dent. J.* **4**, 312–323.

MYERS, H. I. & WYATT, W. P. (1961) Some histopathologic changes in the hamster as the result of a continuously acting orthodontic appliance. *J. dent. Res.* **40**, 846–856.

MYHRE, L., PREUS, H. R. & AARS, H. (1979) Influences of axial load and blood pressure on the position of the rabbit's incisor tooth. *Acta Odont. Scand.* **37**, 153–159.

NESS, A. R. (1954) Measuring the continuous eruption of the rabbit mandibular incisor. *J. Physiol.* **124**, 13–15.

NESS, A. R. (1956) The response of the rabbit mandibular incisor to experimental shortening and to the prevention of its eruption. *Proc. R. Soc.* B **146**, 129–154.

NESS, A. R. (1964) Movement and forces in tooth eruption. In: *Advances in oral biology,* Vol. 1, P. H. STAPLE (ed.), pp. 33–75. London, Academic Press.

NESS, A. R. (1965) Eruption rates of impeded and unimpeded mandibular incisors of the adult laboratory mouse. *Archs. oral Biol.* **10**, 439–451.

NESS, A. R. (1967) Eruption – a review. In: *The mechanisms of tooth support,* D. J. ANDERSON, J. E. EASTOE, A. H. MELCHER & D. C. A. PICTON (eds.), pp. 84–88. Bristol, Wright.

NESS, A. R. (1970) Eruption '70. *Apex J. University College Hosp. dent. Soc.* **4**, 23–27.

NESS, A. R. & SMALE, D. E. (1959) The distribution of mitoses and cells in the tissues bounded by the socket wall of the rabbit mandibular incisor. *Proc. R. Soc.* B **151**, 106–128.

O'BRIEN, C., BHASKAR, S. N. & BRODIE, A. G. (1958) Eruptive mechanism and movement in the first molar of the rat. *J. dent. Res.* **37**, 467–484.

OSBORN, J. W. (1961) An investigation into the interdental forces occurring between the teeth of the same arch during clenching the jaws. *Archs. oral Biol.* **5**, 202–211.

PALCANIS, K. G. (1973) Effect of occlusal trauma on interstitial pressure in the periodontal ligament. *J. dent. Res.* **52**, 903–910.

PALMER, L. G., KATONAH, F. & ANGRIST, A. A. (1951) Comparative effects of ACTH, cortisone, corticosterone, desoxycorticosterone, pregnenolone on growth and development of infant rats. *Proc. Soc. exp. Biol. Med.* **77**, 215–218.

PAYNTER, K. J. (1954) The effect of propylthiouracil on the development of molar teeth of rats. *J. dent. Res.* **33**, 364–376.

PICTON, D. C. A. (1962) Tilting movements of teeth during biting. *Archs. oral Biol.* **7**, 151–159.

PICTON, D. C. A. (1976) Tooth movement as mesial and lateral drift. In: *The eruption and occlusion of teeth,* D. F. G. POOLE & M. V. STACK (eds.), pp. 108–119. London, Butterworths.

PICTON, D. C. A. & MOSS, J. P. (1973) The part played by the trans-septal fibre system in experimental approximal drift of the cheek teeth of monkeys (*Macaca irus*). *Archs. oral Biol.* **18**, 669–680.

PICTON, D. C. A. & MOSS, J. P. (1974) The relationship between the angulation of the roots and the rate of approximal drift of cheek teeth in adult monkeys. *Br. J. Orthod.* **1**, 105–110.

PICTON, D. C. A. & MOSS, J. P. (1978) The effect of reducing cusp height on the rate of approximal drift of cheek teeth in adult monkeys (*Macaca irus*). *Archs. oral Biol.* **23**, 219–223.

PICTON, D. C. A. & MOSS, J. P. (1979) The effect on approximal drift of altering the horizontal component of biting force in *Macaca irus* monkeys. *J. dent. Res.* **58**, Special issue C, 1253.

PICTON, D. C. A. & MOSS, J. P. (1980) The effect on approximal drift of altering the horizontal component of biting force in adult *Macaca irus* monkeys. *J. dent. Res.* **59**, Special issue D, 1800.

PIHLSTROM, B. L. & RAMFJORD, S. P. (1971) Periodontal effect of nonfunction in monkeys. *J. Periodont.* **42**, 748–756.

PINSON, R. R. & STRAHAN, J. D. (1974) The effect on the relapse of orthodontically rotated teeth of surgical division of the gingival fibres – Pericision. *Br. J. Orthod.* **1**, 87–91.

PITARU, S., MICHAELI, Y., ZAJICEK, G. & WEINREB, M. M. (1976) Role of attrition and occlusal contact in the physiology of the rat incisor. IX. The part played by the periodontal ligament in the eruptive process. *J. dent. Res.* **55**, 819–824.

PROCKOP, D. J. & KIVIRIKKO, K. I. (1968) Hydroxyproline and the metabolism of collagen. In: *Treatise on collagen,* Vol. 2, *Biology of collagen,* B. S. GOULD (ed.), pp. 215–246. London, Academic Press.

ROBINS, M. W. (1972) Collagen metabolism in the periodontal ligament of the rat incisor. *J. dent. Res.* **51**, 1246.

ROBINS, M. W. (1979) A photographic method of measuring eruption rates of the mandibular incisors of the mouse. *J. dent. Res.* **58**, Special issue C, 1273.

ROSS, R. (1968) The connective tissue fibre forming cell. In: *Treatise on collagen,* Vol. 2, *Biology of collagen,* B. S. GOULD (ed.), pp. 1–82. London, Academic Press.

RUSSELL, J. D., RUSSELL, S. B. & TRUPIN, K. M. (1978) Differential effects of hydrocortisone on both growth and collagen metabolism of human fibroblasts from normal and keloid tissue. *J. Cell Physiol.* **97**, 221–229.

SARNAT, H. & SCIAKY, I. (1965) Experimental lathyrism in rats: effect of removing incisal stress. *Periodontics* **3**, 128–134.

SCHOUR, I. (1960) *Noyes' oral histology and embryology,* 8th ed. London, Kimpton.

SCHOUR, I. & MASSLER, M. (1942) The teeth. In: *The rat in laboratory investigation,* 2nd ed., E. J. FARRIS & J. Q. GRIFFITH (eds.), pp. 104–165. London, Lippencott Company.

SCHOUR, I. & VAN DYKE, H. B. (1932) Changes in the teeth following hypophysectomy. I. Changes in the incisor of the white rat. *Amer. J. Anat.* **50**, 397–433.

SCHROEDER, H. E. & LISTGARTEN, M. A. (1971) *Fine structure of the developing epithelial attachment of human teeth.* Monographs in developmental biology, Vol. 2, E. WOLSKY (ed.). Basle, Karger.

SCHUBERT, M. & HAMERMAN, D. (1968) *A primer on connective tissue biochemistry.* Philadelphia, Lea and Febiger.

SCHWARZE, C. W. (1972) Langzeitstudie über das sagittale Positionsverhalten der ersten Molaren. *Fortschr. Kieferorthop.* **33**, 93–102.

SCHWARZE, C. W. (1973) Hat die Keimentfernung der Weisheitszähne Einfluss auf Spatform des Zahnbogens? *Fortschr. Kieferorthop.* **34**, 387–400.

SCOTT, J. H. (1948) The development and function of the dental follicle. *Br. dent. J.* **85**, 193–199.

SCOTT, J. H. (1953) How teeth erupt. *Dent. Practnr. dent. Rec.* **3**, 345–350.

SCOTT, J. H. (1967) *Dento-facial development and growth.* Oxford, Pergamon Press.

SCOTT, J. H. & SYMONS, N. B. B. (1977) In: *Introduction to dental anatomy,* 8th ed., pp. 104–105. Edinburgh, Livingstone.

SHORE, R. C. & BERKOVITZ, B. K. B. (1978) Model to explain differential movement of periodontal fibroblasts. *Arch. oral Biol.* **23**, 507–509.

SHORE, R. C. & BERKOVITZ, B. K. B. (1979) An ultrastructural study of periodontal ligament fibroblasts in relation to their possible role in tooth eruption and intracellular collagen degradation in the rat. *Archs. oral Biol.* **24**, 155–164.

SHOSHAN, S. & FINKELSTEIN, S. (1968) Studies on collagen cross-linking *in vivo. Biochem. biophys. Acta* **154**, 261–263.

SHRIMPTON, B. A. (1960) Dynamics of eruption. *N. Z. dent. J.* **56**, 122–124.

SICHER, H. (1942) Tooth eruption: the axial movement of continuously growing teeth. *J. dent. Res.* **21**, 201–210.

SICHER, H. & BHASKAR, S. N. (1972) *Orban's oral histology and embryology* (7th ed.). St. Louis, Mosby.

SICHER, H. & WEINMANN, J. P. (1944) Bone growth and physiologic tooth movement. *Amer. J. Orthod.* **30**, 109–132.

SIERSBAEK-NIELSEN, S. (1971) Rate of eruption of central incisors at puberty: an implant study on eight boys. *Tandlaegebladet.* **75**, 1288–1295.

SILLMAN, J. H. (1951) Serial study of good occlusion from birth to 12 years of age. *Amer. J. Orthod.* **37**, 481–507.

SILLMAN, J. H. (1964) Dimensional changes of the dental arches: longitudinal study from birth to 25 years. *Amer. J. Orthod.* **50**, 824–842.

SMITH, Q. T. & ALLISON, D. J. (1965) Skin and femur collagens and urinary hydroxyproline of cortisone-treated rats. *Endocrinology,* **77**, 785–791.

SMITH, R. G. (1978) A clinical study into the depth of the so-called gingival crevice of some erupting teeth of humans. M.D.S. Thesis, Bristol University.

SODEK, J. (1978) A comparison of collagen and noncollagenous protein metabolism in rat molar and incisor periodontal ligaments. *Archs. oral Biol.* **23**, 977–982.

SPECK, N. T. (1950) A longitudinal study of developmental changes in human lower dental arches. *Angle Orthod.* **20**, 215–228.

STALLARD, H. (1923) The anterior component of the force of mastication and its significance to the dental apparatus. *Dent. Cosmos* **65**, 457–474.

STARLING, E. H. (1909) *The fluids of the body.* Chicago, Keener & Co.

STENVIK, A., IVERSEN, J. & MJÖR, I. A. (1972) Tissue pressure and histology of normal and inflamed tooth pulps in Macaque monkeys. *Archs. oral Biol.* **17**, 1501–1511.

STRAHAN, J. D. & MILLS, J. R. E. (1970) A preliminary report on the severing of gingival fibres following rotation of teeth. *Dent. Practit.* **21**, 101–103.

SVED, A. (1955) The mesial drift of teeth during growth. *Amer. J. Orthod.* **41**, 539–553.

TANZER, M. L. (1965) Experimental lathyrism. In: *International review of connective tissue research,* Vol. 3, D. A. HALL (ed.), pp. 91–112. London, Academic Press.

TAYLOR, A. C. & BUTCHER, E. O. (1951) The regulation of eruption rate in the incisor teeth of the white rat. *J. exp. Zool.* **117**, 165–188.

TEN CATE, A. R. (1971) Physiological resorption of connective tissue associated with tooth eruption. *J. periodont. Res.* **6**, 168–181.

TEN CATE, A. R. (1972) Morphological study of fibrocytes in connective tissue undergoing rapid remodelling. *J. Anat. Lond.* **112**, 401–414.

TEN CATE, A. R. (1976) Tooth eruption. In: *Orban's oral histology and embryology* (8th ed.), S. N. BHASKAR (ed.), p. 365. St. Louis, Mosby.

TEN CATE, A. R., DEPORTER, D. A. & FREEMAN, E. (1976) The fate of fibroblasts in the remodelling of periodontal ligament during physiologic tooth movement. *Amer. J. Orthod.* **69**, 155–168.

THOMAS, N. R. (1965) The process and mechanism of tooth eruption. Ph.D. Thesis, University of Bristol.

THOMAS, N. R. (1967) The properties of collagen in the periodontium of an erupting tooth. In: *The mechanisms of tooth support,* D. J. ANDERSON, J. E. EASTOE, A. H. MELCHER & D. C. A. PICTON (eds.), pp. 102–106. Bristol, Wright.

THOMAS, N. R. (1976) Collagen as the generator of tooth eruption. In: *The eruption and occlusion of teeth,* D. F. G. POOLE & M. V. STACK (eds.), pp. 290–301. London, Butterworths.

THOMPSON, H. E., MYERS, H. I., WATERMAN, J. M. & FLANAGAN, V. D. (1958) Preliminary macroscopic observations concerning the potentiality of supra-alveolar collagenous fibres in orthodontics. *Amer. J. Orthod.* **44**, 485–497.

THOMPSON, J. L. Jr. & KENDRICK, G. S. (1964) Changes in the vertical dimensions of the human male skull during the third and fourth decades of life. *Anat. Rec.* **150**, 209–213.

TOTO, P. D. & SICHER, H. (1966) Eruption of teeth through the oral mucosa. *Periodontics* **4**, 29–32.

TRAUNER, F. (1912) The causes of progressive movement of the teeth towards the front. *Amer. J. Orthod.* **3**, 144–158.

TSURUTA, M., ETO, K. & CHIBA, M. (1974) Effect of daily or 4-hourly administrations of lathyrogens on the eruption rates of impeded and unimpeded mandibular incisors of rats. *Archs. oral Biol.* **19**, 1221–1226.

TYLER, D. W. & BURN-MURDOCH, R. (1976) Tooth movements in an *in vitro* model system. In: *The eruption and occlusion of teeth,* D. F. G. POOLE & M. V. STACK (eds.), pp. 302–304. London, Butterworths.

VAN BEEK, H. (1979) The transfer of mesial drift potential along the dental arch in *Macaca irus*: an experimental study of tooth migration rate related to horizontal vectors of occlusal forces. *Eur. J. Orthod.* **1**, 125–129.

VAN BEEK, H. & FIDLER, V. J. (1977) An experimental study of the effect of functional occlusion on mesial tooth migration in macaque monkeys. *Archs. oral Biol.* **22**, 269–271.

VAN DEN BRENK, H. A. & STONE, M. G. (1974) Actions and interactions of colchicine and cytochalasin B on contraction of granulation tissue and on mitosis. *Nature* **251**, 327–329.

VAN HASSEL, H. J. (1971) Physiology of the human dental pulp. *Oral Surg.* **32**, 126–134.

VAN HASSEL, H. J. & BROWN, A. C. (1969) Effect of temperature changes on intrapulpal pressure and hydraulic permeability in dogs. *Archs. oral Biol.* **14**, 301–315.

VAN HASSEL, H. J. & McMINN, R. G. (1972) Pressure differential favouring tooth eruption in the dog. *Archs. oral Biol.* **17**, 183–190.

VASILIEV, J. M. & GELFAND, I. M. (1976) Effects of colcemid on morphogenetic processes and locomotion of fibroblasts. In: *Cell motility Book A,* R. GOLDMAN, T. POLLARD & J. ROSENBAUM (eds.), pp. 279–304. Cold Spring Harbor Laboratory.

VEGO, L. (1962) A longitudinal study of the mandibular arch perimeter. *Angle Orthod.* **32**, 187–192.

VEIS, A. (1967) Intact collagen. In: *Treatise on collagen,* Vol. 1, *Chemistry of collagen,* G. N. RAMACHAND-RAN (ed.), pp. 367–439. London, Academic Press.

WALKER, T. W., NG, G. C. & BURKE, P. S. (1978) Fluid pressures in the periodontal ligament of the mandibular canine tooth in dogs. *Archs. oral Biol.* **23**, 753–765.

WALLACE, J. S. (1904) *General outline of the causes of irregularities of the teeth* (Chap. 1). London, Dental Manufacturing Co.

WEINSTEIN, S. (1967) Minimal forces in tooth movement. *Amer. J. Orthod.* **53**, 881–903.

WEISS, L. (1973) The cell. In: *Histology* (3rd ed.), R. D. GREEP & L. WEISS (eds.), pp. 56–59. New York, McGraw-Hill.

WESSELS, N. K., SPOONER, B. S. & LUDVENA, M. A. (1973) Surface movements, microfilaments and cell locomotion. In: *Locomotion of tissue cells,* Ciba Symposium 14, pp. 53–77. Amsterdam, Elsevier.

WINDERS, R. V. (1962) Recent findings in myometric research. *Angle Orthod.* **32**, 38–44.

WYNN, W., HALDI, J., HOPF, M. A. & JOHN, K. (1963) Pressure within the pulp chamber of the dog's tooth relative to arterial blood pressure. *J. dent. Res.* **42**, 1169–1177.

YILMAZ, R. S. (1973) Mesial drift of the teeth. M.Sc. Thesis, Bristol University.

YILMAZ, R. S. (1976) Horizontal tooth movement and jaw growth. Ph.D. Thesis, Bristol University.

ZAJICEK, G. (1974) Fibroblast cell kinetics in the periodontal ligament of the mouse. *Cell Tiss. Kinet.* **7**, 479–492.

Chapter 11

THE EFFECTS OF EXTERNAL FORCES ON THE PERIODONTAL LIGAMENT – THE RESPONSE TO AXIAL LOADS

B. J. Moxham and B. K. B. Berkovitz

INTRUSIVE LOADS

Source and nature

MASTICATION

It is commonly assumed that, in the closing phase of a chewing cycle, the teeth cut through the bolus to contact their antagonists in centric occlusion,* thereby transmitting forces axially through the teeth. Despite an early claim by Jankleson, Hoffman and Hendron (1953) that negligible tooth contacts occur during mastication, it has now been demonstrated that, in man, contacts frequently occur (Anderson and Picton, 1957; Graf and Zander, 1963; Adams and Zander, 1964; Ahlgren, 1966; Møller, 1966; Pameijer, Glickman and Roeber, 1968; Ahlgren, 1976; Anderson, 1976). It has been shown, however, that as teeth contact they often glide together in a pathway dictated by cusp morphology and thus do

not usually produce pure axial loads (Hildebrand, 1931; Adams and Zander, 1964; Beyron, 1964; Ahlgren, 1966, 1976; Suit, Gibbs and Benz, 1976; Behrend, 1978). Indeed, that a tooth moves in its socket in a number of different planes during mastication (e.g. Picton, 1962a; Behrend, 1978; Graf, 1978) suggests that masticatory loads on teeth are multidirectional. Studies using intra-oral occlusal telemetry also indicate that teeth do not habitually occlude during chewing in centric occlusion (Graf and Zander, 1963; Kavanagh and Zander, 1965; Glickman, Pameijer and Roeber, 1968; Pameijer, Glickman and Roeber, 1968, 1969; Brion et al., 1969; Pameijer et al., 1970b; Glickman et al., 1974; Bates, Stafford and Harrison, 1975).

Any study undertaken to investigate the functional occlusion of teeth during mastication should take account of the nature of the food and the type of occlusion. Whilst much research has been undertaken to assess such influences, it is difficult to evaluate the results since:

---

*Occlusion with the mandible in centric relation.

1. Comparisons are complicated by important differences in the experimental design. For example, for research involving the measurement of biting loads, transducers have been implanted into natural teeth (e.g. Anderson, 1953), partial dentures (e.g. Glickman *et al.,* 1968; McCall, De Boever and Ash, 1978) or full dentures (e.g. Yurkstas and Curby, 1953).
2. There is considerable variation between subjects and possibly from day to day in the same subject (e.g. De Boever *et al.,* 1978).
3. For many studies, few subjects were used.
4. Psychological factors (e.g. anxiety, motivation, fatigue) may affect results (Marklund and Wennström, 1972) and could differ between studies.
5. Food texture may not match in different investigations even when similar food types are specified.

Despite problems such as these, there is agreement on a number of points.

The number of chewing strokes used to masticate a given test food appears to be relatively constant for any individual, though there is variation between individuals (Anderson, 1953; Eichner, 1964; De Boever *et al.,* 1978). Dahlberg (1946) and De Boever *et al.* (1978) claim that the number of chewing strokes is altered only by extreme changes in the consistency of the test food. When this happens, the changes are related to the length of the early period of chewing when the food is insufficiently reduced to allow the teeth to contact. This effect has been observed also in an experimental animal, the American opossum (*Didelphis marsupialis*), by Hiiemae (1976). Soft food was found to be subjected to only one or two chewing cycles whilst hard food was chewed for several minutes. In view of this, it is conceivable that the type of wear on a tooth is influenced by the consistency of the diet. Berkovitz and Poole (1977) claim to be able to distinguish between the dentitions of wild and laboratory-reared ferrets (*Mustela putorius*) according to the type of wear facets on the teeth, relating this to a difference in the consistency of the diet.

Not only the number of chewing strokes but also the frequency of tooth contact may be dependent upon the character of the food. It has been observed that tooth contacts with soft foods occur with nearly every chewing stroke in man (Anderson and Picton, 1957; Graf and Zander, 1963; Ahlgren, 1966; Møller, 1966). Not surprisingly, chewing cycles without tooth contacts generally occur at the beginning of mastication, though with subsequent reduction in the size of the food particles the number of contacts increases (Anderson and Picton, 1957; Adams and Zander, 1964; Öwall and Møller, 1974; Ahlgren, 1976).

The degree of gliding during tooth contact may also be influenced by the texture of the food. Hildebrand (1931) found a contact glide of 1.75 mm in people with normal occlusion when chewing meat. With carrots, however, Ahlgren (1966) found the contact glide to be smaller (0.9 mm). In Australian aborigines, Beyron (1964) found that the contact glide with meat was long (2.8 mm) and occurred with nearly every chewing movement. This suggests that primitive people have more vigorous grinding movements during mastication.

Less is known about the influence of the type of occlusion on mastication and tooth contacts. Using cinematographic techniques, Beyron (1964) and Ahlgren (1966) have reported that individuals with normal occlusion have regular and co-ordinated masticatory movements. Hildebrand (1931) and Ahlgren (1966, 1967) have shown that masticatory movements are more irregular where there is malocclusion. It was suggested that this irregularity is due to impairment and/or incoordination of proprioception from the periodontium. Hildebrand (1931) found differences in the degree of contact glide in subjects with normal occlusion (1.75 mm) and malocclusion (1.3 mm) when chewing meat. Beyron (1964) has shown that for people with advanced attrition the angle of the contact glide to the occlusal plane during closing is very small (approximately 18°). However, Ahlgren (1976) reported that where there is little attrition this angle is much larger (approximately 37°). He suggested that cuspal guidance is reduced as attrition proceeds and the closing stroke assumes a more horizontal direction. One of the problems of investigating this subject concerns the difficulty of distinguishing between a morphological and functional malocclusion. It can be argued that, even with a morphological malocclusion, the occlusion can be considered functionally normal if a subject can bring the teeth into a position of maximum intercuspation during chewing without muscle pain or periodontal or temporomandibular trauma. This view is supported by the work of Watt (1976). He noted that there may be no masticatory dysfunction or clinical symptoms with malocclusions accompanied by abnormal tooth contacts (as diagnosed by gnathosonic techniques).

The forces which develop between teeth when biting have been measured using two different techniques. One technique employs dynamometers to measure the maximum static isometric closing force the masticatory apparatus can exert. Alternatively, functional forces generated during mastication have been measured using transducers incorporated within crowns or inlays in teeth, or within removable dental prostheses.

Using dynamometers, biting forces of ~ 500 N* can be recorded (e.g. Brekhus, Armstrong and Simon, 1941; Worner and Anderson, 1944; Howell and Manly, 1948). Waugh (1939) recorded a figure as high as ~ 1500 N in Eskimos, though it has been suggested that such values may have been caused by unskilled use of the dynamometer (Jenkins, 1978). Black (1895) and Worner and Anderson (1944) have shown that the maximum biting force is greatest in the region of the first molars. Near the incisors, smaller forces of $\sim 100-200$ N are more usual (Worner and Anderson, 1944; Atkinson and Ralph, 1973; Garner and Kotwal, 1973).

In 1953 Anderson described a technique for measuring biting loads during mastication. A strain gauge incorporated in an occlusal inlay within a molar tooth was arranged in such a way as to measure the biting force in an axial direction. Using this device, maximum axial loads of about $70-150$ N were recorded whilst chewing and swallowing a variety of foods (Anderson, 1956 a and b). Such loads are considerably lower than the maximum forces recorded with dynamometers. Similar work has been undertaken using a variety of force-sensitive devices incorporated into premolars or molars (Nyquist and Öwall, 1968; Ahlgren and Öwall, 1970; Graf, Grassl and Aeberhard, 1974; Graf, 1976), partial dentures (De Boever *et al.,* 1978; McCall *et al.,* 1978) and full dentures (Yurkstas and Curby, 1953; Atkinson and Shephard, 1967; Bearn, 1972). The forces measured

*Where the approximately sign ($\sim$) is used with forces measured in Newtons: ~ 1 N $\equiv 100$ gf.

using these techniques were no higher than those reported by Anderson (1956 a and b). For most of these techniques it is not possible to predict with confidence the precise direction of the forces. However, the techniques of Graf *et al.* (1974) seem to offer the possibility of measuring biting forces in the axial, oro-facial and antero-posterior directions.

Though Anderson (1956a) observed that the forces generally increased as chewing progressed, De Boever *et al.* (1978) have not been able to confirm this. Atkinson and Shephard (1967) and Ahlgren and Öwall (1970) found that the maximum force was reached in the middle of the occlusal phase of the chewing cycle after initial tooth contact had been achieved. This intercuspal phase seems to last between 40 and 170 msec (Ahlgren and Öwall, 1970; Ahlgren, 1976). A number of investigators have reported that masticatory loads are influenced by the consistency of the food (e.g. Yurkstas and Curby, 1953; Anderson, 1956 a and b; Eichner, 1964; De Boever *et al.,* 1978).

Attempts to record forces on the side of the dentition away from the working side have been undertaken by Anderson and Picton (1958), Graf (1976) and De Boever *et al.* (1978). Using bread as a test bolus, Anderson and Picton (1958) claimed that there was a close similarity between the load patterns on the chewing and 'balancing' sides. The findings of Graf (1976) and De Boever *et al.* (1978), however, indicate that the loads on the 'balancing' side are smaller than those on the working side regardless of the test food used.

Research has been conducted to record biting forces on teeth whose occlusal surfaces have been modified. Anderson and Picton (1958) found that the loads with soft foods were markedly reduced where the occlusal surface was lowered by 0.5 mm. On the other hand, Anderson and Picton (1958) and Graf (1976) have shown that masticatory loads were almost doubled where the occlusal surface was raised by $0.2-0.5$ mm.

SOURCES OTHER THAN MASTICATION

The study of tooth contacts in situations other than mastication has been relatively neglected. Teeth may be subjected to axially directed intrusive loads during swallowing, speech and in association with certain habits (e.g. tooth clenching and grinding). Furthermore, whilst it is generally agreed that the teeth are not usually in contact when the mandible is at rest, the concept of a fixed mandibular resting posture is no longer valid (Thompson, 1954; Atwood, 1956; Brill et al., 1959; Bando et al., 1972; Dibdin and Griffiths, 1976) and it is our impression that the teeth contact more frequently when the subject is at rest than has been supposed hitherto. Sources relating to dental therapy (e.g. from orthodontic appliances) are not considered here.

Using miniature transmitters implanted in full dentures, Brewer (1963) claimed that tooth contacts not associated with mastication can occur at rates of up to 1000 per hour! The frequency of swallowing has been determined by several investigators. Frequencies as high as 2400 swallows/day have been reported by Kunvara (1959), Kydd et al. (1963), Kawamura (1968) and Hanson, Logan and Case (1970). Kincaid (1951) observed a wide variation in swallowing frequencies, ranging from 10–138 swallows/h. Flanagan (1964) has reported an average frequency of 800–1200 swallows/day for a group of children aged between 5–12 years. Lear, Flanagan and Moorrees (1965) have calculated a figure for the mean number of swallows considerably less than that determined by other investigators − 585/day ± 208 S.D. Not unexpectedly, they also observed that the swallowing frequency was greatest during eating (mean rate of 296 swallows/h). From telemetric studies in patients with natural dentitions, Graf (1969) calculated that the total time of tooth contacts associated with swallowing during a 24-h period was about 8.5 min. Swallowing contacts during meals accounted for 0.5 min, swallowing between meals during the day accounted for 6.7 min, and the remaining 1.3 min was associated with swallowing during sleep. Not all swallows take place with tooth contacts. Pameijer et al. (1970a) reported that, of 182 swallows recorded during eating and drinking in 6 adult subjects, 16 occurred without tooth contacts. Rix (1953) has claimed that fluids may be swallowed without tooth contacts. Rix (1946, 1953) and Moyers (1971) noted that swallowing in the infant often occurs without tooth contacts. Rix (1946, 1953) reported that the infantile pattern may persist. Indeed, the behavioural characteristic of

'tongue thrusting' between the teeth in school children and young adults in order to obtain an anterior oral seal during swallowing is well known.

Less is known about the frequency of tooth contacts in situations other than swallowing. Attempts have been made to record tooth contacts during sleep in order to investigate bruxism. The frequency and distribution of tooth contacts during sleep in non-bruxists has been studied by Powell and Zander (1965) and Powell (1965). Powell and Zander (1965) calculated that the mean hourly frequency of tooth contacts in seven sleeping subjects ranged from 6– 140. They claimed that such contacts were associated with swallowing. Both Powell and Zander (1965) and Powell (1965) reported that tooth contacts occurred particularly during the periods of lightening of sleep coincident with whole bodily movements (i.e. during the onset of sleep, and waking). However, Reding et al. (1968) reported that tooth contacts during sleep were not noticeable in non-bruxists. Furthermore, where tooth contacts were observed in bruxists they occurred in all phases of sleep. In contrast, Satoh and Harada (1973) found that tooth grinding occurred most frequently during the lighter stages of sleep. Trenouth (1978) reported that a mean of about 360 tooth contacts was observed during a period of approximately 8 hours' sleep in ten non-bruxists. A mean of 1325 tooth contacts was observed for nine bruxists. As far as can be ascertained, no detailed investigations have been undertaken to study tooth contacts during normal speech.

Little is known about the nature of tooth contacts from sources other than mastication. Schärer and Stallard (1965), Pameijer et al. (1970 a and b) and Møller (1976) have shown that tooth contacts during swallowing may also involve gliding movements. Pameijer et al. (1968, 1970 a and b) have reported that tooth contacts during swallowing do not usually occur in centric occlusion. Pameijer et al. (1970a) have shown that the duration of tooth contact during swallowing is longer than during mastication.

Although many studies have been undertaken to measure axial biting loads during mastication, there are but few reports measuring loads during swallowing. The 70–150 N range for biting loads recorded by Anderson (1956 a and b) is said to include forces exerted during swallowing. It is clear from the report of De Boever *et al.* (1978) that forces associated with swallowing have been recorded, but their results have not been published at the time of writing.

Effects on tooth position — the tooth support mechanism

Two approaches have been adopted to investigate the mechanisms of tooth support. One approach involves the study of tooth mobility following the application of axial intrusive loads to teeth whose periodontal tissues are regarded as physiologically normal. Studies of this kind determine the general mechanical properties of the periodontium and ask the sort of question: does the periodontium behave as an elastic/viscoelastic/thixotropic system? The other approach involves studying the effects of intrusive loads on teeth with experimentally altered periodontal tissues in order to provide an explanation for its mechanical properties in biological terms.

PHYSIOLOGICAL TOOTH MOBILITY

Research concerning the effects of axial intrusive loads on tooth mobility was pioneered by Parfitt (1960). His experiments utilized an electronic device for simultaneously recording tooth movement and applied force based upon the principle of inductance. Intrusive loads were applied manually as an increasing force at various rates until the desired peak force was obtained. The teeth studied were human maxillary incisors. The movement transducer incorporated a reference probe which rested on an incisor adjacent to the tooth being investigated. Using springs, a continuous load of ∿ 1 N was placed upon the reference tooth in order 'to ensure its stability'. However, no allowance was made for the possibility that the load on the reference tooth may have influenced the position of the test tooth. Parfitt reported that, if the intrusive force was gradually and evenly increased, the displacement of the tooth showed an initial rapidly rising phase with loads up to about 1 N. With greater loads, the displacement appeared to fade in a logarithmic manner (Fig. 1). To illustrate this point, Parfitt calculated that the mean displace-

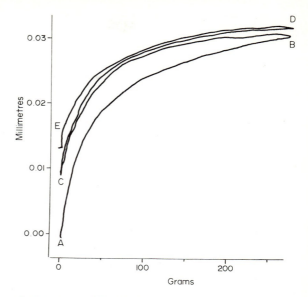

FIG. 1. The axial load/mobility curve for human maxillary incisor. A — Initial position. B — Position at peak force on the first application. C — Return point on removal of force. D — Position at peak force on the second application. E — Return point after the second removal.

ment for a thrust of ∿ 1 N was approximately 20 µm, whilst an increase from ∿ 1 N to ∿ 10 N produced an additional movement of only 8 µm. Parfitt's findings show that the first phase of tooth mobility changes gradually to the second phase, though the change can first be detected at about 0.3 N. When ∿ 5 N peak-loads were maintained on the tooth, intrusion continued by a regular amount with each period of time (approximately 2 µm/min) until a point was reached where no further displacement could be recorded. With repeated intermittent forces of the same order, however, intrusive movements took place beyond the limit reached with the maintained force. The mobility appeared to be influenced by the rate of application of the load and the interval between loads. Less displacement of the tooth was produced if the load was applied rapidly. Where a series of intrusive loads of ∿ 5 N was applied with intervals of 2–5 sec, the tooth did not have sufficient time to return to its original position before the application of the next load (Fig. 2). Indeed, after each successive load the tooth returned slightly less far. Furthermore, the intrusive mobility of the tooth gradually was reduced with each successive load and

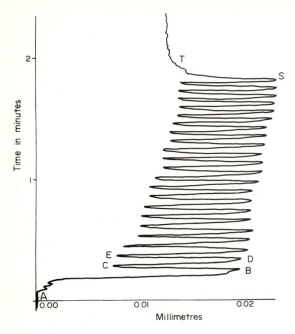

FIG. 2. The axial movement/time curve of a human maxillary incisor tooth. A – Initial position. B – Position at 5 N peak force on the first application. C – First return on removal of force. D – Position at 5 N peak force on the second application. E – Second return on removal of force. S – Position at 5 N peak force on the twenty-second application. T – Return point after the final removal of force.

the tooth appeared to be intruded progressively into the socket as the series continued.

On removing an intrusive load, the tooth was seen to recover its original position in two phases. The first recovery phase showed a rapid return towards its original position in an almost linear manner with time. The second phase involved a slower recovery, there being an apparent logarithmic relationship between movement and time. Full recovery was found to take 1–2 min with an intermittent load. Recovery took longer where the load had been maintained.

In discussing his results, Parfitt was of the opinion that, contrary to the belief at that time, the tooth could not be supported simply by tension through inelastic fibre bundles. He suggested that 'several distinct and independently variable systems' were involved in tooth support. Though it was not possible to demonstrate the precise mechanisms underlying the patterns of tooth displacements, Parfitt suggested that the tooth was supported by fluids related both

to the vascular and tissue fluid systems in the periodontal ligament. This interpretation was based partly upon his observation that tooth movements occurred in synchrony with the arterial pulse wave with intrusive loads less than 0.15 N.

The work of Parfitt has been developed extensively, particularly by Picton and co-workers. Picton (1962b, 1963a) published the results of studies on tooth mobility in human maxillary incisors, mandibular first premolars and maxillary first molars during biting. His apparatus at this time consisted of two movement transducers incorporating resistance-wire strain gauges soldered to the wings of a rubber dam clamp which was placed on the test tooth (Fig. 3a). Metal pointers from the transducers were rested on the teeth immediately adjacent to the test tooth to provide reference points. Biting forces up to ~ 20 N were applied to the test tooth via a dynamometer anchored to teeth in the opposing jaw. Three thrusts were made to each tooth studied, the time interval between thrusts being 30 sec to 1 min. Picton claimed that tilting of the teeth during the biting thrusts could be accounted for. However, he emphasized that since the adjacent reference teeth were also probably displaced by the thrusts, the values obtained for tooth mobility were not to be regarded as absolute. Although considerable variation was sometimes found between consecutive thrusts, the pattern and amount of intrusive tooth movements were similar to those obtained by Parfitt (1960) (Fig. 3b). Thus, the load/tooth mobility curves revealed an initial phase of relatively free movement followed by a second phase of less movement. However, the changeover between the two phases appeared to be rather variable, and tended to occur at the higher load of approximately 4 N.

More recent research suggests that the relationship between intrusive force and displacement is not a simple logarithmic one as suggested by Parfitt (1960). Using more reliable techniques for monitoring tooth displacement, Wills, Picton and Davies (1974, 1976, 1978) showed that on plotting log displacement vs. log force for macaque monkey teeth there is a two-phase parabolic relationship with discontinuity occurring within the force range 0.5–0.8 N (Fig. 4).

In view of Parfitt's (1960) assertion that tooth mobility was influenced by the rate of loading and the time interval between thrusts, further investi-

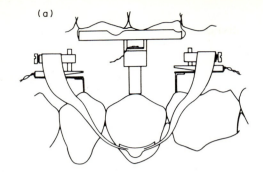

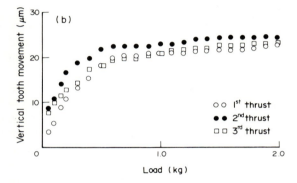

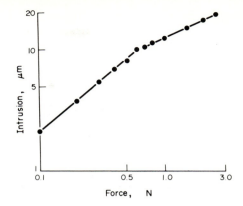

FIG. 4. Log force—log displacement curve for force applied to a maxillary central incisor of a macaque monkey at a rate of 4 N sec^{-1}.

FIG. 3. (a) Diagrammatic representation of apparatus used by Picton to study tooth mobility. Two transducers of movement are fixed to the wings of a rubber dam clamp which is mounted on the tooth to be studied and free of adjacent teeth. A dynamometer fixed to the opposing teeth is used to measure the force applied to the test tooth. (b) Vertical mobility curves obtained for a human maxillary first permanent molar.

gations concerning this have been conducted by Picton (1963b, 1964 a and b) and Wills, Picton and Davies (1978). The first of these studies (Picton, 1963b) was motivated by the need to standardize techniques by reducing the sources of variation observed in previous research (Picton, 1962b, 1963a). Techniques similar to those used for his earlier experiments were employed. However, the next but one tooth on each side of the test tooth were now used as reference teeth. This was done since the teeth immediately adjacent may show movements when force is applied to the test tooth (Picton, 1962a). Axial loads rising from 0 to ∿ 20 N were applied manually to the test tooth and graphic records of the force used to enable the rate of thrust to be controlled. Picton emphasized the need to take care to stabilize the point of application of the

dynamometer on the test tooth and to ensure that the direction of thrust was axial. Variation in the rate of thrust (in the range 0.5—25 sec rise-time) produced no consistent effect on the load/mobility curves. Variation of the time interval between thrusts, however, had an effect. Using standard rise-times, 2- or 5-sec intervals between thrusts caused progressive reduction in mobility and the tooth failed to return to its initial position on removing the load — a finding similar to that observed by Parfitt (1960). Variable effects were seen with longer time intervals between thrusts of 1—2 min. In six out of ten teeth studied, with 1-min intervals between thrusts there was no change (or a slight decrease) in mobility. In seven out of eight teeth studied, no change or a slight increase in mobility was recorded with 1½-min intervals. With 2-min intervals, all teeth (10) showed a progressive increase in mobility. Picton concluded that a time interval of 1—1½ min between thrusts is necessary to ensure repeatable load/mobility curves. Picton interpreted the increased mobility seen with 2-min intervals as the consequence of the tooth adopting an extruded position in the interval between thrusts.

Picton's 1964a experiments generally confirm his 1963b study. However, he observed that, whilst there was a gradual increase in mobility of human maxillary incisors when thrusts of ∿ 2 N or ∿ 20 N were applied at 2-min intervals, there was a more abrupt increase in mobility in the 2 min following twenty thrusts applied with 5-sec intervals. He claimed that rapidly repeated thrusts may thus act as a stimulus for increase in mobility and extrusion. Picton suggested that the possibility that the increase in mobility was the result of passive extrusion (due to lack of restraining forces) was countered by the finding that a series of thrusts applied with intervals of 2 min still produced a *gradual* increase in mobility where there was a 30–60-min rest period prior to applying the thrusts during which the bite was propped open. Whilst his previous experiments (Picton, 1963b) showed that ∿20 N thrusts applied at 5-sec and 2-min intervals resulted respectively in a reduction and an increase in tooth mobility, this difference could not be discerned where a ∿20 N load was maintained on the tooth for up to 5 min prior to experimentation.

The effects of applying axial intrusive thrusts with intervals approximating to those observed during mastication were also studied by Picton (1964b). From the findings of Anderson (1956a) and Graf (1963), he calculated that the mean interval between chewing thrusts is 412 msec. Using this estimate the degree of recovery was studied for some human maxillary central incisors during a series of ∿20 N loads applied at rates of 10 or 60 thrusts per min. The pattern of recovery had characteristics similar to those reported by Parfitt (1960). Picton calculated that the initial linear phase of recovery would have been completed within 412 msec in only five of the ten teeth studied. This implies that a tooth tends to remain in a depressed position in its socket during normal chewing.

Contrary to the findings of Picton's 1963b experiment, the studies of Wills *et al.* (1978) suggest that different loading rates do have a significant effect on tooth mobility. They reported that the rapid application of loads rising to 4 N resulted in less tooth displacement than with loads applied gradually. Apart from differences in the apparatus used to record tooth displacement, a number of differences exist between the 1963b and 1978 experiments:

1. Human teeth were studied in 1963, the teeth of macaque monkeys in 1978.
2. In the 1963 experiment peak thrusts of ∿20 N were applied, the rate of thrust varying from 0.5 to 24 sec rise-time. In the 1978 experiment three rates of loading were applied. The force was applied as a linear ramp function at rates of 4 N per sec or 12 N per sec. The third type

of loading was sufficiently rapid to approximate to a step function, the load being applied within 0.01 sec.
3. In 1978 six preconditioning thrusts of 4 N were applied at 10-sec intervals and the tooth allowed to recover for 2 min.

In discussing their results, Wills *et al.* (1978) did not refer to Picton's 1963b paper and therefore did not reconcile the contrasting results.

The experiments so far described show that the relationship between intrusive force and tooth mobility is 'non-Hookean' and the possibility was raised that the periodontium might have viscoelastic properties. Further studies by Bien and Ayers (1965), Bien (1966), Wills, Picton and Davies (1972) and Picton and Wills (1978) have been undertaken to assess this.

The experiments of Bien and Ayers (1965) and Bien (1966) were conducted on rat maxillary incisors using loads ranging from ∿0.35 N to ∿15 N. Measurement of the displacement of the test tooth was made relative to the adjacent unloaded incisor by means of a microscope fitted with a vernier micrometer eyepiece. Unlike most experiments on tooth mobility, their method involved the sudden application of a deadweight load which was maintained for several minutes and then suddenly removed. Their findings showed a biphasic intrusive response and a biphasic recovery response, the first phase in both being the faster (Fig. 5). Bien (1966) believed the results demonstrated that the periodontal ligament behaved as a viscoelastic gel. He compared the behaviour of the periodontal tissues to various arrangements of mechanical springs and dampers. Figure 6 describes the dimensional changes which would be produced on loading and unloading a variety of mechanical models. Bien suggested that the intrusive and recovery responses of the tooth under load could be represented by a Maxwell element.

Wills *et al.* (1972) analysed the displacement/time curves obtained following the sudden removal of axial intrusive loads of 2.5 N to the incisors of monkeys. Using a technique of exponential curve fitting, they claimed to be able to discern three (occasionally four) phases in the recovery of a tooth. They suggested that their results showed that the periodontium is not analogous to a simple Maxwell element, but should be represented by a series of

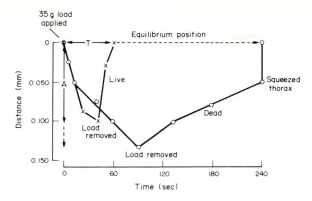

FIG. 5. Displacement of a maxillary incisor of a rat under load. The plottings are diagrammatic representations of the intrusion of the tooth into its socket under load, and its restoration to the equilibrium level after removal of the load. A complete cycle is the period T (abscissa) while the magnitude of the intrusion from the point of equilibrium is the amplitude A (ordinate).

Voigt elements. The use of graphical techniques for curve fitting is open to criticism. For example, because the exact contour of a curve may be difficult to delineate in the face of expected observational errors, the exact number of separate exponential components which comprise it cannot always be established with confidence (Shipley and Clark, 1972). Furthermore, one must have *a priori* grounds for suggesting that the curve consists of a series of

exponentials since other mathematical models can be made to fit. In view of such criticisms, we believe that the more reliable mathematical techniques devised for the analysis of curves (e.g. step-wise regression analysis — Draper and Smith, 1966) are to be preferred to graphical techniques.

Picton and Wills (1978) illustrated records of the pattern of displacement and recovery of a monkey incisor with an intrusive load applied as a ramp function (Fig. 7), likening the response to the force/ displacement relationship of a Voigt element. They also listed five other characteristics of the stressed periodontal ligament which they claimed identified this tissue as viscoelastic:

1. Loads sustained for many seconds or minutes cause creep.
2. There is an inverse relationship between the rate of loading and displacement.
3. The higher the rate of loading, the less is the distinction between early and late phases of displacement.
4. If loadings are repeated at intervals of less than 1½ min, the recovery becomes progressively more incomplete.
5. The rate of recovery is directly related to the loading rate and indirectly related to the duration of the load.

In addition to the models described by Bien

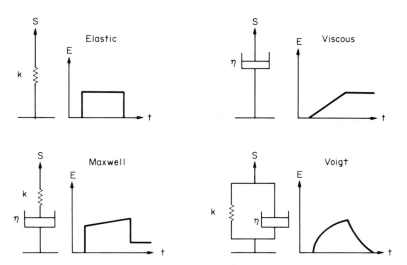

FIG. 6. Four simple rheological analogues and schematic representations of the dimensional changes with time which would be produced on loading and unloading each model.

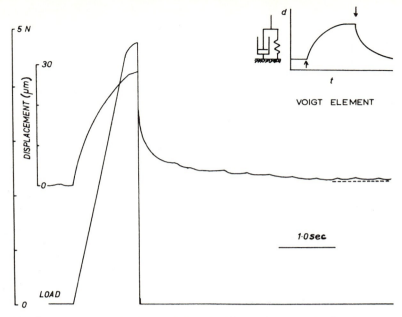

FIG. 7. Record showing the axial load to the maxillary central incisor of a macaque monkey in the lower trace and the intrusion in the upper record. The inset shows how the pattern of displacement and recovery in the upper record can be likened to that of a viscoelastic Voigt element.

(1966), Wills *et al.* (1972) and Picton and Wills (1978), Ross, Lear and DeCou (1976) have suggested that the most suitable model is a three-parameter non-linear spring. It is conceivable that physical characteristics other than viscoelasticity could account for the patterns of tooth displacement observed. For example, the possibility that the periodontal tissues are thixotropic should be considered. A thixotropic material is one which can undergo gel/sol/gel transformations (Pryce-Jones, 1936). In general, a thixotropic system has the following rheological characteristics:

1. An isothermal change in viscosity brought about by pressure alone.
2. When the pressure is removed, the system undergoes a time-dependent recovery and maintains its contours.
3. The flow curve (i.e. the shear stress versus the shear rate) has a hysteresis loop.

Recently, Kardos and Simpson (1979, 1980) have attempted to explain the mechanisms associated with the passage of an erupting tooth through the jaws, orthodontic tooth movement and tooth support on the basis of the periodontal ligament being thixotropic. They reinterpreted the data from the experiments of Parfitt (1960), claiming that the behaviour of a tooth with axial intrusive loads was consistent with the properties of a thixotropic material. At this time, however, care should be taken not to over-speculate since a radical change in our ideas concerning the structure and function of the periodontal ligament would be necessary if it is thixotropic. We believe, therefore, that further research into this matter is required.

Finally, two general comments should be made concerning the interpretations of the findings of the experiments on physiological tooth mobility. Firstly, we should be aware that biting loads during mastication and swallowing are more complex than the loading regimes used in the experiments. Furthermore, even with a unidirectional load, complex multidirectional tooth movements in the socket are produced (e.g. Pryputniewicz and Burstone, 1979). Secondly, whilst some have been tempted to speculate on the significance of their findings in terms of the biology of the periodontal tissues, we are not convinced of the efficacy of this approach. We are of the opinion that this aspect can be elucidated best by research involving the effects of loading on experimentally altered periodontal tissues.

STUDIES CONCERNING THE BIOLOGICAL BASIS OF THE TOOTH SUPPORT MECHANISM

The role of collagen fibres

The classical view of the tooth support mechanism holds that the periodontal ligament is a suspensory ligament. Accordingly, the obliquely orientated collagen fibres transmit axial loads in the form of tension to the alveolar bone. This concept has been elaborated upon in the light of Harkness' (1968) observation that unstressed collagen fibres are wavy. Thus, it can be envisaged that the collagen fibres gradually straighten out with intrusive loads. This idea, together with other details of the biophysical properties of the collagen fibres of the periodontal ligament, are described in Chapter 5, pages 110–114. In Chapter 3, Sloan has argued that the organization of the periodontal collagen reflects the magnitude and direction of the masticatory forces.

Some early dissenting voices against the tensional hypothesis were those of Synge (1933 a and b) and Gabel (1956). More recently, studies on physiological tooth mobility have shown that the relationship between tooth displacement and axial load is not entirely consistent with the tensional hypothesis (see preceding section).

Picton (1965) and Picton and Davies (1967) conducted experiments to evaluate the relative importance of tension and compression in the tooth support mechanism. These involved examining the distortion of the alveolar margins when axial intrusive loads and horizontal loads were applied to the teeth of monkeys. Picton (1965) observed that intrusive thrusts caused dilation of the socket in 80% of cases, little or no distortion in 12% of cases and constriction in the remaining 8%. Picton and Davies (1967) obtained similar results. It was concluded that the periodontal tissues act, at least in part, as a compressive system in resisting axial loads since convergence of the alveolar margins was predicted if a tensional system had been involved. However, the

experiments do not prove that collagen fibres in the periodontal ligament are not placed under tension, especially since no direct observations of the tissue under load were made. Indeed, the possibility that a tooth might be supported by both compressive and tensional reactions in different parts of the periodontal ligament was considered by Picton (1965). That tension may be of importance was shown by the finding that horizontal force to a tooth displaced the alveolar crest a similar distance with force directed towards or away from the palate (Picton, 1965). Furthermore, Picton and Slatter (1972) observed that cutting the gingiva and periodontal ligament with a thin steel blade produced a similar increase in horizontal mobility when the tooth was pushed towards or away from the site of trauma. Further evidence that the periodontal tissues may be put in a tensional mode with intrusive loads has been obtained from the work of Gathercole and Keller (see Chapter 5, pages 113, 114).

One criticism that may be levelled at the experiments of Picton (1965) and Picton and Davies (1967) concerns the possibility that surgical trauma of the periodontium, produced in order to expose the alveolar margins, caused disturbance to the tooth support mechanism. Whilst this possibility was acknowledged, Picton and Davies (1967) claimed that the trauma was minimal. Indeed, Picton (1967) claimed that axial tooth mobility was only slightly increased by surgical trauma to the mesial and distal regions of the periodontium. He concluded that limited areas of the periodontal ligament may be traumatized without gross disturbance to the support mechanism.

To date, few experiments have been conducted to assess how experimental changes to the collagen fibres affect the reaction of the tooth to intrusive loads. Parfitt (1967) claimed to have shown that collagenases altered the characteristics of the movement of teeth *in vitro* with intrusive loads. However, it is not possible to properly assess this work since details of the experiment were not published. That collagen does play a role in the tooth support mechanism can be deduced from experiments in which collagen cross-linking was inhibited by the administration to rats of the lathyritic agent β-aminoacetonitrile bisulphate (e.g. Berkovitz, Migdalski and Solomon, 1972). Considerable dilaceration of the roots of maxillary incisor teeth maintained in occlusion was observed. Teeth relatively free of the occlusion showed no such disturbance. That the lathyrogen had produced an effect on the collagen of the periodontal ligament was evidenced by the ease with which teeth could be extracted manually.

The role of the periodontal vasculature and interstitial fluid

Boyle (1938) initially implicated the vascular system in the tooth support mechanism. Parfitt (1960) attempted to interpret his findings on physiological tooth mobility in terms of fluid movements in both the blood vessels and ground substance of the periodontal ligament.

From experiments conducted by Bien and Ayers (1965), Bien (1966) proposed a haemodynamic hypothesis of tooth support. This was based upon the pattern of recovery of a maxillary incisor in a recently killed rat after the removal of an intrusive load. It was reported that complete recovery to the preloading position was not spontaneous but required thoracic massage (Fig. 5). Because of the biphasic response to axial loading, Bien (1966) claimed that two fluid-damping effects were implicated in the tooth support mechanism. The first damping effect was thought to involve a squeeze film. This is analogous to a thin film of lubricant between load-bearing surfaces in which the fluid under pressure is squeezed to the edges of the plate in order to cushion the load. The second damping effect was thought to involve vascular changes within the periodontal tissues. Ballooning of small blood vessels to produce cirsoid aneurisms was said to occur as a result of constriction of the vessels by intervening fibres of the ligament. Bien claimed that cirsoid aneurisms, as minute flexible-walled sacs of fluid, act as minute springs. He further considered that they replenish the squeeze film and dissipate kinetic energy by forcing fluid through the vessel walls. Interesting as these concepts are, there is little evidence to support them. With regard to the role of periodontal fluid in tooth support, we know too little about its distribution and behaviour within the periodontal ligament to enable us to predict the effects of loading upon it. For example, is the distinction between

bound and unbound water of significance? Furthermore, movement of water between the vascular and extra-vascular components, between one part of the ligament and another, and even between the ligament and alveolar bone seems likely to influence the behaviour of the tooth under loading. With regard to the contribution of the cirsoid aneurisms, there is no evidence to support their formation. Despite these criticisms, the work of Bien and Ayers (1965) and Bien (1966) demonstrates the importance of the vascular system in the tooth support mechanism by providing a mechanism by which there is recovery of position after intrusive loads are removed.

That tooth position is influenced by the periodontal vasculature has been shown by a number of investigations. Parfitt (1960), Körber and Körber (1967), Körber (1970, 1971), Slatter and Picton (1972), Packman, Shoher and Stein (1977) and Burn-Murdoch and Picton (1978) have observed that teeth show pulsatile movements which are synchronous with the arterial pulse. Parfitt (1960) reported that systemically administered atropine given to a human subject resulted in slight extrusion of a maxillary incisor. Wills and Picton (1978) reported changes in the resting position of incisor teeth in macaque monkeys following submucosal injections of saline and water. In nearly every case, water caused an extrusion, but there was a more frequent intrusion following saline injection. Moxham (1978, 1979), in studying the influence of the vascular system on tooth eruption in rabbit incisors, has reported that hypotensive drugs, noradrenaline, acetylcholine and section and stimulation of the sympathetic trunk have marked effects on tooth position (see also Chapter 10, pages 233–235).

Investigations have been undertaken to assess the influence of vascular/fluid systems of the periodontium on tooth mobility. Wills, Picton and Davies (1976) have observed that the intravenous administration of angiotensin resulted in a reduced displacement with intrusive loads in the teeth of macaque monkeys. Similar changes in mobility have been observed following the submucosal injection of noradrenaline at sites both near and at a distance from the test tooth (Slatter and Picton, 1972; Wills *et al.*, 1976). A consistent pattern was not seen, however, when the noradrenaline solution was injected near the test tooth. It was suggested that in these circumstances there might be distinct vaso-constrictor and volume effects of the carrier solution. Wills *et al.* (1976) also reported a reduction in mobility following exsanguination. A trend towards a return to normal mobility was observed after exsanguination when the thorax was squeezed. Wills and Picton (1978) reported that submucosal injection of water caused an increased mobility with intrusive loads. However, conflicting effects have been reported with saline. Wills *et al.* (1976) claimed that submucosal injections of saline gave a considerable increase in displacement whilst Wills and Picton (1978) have shown that a decrease in mobility can result.

Whilst the experiments involving submucosal injections of solutions seem to confirm the importance of the vasculature and fluids of the periodontal ligament in the tooth support mechanism, care must be taken in interpreting the findings. Firstly, we know too little of the physical, chemical and biological properties of the ligament to predict with confidence the effects of such solutions. For example, if the ligament is thixotropic, the changes in mobility observed following the addition of fluids could be interpreted in terms of gel/sol transformations (Kardos and Simpson, 1980). Secondly, injected solutions may have more than one effect. For example, it has already been mentioned that noradrenaline may have a vasoconstrictor effect and an effect related to the carrier solution. In addition, Wills and Picton (1978) suggest that saline and water may not only produce volume changes within the periodontal tissues but may also affect the biochemistry of the collagen and ground substance.

Another approach to study the role of the vasculature in the tooth support mechanism involves assessing the effects of loading on blood flow through the periodontal ligament. However, as discussed in Chapter 7 by Edwall, reliable techniques for measuring periodontal ligament blood flow are not yet available. Packman *et al.* (1977) attempted to investigate the effects of both axial and horizontal loads on the periodontal microcirculation using photoelectric plethysmography. Whilst they reported that significant changes in blood flow could be discerned during loading, it is not possible to evaluate how much of the change also related to circulatory changes in the alveolar bone and gingiva.

Walker, Ng and Burke (1978) have recorded changes in fluid pressures in the periodontal ligaments of the canine teeth of dogs during and following the application of loads up to 5 N. They reported that on applying a load there was an immediate increase in pressure which decayed rapidly (halving time less than 1 sec). Removal of the load produced an inverse pattern (but with a reduced peak pressure and a longer halving time). However, since the pressure changes were small compared with the loads applied, they concluded that the free fluids of the periodontal ligament only make a minor contribution to tooth support. They wrote that the major contribution is provided by 'the solid (collagen fibres) and semi-solid (ground substance) compartments of the ligament, acting in conjunction with the periodontal vasculature'. In considering the significance of their findings, the well-known difficulties of recording tissue fluid pressures reliably (e.g. Guyton, 1963; Brown, 1968; Stromberg and Wiederheilm, 1977) must be borne in mind.

The role of ground substance

As indicated in Chapter 6, little is known about the ground substance of the periodontal ligament. However, two major constituents are water (bound and free) and glycoproteins. Experiments designed to determine the significance of periodontal fluids in the tooth support mechanism have already been described. Wills and Picton (1980) have studied the effect on axial tooth mobility of submucosal injections of hyaluronidase in macaque monkeys. The solvent used was water. They reported that injections of water alone produced a transient increase in mobility within 30 min which was still apparent at 1 h. Following injections of hyaluronidase there was a marked increase in mobility after 20 min for a single thrust, with a subsequent rapid return towards the mobility of control teeth. No such increase in mobility was recorded when a sixteen-thrusts regimen was used. Previous work had indicated a reduction in mobility following injections of hyaluronidase with saline (Picton, 1976).

The role of alveolar bone

It has been demonstrated that forces applied to teeth

cause distortion of adjacent bone, which tends to spread to the rest of the jaw (e.g. Jung, 1952; McDowell and Regli, 1961; Picton, 1962c). Using horizontal loads on macaque monkey teeth, Picton and Davies (1967) noted that displacement of the bone of the tooth socket was mainly in the same direction as the thrust. However, with some thrusts the bone was seen to be displaced in the direction opposite to the root. This might suggest that distortion of the bone was produced by the spread of stress from elsewhere in the alveolus (Picton, 1969). Picton (1965) and Picton and Davies (1967) have observed that the alveolar margins are dilated under axial loads. Picton (1969) and Picton *et al.* (1974) have suggested that the fast initial phase of recovery following removal of an intrusive load may be accounted for by recoil of bone.

SUMMARY

The following general conclusions about the tooth support mechanism can be drawn from the experiments conducted to investigate the effects of axially directed intrusive loads on normal and experimentally altered periodontal tissues:

(a) The weight of evidence suggests that the periodontal ligament does not behave as a suspensory ligament in the classical sense of the term. This conclusion is based upon the findings that:
  1. the relationship between force and displacement has 'non-Hooke-type' characteristics, being non-linear and multiphasic;
  2. there is evidence that both tension and compression of the periodontal ligament occur with loading.

(b) The characteristics of physiological tooth mobility with axial loads are considered to be consistent with the view that the periodontal tissues are viscoelastic. However, interpretations based upon other physical properties (e.g. thixotropy) cannot be discounted.

(c) Experiments which have attempted to produce selective changes within the periodontal ligament have not been able to establish that any single element within the tissue is responsible for the tooth support mechanism. This

mechanism is conceivably a function of the periodontal tissues as a whole.

EXTRUSIVE LOADS

Much less is known about the source and nature of extrusive loads and their effects upon tooth position and the periodontal tissues than is known about intrusive loads. Using a technique for continuously recording tooth movements, it has been shown that extrusive loads as small as 0.01 N are sufficient to produce changes in position of rabbit mandibular incisors (Moxham and Berkovitz, 1979) and of ferret mandibular canines (Moxham and Berkovitz, unpublished data). It is possible, therefore, that oral soft tissues, gravity and sticky foods produce extrusive movements. Extrusive loads may also be applied to the teeth in association with certain habits (e.g. tooth picking) and with some orthodontic procedures.

Parfitt (1960) reported that tractional forces of ~ 0.15 N and ~ 0.3 N caused a human maxillary central incisor to extrude by 6 μm and 8 μm respectively. Heners (1974) claimed that human maxillary central incisors extruded by about 20 μm with ~ 5 N loads. Recently, some preliminary reports have been published using holographic techniques to measure tooth movement which promise to provide very accurate information about the displacement of human teeth in three dimensions with extrusive loads (Every, Burstone and Pryputniewicz, 1978, 1979).

The pattern of tooth movement during, and following, the application of extrusive loads has been described by Moxham and Berkovitz (1979) for the rabbit mandibular incisor. Figure 8 illustrates diagrammatically the method of applying loads and the displacement transducer used to monitor tooth position continuously. Figure 9 shows the typical responses of a rabbit incisor to the sudden application of an extrusive load which is maintained for 5 min and then suddenly removed. To date, responses of this kind have been observed for loads varying between 0.01 – 2 N. On applying the load a biphasic response is seen. During the first phase, there is a rapid, instantaneous extrusion of the tooth. The second phase involves a more gradual extrusion.

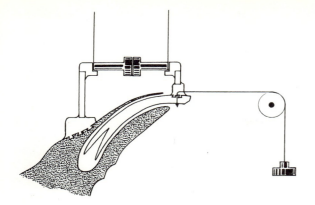

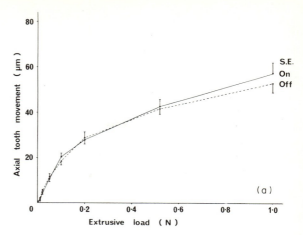

FIG. 8. Diagrammatic representation showing an extrusive load being applied over a pulley to a rabbit mandibular incisor on to which a variable capacitance displacement transducer has been placed.

A similar, but intrusive, biphasic recovery response is observed on removing the load. The amount of displacement of the tooth during the first phase of both the extrusive and recovery cycles is similar. However, the second phase of the extrusive cycle is generally greater than that of the recovery cycle. Thus, the tooth does not return to its resting position but shows a slightly extruded position. Similar biphasic responses to extrusive loads have been observed for ferret mandibular canines (Moxham and Berkovitz, unpublished data) and for rat maxillary incisors (Burn-Murdoch, personal communication).

A quantitative assessment of the effects of extrusive loads on the rabbit mandibular incisor was subsequently undertaken by Moxham and Berkovitz (in press). Figure 10 summarizes the results obtained. These show that, whilst both first and second phases of the extrusive and recovery cycles are force-depen-

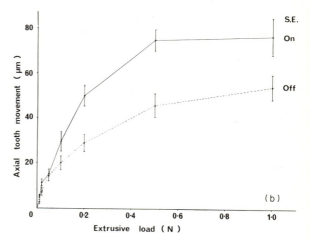

FIG. 10. Graphs showing axial movements of rabbit mandibular incisors (right) in response to extrusive loads. Each point represents the mean movement for the incisors of twelve animals (± 1 S.E.). (a) First phase of movement with load on and off. (b) Second phase of movement with load on and off. See Fig. 9 and text for explanation of the phases.

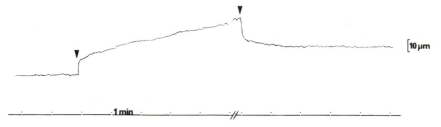

FIG. 9. Pen recorder trace illustrating the effects on tooth position of applying an extrusive load to a rabbit mandibular incisor. The first arrow indicates application and the second removal of the load. In this instance a load of 0.05 N was applied.

dent, they are not linearly graded. This indicates that the responses do not have Hooke-type characteristics and may support the view that the periodontal tissues behave as a viscoelastic system. However, the authors were of the opinion that an interpretation of their findings in biological terms should wait until experiments have been conducted which involve an assessment of the effects of extrusive loads following selective changes to the periodontal tissues.

Comparing the reactions of the rabbit mandibular incisor to extrusive loads with the reactions of the rat maxillary incisor to intrusive loads (Bien and Ayers, 1965; Bien, 1966), the following differences are notable:

(i) Whereas an instantaneous elastic displacement of the rabbit incisor to the sudden application of an extrusive load was observed, the first response of the rat incisor to an intrusive load was more gradual.

(ii) Whereas the rat incisor returned to its original

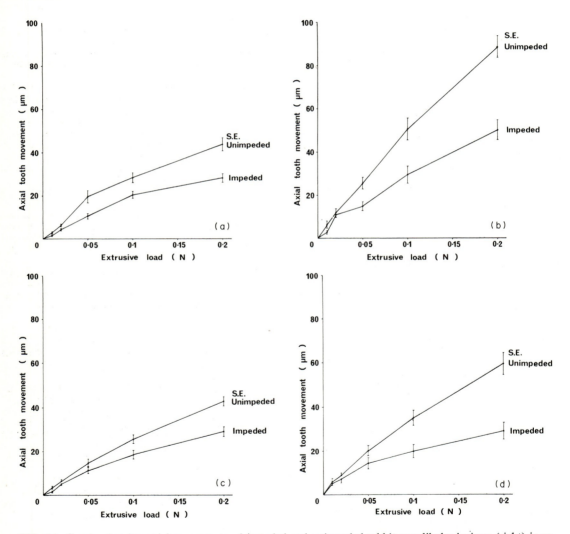

FIG. 11. Graphs showing axial movements of impeded and unimpeded rabbit mandibular incisors (right) in response to extrusive loads. Each point represents the mean movement for the incisors of twelve animals (± 1 S.E.). (a) First phase of movement with load on. (b) Second phase of movement with load on. (c) First phase of movement with load off. (d) Second phase of movement with load off. See Fig. 9 and text for explanation of the phases.

resting position within minutes of the intrusive load being removed, at the end of the extrusive recovery cycle the rabbit incisor showed a slightly extruded position.

(iii) The responses of the rat incisor to intrusive loads changed significantly after death, the tooth only returning to its resting position after the load had been removed when the thorax was squeezed. However, in both the live and dead rabbits it was possible to observe similar reactions to extrusive loads.

Thus, although there are similarities in the responses of a continuously growing incisor to intrusive and extrusive loads, the differences suggest that these loads may be resisted by different mechanisms in the periodontal tissues. Alternatively, the differences may be related to differences in the periodontal tissues of the experimental animals used. Wills and Manderson (1977) have reported responses to static intrusive loading of the palates of macaque monkeys similar to the responses of the periodontal tissues following extrusive loading. Since the tissues of the palate differ markedly from the periodontal tissues in structure, composition and tissue dynamics, the explanation of the mechanism(s) underlying the reaction of the periodontal tissues to loading may be elusive.

Experiments involving the application of extrusive loads should provide information not only about the biomechanical properties of the periodontal ligament but also about other characteristics of this tissue (for example, the eruptive mechanism). Moxham and Berkovitz (in press) have investigated differences in the reactions to extrusive loads of impeded and unimpeded rabbit mandibular incisors erupting at different rates. The unimpeded teeth were cut out of the bite and maintained so for 5 days prior to experimentation, whereas the impeded teeth were left in occlusion. Figure 11 summarizes the results obtained. They show that there is a significant reduction in the resistance of the unimpeded rabbit mandibular incisor to extrusive forces. Thus, it is conceivable that changes in eruption rates may be associated with changes in resistance to eruption rather than with changes in the mechanism(s) responsible for generating eruptive forces. This highlights the difficulty of interpreting experimentally produced changes in eruption rates (see also Chapter 10).

ACKNOWLEDGEMENTS

The authors gratefully acknowledge the financial assistance obtained from the Medical Research Council.

REFERENCES

ADAMS, S. H. & ZANDER, H. A. (1964) Functional tooth contacts in lateral and centric occlusion. *J. Amer. dent. Assoc.* **69**, 465–473.

AHLGREN, J. (1966) Mechanisms of mastication. *Acta odont. Scand.* **24**, Suppl. 44.

AHLGREN, J. (1967) Patterns of chewing and malocclusion of teeth. A clinical study. *Acta odont. Scand.* **25**, 3–13.

AHLGREN, J. (1976) In: *Mastication*, D. J. ANDERSON & B. MATTHEWS (eds.), pp. 119–127. Bristol, Wright.

AHLGREN, J. & ÖWALL, B. (1970) Muscular activity in chewing force: a polygraphic study of human mandibular movements. *Archs. oral Biol.* **15**, 271–280.

ANDERSON, D. J. (1953) A method for recording masticatory loads. *J. dent. Res.* **32**, 785–789.

ANDERSON, D. J. (1956a) Measurement of stress in mastication. I. *J. dent. Res.* **35**, 664–670.

ANDERSON, D. J. (1956b) Measurement of stress in mastication. II. *J. dent. Res.* **35**, 671–673.

ANDERSON, D. J. (1976) The incidence of tooth contacts in normal mastication and the part they play in guiding the final stage of mandibular closure. In: *Mastication*, D. J. ANDERSON & B. MATTHEWS (eds.), pp. 237–240. Bristol, Wright.

ANDERSON, D. J. & PICTON, D. C. A. (1957) Tooth contact during chewing. *J. dent. Res.* **36**, 21–26.

ANDERSON, D. J. & PICTON, D. C. A. (1958) Masticatory stresses in normal and modified occlusion. *J. dent. Res.* **37**, 312–317.

ATKINSON, H. F. & RALPH, W. J. (1973) Tooth loss and biting force in man. *J. dent. Res.* **52**, 225–228.

ATKINSON, H. F. & SHEPHARD, R. W. (1967) Masticatory movements and the resulting force. *Archs. oral Biol.* **12**, 195–202.

ATWOOD, D. A. (1956) A cephalometric study of the clinical rest position of the mandible. Part I: The variability of the clinical rest position following the removal of occlusal contacts. *J. Prosthet. Dent.* **6**, 504–519.

BANDO, E., FUKUSHIMA, S., KAWABATA, H. & KOHNO, S. (1972) Continuous observations of mandibular positions by telemetry. *J. Prosthet. Dent.* **28**, 485–490.

BATES, J. F., STAFFORD, G. D. & HARRISON, A. (1975) Masticatory function — a review of the literature. II. Speed of movement of the mandible, rate of chewing and forces developed in chewing. *J. oral Rehab.* **2**, 349–361.

BEARN, E. M. (1972) Some masticatory force patterns produced by full denture wearers. *Dent. Pract.* **22**, 342–346.

BEHREND, D. A. (1978) Patterns of tooth displacement in

simulated chewing cycles in man. *Archs. oral Biol.* **23**, 1089–1093.

BERKOVITZ, B. K. B., MIGDALSKI, A. & SOLOMON, M. (1972) The effect of the lathyritic agent amino-acetonitrile on the unimpeded eruption rate in normal and root-resected rat lower incisors. *Archs. oral Biol.* **17**, 1755–1763.

BERKOVITZ, B. K. B. & POOLE, D. F. G. (1977) Attrition of the teeth in ferrets. *J. Zool., Lond.* **183**, 411–418.

BEYRON, H. (1964) Occlusal relations and mastication in Australian aborigines. *Acta odont. Scand.* **22**, 597–678.

BIEN, S. M. (1966) Fluid dynamic mechanisms which regulate tooth movement. In: *Advances in oral biology*, Vol. 2, P. H. STAPLE (ed.), pp. 173–201. London, Academic Press.

BIEN, S. M. & AYERS, H. D. (1965) Responses of rat maxillary incisors to loads. *J. dent. Res.* **44**, 517–520.

BLACK, G. V. (1895) An investigation of the physical characteristics of the human teeth in relation to their diseases, and to practical dental operations, together with the physical characters of filling materials. *Dent. Cosmos.* **37**, 469–484.

BOYLE, P. E. (1938) Tooth suspension. A comparative study of the paradental tissues of man and of the guinea pig. *J. dent. Res.* **17**, 37–46.

BREKHUS, P. J., ARMSTRONG, W. D. & SIMON, W. J. (1941) Stimulation of the muscles of mastication. *J. dent. Res.* **20**, 87–92.

BREWER, A. (1963) Prosthodontic research at the school of aerospace medicine. *J. Prosthet. Dent.* **13**, 49–54.

BRILL, N., LAMMIE, G. A., OSBORNE, J. & PERRY, H. T. (1959) Mandibular positions and mandibular movements. *Br. dent. J.* **106**, 391–400.

BRION, M. A. M., PAMEIJER, J. H. N., GLICKMAN, I. & ROEBER, F. W. (1969) Recent intraoral telemetry findings and their developments in the study of occlusion. *Int. dent. J.* **19**, 541–552.

BROWN, A. C. (1968) Pulp tissue pressure and blood flow. In: *Biology of the dental pulp organ*, S. B. FINN (ed.), pp. 381–395. Alabama, University of Alabama Press.

BURN-MURDOCH, R. A. & PICTON, D. C. A. (1978) A technique for measuring eruption rates in rats of maxillary incisors under intrusive loads. *Archs. oral Biol.* **23**, 563–566.

DAHLBERG, B. (1946) The masticatory habits. An analysis of the number of chews when consuming food. *J. dent. Res.* **25**, 67–72.

DE BOEVER, J. A., McCALL, W. D., HOLDEN, S. & ASH, M. M. (1978) Functional occlusal forces: an investigation by telemetry. *J. Prosthet. Dent.* **40**, 326–333.

DIBDIN, G. H. & GRIFFITHS, M. J. (1976) Observations on the resting posture of the mandible using telemetry. In: *Mastication*, D. J. ANDERSON & B. MATTHEWS (eds.), pp. 100–104. Bristol, Wright.

DRAPER, N. R. & SMITH, H. (1966) *Applied regression analysis.* New York, Wiley.

EICHNER, K. (1964) Auf Schlüsse über den Kanvorgang durch elektronische Kankraftmessungen. *Deutsche zahnärztl. Z.* **19**, 415–426.

EVERY, T. W., BURSTONE, C. J. & PRYPUTNIEWICZ, R. J. (1978) Holographic measurement of incisor extrusion. *J. dent. Res.* **57**, Special Issue A. Abst. 164.

EVERY, T. W., BURSTONE, C. J. & PRYPUTNIEWICZ, R. J. (1979) Holographic analysis of tooth movement resulting from known axial loads. *J. dent. Res.* **58**, Special Issue A. Abst. 1243.

FLANAGAN, J. B. (1964) Observations on the incidence of deglutition in man and measurement of some accompanying forces exerted on the dentition by perioral and lingual musculature. Master's Thesis, Harvard University.

GABEL, A. B. (1956) A mathematical analysis of the function of the fibres of the periodontal membrane. *J. Periodont.* **27**, 191–198.

GARNER, L. D. & KOTWAL, N. S. (1973) Correlation study of incisive biting forces with age, sex and anterior occlusion. *J. dent. Res.* **52**, 698–702.

GLICKMAN, I., HADDAD, A. W., MARGIGNONI, M., MEHTA, N., ROEBER, F. W. & CLARK, R. E. (1974) Telemetric comparison of centric relation and centric occlusion reconstructions. *J. Prosthet. Dent.* **31**, 527–536.

GLICKMAN, I., PAMEIJER, J. H. N. & ROEBER, F. W. (1968) Intraoral occlusal telemetry. Part 1. A multifrequency transmitter for registering tooth contacts in occlusion. *J. Prosthet. Dent.* **19**, 60–68.

GRAF, H. (1963) Occlusal contact patterns in mastication. M.S. Thesis, University of Rochester, N.Y. (quoted by PICTON, D. C. A., 1964b).

GRAF, H. (1969) Bruxism. *Dent. Clin. N. Amer.* **13**, 659–665.

GRAF, H. (1976) In: *Mastication*, D. J. ANDERSON & B. MATTHEWS (eds.), pp. 256–257. Bristol, Wright.

GRAF, H. (1978) Occlusal forces and mandibular movements. In: *Oral physiology and occlusion*, J. H. PERRYMAN (ed.), pp. 17–21. Oxford, Pergamon Press.

GRAF, H., GRASSL, H. & AEBERHARD, H. J. (1974) A method for measurement of occlusal forces in three directions. *Helv. Odont. Acta* **18**, 7–11.

GRAF, H. & ZANDER, H. A. (1963) Tooth contact pattern in mastication. *J. Prosthet. Dent.* **13**, 1055–1066.

GUYTON, A. C. (1963) A concept of negative interstitial pressure based on pressures in implanted capsules. *Circ. Res.* **12**, 399–414.

HANSON, M. L., LOGAN, W. B. & CASE, J. L. (1970) Tongue thrust in pre-school children. *Am. J. Orthod.* **57**, 15–22.

HARKNESS, R. D. (1968) Mechanical properties of collagenous tissues. In: *Treatise on collagen*, Vol. 2: *Biology of collagen*, Part A, B. S. GOULD (ed.), pp. 248–310. London, Academic Press.

HENERS, M. (1974) Syndesmotic limiting movement of the periodontal ligament. *Int. dent. J.* **24**, 319–327.

HIIEMAE, K. M. (1976) Masticatory movements in primitive mammals. In: *Mastication*, D. J. ANDERSON & B. MATTHEWS (eds.), pp. 105–117. Bristol, Wright.

HILDEBRAND, G. Y. (1931) Studies in the masticatory movements of the human lower jaw. *Scand. Arch. Physiol.* Suppl. 61.

HOWELL, A. H. & MANLEY, R. S. (1948) An electronic strain gauge for measuring oral forces. *J. dent. Res.* **27**, 705–712.

JANKLESON, B., HOFFMAN, G. M. & HENDRON, J. A. (1953) The physiology of the stomatognathic system. *J. Amer. dent. Assoc.* **46**, 375–386.

JENKINS, G. N. (1978) *The physiology and biochemistry of the mouth*, 4th ed. Oxford, Blackwell.

JUNG, F. (1952) Die Elastizität der Skeletteile des Gebissystems. *Stoma* **5**, 74–93.

KARDOS, T. B. & SIMPSON, L. D. (1979) A theoretical consideration of the periodontal membrane as a collagenous thixotropic system and its relationship to tooth eruption. *J. Periodont. Res.* **14**, 444–451.

KARDOS, T. B. & SIMPSON, L. D. (1980) A new periodontal membrane biology based upon thixotropic concepts. *Amer. J. Orthod.* **77**, 508–515.

KAVANAGH, D. & ZANDER, H. A. (1965) A versatile recording system for studies of mastication. *Med. Biol. Eng.* **3**, 291–300.

KAWAMURA, Y. (1968) Dental significance of four oral physiological mechanisms. *J. Canad. dent. Ass.* **34**, 582–590.

KINCAID, R. M. (1951) The frequency of deglutition in man: its relationship to overbite. *Angle Orthod.* **21**, 34–43.

KÖRBER, K. H. (1970) Periodontal pulsation. *J. Periodont.* **41**, 686–708.

KÖRBER, K. H. (1971) Electronic registration of tooth movements. *Int. dent. J.* **21**, 466–477.

KÖRBER, K. H. & KÖRBER, E. (1967) Patterns of physiological movement in tooth support. In: *Mechanisms of tooth support*, D. J. ANDERSON, J. E. EASTOE, A. H. MELCHER & D. C. A. PICTON (eds.), pp. 148–153. Bristol, Wright.

KUNVARA, B. (1959) Muscular forces of the tongue: Influence of tongue movements on the development of dental arches, jaws and palate. *Dent. Abr. (Chic.)* **4**, 10–11.

KYDD, W. L., AKAMINE, J. S., MENDEL, R. A. & KRAUS, B. S. (1963) Tongue and lip forces exerted during deglutition in subjects with and without an anterior open bite. *J. dent. Res.* **42**, 858–866.

LEAR, C. S. C., FLANAGAN, J. B. & MOORREES, C. F. A. (1965) The frequency of deglutition in man. *Archs. oral Biol.* **10**, 83–89.

MARKLUND, G. & WENNSTRÖM, A. (1972) A pilot-study concerning the relation between manifest anxiety and bite force. *Sven Tandlak Tidskr.* **65**, 107–110.

McCALL, W. D., DE BOEVER, J. A. & ASH, M. M. (1978) Telemetry system to study functional occlusal forces. *J. Prosthet. Dent.* **40**, 98–102.

McDOWELL, J. A. & REGLI, C. P. (1961) A quantitative analysis of the decrease in width of the mandibular arch during forced movements of the mandible. *J. dent. Res.* **40**, 1183–1185.

MØLLER, E. (1966) The chewing apparatus: an electromyograph study of the action of the muscles of mastication and its correlation to facial morphology. *Acta Physiol. Scand.* **69**, Suppl. 280.

MØLLER, E. (1976) Human muscle patterns. In: *Mastication and swallowing: Biological and clinical correlates*, B. J. SESSLE & A. G. HANNAM (eds.), pp. 128–141. Toronto, University of Toronto Press.

MOXHAM, B. J. (1978) An assessment of the vascular or tissue hydrostatic pressure hypotheses of eruption using a continuous recording technique for monitoring movements of the rabbit mandibular incisor. Ph.D. Thesis, University of Bristol.

MOXHAM, B. J. (1979) The effects of some vaso-active drugs on the eruption of the rabbit mandibular incisor. *Archs. oral Biol.* **24**, 681–688.

MOXHAM, B. J. & BERKOVITZ, B. K. B. (1979) The effects of axially-directed extrusive loads on movements of the mandibular incisor of the rabbit. *Archs. oral Biol.* **24**, 759–763.

MOXHAM, B. J. & BERKOVITZ, B. K. B. (in press) A quantitative assessment of the effects of axially-directed extrusive loads on displacement of the impeded and unimpeded rabbit mandibular incisor. *Archs. oral Biol.*

MOYERS, R. E. (1971) Postnatal development of orofacial musculature. *ASHA Reports*, No. 6, 38–47.

NYQUIST, C. & ÖWALL, B. (1968) Masticatory load registrations during function. A methodological study. *Odontol. Revy.* **19**, 45–54.

ÖWALL, B. & MØLLER, E. (1974) Oral tactile sensibility during biting and chewing. *Odontol. Revy.* **25**, 327–346.

PACKMAN, H., SHOHER, I. & STEIN, R. S. (1977) Vascular responses in the human periodontal ligament and alveolar bone detected by photoelectric plethysmography: the effect of force application to the tooth. *J. Periodont.* **48**, 194–200.

PAMEIJER, J. H. N., BRION, M., GLICKMAN, I. & ROEBER, F. W. (1970a) Intraoral occlusal telemetry. Part IV. Tooth contact during swallowing. *J. Prosthet. Dent.* **24**, 396–400.

PAMEIJER, J. H. N., BRION, M., GLICKMAN, I. & ROEBER, F. W. (1970b) Intraoral occlusal telemetry. Part V. Effect of occlusal adjustment upon tooth contacts during chewing and swallowing. *J. Prosthet. Dent.* **24**, 492–497.

PAMEIJER, J. H. N., GLICKMAN, I. & ROEBER, F. W. (1968) Intraoral telemetry. Part II. Registration of tooth contacts in chewing and swallowing. *J. Prosthet. Dent.* **19**, 151–159.

PAMEIJER, J. H. N., GLICKMAN, I. & ROEBER, F. W. (1969) Intraoral occlusal telemetry. Part III. Tooth contacts in chewing, swallowing and bruxism. *J. Periodont.* **40**, 253–258.

PARFITT, G. J. (1960) Measurement of the physiological mobility of individual teeth in an axial direction, *J. dent. Res.* **39**, 608–618.

PARFITT, G. J. (1967) The physical analysis of the tooth-supporting structures. In: *Mechanisms of tooth support*, D. J. ANDERSON, J. E. EASTOE, A. H. MELCHER & D. C. A. PICTON (eds.), pp. 154–156. Bristol, Wright.

PICTON, D. C. A. (1962a) Tilting movements of teeth during biting. *Archs. oral Biol.* **7**, 151–159.

PICTON, D. C. A. (1962b) A study of normal tooth mobility and the changes with periodontal disease. *Dent. Practit.* **12**, 167–173.

PICTON, D. C. A. (1962c) Distortion of the jaws during biting. *Archs. oral Biol.* **7**, 573–580.

PICTON, D. C. A. (1963a) Vertical movement of cheek teeth during biting. *Archs. oral Biol.* **8**, 109–118.

PICTON, D. C. A. (1963b) The effect on normal vertical tooth mobility of the rate of thrust and time interval between thrusts. *Archs. oral Biol.* **8**, 291–299.

PICTON, D. C. A. (1964a) The effect of repeated thrusts on normal axial tooth mobility. *Archs. oral Biol.* **9**, 55–63.

PICTON, D. C. A. (1964b) Some implications of normal tooth mobility during mastication. *Archs. oral Biol.* **9**, 565–573.

PICTON, D. C. A. (1965) On the part played by the socket in tooth support. *Archs. oral Biol.* **10**, 945–955.

PICTON, D. C. A. (1967) The effect on tooth mobility of trauma to the mesial and distal regions of the periodontal membranes in monkeys. *Helv. Odont. Acta* **11**, 105–112.

PICTON, D. C. A. (1969) The effect of external forces on the periodontium. In: *Biology of the periodontium*, A. H. MELCHER & W. H. BOWEN (eds.), pp. 363–419. London, Academic Press.

PICTON, D. C. A. (1976) Discussion in: *The eruption and occlusion of teeth*, D. F. G. POOLE & M. V. STACK (eds.), pp. 224. London, Butterworths.

PICTON, D. C. A. & DAVIES, W. I. R. (1967) Distortion of the socket with normal tooth movement. In: *Mechanisms of tooth support*, D. J. ANDERSON, J. E. EASTOE, A. H. MELCHER & D. C. A. PICTON (eds.), pp. 157–161. Bristol, Wright.

PICTON, D. C. A., JOHNS, R. B., WILLS, D. J. & DAVIES, W. I. R. (1974) The relationship between the mechanisms of tooth and implant support. In: *Oral Sciences Review*, Vol. 5, A. H. MELCHER & G. A. ZARB (eds.), pp. 3–22. Copenhagen, Munksgaard.

PICTON, D. C. A. & SLATTER, J. M. (1972) The effect on horizontal mobility of experimental trauma to the periodontal membrane in regions of tension or compression in monkeys. *J. periodont. Res.* **7**, 35–41.

PICTON, D. C. A. & WILLS, D. J. (1978) Viscoelastic properties of the periodontal ligament and mucous membrane. *J. Prosthet. Dent.* **40**, 263–272.

POWELL, R. N. (1965) Tooth contact during sleep. Association with other events. *J. dent. Res.* **44**, 959–967.

POWELL, R. N. & ZANDER, H. A. (1965) The frequency and distribution of tooth contact during sleep. *J. dent. Res.* **44**, 713–717.

PRYCE-JONES, J. (1936) Some fundamental aspects of thixotropy. *J. Oil and Colour Chem. Assoc.* **19**, 295–337.

PRYPUTNIEWICZ, R. J. & BURSTONE, C. J. (1979) The effect of time and force magnitude on orthodontic tooth movement. *J. dent. Res.* **58**, 1754–1764.

REDING, G. B., ZEPELIN, H., ROBINSON, J. E. Jr., ZIMMERMAN, S. O. & SMITH, V. H. (1968) Nocturnal teeth-grinding: all-night psychophysiologic studies. *J. dent. Res.* **47**, 786–797.

RIX, R. E. (1946) Deglutition and the teeth. *Dent. Rec.* **66**, 103–108.

RIX, R. E. (1953) Some observations upon the environment of the incisors. *Dent. Rec.* **73**, 427–441.

ROSS, G. G., LEAR, C. S. & DECOU, R. (1976) Modeling the lateral movement of teeth. *J. Biomechanics* **9**, 723–734.

SATOH, T. & HARADA, Y. (1973) Electrophysiological study on tooth-grinding during sleep. *Electroenceph. Clin. Neurophysiol.* **35**, 267–275.

SCHÄRER, P. & STALLARD, R. E. (1965) The use of multiple radio transmitters in studies of tooth contact patterns. *Periodontics* **3**, 5–9.

SHIPLEY, R. A. & CLARK, R. E. (1972) *Tracer methods for in vivo kinetics*, p. 72. London, Academic Press.

SLATTER, J. M. & PICTON, D. C. A. (1972) The effect on intrusive tooth mobility of noradrenaline injected locally in monkeys (*Macaca irus*). *J. Periodont. Res.* **7**, 144–150.

STROMBERG, D. D. & WIEDERHIELM, C. A. (1977) Intravascular and tissue space oncotic and hydrostatic pressure. In: *Microcirculation*, G. KALEY & B. M. ALTURA (eds.), pp. 187–196. Baltimore, University Park Press.

SUIT, S. R., GIBBS, C. G. & BENZ, S. T. (1976) Study of gliding tooth contacts during mastication. *J. Periodont.* **47**, 331–334.

SYNGE, J. L. (1933a) The lightness of teeth, considered as a problem concerning the equilibrium of a thin incompressible elastic membrane. *Phil. Trans. R. Soc. Lond.* **231A**, 435–477.

SYNGE, J. L. (1933b) The equilibrium of a tooth with a general conical root. *Phil. Mag.* **15**, 969–973.

THOMPSON, J. R. (1954) Concepts regarding function of the stomatognathic system. *J. Amer. dent. Assoc.* **48**, 626–637.

TRENOUTH, M. J. (1978) Computer analysis of nocturnal tooth-contact patterns in relation to bruxism and mandibular joint dysfunction in man. *Archs. oral Biol.* **23**, 821–824.

WALKER, T. W., NG, G. C. & BURKE, P. S. (1978) Fluid pressures in the periodontal ligament of the mandibular canine tooth in dogs. *Archs. oral Biol.* **23**, 753–765.

WATT, D. M. (1976) The incidence of abnormal tooth contacts and their detection. In: *Mastication*, D. J. ANDERSON & B. MATTHEWS (eds.), pp. 242–249. Bristol, Wright.

WAUGH, L. M. (1939) Dental observations among Eskimo. VII. *J. dent. Res.* **15**, 355–356.

WILLS, D. J. & MANDERSON, R. D. (1977) Biomechanical aspects of the support of partial dentures. *J. Dentistry* **5**, 310–318.

WILLS, D. J. & PICTON, D. C. A. (1978) Changes in the mobility and resting position of incisor teeth in macaque monkeys. *Archs. oral Biol.* **23**, 225–229.

WILLS, D. J. & PICTON, D. C. A. (1980) The effect on axial tooth mobility of submucosal injections of hyaluronidase in adult *Macaca irus* monkeys. *J. dent. Res.* **59**, Special Issue D, 1841.

WILLS, D. J., PICTON, D. C. A. & DAVIES, W. I. R. (1972) An investigation of the viscoelastic properties of the periodontium in monkeys. *J. periodont. Res.* **7**, 42–51.

WILLS, D. J., PICTON, D. C. A. & DAVIES, W. I. R. (1974) The effect of the rate of application of force on the intrusion of central incisors in adult monkeys (*Macaca irus*). *J. dent. Res.* **53**, 1054.

WILLS, D. J., PICTON, D. C. A. & DAVIES, W. I. R. (1976) A study of the fluid systems of the periodontium in macaque monkeys. *Archs. oral Biol.* **21**, 175–185.

WILLS, D. J., PICTON, D. C. A. & DAVIES, W. I. R. (1978) The intrusion of the tooth for different loading rates. *J. Biomechanics* **11**, 429–434.

WORNER, H. K. & ANDERSON, M. N. (1944) Biting force measurements on children. *Aust. J. Dent.* **48**, 1–12.

YURKSTAS, A. & CURBY, W. A. (1953) Force analysis of prosthetic appliances during function. *J. Prosthet. Dent.* **3**, 82–87.

Chapter 12

THE EFFECTS OF EXTERNAL FORCES ON THE PERIODONTAL LIGAMENT – THE RESPONSE TO HORIZONTAL LOADS

P. Rygh, B. J. Moxham and B. K. B. Berkovitz

Section A.   B. J. Moxham and B. K. B. Berkovitz

INTRODUCTION

A load is termed horizontal (or lateral) if it acts more or less perpendicular to the tooth's longitudinal axis. Horizontal loads are generated physiologically from the oral musculature (lips, cheeks and tongue) and from neighbouring and antagonistic teeth. Indeed, these loads are thought by some to be responsible for producing approximal drifting of teeth (see Chapter 10, pages 237–240). Some estimates are available of the horizontal pressures produced by the tongue and perioral musculature at rest and during various oral functions (e.g. Feldstein, 1950; Winders, 1956, 1958, 1962; Kydd, 1957; Sims, 1958; Gould and Picton, 1964; Proffit et al., 1964; Proffit, Chastain and Norton, 1969; Luffingham, 1968, 1970; Proffit and Norton, 1970; Posen, 1972; Proffit, 1972; Proffit, McGlone and Barrett, 1975; Sakuda et al., 1975; Christiansen, Evans and Sue, 1979). Only small pressures are exerted at rest (less than 0.1 N/cm^2). During speech, swallowing and mastication the pressures increase significantly. Gould and Picton (1964) have recorded pressures as high as 3 N/cm^2 during sip swallowing. It is generally agreed that the lingual musculature is the most active during function and that the maximum loads that can be exerted by the tissues are markedly higher than those produced during normal function. However, there is doubt about the data so far reported since the size and position of the transducers are known to influence the results (Gould and Picton, 1963; Lear et al., 1965; Christiansen et al., 1979). Another common source of horizontal loads is associated with clinical treatment (e.g. from appliances designed for orthodontic purposes). Such loads essentially differ from those produced from physiological sources in that they are continuous.

THE RESPONSE TO HORIZONTAL LOADS OF SHORT DURATION

Horizontal tooth mobility

Experiments on tooth mobility using horizontal loads of short duration are similar in concept and technique to those using axial intrusive loads (Chapter 11). With one exception, the studies described here have used loads in bucco-lingual directions. In all cases the loads were applied to the crowns of the teeth, producing tipping movements.

In 1951 Mühlemann reported a method for measuring horizontal tooth mobility. He employed an intra-orally attached dial indicator to record tooth displacement and a hand-held dynamometer to apply loads. He subsequently published a series of papers describing mobility of Rhesus monkey teeth (Mühlemann, 1954a, b, c; Mühlemann and Zander, 1954). In these, loads ranging from ~0.5 to ~5 N* were applied for 2 sec. It was observed that the mobility for both single and multirooted teeth did not increase linearly with increasing load but showed a 'quasi-logarithmic' relationship (Fig. 1). Initially, there was a relatively marked change in mobility with increasing load. Above ~1 N, a load increase did not have so great an effect. As an example, for the tooth illustrated in Fig. 1 a load of ~1 N produced a displacement of approximately 150 μm. A ~5 N load produced only a further 50 μm displacement. Molars seemed to show slightly less mobility than incisors. If a load was rapidly repeated or was prolonged, an increase in mobility was seen (mainly for loads in the 'initial phase'). The original load/tooth mobility curve was restored after 25 min rest.

*Where the approximately sign (~) is used with forces measured in Newtons : ~1 N ≡ 100 gf.

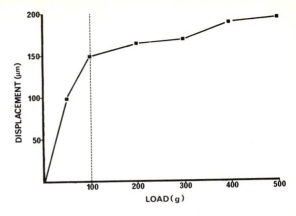

FIG. 1. Graph showing the relationship between horizontal tooth displacement and load for Rhesus monkey teeth. The broken vertical line delineates the initial phase of tooth mobility from the secondary phase.

This pattern of mobility has been confirmed by other workers using a variety of teeth and techniques (e.g. Mühlemann, 1960; Parfitt, 1961; Picton, 1964; Mühlemann, Savdir and Rateitschak, 1965; Picton, 1965; Picton and Davies, 1967; Picton, 1967; Picton, 1969; Christiansen and Burstone, 1969; Picton and Slatter, 1972). Furthermore, as noted by Picton (1969), it resembles the reactions described for axial intrusive loads (see page 253). It is usually claimed, however, that axial loads induce much smaller displacements than horizontal thrusts (e.g. Mühlemann, 1967; Heners, 1974).

The recovery of a tooth on removal of a horizontal load was described by Picton (1964). He studied human maxillary central incisors and first premolars following horizontal thrusts of ~10 N applied at rates of about 10 and 60 per min. He reported that the recovery was in two phases. Initially, there was a fast return of the tooth towards its starting position (in a linear manner with time). As the tooth approached the starting position, a second and logarithmic phase developed. The biphasic recovery response has been reported by others (e.g. Hofmann, 1963; Mühlemann et al., 1965; Körber and Körber, 1967; Körber, 1971; Picton et al., 1974; Ross, Lear and DeCou, 1976).

It has been established that tooth displacement during the application of a horizontal load is time dependent (e.g. Körber, 1971; Ross et al., 1976; Burstone, Pryputniewicz and Bowley, 1978). Figure 2 illustrates the pattern for a human maxillary central

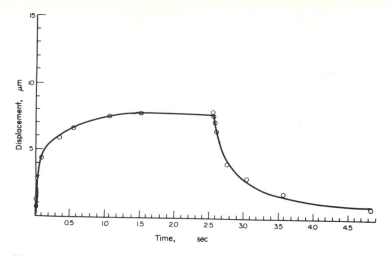

FIG. 2. Graph illustrating the relationship between horizontal tooth displacement and time following the sudden application (and sudden removal) of a lingually directed load of ~0.05 N to a human maxillary central incisor.

incisor following the sudden application and sudden removal of a load observed by Ross *et al.* (1976). Thus, on applying the load there is an initial rapid displacement away from the force, followed by a phase of more gradual displacement. Note also the biphasic response on removal of the load. These responses also show similarities with those obtained with an axial load (see Chapter 11, pages 256 and 262). As for axial loads, attempts have been made to describe the responses in terms of rheological models. The resistance of the periodontal tissues to horizontal loading cannot be explained in terms of a simple linear mechanical model. Whilst the pattern shown in Fig. 2 might suggest a viscoelastic system composed of Maxwell or Voigt elements (springs and dampers in series or in parallel – see page 257 for further explanation), Ross *et al.* (1976) proposed a three-parameter non-linear spring model for the periodontal tissues. As for the attempts to model responses to axial loads, however, further work is necessary to show the biological significance. Furthermore, other physical properties (e.g. thixotropy) may complicate the issue.

Lear, Mackay and Lowe (1972) and Lear, DeCou and Ng (1974) investigated the threshold levels for displacement of human maxillary central incisors and first premolars in response to horizontal forces. For thrusts lasting 100 msec, the threshold was approximately 0.01 N. The thresholds, however, were related to the duration of force. When loads were applied for

25 msec, the threshold was raised to 0.03 N. It is noteworthy that to date most investigators have used horizontal loads much above threshold values.

Whilst the pattern of displacement with horizontal loads of short duration is of significance for appreciating the general mechanical characteristics of the periodontal tissues, the amount of displacement is probably more relevant for assessing the clinical state of the periodontium. However, though there is agreement about the basic pattern, data about amounts of displacement are unreliable because of problems of comparing results from different experiments. Some of these problems are:

1. A variety of teeth and experimental animals have been used.

2. The root length and degree of tilt in the alveolus have not always been considered.

3. There has been no standard loading regime (in terms of the range of loads and duration of application).

4. Different techniques of applying loads and recording displacement have been used. These differ both in terms of sensitivity and in basic principle of design. For example, Mühlemann's (1951) mechanical displacement transducer recorded in units of 10 μm whilst the non-invasive, holographic technique of Burstone and Pryputniewicz (1980) has a stated accuracy of 0.5 μm.

5. As for axial intrusive loads, it has been shown that horizontal mobility is influenced by the rate of loading (Körber and Körber, 1967; Körber, 1971; Lear *et al.*, 1972). Indeed, a marked change can be recorded even for small differences in rate. Körber (1971) reported that for a human maxillary incisor a rate of 500 gf/0.25 sec produced a displacement of about 7 μm, a rate of 500 gf/1 sec a displacement of 36 μm and a rate of 500 gf/2 sec a displacement of 58 μm. As it is not always clear in most reports whether loading was instantaneous, complications in comparing data might arise if even slight differences in loading rate occurred.

6. Most studies have applied loads in bucco-lingual directions. Picton and Slatter (1972) studied the effects of mesio-distally directed loads following removal of contact points. Even with bucco-lingual loads, the presence of tooth contacts may influence the results. Mühlemann (1954b) reported that removal of contact points can produce an increase in mobility. Thus, in the absence of comment about tooth contacts in most reports should we assume that all the teeth were able to move in a similar unrestricted manner?

7. It is reasonable to assume that the functional state of the tooth influences mobility. It has been shown that the previous loading history affects tooth mobility. Indeed, some studies using axial intrusive loads employ a standard series of conditioning thrusts prior to the experiment proper (e.g. Wills, Picton and Davies, 1978). The work of Mühlemann (1954b) and Körber (1971) suggests that there is also a change in mobility if experiments using horizontal loads are preceded by priming thrusts. Mühlemann (1960, 1967) stated that mobility is greater in children and young adults, in females, and during pregnancy. Himmel *et al.* (1957) and O'Leary, Rudd and Nabers (1966) claim that mobility is lowest in the evening and highest in the morning on awaking. O'Leary *et al.* (1966) also showed that lack of occlusal contact can affect tooth mobility. Mühlemann (1954a) has reported that erupting teeth have greater mobility than erupted teeth. In most studies on horizontal mobility the functional state of the teeth is not considered and conceivably there could be markedly different states in different studies.

8. Since horizontal loads produce tipping movements, it is important to have a standardized point both for applying loads and for measuring displace-ment. Details of the placement of the apparatus are not always given, and it is unlikely that such points correspond in different studies.

Recently, holography has been employed to study horizontal mobility (Bowley *et al.*, 1974; Pryputnie-wicz, Burstone and Bowley, 1978; Burstone *et al.*, 1978; Pryputniewicz and Burstone, 1979; Burstone and Pryputniewicz, 1980). Because of its sensitivity, such a technique seems likely to provide many precise data about the force–displacement characteristics of human teeth. Burstone and Pryputniewicz (1980) claim that previous work is unreliable primarily because the experiments used techniques which were relatively inaccurate, could not measure three-dimensional displacements and, being invasive, influenced the tooth movement. Figure 3 shows an example of the relationship between displacement and time observed with a labially directed ∼ 3 N load reported by Burstone *et al.* (1978). Whilst the largest motion is as expected in the lingual–labial direction, there is also an extrusion and displacement mesio-distally.

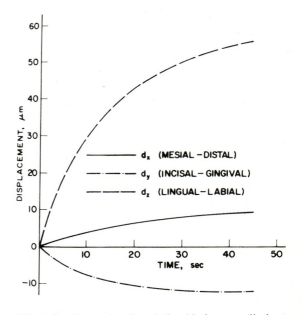

FIG. 3. Graph showing the relationship between displacement (in three dimensions) and time from the instant of the application of a force (∼ 3 N in lingual–labial direction, parallel to the occlusal plane) for a human maxillary central incisor.

The centre of rotation with horizontal loads

A horizontal load applied to the crown of a tooth will tip the tooth around a centre of rotation. Mühlemann (1951) suggested that this centre varied in position according to the size and angulation of the load. Mühlemann and Houglum (1954) and Mühlemann and Zander (1954) described techniques for estimating rotation centres in single-rooted teeth. The latter study indicated that the rotation centre varied with the size of the load and the type of tooth. However, Haack and Weinstein (1963) claim that a force directed at a given point in a given direction produced the same rotation centre regardless of magnitude.

Christiansen and Burstone (1969) determined the centres of rotation of human maxillary central incisors using lingual, labial and mesial tipping loads ranging from about 0.2 N to about 7 N. They reported that the centre is related not to the magnitude of load but to the moment-to-force ratio. A theoretical rotation centre was calculated based upon a formula devised according to the concepts of Burstone (1962): Moment-to-force ratio $= 0.068h^2/y$ where h is alveolar crest to root apex distance, y is the distance between the centre of rotation and the 'centoid' (a point 40% of the distance apical to the distance between the alveolar crest and the root apex). The formula assumes that the tooth is in equilibrium, that the stress distribution is uniform along the root, and that the stress/strain ratio is uniform or linear. The theoretical rotation centre was found by Christiansen and Burstone to be about 55% of the distance from the apex to the alveolar crest. The theoretical centre was compared with experimentally determined centres for the incisors of six subjects. For three subjects, the experimental centre closely approximated the theoretical centre with loads above 0.5 N.

A tooth-periodontium model based upon plane elasticity theory and plane photoelasticity has been devised by Nikolai (1974) to enable determination of the location of rotation centres in single-rooted teeth with horizontal crown loading. It was assumed that the periodontal ligament is homogeneous and isotropic, exhibits Hookean behaviour, is residual stress-free, and that the crown load is transferred totally and in a continuously-distributed manner across the root–ligament boundary. It was claimed that the rotation centres determined using the model were located only slightly occlusal to that predicted according to the concepts of Burstone (1962). However, this model (like Burstone's) is two-dimensional and some of the assumptions seem erroneous. Furthermore, the time-dependent behaviour of the tissues is not considered.

Using holography, Burstone *et al.* (1978) and Pryputniewicz and Burstone (1979) determined rotation centres for some human maxillary incisors with labially directed loads of ~ 3 N or ~ 5 N. Pryputniewicz and Burstone (1979) reported that, with a slight modification to the formula used by Christiansen and Burstone (1969), the theoretical centre fitted reasonably with the experimentally determined centre. They also reported differences in the rotation centre with ~ 3 N and ~ 5 N loads. However, unlike previous views that higher loads moved rotation centres coronally, the centre for the higher load was moved apically. The results also showed that the longer the root the further apical the rotation centre. Despite the apparent errors and/or conceptual limitations involved in formulating theoretical models, it is remarkable that the experimental data from this study should still show reasonable fit. Pryputniewicz and Burstone (1979) were of the opinion that the minor discrepancies could be attributed to differences between a two-dimensional model with linear properties of the periodontal ligament and a three-dimensional *in vivo* situation with a ligament having non-linear characteristics.

The biological mechanisms involved in the support against horizontal loads

Since the pattern of mobility with horizontal loads has similarities with that for axial loads, it is likely that the mechanisms involved in the resistance of the periodontal tissues to these loads are similar.

Mühlemann (1951) noted that the biphasic pattern of mobility was lost in human ankylosed teeth. He concluded that the normal pattern for horizontal mobility was a function of the periodontal ligament. From light microscopic observations, Mühlemann (1954a) and Mühlemann and Zander (1954) claimed that the amount of initial tooth mobility was related to the degree of organization of the periodontal ligament. A loosely structured ligament appeared to show more mobility than one with densely organized collagen fibres. Mühlemann and Zander (1954) stated that the first phase of mobility with loads below 1 N is due to an intra-alveolar tipping of the tooth with reorientation of the fibre bundles. With a load at the transition between the first and second phase (~ 1 N), they claimed that the already stretched fibre bundles on the tension side resisted any further root displacement and prevented a further increase of the periodontal width on that side. Higher loads were thought to lead to distortion and compression of the periodontium with deformation of the alveolar bone.

The role of the periodontal tissues in resisting horizontal loads has been evaluated further by observations of the displacement of the alveolar margins (Picton, 1965) and by tooth-mobility studies following surgical trauma to the gingival and periodontal tissues (Picton, 1967, Picton and Slatter, 1972). All three investigations were conducted on monkey teeth.

Picton (1965) reported that, with loads of ~ 2.5 N applied labially or lingually, the lingual and labial alveolar margins were usually displaced in the same direction as the applied force. The amount of displacement was similar for both margins. He thus confirmed that horizontal loads produced a combination of compression and tension in different regions of the periodontium. Unlike Mühlemann and Zander (1954), Picton noted that bone distortion occurred with loads less than 1 N (often with loads as low as ~ 0.5 N).

Picton (1967) studied the effects of traumatizing the periodontal tissues on the mesial and distal surfaces of maxillary incisor teeth subjected to loads in labio-palatal directions. Little change in tooth mobility was seen (though forces applied labially seemed to show a slight increase). He concluded that limited areas of the periodontal ligament tangential to the load may be traumatized without gross disturbance of the mechanisms of tooth support.

Picton and Slatter (1972) assessed the effects of traumatizing the periodontal tissues on the mesial or distal surfaces of incisors subjected to loads applied in mesial and distal directions. They reported an increase in mobility whether the tooth was displaced towards or away from the site of trauma. They again concluded that tension and compression operate when a horizontal load is applied to a tooth, both appearing to be of equal importance.

As for axial loads, we believe that a biological interpretation of the patterns of horizontal mobility is speculative unless supported by experiments involving observations of the consequences of imposing selective changes to the periodontium. However, little work has been conducted using this approach. Mühlemann (1954c) studied the effects of heat or formalin treatment on teeth in dissected monkey jaws. He claimed that these treatments abolished the initial phase of tooth mobility and reduced the amount of secondary mobility. He suggested that these results could be explained in terms of an alteration in the periodontal fibres. The unphysiological nature of these *in vitro* experiments cast doubt on this interpretation, especially since it has been shown that tissue fluids and vasculature play a role in the tooth support mechanism (see pages 260, 261). Indeed, Körber (1962) has reported that hyperaemia and the local injection of vasoconstrictors influence horizontal tooth mobility. Furthermore, the experiments of Packman, Schoher and Stein (1977) suggest that horizontal loading can affect blood flow in the periodontal ligament (see Chapter 7, page 162). It was concluded in Chapter 11 that the support mechanism for axial loads was likely to be a function of the periodontal tissues as a whole and was not reliant upon any single element. In view of the many similarities between the responses of a tooth to axial and horizontal loads, it is tempting to deduce a similar conclusion for the support mechanism for horizontal loads.

THE EFFECTS OF HORIZONTAL ORTHODONTIC LOADS ON TOOTH DISPLACEMENT

The histological changes occurring within the periodontal ligament following orthodontic loading is discussed in detail in the succeeding section. Here we will describe briefly the pattern of tooth movements in response to orthodontic loads of long duration which produce tilting. Little information is available concerning the threshold force for such movements. Bass and Stephens (1970) suggest that orthodontic movements are unlikely to occur with forces below 0.1 N. (This compares with the 1.5 N to 3 N loads which are necessary to move a tooth bodily (Storey and Smith, 1952).)

Crabb and Wilson (1972) determined the rate of space closure between maxillary canines and second premolars following extraction of the maxillary first premolars. The forces applied to the canines were in the range of 0.3 N to 0.5 N. The springs were reactivated every 28 days. The results indicate a mean rate of space closure of about 1 mm/28 days.

Reitan (1975) has described several phases associated with orthodontic tooth movement (Fig. 4). With light, continuous, orthodontic loads, it seems to take on average 5 days before the periodontal tissues are compressed to the point where there is a cessation of tooth movement. This period is shortened with excessive loads. There then follows a period of about 2 to 3 weeks during which the tooth shows only minor changes in position. However, a secondary period of tooth movement occurs after undermining of the bone. The pattern shown in Fig. 4 is typical of the reactions which occur when the load is not regularly reactivated. Figure 5 shows the pattern which occurs when a load is strictly maintained with frequent reactivation.

Following the removal of an orthodontic load, there is a period of recovery or relapse. Figure 6

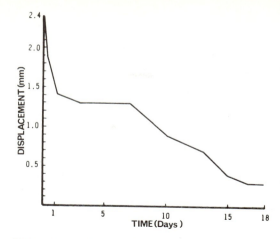

FIG. 6. Graph showing the relationship between the degree of relapse and time, following labial tipping of a maxillary lateral incisor with a force of ~ 0.4 N.

illustrates a case of relapse reported by Reitan (1967). Note that in this instance there was considerable relapse during the first day after the orthodontic appliances had been removed. Thereafter, relapse may be prevented for a short while by periodontal changes or new bone formation.

Section B.   P. Rygh

THE HISTOLOGICAL RESPONSES OF THE PERIODONTAL LIGAMENT TO HORIZONTAL ORTHODONTIC LOADS

Introduction

A load acting more or less perpendicular to the longitudinal axis of a tooth produces wide areas of pressure on one side of the root and corresponding areas of tension on the other. If the force could be placed near the centre of the root (through its centre of resistance) a translation or bodily movement of the tooth would be produced, with a relatively uniform distribution of pressure on one side of the root and of tension on the other (Fig. 7a). In practice, to produce translation for orthodontic treatment forces have to be applied against the crown of the tooth via some system that will ensure a two point contact (e.g. as seen in the edgewise technique where brackets or tubes allow closely fitting rectangular arches to produce the necessary

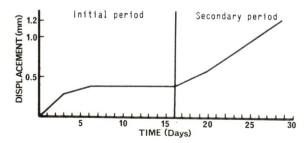

FIG. 4. Graph illustrating the relationship between tooth displacement and time following the application of a light orthodontic load.

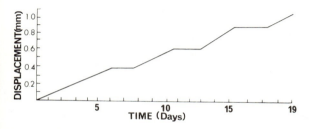

FIG. 5. Graph showing the relationship between tooth displacement and time following the application of an orthodontic load which was frequently reactivated.

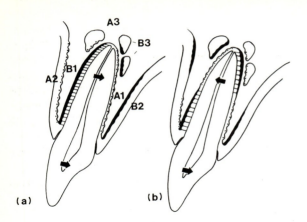

FIG. 7. (a) Translation of tooth with uniform distribution of pressure on one side of the root. Bone resorption occurs along the alveolar surface (A1) on the pressure side, on the labial surface of the alveolar process (A2), and in marrow spaces (A3). Bone deposition occurs along the alveolar surface (B1) on the tension side, on the lingual surface of the alveolar process (B2) and in marrow spaces (B3). (b) Tipping of tooth with pressure and tension zones on both sides of the root.

couple). A tipping movement can easily occur as a result of the application of a horizontal force unless special precautions are taken. The point of rotation for such movement varies, depending on the site of force application, the shape of the tooth and the architecture of the tooth's supporting system. The result is that crown and root tip in opposite directions (Fig. 7b), producing pressure and tension zones on either side of the root and a varying distribution of stress. This means that the load produced is concentrated in localized areas of the periodontal ligament. There are two major advantages to using horizontal forces for orthodontic purposes which produce bodily movement of the tooth as opposed to forces which produce tipping movements. Firstly, the end result appears to be more stable (e.g. Reitan, 1975). Secondly, since in producing translation loads are dissipated over the entire side of the tooth, there is greater control of the applied forces. On the other hand, the magnitude of the force is difficult to control with tipping because of the localized concentration of stresses in the periodontal ligament.

By applying horizontal forces to a tooth, pressure and tension areas are induced along the root surfaces. In such zones, it is reasonable to assume that the fibrous part of the periodontal ligament and the 'viscoelastic' shock-absorbing system are not being activated uniformly and that the resulting morphological changes within the periodontal ligament will differ where the tooth is pressed against the alveolar wall and where it is drawn away from it.

Responses on the tension side

When a horizontal force of 15 g or more is applied to the crown of a tooth, the periodontal space will become wider on the side where the tooth is drawn away from the alveolar bone. Bundles of fibres are stretched and the alveolar crest is pulled in the same direction (Fig. 7a).

If the tooth is stabilized in the new position by a continuous force, a number of cellular processes are activated within the periodontal ligament. There is an increase in the number of connective tissue cells by cell division. For young humans, incipient cell proliferation is seen after 30–40 hours, particularly near the socket wall. Shortly after, osteoid tissue will be deposited on the wall (Fig. 8). Where the fibrous bundles are thick, new bone appears to be deposited along them. If the bundles are thin, a more uniform layer is deposited along the root surface (Reitan, 1951). Calcification in the deeper layers of the osteoid starts shortly after, while the superficial part remains uncalcified.

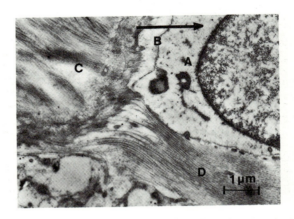

FIG. 8. Electron micrograph of the periodontal ligament on the tension side of a rat first molar following experimental movement in direction of arrow for 7 days. Osteoblast (A) deposits osteoid (B) on the surface of the alveolar bone (C). Collagen fibre (D) inserts into the new bone. ×9000.

Metabolic activity during experimental tooth movement has been studied autoradiographically. Crumley (1964) observed that incorporation of ^{3}H-proline was increased slightly on the tension side of rat molars, while Baumrind and Buck (1970) found an initial decline in the uptake of this labelled amino acid.

The blood vessels appear to be distended. In longitudinal sections of the tooth, fibroblasts in the periodontal ligament are oriented in the same direction as the principal fibres: in the direction of strain. The fibroblasts appear spindle-shaped. The cells adjacent to the alveolar wall often appear more spherical (Fig. 9).

It has been thought that periodontal ligament fibres at the alveolar bone surface became entrapped passively by the advancing front of new bone formation to form Sharpey's fibres (e.g. Kraw and Enlow, 1967). However, recent findings suggest that new Sharpey's fibres are secreted simultaneously with new bone deposition. As the fibroblasts migrate from the bone, they may deposit either entirely new Sharpey's fibres or new fibrils which are incorporated into existing fibres (Garant and Cho, 1979).

Techniques have recently been developed to differentiate older from newer collagen. Such techniques rely upon the combination of oxidation and staining of specimens by aldehyde fuchsin (e.g. Halmi) similar to the procedures which are used for the identification of oxytalan (Rygh, in preparation). Preliminary findings suggest that, with slow physiological tooth movement, there is entrapment of older, 'mature', Sharpey's fibrils by the advancing bone front (Fig. 10). With orthodontic loads, however, in the tension zone there is both an incorporation of pre-existing collagen fibres into new osteoid and a considerable production of new collagen fibres near the advancing bone front (Fig. 11). It can be argued that such features reflect the need for more rapid remodelling in this situation. Whilst part of the newly synthesized collagen will be incorporated into the new osteoid, some will be incorporated into the periodontal ligament (Fig. 12), perhaps associated with the increase in width on the tension side (Rygh, 1976). Lengthening of fibres

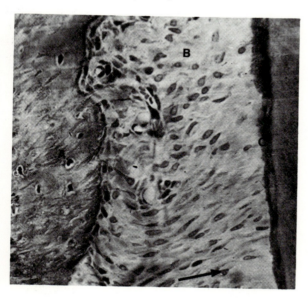

FIG. 9. Longitudinal section of periodontal ligament under tension on the buccal side of a rat first molar moved by continuous force for 28 days. The region is close to the alveolar crest. A, Alveolar bone. B, Periodontal ligament. C, Cementum. In this plane, the fibroblasts are spindle-shaped and oriented in the direction of pull (arrow) while the cells adjacent to the alveolar wall are more rounded. ×350.

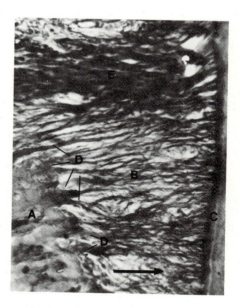

FIG. 10. Longitudinal section of periodontal ligament at the alveolar crest region of a rat first molar undergoing physiological movement in direction of arrow. A, Alveolar bone. B, Periodontal ligament. C, Cementum. Note entrapment of Sharpey's fibres (D) by advancing bone front. Transseptal fibres (E) are more heavily stained than the dentoalveolar fibres. (Aldehyde-fuchsin Halmi after oxidation. ×270.)

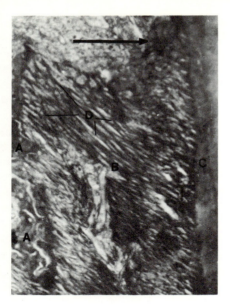

FIG. 11. Longitudinal section of inter-radicular periodontal ligament on the tension side of rat first molar 21 days after being moved experimentally by a continuous force. Arrow, direction of force. A, Alveolar bone. B, Periodontal ligament. C, Cementum. Darkly stained stretched dentoalveolar fibres (D) are remodelled without being removed. (Compare pressure side Fig. 15.) (Aldehyde-fuchsin Halmi after oxidation. × 270.)

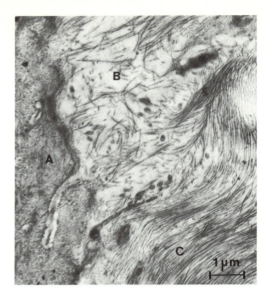

FIG. 12. Electron micrograph of the tension side of rat periodontal ligament adjacent to alveolar bone (A) 15 days after being moved experimentally by a continuous force. Note the loosely arranged un-oriented collagen fibrils (B) as well as the fibre bundle (C). × 9000.

seems also to occur by incorporation of new fibrils into existing fibres (even at some distance from the alveolar bone wall).

There is no evidence that an extensive breakdown of the collagen fibres occurs on the tension side of the periodontal ligament in an intermediate zone (see Fig. 11). Furthermore, Freeman and Ten Cate (1978) did not discern any localized concentration of fibro-blasts with intracellular collagen profiles on the tension side of the periodontal ligament of rat molars. The reason may be that the need for reorientation is small in areas where the tooth is to be moved in the same direction as the fibres are orientated.

Responses on the pressure side

On the side of the periodontal ligament towards which

a tooth is moved, the periodontal space becomes narrower. The crest of the alveolar bone is slightly deformed. Assuming the applied force is sufficiently strong and is maintained for long enough, certain cell processes will occur within the periodontal ligament and on the surfaces of the alveolar bone.

Similarities exist between changes elicited by experimental, orthodontic-like forces and the remodel-ling changes of the supporting tissues of teeth with physiological migration. Histological studies of the periodontal ligaments of such teeth show resorption of the alveolar bone surface on the side towards which the tooth is moving (e.g. Reitan, 1951; Kraw and Enlow, 1967). However, whereas with physio-logical migration the number of osteoclasts is usually low (indicating a rather slow process), orthodontic-like forces elicit more dramatic changes. Such changes can be categorized broadly into 'direct resorption' where the pressure is relatively light and 'hyalinization' where the pressure is large enough to produce degenera-tive changes.

DIRECT RESORPTION

Some hours after the application of a horizontal orthodontic force of the order of 30—100 g to a human premolar, osteoclasts can be seen in the periodontal ligament along the alveolar bone surface. In children aged between 10—13 years, Reitan (1951) occasionally found evidence of resorption after 12 hours, though invariably by 40 hours. With optimum force after 3—4 days, numerous osteoclasts are present along the alveolar wall. In light-microscopical sections a clear zone often separates resorbing cells from the bone (Fig. 13). This artefact appears to be related to the destruction of both alveolar bone and Sharpey's fibres. With the electron microscope, however, the ruffled border of osteoclasts is seen to be in close contact with the resorbing bone surface (Fig. 14) and both crystals and collagen fibres may be found between the cell processes. Garant (1976) has observed fibro-

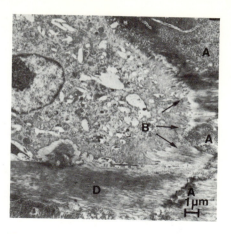

FIG. 14. Detail of pressure area corresponding to Fig. 13. Alveolar bone (A) is resorbed by osteoclast (B). Note intimate contact between bone and the osteoclast's ruffled border area (arrows). The adjacent Sharpey's fibre (D) does not seem to be affected by the osteoclast. (Electron micrograph of demineralized section. ×2800.)

blasts with increased amounts of intracellular collagen profiles near osteoclasts in the periodontal ligaments of rat molars and the question remains as to whether such fibroblasts may also play a role in bone resorption.

As revealed by the special staining techniques previously referred to (Rygh, in preparation), there is extensive remodelling of collagen throughout the periodontal ligament (with the possible exception of Sharpey's fibres at the root surface (Fig. 15)). At the same time there is formation of new collagen which becomes attached to the alveolar bone by localized bone apposition (Fig. 16). Collagen detached from alveolar bone during resorptive activity may become reattached to bone or to pre-existing periodontal collagen fibres by the local activity of osteoblasts or fibroblasts respectively (Beertsen, 1975, 1979).

The precise pathway whereby degraded collagen is removed has still to be determined. Freeman and Ten Cate (1978) implicate periodontal fibroblasts because of the presence within many of these cells of intracellular collagen profiles. However, compressed collagen in hyalinized zones is probably removed by macrophages (Rygh, 1974).

During physiological migration, resorption of collagen may occur in a selective manner. It is possible

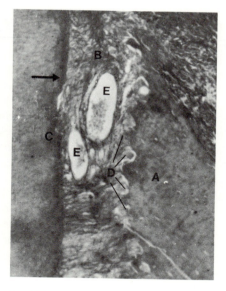

FIG. 13. Longitudinal section of the pressure (mesial) side of the periodontal ligament of a rat first molar moved experimentally by a continuous force for 3 weeks, near the alveolar crest region. Arrow, direction of force. A, Alveolar bone. B, Periodontal ligament (note width). C, Cementum. Direct resorption by osteoclasts (D). E, Blood vessels. Note the clear zone between the osteoclasts and the surface of the alveolar bone. (Aldehyde-fuchsin Halmi after oxidation. ×230.)

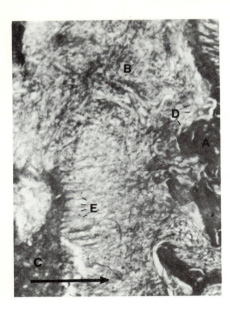

FIG. 15. Longitudinal section of inter-radicular periodontal ligament on the pressure side of a rat first molar 21 days after being moved experimentally by continuous force. Arrow, direction of force. A, Alveolar bone. B, Periodontal ligament. C, Cementum. Resorption by osteoclasts (D) of alveolar wall. Note the relative absence of principal fibre bundles of Sharpey's fibres throughout the periodontal ligament as indicated by the lighter staining of the majority of the fibres (compare Fig. 11). Some denser staining structures (E) indicate older fibres inserting into the cementum. (Aldehyde-fuchsin Halmi after oxidation. ×270.)

The rich supply of blood vessels within the periodontal ligament may play a role in the mechanisms of tooth support (see Chapter 11), though little is known concerning their reaction to moderate pressure. However, unless an adequate vascular supply is present, the differentiation of specialized cells will not take place. The periodontal vasculature ought to be capable, therefore, of compensating for any increased pressure associated with the initial narrowing of the periodontal ligament.

The width of the periodontal space seems to be important in determining the reactions of the ligament to load and is itself directly related to the functional state of the tooth. Recently erupted teeth in children have a wider periodontal ligament than those in adults (and particularly those not in function such as impacted teeth where the width of the ligament may only be one-third of that seen in erupted teeth (Coolidge, 1937)) and this may help explain why children's teeth are more easily moved orthodontically. Under non-pathological conditions, the width of the periodontal ligament will give an indication of its capacity for remodelling during the initial phase of increased loading of the tooth. With extensive direct resorption of the socket wall as the result of the application of orthodontic forces, the width of the ligament is increased (Fig. 13). Only during the initial phase of orthodontic tooth movement and after reactivation of an applied force is there a narrowing of the ligament on the pressure side.

HYALINIZATION

Increased pressure in a localized region of the periodontal ligament can exceed easily the optimum and inhibit the differentiation of osteoclasts. As a result, the direct resorption of alveolar bone that would 'relieve' the pressure in the ligament cannot occur. Instead, a series of degenerative tissue reactions take place, commencing within a few hours. The term 'hyalinization' is used to describe these tissue reactions, owing to the fact that the degenerated tissue has a glass-like appearance in routine histological sections. The presence of hyalinization has been interpreted by Kardos and Simpson (1980) as representing a change in consistency of the collagenous matrix rather than its degeneration, and providing evidence

that this ensures that at any given time most of the supporting apparatus of the tooth remains intact.

Little is known about the reaction of the ground substance of the periodontal ligament in areas subjected to pressure of long duration. The ground substance appears to be the major water-binding constituent of connective tissues (Schubert and Hamerman, 1968). Even though it is presumed that both bound and unbound water are present in the periodontal ligament, it is not known whether there is movement of water between the vascular and extra-vascular compartments during loading and unloading of a tooth (Melcher and Walker, 1976). The question of whether ground substance will flow (and under what conditions) is still unanswered.

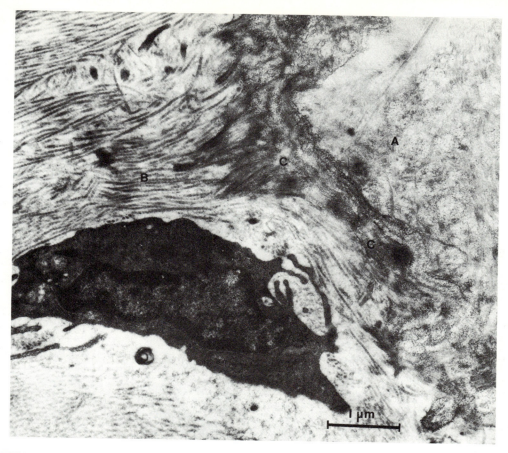

FIG. 16. Electron micrograph of rat periodontal ligament on the pressure side 21 days after being moved experimentally by continuous force. A, Alveolar bone. B, New periodontal collagen fibrils becoming attached by deposition of new bone (C). (Decalcified section. ×18,000.)

that the periodontal ligament has the properties of a thixotropic gel.

With experimental labial tipping of, for example, a human incisor or premolar, a pronounced pressure zone in the periodontal ligament is seen after 2 days. Tissue changes within the periodontal ligament (Fig. 17) are characterized by oedema, gradual obliteration of blood vessels and the breakdown of vein walls. The vascular changes are followed by leakage of blood constituents into the extravascular space.

Changes in the fibroblasts are also seen. These often begin with moderate swelling of the endoplasmic reticulum (Fig. 18a). More extensive swelling and the formation of vacuoles occur later (Fig. 18b), followed by rupture of the cytoplasmic membrane and loss of

cytoplasm (Rygh, 1972b). This leaves isolated nuclei which undergo lysis over a period of several weeks (Fig. 18c).

Rygh (1973b) has shown that after 3–5 weeks some of the collagen fibrils undergo a longitudinal splitting. However, most collagen retains its typical banded appearance and is altered less than was assumed previously (e.g. Kvam, 1972).

It is not known what happens to the ground substance in a hyalinized zone. It is possible that, as long as ground substance remains in the periodontal ligament, the tissue will show its glass-like appearance. With long-acting, heavy compression, the ground substance and tissue fluid can be squeezed out of the compressed zone, reducing the distance between the

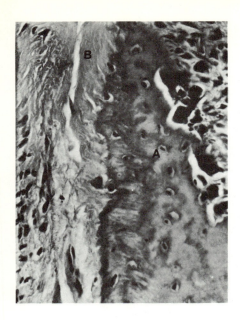

FIG. 17. Longitudinal section of dog periodontal ligament in region of alveolar crest
21 days after application of continuous force.
A, Indirect resorption of buccal alveolar bone
from external surface. B, Hyalinized area.
×360.

tooth and alveolar wall to 5−10 μm (Rygh, 1977).

The degenerative processes of the different tissue components persist as long as the pressure is maintained and, in so doing, prevent recolonization of the damaged tissue by cells from the adjacent, undamaged periodontal ligament (Rygh, 1972a). With time, accumulated erythocyte breakdown products in the pressure region may undergo crystallization (Fig. 19).

All tooth movement stops until the adjacent bone is resorbed by cells that differentiate on its spongiosa surface or subperiosteally where there is no cancellous bone between the lamina dura and the external cortical bone (Fig. 17). This indirect or 'undermining' resorption occurs simultaneously with the invasion of phagocytosing cells from the peripheral undamaged ligament. All tissue components (including collagen) damaged during compression are removed eventually (Fig. 20).

These observations may contribute to our understanding of root resorption which may occur following the application of orthodontic loads (Rygh, 1976). In such situations, there is hyalinization of areas of periodontal ligament. This is followed not only by

removal of the damaged hyalinized tissue, but also of the adjacent unmineralized cementoid. Thus, there is loss of tissues which protect the root surface against resorbing cells.

Hyalinization occurs commonly during the initial phase following application of an orthodontic force. It is important to stress that tooth movement will not occur until undermining resorption of the alveolar bone has been accomplished. During tipping movements, an area of compression (as seen in the alveolar crestal regions) can act as a fulcrum (Fig. 7b).

Hyalinized areas are normally removed after a 3−5-week period, provided that if any further force is to be applied there is only gentle reactivation. The 'post-hyalinized' periodontal ligament under pressure is markedly wider than before, presumably in order to withstand the greater mechanical influences. If the orthodontic loads are now removed, the original width is rapidly attained.

Reitan (1961) has studied the behaviour of epithelial cell rests in teeth subjected to orthodontic loads. He observed that there was no regeneration of the epithelial cells following regeneration of hyalinized connective tissue.

With the moderate orthodontic forces now used clinically, hyalinized zones usually are confined to only a localized area of the periodontal ligament, about 1−2 mm in length.

Reactions on other root surfaces

In addition to the pressure and tension sides of the root, there are two lateral root surfaces of the tooth to consider. Figure 21 diagrammatically shows the changes occurring in these regions during tooth movement. In the areas of the periodontal ligament corresponding to such lateral surfaces, extensive reorientation of collagen fibres occurs (Rygh, in preparation). Furthermore, the insertion of these fibres into alveolar bone (and presumably the arrangement of the ground substance) is undergoing restructuring and reorientation. Such remodelling may be needed to ensure stability after orthodontic tooth movement. It is likely that this point has been underestimated with regard to the tendency for relapse.

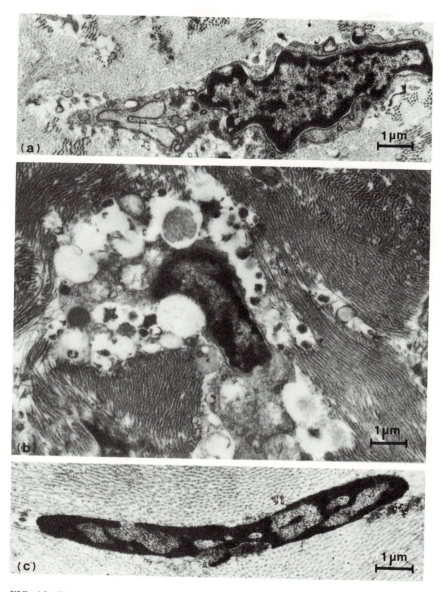

FIG. 18. Electron micrograph showing degenerative changes within periodontal fibroblasts during hyalinization of the periodontal ligament following application of continuous force of 10 g: (a) swelling of endoplasmic reticulum (duration of force 30 min); (b) advanced swelling with formation of vacuoles (duration of force 2 h); (c) cell nucleus during breakdown (duration of force 2 h). ×9000.

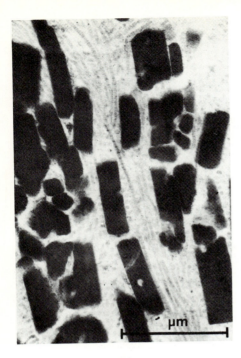

FIG. 19. Electron micrograph of periodontal ligament showing formation of crystals during breakdown of erythrocytes in hyalinized zone following application of continuous force for 2 days. ×29,000.

Some reactions in other supporting tissues

The remodelling of the periodontal ligament is only one aspect of the alteration of the tooth-supporting tissues under load. The pattern of reactions in the periodontal ligament is dependent on the architecture of the surrounding structures and must therefore be seen in relation to the response in these tissues. When a tooth moves into a new position as a response to a change in its environment, the supporting structures move with it. The architecture of the supporting structures (i.e. gingiva, periodontal ligament and the alveolar bone) is under continuous adjustment, according to functional demands.

ALVEOLAR BONE

On both the pressure and tension side, one sees resorption and deposition processes occurring on both the endosteal and the periosteal aspects.

Generally, direct resorption of the alveolar wall is accompanied by deposition of bone on the opposite surface. In this way constant dimensions of the alveolar bone are maintained (Fig. 7a). The alveolar wall adjacent to a hyalinized area of periodontal ligament is resorbed from the spongiosa aspect. However, where the bone is of a more compact nature, it resorbs directly from its external surface (Figs. 7b, 17). At the same time, osteoclasts differentiate from the relatively normal periodontal ligament tissue at the periphery of the hyalinized zone (Reitan, 1951; Rygh, 1973a). Such osteoclasts resorb alveolar bone and allow some relocation of the tooth.

Since remodelling of bone by resorption and deposition is mediated by cells situated on bone surfaces, the architecture of the bone will have an important bearing on the rate of tooth movement following loading. Thus, in cancellous bone with thin trabeculae and a large number of osteogenic cells, the greater cell surface area will provide a favourable environment for rapid remodelling and therefore rapid tooth movement. This is especially evident with teeth that are moved into new extraction sites. In the cell-rich tissue that fills and re-establishes the alveolus, orthodontic remodelling occurs very quickly. For example, under optimal conditions a maxillary canine can be moved by translation a full tooth's breadth into the extraction space of a first premolar within 100 days.

In compact (cortical) bone, resorption must occur either from the inner alveolar or outer periosteal surfaces (Fig. 7b). If the endosteal surface of cortical bone bordering a hyalinized zone is thick, direct resorption from the outer alveolar side can take a considerable time (Reitan, 1951). In this situation, compensatory bone deposition may not occur, the overall result being a loss of some alveolar bone. Such a problem arises with labial movement or extrusion of teeth when using large forces. It has been claimed that compensatory deposition does not occur on the bony aspect adjacent to hyalinized areas (Melcher, 1976). Nevertheless, deposition of bone may be observed close to compressed areas (Fig. 22). This may be due to rapid development of excessive pressures changing the situation or, in young individuals, compensatory strengthening of the alveolar bone.

In orthodontic treatment where a pronounced horizontal tooth movement is desired, one ought to

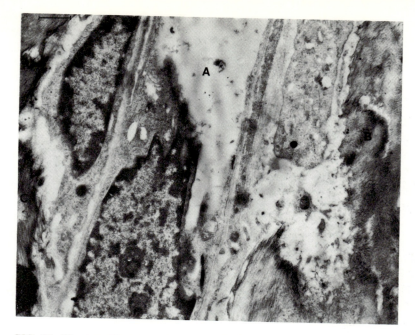

FIG. 20. Electron micrograph showing a blood vessel (A) invading a hyalinized zone and occupying the entire space between the alveolar bone (B) and cementum (C) 5 days following application of continuous force. All periodontal structures have been removed. ×8000.

use moderate forces that will be distributed as evenly as possible over the pressure side. This will ensure that direct resorption can occur. During treatment planning, the means by which the force is to be applied (as well as the amount) should be considered carefully with respect to the shape of the tooth and to the structure of the surrounding supporting tissues.

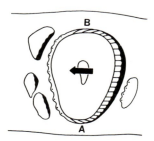

FIG. 21. Diagram illustrating the extensive reorientation of fibrous and other elements on the lingual (A) and buccal (B) aspects of the periodontal ligament during tooth movement.

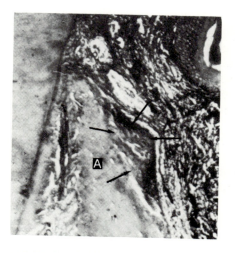

FIG. 22. Longitudinal section of periodontal ligament of rat first molar near the alveolar crest 14 days after application of continuous force. Note the compensatory bone deposition (arrows) on the external surface of the buccal alveolar bone (A). (Aldehyde-fuchsin Halmi oxidation. ×180.)

It is often possible to move a tooth through cancellous bone instead of cortical bone, providing such factors are considered.

GINGIVA

In certain types of orthodontic tooth movement relapse to the original position is thought to involve the supra-alveolar structures. Reitan (1959) found that after rotation of maxillary lateral incisors in the dog, the gingival fibre bundles remained stretched and displaced 33 weeks later. However, the principal fibres of the periodontal ligament readjusted very rapidly. Furthermore, it has been shown that gingivectomy and surgical circumferential incision of gingival fibres may reduce relapse to a considerable extent (e.g. Edwards, 1968). Pinson and Strahan (1974) reduced relapse after rotation by approximately 50% following surgical division of the gingival fibres.

It has been suggested that the slower remodelling of gingival structures is due to slower collagen turnover in gingival tissue than in the periodontal ligament (Skougaard, Levi and Simpson, 1969; Sodek, 1977). Further evidence for differences between gingival and periodontal ligament collagen fibres has been derived from special staining techniques (Fig. 10). The reasons for such differences remain unknown. One possibility may relate to the fact that many gingival fibres are not attached into alveolar bone. Among the important groups of gingival fibres are the transseptal fibres which, by some as yet unknown mechanism, have been implicated in the process of approximal drift (see Chapter 10).

Transmission of mechanical influences into cellular reactions

Many hypotheses have been put forward to explain the increased mitotic activity and differentiation into specialized cells of mesenchymal cells in the periodontal ligament of a tooth that has been exposed to an external force. Alterations in the availability of circulating hormones or alterations in the surface properties of the cells could occur. Calcium ions and cyclic AMP are known to influence mitosis as do inhibitors secreted by the cells themselves (Melcher, 1976). Oxygen tension and pH in the microenvironment influence resorption and deposition of bone. Melcher (1976) postulates that cells of the periodontal tissues secrete substances capable of stimulating differentiation of osteoclasts and osteoblasts in response to appropriate stimuli. However, there is evidence to show that osteoclasts are derived from haemopoietic cells and transported via the circulation. This, together with details concerning cell kinetics within the periodontal ligament, is considered in Chapter 2.

The changes in alveolar bone that occur during tooth movements have been interpreted in relation to strain-generated potentials within the bone (sometimes referred to as a piezo-electric effect). These potentials arise as a result of deformation of the collagen and/or hydroxyapatite and by streaming of fluid throughout the tissue. The electrical charges which result when a bone is deformed have been assumed to affect bone remodelling (e.g. Bassett, 1971; Zengo, Pawluk and Bassett, 1973; Zengo et al., 1974). Davidovitch et al. (1980a) have reported that electrical stimulation enhances cellular enzymatic phosphorylation activities in the periodontal tissues of cat maxillary canines. The characteristics of the applied force, architecture of the bone and individual patient reaction may influence strain-generated potentials and further research is required to clarify possible relationships between such potentials and tooth movement. However, Davidovitch et al. (1980b) have recently investigated the usefulness of exogenous electric currents in accelerating orthodontic tooth movement in cat maxillary canines tipped by a force of 80 g. They observed that teeth treated by force and electricity moved significantly faster than those treated by force alone.

Some variables which influence the response in the supporting tissues

NATURE OF THE LOAD

Duration of the force seems to be of paramount importance. Observations suggest that long-acting small forces may summate over a certain period and produce similar reactions to large forces which act for only brief periods. It is difficult, however, to characterize the tissue responses elicited by very small intermittent forces since the number of osteoclasts is small and the rate of bone deposition slow.

All natural stimuli are intermittent in character. The inter-relationship between the force, its duration and its frequency, determine whether tooth movement or compensatory strengthening of the supporting apparatus will occur. It has been claimed that no orthodontic movement will take place if the force duration does not exceed 6 hours per day (Proffit, personal communication).

If one applies a very small, but continuous, horizontal force to a tooth, the normal stimuli from occlusal function (chewing, swallowing, etc.) will cause an additional intermittent force. When this continuous force is increased beyond a certain limit, the tooth will be unable to recoil from the alveolar wall against which it is being pressed. In the case of intermittent loads, each time the application of a force is interrupted the tooth tends to return to its original position. On the pressure side, the vasculature is disturbed less easily and hyalinization occurs to a lesser degree and over a smaller area than with a continuous force. One sees large numbers of cells associated with an increased width of the periodontal ligament, on both the pressure and tension sides. In relation to the maintenance or even increase of functional stimuli as seen with certain removable appliances (such as activators, monoblocs, Bimler plates, etc.), the number of cells in the periodontal ligament will also increase. These cell numbers are greater than those seen in response to continuous forces of the same magnitude (e.g. Reitan, 1951).

Bone deposition on the tension side is dependent on the time for which the force is applied and occurs faster during an active stretching period. If the rest periods between force application are too long (or too frequent) bone deposition is limited (Reitan and Rygh, 1979). When bodily tooth movement is required over a considerable distance, therefore, a continuous force (or a continuous force interrupted only by short intervals) is advantageous.

AGE

Age is an important determinant of the periodontal

response to forces. The capacity for adaptation is greatest during the period of active growth. In the periodontal ligament of a child there are more fibroblasts and less collagen than in the adult and the alveolar bone surface is lined with osteoblasts in contrast to their more sparse distribution in adults (Reitan, 1954). (Cellular age changes are considered further in Chapter 2.) Alveolar bone in a young person contains more marrow spaces than in an adult. In young dogs, a considerable increase in the number of cells is seen on the tension side after 12 hours (Gottlieb and Orban, 1931). In children, fibroblast proliferation is seen on the tension side 30–40 hours after applying a horizontal load (Reitan, 1951). On the other hand, in adults it occurs only after several days (Reitan, 1954). Indeed, perhaps it is the delayed cellular response in adults that is associated with the greater stability of adult teeth. During orthodontic treatment growth may be utilized by respectively inhibiting and stimulating the sagittal and vertical development of the jaws to reduce or eliminate any discrepancy between upper and lower dental arches; in such cases little tooth movement may be needed.

The healthy supporting tissues of an adult tooth provides resistance to changing demands in the occlusion. With age, however, the periodontium appears to undergo some degenerative change. For example, the amount of newly formed bone per unit time is less in the elderly (Melsen and Melsen, 1979). The effect of these changes is to reduce the ability of the periodontium to resist displacement of the tooth under occlusal loads.

THE ARCHITECTURE OF THE PERIODONTIUM

This may vary from individual to individual, even in children. For example, bone density and the nature of the fibre system may produce varying degrees of resistance to given environmental forces. Perhaps such variation may account for the different tendencies of the teeth in patients to relapse after orthodontic treatment.

HORMONAL BALANCE

The hormonal balance and related factors — such as medication (e.g. cortisone), the presence of an allergy or general disease (e.g. osteomalacia, epilepsy) — may influence the tissue reponse to orthodontic tooth movement (Melsen, Melsen and Mosekilde, 1976). However, the precise mechanisms remain unknown; though it is conceivable that altered rates of turnover of the tooth-supporting tissues or factors relating to bone metabolism may be involved.

REFERENCES

BASS, T. P. & STEPHENS, C. D. (1970) Some experiments with orthodontic springs. *Dent. Practnr.* **21**, 21–36.

BASSETT, C. A. L. (1971) Biophysical principles affecting bone structure. In: *The biochemistry and physiology of bone,* Vol. III, G. H. BOURNE (ed.), pp. 1–76. London, Academic Press.

BAUMRIND, S. & BUCK, D. L. (1970) Rate changes in cell replication and protein synthesis in the periodontal ligament incident to tooth movement. *Amer. J. Orthod.* **57**, 109–131.

BEERTSEN, W. (1975) Migration of fibroblasts in the periodontal ligament of the mouse incisor as revealed by autoradiography. *Archs. oral Biol.* **20**, 659–666.

BEERTSEN, W. (1979) Remodelling of collagen fibers in the periodontal ligament and the supra-alveolar region. *Angle Orthod.* **49**, 218–224.

BOWLEY, W. W., BURSTONE, C. J., KOENIG, H. A. & SIATKOWSKI, R. (1974) Prediction of tooth displacement using laser holography and finite element technique. *Proceedings of the Symposium of Commission V, International Society for Photogrammetry, Washington,* pp. 241–273.

BURSTONE, C. J. (1962) The biomechanics of tooth movement. In: *Vistas in orthodontics,* B. S. KRAUS & R. A. RIEDEL (eds.), pp. 197–213. Philadelphia, Lea and Febiger.

BURSTONE, C. J. & PRYPUTNIEWICZ, R. J. (1980) Holographic determination of centers of rotation produced by orthodontic forces. *Amer. J. Orthod.* **77**, 396–409.

BURSTONE, C. J., PRYPUTNIEWICZ, R. J. & BOWLEY, W. W. (1978) Holographic measurement of tooth mobility in three dimensions. *J. periodont. Res.* **13**, 283–294.

CHRISTIANSEN, R. L. & BURSTONE, C. J. (1969) Centers of rotation within the periodontal space. *Amer. J. Orthod.* **55**, 353–369.

CHRISTIANSEN, R. L., EVANS, C. A. & SUE, S. K. (1979) Resting tongue pressures. *Angle Orthod.* **49**, 92–97.

COOLIDGE, E. D. (1937) The thickness of the human periodontal membrane. *J. Amer. dent. Assoc. Cosmos.* **24**, 1260–1270.

CRABB, J. J. & WILSON, H. J. (1972) The relation between orthodontic spring force and space closure. *Dent. Practnr.* **22**, 233–240.

CRUMLEY, P. J. (1964) Collagen formation in the normal and stressed periodontium. *Periodontics* **2**, 53–61.

DAVIDOVITCH, Z., FINKELSON, M. D., STEIGMAN, S., SHANFELD, J. L., MONTGOMERY, P. C. & KOROSTOFF, E. (1980a) Electric currents, bone remodel-

ling, and orthodontic tooth movement. 1. The effect of electric currents on periodontal cyclic nucleotides. *Amer. J. Orthod.* **77**, 14–32.

DAVIDOVITCH, Z., FINKELSON, M. D., STEIGMAN, S., SHANFELD, J. L., MONTGOMERY, P. C. & KOROSTOFF, E. (1980b) Electric currents, bone remodelling, and orthodontic tooth movement. II. Increase in rate of tooth movement and periodontal electric current. *Amer. J. Orthod.* **77**, 33–47.

EDWARDS, J. G. (1968) A study of the periodontium during orthodontic rotation of teeth. *Amer. J. Orthod.* **54**, 441–459.

FELDSTEIN, L. (1950) An instrument for measuring muscular forces acting on the teeth. *Amer. J. Orthod.* **36**, 856–859.

FREEMAN, E. & TEN CATE, A. R. (1978) Early ultrastructural changes in the periodontal ligament during orthodontic tooth movement. *J. dent. Res.* **57**: Special Issue A, 138.

GARANT, P. R. (1976) Collagen resorption by fibroblasts. A theory of fibroclastic maintenance of the periodontal ligament. *J. Periodontol.* **47**, 380–390.

GARANT, P. R. & CHO, M. I. (1979) Autoradiographic evidence of the coordination of the genesis of Sharpey's fibers with new bone formation in the periodontium of the mouse. *J. periodont. Res.* **14**, 107–114.

GOTTLIEB, B. & ORBAN, B. (1931) *Die Veränderungen der Geurebe bei übermässigen Beanspruchung der Zähne.* Leipzig, Thieme.

GOULD, M. S. E. & PICTON, D. C. A. (1963) An evaluation of a method of measuring forces exerted by the tongue on the teeth. *Br. dent. J.* **114**, 175–180.

GOULD, M. S. E. & PICTON, D. C. A. (1964) A study of pressures exerted by the lips and cheeks on the teeth of subjects with normal occlusion. *Archs. oral Biol.* **9**, 469–478.

HAACK, D. C. & WEINSTEIN, S. (1963) Geometry and mechanics as related to tooth movement studied by means of two-dimensional model. *J. Amer. dent. Assoc.* **66**, 157–164.

HENERS, M. (1974) Syndesmotic limiting movement of the periodontal ligament. *Int. dent. J.* **24**, 319–327.

HIMMEL, G. K., MARTHALER, T. M., RATEITSCHAK, K. H. & MÜHLEMANN, H. R. (1957) Experimental changes of diurnal periodicity in the physical properties of periodontal structures. *Helv. Odont. Acta* **1**, 16–18.

HOFMANN, M. (1963) Zahnbeweglichkeit — Bestimmung und Analyse. *Dtsch. zahnärztl. Zs.* **18**, 924–933.

KARDOS, T. B. & SIMPSON, L. O. (1980) A new periodontal membrane biology based upon thixotropic concepts. *Amer. J. Orthod.* **77**, 508–515.

KÖRBER, K. H. (1962) Elektronisches Messen der Zahnbeweglichkeit. *Dtsch. Zahnärztebl.* **16**, 605.

KÖRBER, K. H. (1971) Electronic registration of tooth movements. *Int. dent. J.* **21**, 466–477.

KÖRBER, K. H. & KÖRBER, E. (1967) Patterns of physiological movement in tooth support. In: *The mechanisms of tooth support,* D. J. ANDERSON, J. E. EASTOE, A. H. MELCHER & D. C. A. PICTON (eds.), pp. 148–153. Bristol, Wright.

KRAW, A. G. & ENLOW, D. H. (1967) Continuous attachment of the periodontal membrane. *Amer. J. Anat.* **120**, 133–148.

KVAM, E. (1972) Scanning electron microscopy of tissue

changes on the pressure surface of human premolars following tooth movement. *Scand. J. dent. Res.* **80**, 357–368.

KYDD, W. L. (1957) Maximum forces exerted on the dentition by the perioral and lingual musculature. *J. Amer. dent. Assoc.* **55**, 646–651.

LEAR, C. S. C., CATZ, J., GROSSMAN, R. C., FLANAGAN, J. B. & MOORREES, C. F. A. (1965) Measurement of lateral muscle forces on the dental arches. *Archs. oral Biol.* **10**, 669–689.

LEAR, C. S. C., DECOU, R. E. & NG, D. H. P. (1974) Threshold levels for displacement of human maxillary central incisors in response to lingually directed forces. *J. dent. Res.* **53**, 942.

LEAR, C. S. C., MACKAY, J. S. & LOWE, A. A. (1972) Threshold levels for displacement of human teeth in response to laterally directed forces. *J. dent. Res.* **51**, 1478–1482.

LUFFINGHAM, J. K. (1968) Pressure exerted on teeth by the lips and cheeks. *Dent. Practnr.* **19**, 61–64.

LUFFINGHAM, J. K. (1970) A study of the buccal forces exerted upon the teeth during finger-sucking. *Br. Soc. Study Orthod.* **56**, 85–89.

MELCHER, A. H. (1976) Biological processes in tooth eruption and tooth movement. In: *Scientific foundations of dentistry*, B. COHEN & I. R. H. KRAMER (eds.), pp. 417–426. London, Heinemann.

MELCHER, A. H. & WALKER, T. W. (1976) The periodontal ligament in attachment and as a shock absorber. In: *The eruption and occlusion of teeth*, D. F. G. POOLE & M. V. STACK (eds.), pp. 183–192. London, Butterworths.

MELSEN, B. & MELSEN, F. (1979) Generelle fahtorers indflydelse pa vevsreaksjoner. In: *Nordisk Klinisk Odontologi*, J. J. HOLST (ed.), Chapter 15, IV, 12.

MELSEN, B., MELSEN, F. & MOSEKILDE, L. (1976) Bone changes of importance in the orthodontic patient with epilepsy. *Trans. Eur. Orthod. Soc.* 227–233.

MÜHLEMANN, H. R. (1951) Periodontometry; a method for measuring tooth mobility. *Oral Surg. Oral Med. Oral Path.* **4**, 1220–1233.

MÜHLEMANN, H. R. (1954a) Tooth mobility: The measuring method. Initial and secondary tooth mobility. *J. Periodont.* **25**, 22–29.

MÜHLEMANN, H. R. (1954b) Tooth mobility (II). Role of interdental contact points and of activation on tooth mobility. *J. Periodont.* **25**, 125–128.

MÜHLEMANN, H. R. (1954c) Tooth mobility (IV). Tooth mobility changes through artificial alterations of the periodontium. *J. Periodont.* **25**, 198–202.

MÜHLEMANN, H. R. (1960) Ten years of tooth mobility measurements. *J. Periodont.* **31**, 110–122.

MÜHLEMANN, H. R. (1967) Tooth mobility: a review of clinical aspects and research findings. *J. Periodont.* **38**, 686–708.

MÜHLEMANN, H. R. & HOUGLUM, M. W. (1954) The determination of the tooth rotation center. *Oral Surg. Oral Med. Oral Path.* **7**, 392–394.

MÜHLEMANN, H. R., SAVDIR, S. & RATEITSCHAK, K. H. (1965) Tooth mobility — Its causes and significance. *J. Periodont.* **36**, 148–153.

MÜHLEMANN, H. R. & ZANDER, H. A. (1954) Tooth mobility (III). The mechanism of tooth mobility. *J. Periodont.* **25**, 128–137.

NIKOLAI, R. J. (1974) Periodontal ligament reaction and displacements of a maxillary central incisor subjected to transverse crown loading. *J. Biomechanics* **7**, 93–99.

O'LEARY, T. J., RUDD, K. D. & NABERS, C. L. (1966) Factors affecting horizontal tooth mobility. *Periodontics* **4**, 308–315.

PACKMAN, H., SCHOHER, I. & STEIN, R. S. (1977) Vascular responses in the human periodontal ligament and alveolar bone detected by photoelectric plethysmography: the effect of force application to the tooth. *J. Periodont.* **48**, 194–200.

PARFITT, G. J. (1961) The dynamics of a tooth in function. *J. Periodont.* **32**, 102–107.

PICTON, D. C. A. (1964) Some implications of normal tooth mobility during mastication. *Archs. oral Biol.* **9**, 565–573.

PICTON, D. C. A. (1965) On the part played by the socket in tooth support. *Archs. oral Biol.* **10**, 945–955.

PICTON, D. C. A. (1967) The effect on tooth mobility of trauma to the mesial and distal regions of the periodontal membranes in monkeys. *Helv. Odont. Acta* **11**, 105–112.

PICTON, D. C. A. (1969) The effect of external forces on the periodontium. In: *Biology of the periodontium*, A. H. MELCHER & W. H. BOWEN (eds.), pp. 363–419. London, Academic Press.

PICTON, D. C. A. & DAVIES, W. I. R. (1967) Dimensional changes in the periodontal membrane of monkeys (*Macaca irus*) due to horizontal thrusts applied to the teeth. *Archs. oral Biol.* **12**, 1635–1643.

PICTON, D. C. A., JOHNS, R. B., WILLS, D. J. & DAVIES, W. I. R. (1974) The relationship between the mechanisms of tooth and implant support. In: *Oral Science Review*, 5, A. H. MELCHER & G. A. ZARB (eds.), pp. 3–22. Copenhagen, Munksgaard.

PICTON, D. C. A. & SLATTER, J. M. (1972) The effect on horizontal tooth mobility of experimental trauma to the periodontal membrane in regions of tension or compression in monkey. *J. periodont. Res.* **7**, 35–41.

PINSON, R. R. & STRAHAN, J. D. (1974) The effect on the relapse of orthodontically rotated teeth of surgical division of the gingival fibres — pericision. *Br. J. Orthod.* **1**, 87–91.

POSEN, A. L. (1972) The influence of maximum perioral and tongue force on the incisor teeth. *Angle Orthod.* **42**, 285–309.

PROFFIT, W. R. (1972) Lingual pressure patterns in the transition from tongue thrust to adult swallowing. *Archs. oral Biol.* **17**, 555–564.

PROFFIT, W. R., CHASTAIN, B. B. & NORTON, L. A. (1969) Linguopalatal pressure in children. *Amer. J. Orthod.* **55**, 154–166.

PROFFIT, W. R., KYDD, W. L., WILSKIC, G. H. & TAYLOR, D. T. (1964) Intraoral pressures in a young adult group. *J. dent. Res.* **43**, 555–562.

PROFFIT, W. R., McGLONE, R. E. & BARRETT, M. J. (1975) Lip and tongue pressures related to dental arch and oral cavity size in Australian aborigines. *J. dent. Res.* **54**, 1161–1172.

PROFFIT, W. R. & NORTON, L. A. (1970) The tongue and oral morphology: influences of tongue activity during speech and swallowing. *ASHA Reports,* No. 5, 106–115.

PRYPUTNIEWICZ, R. J. & BURSTONE, C. J. (1979) The

effect of time and force magnitude on orthodontic tooth movement. *J. dent. Res.* **58**, 1754–1764.

PRYPUTNIEWICZ, R. J., BURSTONE, C. J. & BOWLEY, W. W. (1978) Determination of arbitrary tooth displacements. *J. dent. Res.* **57**, 663–674.

REITAN, K. (1951) The initial tissue reaction incident to orthodontic tooth movement as related to the influence of function. *Acta Odont. Scand.* Suppl. 6, 1–240.

REITAN, K. (1954) Tissue reaction as related to the age factor. *Dent. Rec.* **74**, 271–278.

REITAN, K. (1959) Tissue rearrangement during retention of orthodontically rotated teeth. *Angle Orthod.* **29**, 105–113.

REITAN, K. (1961) Behaviour of Malassez epithelial rests during orthodontic tooth movement. *Acta Odont. Scand.* **19**, 443–468.

REITAN, K. (1967) Clinical and histologic observations on tooth movement during and after orthodontic treatment. *Amer. J. Orthod.* **53**, 721–745.

REITAN, K. (1975) Biomechanical principles and reactions. In: *Current orthodontic concepts and techniques*, Vol. 1 (2nd ed.), T. M. GRABNER & B. F. SWAIN (eds.), pp. 111–229. Philadelphia, Saunders.

REITAN, K. & RYGH, P. (1979) Vevsreaksjoner ved ortodontisk terapi. In: *Nordisk klinisk odontologi*, J. J. HOLST (ed.). Chapter 15, III, 3.

ROSS, G. G., LEAR, C. S. & DECOU, R. (1976) Modeling the lateral movements of teeth. *J. Biomechanics* **9**, 723–734.

RYGH, P. (1972a) Ultrastructural vascular changes in pressure zones of rat molar periodontium incident to orthodontic tooth movement. *Scand. J. dent. Res.* **80**, 307–321.

RYGH, P. (1972b) Ultrastructural cellular reactions in pressure zones of rat molar periodontium incident to orthodontic tooth movement. *Acta Odont. Scand.* **30**, 575–593.

RYGH, P. (1973a) Ultrastructural changes in pressure zones of human periodontium incident to orthodontic tooth movement. *Acta Odont. Scand.* **31**, 109–122.

RYGH, P. (1973b) Ultrastructural changes in the periodontal fibers and their attachment in rat molar periodontium incident to orthodontic tooth movement. *Scand. J. dent. Res.* **81**, 467–480.

RYGH, P. (1974) Elimination of hyalinized periodontal tissues associated with orthodontic tooth movement. *Scand. J. dent. Res.* **82**, 57–73.

RYGH, P. (1976) Ultrastructural changes in tension zones of rat molar periodontium incident to orthodontic tooth movement. *Amer. J. Orthod.* **70**, 269–281.

RYGH, P. (1977) Orthodontic root resorptions studied by electron microscopy. *Angle Orthod.* **47**, 1–16.

RYGH, P. (in preparation) Remodelling of periodontal fibers incident to experimental tooth movement.

SAKUDA, M., YOSHIDA, K., WADA, K., KURODA, Y. & HAYASHI, I. (1975) Changes of cheek pressure during swallowing following expansion of the maxillary dental arch in repaired cleft palates. *J. oral Rehab.* **2**, 145–156.

SCHUBERT, M. & HAMERMAN, D. (1968) *A primer on connective tissue biochemistry.* Philadelphia, Lea & Febiger.

SIMS, F. W. (1958) The pressure exerted on maxillary and mandibular central incisors by the perioral and lingual musculature. *Amer. J. Orthod.* **44**, 64–65.

SKOUGAARD, M. R., LEVI, B. M. & SIMPSON, J. (1969) Collagen metabolism in skin and periodontal membrane of the marmoset. *J. periodont. Res.* **4**, 28–29.

SODEK, J. (1977) A comparison of the rates of synthesis and turnover of collagen and non-collagen proteins in adult rat periodontal tissues and skin using a micro-assay. *Archs. oral Biol.* **22**, 655–666.

STOREY, E. & SMITH, R. (1952) Force in orthodontics and its relation to tooth movement. *Aust. J. Dent.* **56**, 11–18.

WILLS, D. J., PICTON, D. C. A. & DAVIES, W. I. R. (1978) The intrusion of the tooth for different loading rates. *J. Biomechanics* **11**, 429–434.

WINDERS, R. V. (1956) A study of the development of an electronic technique to measure the forces exerted on the dentition by the perioral and lingual musculature. *Amer. J. Orthod.* **42**, 645–657.

WINDERS, R. V. (1958) Forces exerted on the dentition by the perioral and lingual musculature during swallowing. *Angle Orthod.* **28**, 226–235.

WINDERS, R. V. (1962) Recent findings in myometric research. *Angle Orthod.* **32**, 38–43.

ZENGO, A. N., PAWLUK, R. J. & BASSETT, C. A. L. (1973) Stress-induced bioelectric potentials in the dentoalveolar complex. *Amer. J. Orthod.* **64**, 17–27.

ZENGO, A. N., BASSETT, C. A. L., PAWLUK, R. J. & PROUNTZOS, G. (1974) *In vivo* bioelectric potentials in the dentoalveolar complex. *Amer. J. Orthod.* **66**, 130–139.

Chapter 13

DEVELOPMENTAL ANOMALIES AND PERIODONTAL DISEASES

A. H. Brook

INTRODUCTION

In discussing developmental anomalies and periodontal disease it is necessary to consider whether there is a genetic component in common periodontal disease and, if one is discernible, by which of the known genetic mechanisms is it mediated? Secondly, are there any specific conditions confined to the periodontal ligament which are at least partially genetically determined? Thirdly, what conditions of abnormal development of the dento-alveolar structures predispose to or modify the development of chronic inflammatory periodontal disease? Finally, which developmentally determined generalized diseases are frequently accompanied by periodontal pathology?

GENETIC FACTORS IN INFLAMMATORY PERIODONTAL DISEASE

That genetic factors can exert a considerable influence on the periodontium is shown by several conditions, e.g. acatalasia, hypophosphatasia and cyclic neutropenia caused by single mutant genes in which severe periodontitis is a constant and striking finding. These genes have their effect on periodontal structures in all environments and so illustrate the marked periodontal pathology that inherited characteristics can produce. However, these conditions are systemic diseases with a periodontal component and will be discussed later. First of all, the role of genetic factors in common periodontal disease must be considered.

Chronic inflammatory periodontal disease (CIPD)

Common periodontal disease clearly has a complex aetiology in which it seems possible to distinguish a genetic component (Gorlin, Stallard and Shapiro, 1967). Unfortunately, the evidence for the extent and nature of this genetic component is still limited since there have been relatively few population, family or twin studies.

The tendency of various racial groups to exhibit differing severity of CIPD has been discussed by several authors. Zimmerman and Baker (1960) noted a higher incidence of gingival disease in Negro than in White children. Chung et al. (1970) carried out a genetic and epidemiological study in 9912 Hawaiian school children, aged 12–18 years. After allowance was made for the effects of epidemiologic factors and variation in oral hygiene, they found a non-additive racial effect on periodontal disease, discernible when racial crossing was between major racial groups. Children of Hawaiian ancestry had a distinctly greater severity of disease than other racial groups. Children of mixed race had an average periodontal score closer to the parental race with the lower mean. Furthermore, the significant effect of the hybridity of the child when major racial crosses were involved suggests an important role of recessive gene(s) in the aetiology of CIPD.

Witkop et al. (1966) considered the effects of inbreeding on periodontitis, in a study of 2821 individuals from an inbred population, the Brandy-wine triracial isolate (Negro–White–Indian) of southern Maryland. They found that the periodontal indices by age and sex were very similar to those of Baltimore Negroes, but approximately 50% higher than Baltimore Whites by age. Males showed approximately 40% more disease than females. Both gingivitis and periodontal pocketing increased with the degree of inbreeding. The authors considered that there could have been a socio-economic effect, but since there was no difference between the socio-economic scores of the three groups the effect is more likely to have been genetic. Niswander (1975) suggests that recessive genes may be involved in the aetiology of CIPD. However, the results of these population and family studies are also compatible with a polygenic influence, itself part of a multi-factorial aetiology.

Another method of studying the genetic basis of common disease is to investigate the incidence of the disease in groups characterized by specific genes, such as those for blood groups. If a disease occurs at a significantly higher rate in individuals with a particular blood group, a genetic mechanism may well be involved. Polevitzky (1929) studied CIPD

in relation to blood grouping and found a slight increase in persons having blood group A and a slight decrease in those of blood group B. In contrast, Carmichael (1965) found no significant correlation between ABO blood groups and periodontal disease. Pradhan et al. (1971) suggested that Carmichael's findings could have been influenced by sample size and the groups being heterogenous with regard to age, socio-economic factors and oral hygiene habits. They claimed that their own study group of medical students were homogenous in age, dietary habits, living conditions and oral hygiene habits. They reported a broad correlation between periodontal disease and blood groups, but none with secretor status for group-specific substances in saliva. Groups O and AB were more frequently associated with severe degrees of periodontal involvement. Malena (1972) found a lower than expected number of subjects with the A blood group among gingivitis patients. Kaslick, West and Chasens (1980) showed a somewhat lower percentage of group A subjects but primarily a higher percentage of AB patients and a lower percentage of subjects with blood group O compared to their general population controls. Their periodontitis group was not significantly different from either the normal study group or the general population control in terms of ABO grouping. This result agrees with those of Barros and Witkop (1963) and Carmichael (1965) but not with Polevitzky (1929) or Pradhan et al. (1971).

Specific immune responses are also under genetic control. It has been shown that genes responsible for specific immune responses are placed close to each other and to the histocompatibility locus. The 'histocompatibility' antigens are the expression of 'histocompatibility' genes, and certain HL-A antigens have been associated with particular diseases. Kaslick et al. (1980) examined the association between ABO blood groups (see above), HL-A antigens and periodontal disease in young adults. Two hundred and thirty-eight Caucasians were divided into normal, necrotizing ulcerative gingivitis, chronic gingivitis, juvenile periodontitis and periodontitis groups. Results showed that, compared to the normal group, there was a significant reduction in HL-A2 antigen frequency in the periodontitis group, a trend toward HL-A2 frequency reduction in the juvenile periodontitis group and a significant reduction in the HL-A2 frequency when both of these bone loss groups were combined into one group. When only those individuals under 25 years of age were studied in the combined bone-loss group there was more of a reduction in HL-A2 frequency.

Alpha-antitrypsin is a serum protease inhibitor produced by the liver with an established role in the response to destructive inflammatory disease. It exhibits inheritable genetic polymorphism (Pi types). Peterson and Marsh (1979) reported that certain Pi types appear to be related to increased susceptibility to chronic periodontitis. The periodontitis population they observed varied significantly from the control population; the presence of the Z gene in the MZ Pi type appeared to increase in individuals susceptible to chronic inflammatory periodontal disease.

Regarding genetic factors in CIPD as assessed from animal experiments, Baer and Lieberman (1959) found one mouse strain susceptible to CIPD while another two strains were relatively resistant. The trabecular pattern of the alveolar bone was said to be distinct for each strain and was not altered by the diet. They concluded that neither the physical consistency of the diet, the width of the maxilla nor the weight of the mandible were important aetiological factors in CIPD in these mice strains.

From the above information it is apparent that genetic factors in periodontal disease are complex and that the isolation of these factors is difficult. There does seem, however, to be a genetic component in common periodontal disease but we cannot yet quantify it or confidently identify the inheritance pattern.

Juvenile periodontitis/periodontosis

Baer (1971) described periodontosis/juvenile periodontitis as 'a disease of the periodontium occurring in an otherwise healthy adolescent characterised by a rapid loss of alveolar bone about more than one tooth of the permanent dentition. There are two basic forms in which it occurs. In one form the teeth affected are the incisors and the first molars. In the other, more generalized form, most of the dentition can be affected. The amount of destruction manifested is not commensurate with the amounts of local irritants present.'

The role of plaque and of the host response, as well as the histopathology of the ligament, are considered in Chapter 15. Here will be considered both direct and indirect evidence for the role of genetic factors in the aetiology of juvenile periodontitis. The direct evidence relates to the familial occurrence of juvenile periodontitis. The indirect evidence arises from a consideration of the part played in the aetiology by the immune system, and the distribution of the blood groups and antigen types.

In considering the more direct evidence for genetic factors, there is a suggestion that juvenile periodontitis occurs more frequently among relatives of affected patients than in the general population. The familial occurrence of juvenile periodontitis has been reported by Cohen and Goldman (1960); Benjamin and Baer (1967); Butler (1969); Mühlemann (1972); Jorgenson *et al.* (1975) and Kirkham (1977). Rao and Tewani (1968) also noticed a familial occurrence in forty-nine cases out of eighty-nine. Benjamin and Baer (1967) found juvenile periodontitis in siblings, identical twins, 'parents-offspring', and first cousins. In Butler's (1969) family of five children, a 15-year-old boy and his sister aged 12 years had juvenile periodontitis and a maternal aunt and grandfather had lost their teeth at an early age. A case of juvenile periodontitis spanning three generations has been reported (Sussman and Baer, 1978). In a Danish study of about 150 cases of juvenile periodontitis (Frandsen, 1978) there were three pairs of identical twins affected by the disease (although the bone loss was not similar in the twins).

From such evidence it seems likely that inheritance plays a considerable part in the aetiology of juvenile periodontitis. The point to consider next is by which of the known genetic mechanisms this is mediated.

Melnick, Shields and Bixler (1976) carried out a segregation analysis on the pedigrees already available in the literature. They claimed that a dominant trait with 78% penetrance was the model that best fitted the available data. Since there was a preponderance of females among those affected, they conclude that it is an x-linked dominant trait with decreased penetrance. Melnick *et al.* (1976) also reported that all of the suggested clinical types of juvenile periodontitis had appeared in a single family.

Thus, there may not be separate types of juvenile periodontitis but rather variations in the expression of a single gene.

Rather than a dominant trait, Fourel (1972) and Jorgenson *et al.* (1975) have suggested an autosomal recessive mode of inheritance. Each study examined only one family, although that investigated by Fourel involved more than twenty individuals. In addition to the family study, both authors based their views on other reported families, on reported consanguinity and on the higher frequency of juvenile periodontitis in isolates. However, when Fourel refers to consanguinity, it is in relation to the Papillon—Lefèvre syndrome, which is an autosomal recessive condition (see page 303). In rare, recessive disorders the disease is encountered in siblings only (in whom the risk of homozygosity is 25%). Usually the parents are healthy, being heterozygotes. Additional cases are not often seen in second-degree relatives aunts or uncles nor among the first or more remote cousins. Accordingly, there will always be a proportion of sporadic cases without any siblings, and a good proportion of families where all the siblings are healthy, the more so with small family size.

Saxen (1980) examined the appearance of the affected individuals in different generations. From a total of sixty-two parents of thirty-one propositi, all but two were examined. No affected parent was found. This is strong evidence against the dominant mode of Mendelian inheritance. This, and the fact that the first-degree relatives were unable to report probable cases in second-degree relatives, also reduces the likelihood of a polygenic or multifactorial mode of inheritance. Of the sixty-four siblings examined, eleven were affected. By calculating the genetic ratio, Saxen showed that her results were compatible with an autosomal recessive mode of inheritance. The sex ratio among the propositi, twenty females and eleven males, could be attributed either to chance or to self-selection with females attending the dentist more frequently. This should not be reflected in the affected siblings. The small number of affected siblings, (11), does not permit conclusions in any direction although the ratio of 7 : 4 was similar to that among the propositi. The lack of affected remote relatives reduces the probability of an x-linked recessive mode of inheritance.

The report of Sussman and Baer (1978) on juvenile periodontitis in three generations appears to be contrary to an hypothesis of recessive inheritance. They reported a 17-year-old girl, her 30-year-old mother and 50-year-old grandmother as having juvenile periodontitis. Bearing in mind the criteria for juvenile periodontitis the disease of a 50-year-old individual with almost all the natural teeth remaining, and only some 2—3 mm bone loss in the maxilla, is difficult to diagnose as juvenile periodontitis, even though the gingival tissues appear normal. It is compatible with recessive inheritance for the mother and the daughter to have the disease, provided that the father was a heterozygote for this gene.

If juvenile periodontitis is transmitted recessively, its gene frequency would be rather high, i.e. (0.03 or 3%) (Saxen, 1980). Lack of certainty concerning the sex ratio of affected individuals is an important factor preventing agreement on the mode of inheritance. The actual basis of the disease, i.e. the primary defect(s), remains unexplained (Saxen, 1980).

As for chronic marginal periodontitis the ABO-blood groups have been analysed in juvenile periodontitis. Kaslick, West and Chasens (1980) found many patients to be of blood group B and a smaller number than expected to be of group O. Their conclusion was that a genetic factor played a role in the aetiology of juvenile periodontitis. Malena's (1972) results suggested that the blood-phenotype A was more susceptible to the disease than phenotypes A_2, B, AB and O.

The association between periodontal disease and HLA-A2 antigen has been investigated. Kaslick *et al.* (1975) found that only 25% of patients with juvenile periodontitis were HLA-A2 antigen positive whereas 61% of the normal controls were positive. The corresponding figure for patients with chronic marginal periodontitis was 21%. Reinholdt, Bay and Svejgaard (1977) also found a low frequency of HLA-A2 antigen in patients with juvenile periodontitis but not in a chronic periodontitis group. These authors reported that the tissue-type specificities HLA-A9, HLA-A28 and HLA-BW15 were of significantly higher frequency in the juvenile periodontitis group.

In view of the familial incidence and the possibility of immunological mechanisms being involved in juvenile periodontitis, Cullinan *et al.* (1980) undertook a study to determine whether the familial susceptibility was dependent on genes within the MHC and could be associated with the expression of a particular association between juvenile periodontitis and HLA among unrelated individuals or in families. They found no such association and no support for the possibility of 'molecular mimicry' of the Gram-negative micro-organisms which could be linked with ·juvenile periodontitis and a particular HLA antigen.

Data have also been reported which indicate that the host defence seems to be impaired in individuals with juvenile periodontitis (see Chapter 15). In juvenile periodontitis the inability of lymphocytes to respond to some Gram-negative bacteria and plaque antigens is manifested early in life, whereas in chronic marginal periodontitis this defect develops later in life (Liljenberg and Lindhe, 1980). In two groups, the juvenile and the 'post-juvenile' periodontitis group, the same cell-mediated immunodeficiency and increased serum immunoglobulin concentration were found (Lehner et al., 1974). Bacterial antigens isolated from periodontal pockets of juvenile periodontitis cases failed to induce blastogenesis of peripherally derived circulating blood lymphocytes (primarily T-type) of the patients when they were co-incubated in in vitro cell culture systems. The possibilities exist that the patients' lymphocytes (in vivo) are unable to recognize the foreign nature of the bacterial antigens (and are therefore non-reactive), suffer from blastogenic defects, or have been deprived of the active and appropriate intercession of macrophages for processing of the antigen or its disposal. In the latter instance, macrophage processing of the antigen may be required as a precursor phenomenon, modifying the antigenic material so that it is capable of eliciting lymphocyte reactivity. A macrophage defect could also exist relative to appropriate processing of the bacterial antigens peculiar to juvenile periodontitis.

Clinically detectable lymphadenopathy has been found in some patients with juvenile periodontitis and may be involved in an immune response to the plaque microorganisms (Manson and Lehner, 1974; Manson, 1977). Friedman et al. (1976) using scanning electron microscopy found that most of the lymphocytes from the periodontal lesions showed a smooth surface indicating that they were not activated, in contrast to normal villous-covered activated cells.

However, two studies on abnormalities in the immune system in patients with juvenile periodontitis have suggested that such findings could be a secondary consequence of the chronic periodontal inflammation rather than a primary causative factor (Budtz-Jorgensen et al., 1978; Jacobson, Svärdström and Danielsson, 1978).

Clark, Page and Wilde (1977) demonstrated that patients with juvenile periodontitis frequently had a defective neutrophil chemotactic response. Furthermore, serum from several of the patients contained a factor which markedly inhibited neutrophil chemotaxis. Similar findings, including defective phagocytosis, have been reported by Cianciola et al. (1977) and Lavine et al. (1979). Monocyte function remained unaffected. The question of whether this reduction in the patient's protective response precedes or is a result of the disease remains to be determined. It is possible that the development of juvenile periodontitis requires both neutrophil dysfunction and a specific bacterial flora. The siblings of patients with juvenile periodontitis that do not have the disease themselves might have the neutrophil dysfunction but not the right kind of bacteria (Nisengard, Myers and Newman, 1977). Nisengard et al. (1977) studied the antibody titres to the microbiota associated with juvenile periodontitis. They found there was a disease-specific group of Gram-negative anaerobic rods and also demonstrated a spectrum of humoral responses to the microbiota.

Van Swol et al. (1980) determined IgA, IgG, and IgM concentrations in the granulation tissue removed from deep infrabony pockets of patients with juvenile periodontitis and advanced periodontitis. Comparison of mean immunoglobulin levels between the juvenile periodontitis and advanced periodontitis groups revealed a significant increase ($P<0.05$) for IgG in the granulation tissue from the juvenile periodontitis group. There was also an increased detection rate of IgM in the juvenile periodontitis granulation tissues, which may represent an enhanced response to the Gram-negative bacteria in the area of periodontal destruction. Possible protective effects of IgM against Gram-negative organisms, however, may be offset by a dysfunction of polymorphonuclear leukocytes manifested by a reduction in phagocytosis and a diminished response to chemotactic stimuli. IgM may be a more efficient activator of complement than IgG (Van Swol *et al.*, 1980), and there-fore more efficient in killing Gram-negative organisms. If so this would support the concept of a normal production rate of immunoglobulins in patients with juvenile periodontitis, but a deficient cellular immune response.

Raised serum alkaline phosphatase levels in affected patients were noted by Melnick, Shields and Bixler (1976), and a defect of citric acid metabolism has been suggested by Tsunemitsu *et al.* (1964). Reisel (1971) has suggested that juvenile periodontitis is an early manifestation of juvenile skeletal osteoporosis. However, these suggestions await further investiga-tion as regards possible primary bone defects in perio-dontosis.

Third molar germs were transplanted into sockets of freshly extracted first molars from periodontosis patients with resultant complete healing of the bone (Baer and Gamble, 1966). A similar result was reported by Borring-Møller and Frandsen (1978) who per-formed tooth transplantations in eight patients with juvenile periodontitis and followed the cases for 7 years. No pocket depths over 3 mm were found nor was there any abnormal mobility of the transplanted teeth. Both these studies make doubtful any primary role of the bone in this disease.

It may be concluded that a genetic basis for the disease is now widely accepted although there is still uncertainty as to the exact genetic mechanism.

ABNORMAL DEVELOPMENTS OF THE DENTO-ALVEOLAR COMPLEX: THEIR IMPORTANCE IN CHRONIC INFLAM-MATORY PERIODONTAL DISEASE

A number of developmental factors may contribute to the initiation and progression of chronic inflam-matory periodontal disease (CIPD). The influence of tooth morphology and structure is discussed here.

Tooth morphology

Some developmental variations of tooth morphology may provide shelter for accumulation and retention of plaque, thus predisposing the tooth to a localized periodontal lesion (Shiloah and Kopczyk, 1979).

Morphological defects of the dentition can be regarded as a predisposing cause of CIPD. Buccal gingival contours, marginal ridges on the occlusal surfaces of posterior teeth, and normal contact areas all play a part in the food-shedding mechanism to protect the marginal gingiva and the gingival crevice (Lee, Lee and Poon, 1968). Excessive contours and concavities can hamper efforts to remove plaque (Shiloah and Kopczyk, 1979).

As the pathologic process advances on multi-rooted teeth, areas of the cement–enamel junction and of the root furcations become exposed. Furca-tion morphology takes many forms. Some roots are splayed; others are fused, leaving a concavity or groove but no separation of roots. Most furcations are between such extremes. The more constricted the furcation, the more difficult it is to clean. Varia-tion in the level of the furcation may well influence the progress of the periodontal lesion, as in the rare condition of taurodontism (Holt and Brook, 1979).

In taurodontism, the body of the tooth is enlarged at the expense of the roots (Keith, 1913). The pulp chamber appears large and often extends below the level of the alveolar crest. The usual constriction at the level of the amelo-cemental junction is frequently absent (Hamner, Witkop and Metro, 1964). Depending on the level of the furcation, the affected teeth have been termed hypo-, meso- and hypertaurodont: in the latter the pulp chamber extends nearly to the apex with little division of the root. The more apical location of the furcation in taurodont teeth miti-gates against early involvement of the latter in perio-dontitis.

Taurodontism is seen in some patients with amelogenesis imperfecta, e.g. in the mixed type of enamel defect in which there is both hypocalcification and hypoplasia. A similar association is present as part of the Tricho-dento-osseous syndrome (Witkop, 1975) where, in addition to enamel defects and tauro-dontism, there is also tight curly hair and sclerosis of bone. The condition has also been seen in patients with polypoidy of the X-chromosome in males, e.g. Klinefelter's syndrome (XXY) (Sauk, 1980).

Taurodontism is thought to originate from a defect in Hertwig's root sheath, which fails either to invaginate at the usual horizontal level or to achieve union of the flaps which determine root morpho-differentiation (Holt and Brook, 1979).

Enamel projections are irregularities of the enamel margin in deciduous and permanent molars, that may extend from the cement—enamel junction in molars toward and, perhaps, into the furcation. This phenomenon has been correlated with furcation involvement in CIPD. Teeth with this anomaly may have a cul-de-sac of unattached gingiva which accumulates dental plaque. They also occur on taurodont teeth. The projections have been classified into three groups:

Class 1 — a distinct change in the cement—enamel junction with enamel projecting towards the furcation.

Class 2 — enamel projecting further towards but not involving the furcation.

Class 3 — extending to involve the furcation. Class 3 projections occur more often on mandibular than maxillary teeth, especially on the buccal aspect (Masters and Hoskins, 1964). Indeed, their clinical observations seemed to associate enamel projections with approximately 90% of isolated bifurcational involvements (Leib, Berdon and Sabes, 1967). Bissada and Abdelmalek (1973) reported a 50% correlation between cervico-enamel projection and furcation involvement. In other studies, however, no statistically significant association between enamel extensions and furcation involvements has been shown (Holt, 1976). Estimates of their frequency in the deciduous dentition are not available. Microscopic studies of extracted permanent teeth suggest a range of 6—24% for the Grade 3 projections. There appears to be a higher prevalence in persons of Mongoloid origin than in Caucasians (Masters and Hoskins, 1964; Holt, 1976).

Enamel pearls are isolated, round or oval deposits composed of enamel only or containing a dentine core, which may also enclose an extension of pulpal tissue. They have not been found in the deciduous dentition. Most reports of pearls in the permanent dentition have been confined to molars, but they have also been seen on incisors and premolars, although not on canines. They tend to occur distally on upper molars and buccally on lower molars, often being bilaterally symmetrical. On extracted teeth examined macroscopically, the overall incidence ranged from 1 to 7% (Holt, 1976). Pearls may occur singly or as multiples on one tooth. Kerr (1961) suggested, because of the frequency with which they occur in bifurcations, that enamel pearls may influence the development and progress of a pocket in that region. He postulated that the periodontal ligament fibres had no true attachment to the tooth in the area of the cervico-enamel projection or the enamel pearl.

Enamel pearls are probably indicative of some disturbance in the function of Hertwig's root sheath. There is some evidence from work on rodents and in man that some may be due to trauma (Holt, 1976).

Grooving of the crown and root surfaces is a structural variation in many teeth. Lee, Lee and Poon (1968) describe developmental grooves on the palatal surface of maxillary incisor teeth, commencing at the junction of the cingulum and the lateral marginal ridges, and extending on to the root surface. They may continue for variable distances along the length of the distolingual aspect of the root. The defect is in communication with the gingival crevice. The epithelial attachment in this area is frequently diseased, forming a ready pathway for the ingress of bacterial metabolites and the formation of an infrabony periodontal pocket. Everett and Kramer (1972) found grooves in 1% of maxillary lateral incisors. Lee *et al.* (1968) described thirteen cases of palato-gingival grooving in teeth of individuals of both Chinese and Indian origin. These grooves are thought to result from an infolding or invagination of Hertwig's sheath, as in dens invaginatus (Lee *et al.*, 1968).

Deep lingual or buccal grooves marking the site of incomplete root bifurcations are found particularly in mandibular second molars. They have also been described in mandibular first premolars (Holt, 1976), and lingual grooves from the occlusal surface of these teeth extending towards the gingival margin have been observed by Berry (1978).

In addition to those invaginations whose primary site of origin is the tooth crown, invaginations have been described by several authors in which the apparent site of origin is the tooth root (Oehlers, 1958). Provided the opening of the invagination has no connection with the oral cavity no complications need ensue. With loss of gingival attachment, however, infection and necrosis of the pulp could ensue in the same manner as with a coronal invagination.

There are instances of double teeth where adventitious furcations can form surface projections of cervical enamel and create an obvious periodontal ligament problem (Brook and Winter, 1970).

Boyde and Jones (1972) carried out a scanning electron microscope study of completed enamel surfaces of unerupted human teeth. They speculated that cervical enamel surface projections could serve as plaque-retaining features.

It may be concluded that there exist a variety of root forms and cervical enamel projections which may predispose teeth to involvement in severe or complicated CIPD.

Tooth structure

Many anomalies of enamel structure, both genetic and environmental, may allow plaque to accumulate due to surface roughness, pitting or grooving. The poor appearance and the lack of improvement to be achieved by tooth-brushing mean that there is little motivation for good hygiene. Extreme discomfort may be experienced by children with hypocalcified enamel when ingesting a wide variety of foods and drink. In some defects, the enamel may break off as large flakes to expose wide areas of sensitive dentine. Poor masticatory function and inadequate oral hygiene may result.

DENTINE DYSPLASIA. SHIELDS TYPE I

This condition has previously been termed rootless teeth, non-opalescent and opalescent dentine, and radicular dentine dysplasia. The teeth have clinically normal crown form but short roots, abnormal root form and at least partial absence of pulp chamber and canals. Both dentitions are affected. The teeth are often malpositioned and very mobile and therefore easily displaced, even by minor trauma. The disease is inherited as an autosomal dominant trait with a frequency of about 1 : 100,000. Teeth affected by this condition tend to migrate and be exfoliated early, even though there is usually little associated gingivitis (Sedano, Sauk and Gorlin, 1977).

SYSTEMIC DEVELOPMENTAL DISORDERS WITH PERIODONTAL LIGAMENT INVOLVEMENT

Diseases affecting tooth eruption

Developmental disturbances to the eruption of teeth may arise directly by influencing the mechanism(s) responsible for generating eruptive forces or indirectly by structures presenting a barrier in the pathway of the erupting tooth. Although the eruptive mechanism is as yet unknown (see Chapter 10) it is thought to reside within the periodontal ligament. Few abnormalities seem to affect the eruptive mechanism directly. Cleidocranial dysostosis results in a generalized failure of tooth eruption throughout the jaws. It is transmitted as an autosomal dominant condition (Gorlin, Pindborg and Cohen, 1976). Other conditions where there may be a generalized failure in tooth eruption relate to hormonal disturbances and these are described in Chapter 20. With respect to indirect factors, Di Biase (1976) has reviewed dental abnormalities which may affect eruption. It can also be envisaged that abnormal changes within the mucosa overlying a developing tooth, as in hereditary fibromatosis gingivae, could increase the resistance to eruption, with the result that the tooth may be prevented from erupting. Since in these situations eruption will occur once the overlying tissue is surgically removed (Duckworth, 1962; Howard, 1966; Johnston, 1969; Di Biase, 1971) it may be that the periodontal ligament is unaffected.

Down's Syndrome

Many Down's Syndrome patients have periodontal disease (Cohen *et al.,* 1961). Dow (1951) found that over 90% of 8—12-year-old 'mongolian' children had periodontal disease. Cutress (1971) reported that the severe periodontal disease commonly found in subjects with Trisomy 21 started at an early age, 5 years or younger, and progressed at such a rate that some teeth were lost by the age of 10 to 11 years. Examining patients aged 19 to 25 years of age,

Kisling and Krebs (1963) found the prevalence of gingivitis to be 100%. Cohen (1960) observed severe periodontal disease in over 90% of a group of mongoloid patients. Similar findings were reported by Johnson and Young (1963).

Periodontal disease in these patients does not seem to affect all areas of the mouth. Cohen (1960) found radiographically that the most frequent sites of bone loss were the anterior regions of both jaws. Johnson and Young (1963) also reported that the anterior region of the mandible had more severe periodontal destruction. Although the alveolar bone loss occurs in both dentitions, it is more common around permanent teeth (Cohen, 1960; Johnson and Young, 1963). There is some suggestion that males are affected more severely than females (McMillan and Kashgarian, 1961).

In an attempt to consider whether there is truly a systemic factor predisposing Down's Syndrome patients to periodontal disease, or whether the levels of disease could be attributed entirely to environmental effects, comparison has been made of Trisomy 21 patients with other congenitally mentally retarded patients. Johnson and Young (1963) reported that the severity of periodontal disease in Down's Syndrome patients was about twice that in other congenitally mentally retarded patients. They found no cases with severe alveolar bone loss in non-mongoloid children. Sznajder *et al.* (1968) found that both mongoloid and cerebral palsy children had poor oral hygiene and similar plaque indices. However, cerebral palsy children did not have advanced periodontal disease with pocket formation, as did the mongoloid children. Cutress (1971) found that extractions for periodontal disease in a large group of subjects aged 10 to 24 years were largely confined to Down's Syndrome patients. Few of the other mentally retarded subjects in his study had extractions for periodontal disease, and none of the normal subjects had required such treatment.

Swallow (1964) and Cutress (1971) reported a higher prevalence of periodontal disease in institutionalized patients with Down's Syndrome than in those living at home. This suggests that both the genetic background of the patient and the environment in which he lives influence the level of CIPD. The relatively low severity of CIPD in Down's Syndrome patients resident at home suggests that oral hygiene practices may be different. However, Cutress (1971) reported that the oral hygiene scores for institutionalized and home groups of Down's Syndrome patients did not differ significantly. Moreover, the greater severity of periodontal disease in Trisomy subjects cannot be explained by the amount of calculus present, because calculus scores were similar for both Down's Syndrome patients and other mentally retarded institutionalized subjects. Local factors, such as tongue abnormalities, dental morphological abnormalities, malocclusion and poor masticatory function may be important. Cohen (1960) suggested that there was reduced resistance to 'local irritation'. No evidence has been found for differences in the microbiology of plaque samples in Down's Syndrome, other mentally retarded and normal subjects (Cutress, Brown and Guy, 1970).

Regarding other factors in the periodontal problems of patients with Down's Syndrome, Sobel and co-workers (1958) showed that they exhibited a lower absorption of vitamin A, lower serum calcium and albumin. Severity of CIPD in Down's Syndrome patients may therefore depend on a combination of genetic and environmental factors, although the precise nature of these is still not clear.

Immunodeficiency diseases

Immunodeficient patients, characterized primarily by dysfunction of the secretory IgA system, have been reported to show less periodontal inflammation than immunocompetent subjects matched in age and Plaque Index (Robertson *et al.*, 1980). In addition, the immunodeficiency disease did not seem to predispose to acute pathology involving the gingiva or other oral soft tissues. The findings with respect to gingival inflammation agree with previous studies of immunodeficient patients (Robertson and Cooper, 1974) and studies of patients receiving immunosuppressive agents (Tollefsen, Saltvedt and Koppang, 1978). Thus the salivary immunoglobulins probably do not play a major protective role in the early periodontal lesion.

Diminished levels of gingival inflammation in these patients allow speculation of either a qualitative difference in the oral microflora or an impairment in host ability to react to plaque. Some differences have been reported in the microbial composition of plaque obtained from patients with abnormalities of the immune system (Brown, 1978). With respect to the host response, the nature of the cellular infiltrate in the local periodontal lesions may be important (see Chapter 15).

Haematological diseases

Many neutrophil disorders and histiocytosis are developmental in origin. They are considered in Chapter 17 which deals with blood and lymphoreticular diseases as they affect the periodontal ligament.

Connective tissue diseases
(See also Chapter 19.)

EHLERS—DANLOS SYNDROMES

Ehlers—Danlos syndromes consist of varying degrees of hyperelastic skin, skin haemorrhages, loose-jointedness and cutaneous pseudotumours. Seven entities have been recognized on the basis of genetics, clinical findings and pathogenesis.

Three variants are autosomal dominant traits (Types I, II, III), three autosomal recessive traits (Types IV, VI, VII) and one is x-linked Type V. Known basic defects are: Type IV — type 3 collagen deficiency; Type V — lysyloxidase deficiency; Type VI — hydroxylysine deficiency; Type VII — procollagen peptidase deficiency (Gorlin, 1976).

The oral mucosa is fragile and easily bruised. Gorlin (1976) noted that gingivae and periodontium are susceptible to injury and to destructive periodontal disease at an early age. Barabas (1969) reported that in the molar teeth examined the cementum seemed disorganized and contained organic inclusions. No periodontal ligament changes have been reported.

MUCOPOLYSACCHARIDOSES AND MUCOLIPIDOSES

The mucopolysaccharidoses (MPSs) and mucolipidoses (MLs) comprise a heterogeneous group of approximately twenty rare, phenotypically similar but genetically distinct, inborn errors of metabolism. Most of these disorders culminate in severe disability over many years, and only seldom result in death in infancy. Specific enzyme deficiencies recently have been discovered for the majority of the mucopolysaccharidoses and also for a few of the mucolipidoses (Gorlin, 1976).

The mucopolysaccharidoses and mucolipidoses are good examples of genetic heterogeneity (multiple genetic causes of a similar phenotype) and pleiotropism (a single gene resulting in several different phenotypic manifestations). For many of these diseases, the genotype can be determined directly by measuring the gene product.

The pattern of inheritance for all these diseases is autosomal recessive with the exception of mucopolysaccharidosis II, which is x-linked (Goodman and Gorlin, 1977). The total incidence of the MPSs has been estimated as approximately 4 : 100,000 (Legum, Schorr and Berman, 1976).

It would seem that tooth eruption is delayed in at least 50% of gargoyle patients (Cawson, 1962). The gingivae are described as hyperplastic, hypertrophic or broad and thick. Ligament changes are not reported, although a prominent feature of the histology of idiopathic gingival hyperplasia was the accumulation of mucoid material among the collagen fibres (Rushton, 1957).

Delay in the appearance of teeth, especially the secondary dentition, is frequent in Hurler syndrome and the teeth may be of an abnormal size and shape. Gingival hypertrophy leads to wide alveolar margins and encroachment of the gums onto the crowns of the teeth (Cawson, 1962). Localized bone destruction resembling dentigerous cysts is common in the mandibular molar region by the age of 3 years. Sedano, Sauk and Gorlin (1977) believed these bone lesions represent hyperplastic dental follicles engorged by dermatan sulphate.

The basis of Maroteaux—Lamy Disease (MPS W) (Polydystrophic Dwarfism) appears to be a deficiency of arylsulphatase B. The permanent mandibular molars are usually delayed in eruption and may be surrounded by radiolucent areas which possibly represent accumulations of dermatan sulphate (Sedano, Sauk and Gorlin, 1977).

The fibroblasts of mucolipidosis II (I-cell disease) contain in their cytoplasm numerous granular inclusions believed to be altered lysosomes. The gingivae are greatly enlarged and may cover the teeth or interfere with eruption. Storage material may occur around unerupted teeth, particularly molars (Gorlin, 1976).

Metabolic disorders

ACATALASIA

Catalase generates oxygen by rapidly decomposing hydrogen peroxide. The physiological role of catalase is not clear. It provides a pathway for breaking down hydrogen peroxide which might otherwise accumulate within the cell. Liberated catalase usually protects surrounding tissues from hydrogen peroxide generated by polymorphonuclear leukocytes during phagocytosis. Acatalasic patients are unable to degrade exogenous or endogenous hydrogen peroxide which accumulates in the periodontal tissues, deprives them of oxygen and causes ulceration and necrosis of the soft and hard tissues (Delgado and Calderon, 1979). The clinical manifestations of catalase deficiency are confined to the oral tissues, specifically to the periodontium. The main oral findings in two Peruvian brothers with acatalasia examined by Delgado and Calderon (1979) were gingival necrosis and severe alveolar bone destruction; otherwise the patients were in good health.

The lesions may appear as soon as the deciduous and permanent teeth erupt. They may begin on the interdental papilla of the incisors and progress to the rest of the teeth. Ulceration and necrosis of the gingivae, vestibular fistulas, migration of teeth, and denuded root surfaces may follow.

Where teeth are absent, the alveolar mucosa is normal; after extractions, wound sockets heal normally. Antibiotic therapy and removal of dental plaque limits the progression of the gingival lesions. Gingival damage perhaps results from a lack of catalase activity in the gingiva, permitting proliferation of bacteria in dental plaque and gingival inflammation. The absence of catalase allows accumulation of hydrogen peroxide in gingival tissues. Most of the cultures obtained from necrotic gingival tissues and from dental plaque showed a predominance of catalase-negative pneumococci which are also known to be hydrogen peroxide producers (Delgado and Calderon, 1979). *Lactobacillus acidophilus* and streptococci also generate hydrogen peroxide. Hydrogen peroxide production during the gingival inflammatory process results from phagocytosis by the polymorphonuclear leukocyte. Thus, it is postulated that the gingival lesions resulted from damage to tissue from hydrogen peroxide generated by organisms in gingival plaque. Some patients with acatalasia, however, do not develop gingival lesions. This could be due to their peculiar oral flora, salivary composition, immunologic status, or tooth composition.

Takahara (1952) proposed that acatalasia was inherited as an autosomal recessive trait. Individuals homozygous for the disorder have little or no catalase activity (Aebi and Wyss, 1978). Using spectrophotometric methods to determine the catalase activity in red blood cells, Delgado and Calderon (1979) were able to show three phenotypes: acatalasic, hypocatalasic and normal. All carriers of acatalasia were hypocatalasic. Thirteen hypocatalasemic (carrier) individuals, including both parents, were found among twenty-nine relatives of the probands examined from four generations. No other acatalasemic individuals were found. Hypocatalasic relatives of the probands did not have oral lesions, and no other abnormalities were detected. The parents of the affected children were not known to be related; however, both parents and their families come from the same small rural community. The inheritance pattern in the kindred was compatible with an autosomal recessive mode of inheritance for the disorder (Delgado and Calderon, 1979).

HYPOPHOSPHATASIA

Hypophosphatasia is a disease complex in which bone fails to mineralize properly. The disease may be either primary or secondary to hypothyroidism, gross anaemia, scurvy, kwashiorkor, achondroplasia, cretinism or the incorporation of radioactive material in bone. It is the primary disease which is considered here.

The condition is characterized usually by subnormal serum alkaline phosphatase values, the presence of phosphoethanolamine in plasma and urine, skeletal abnormalities, and premature loss of teeth. The clinical phenotype of hypophosphatasia may be attributed to defects in the formation of either bone or cementum.

At least three clinical forms of primary disease are seen (Fraser, 1957):

1. The infantile type. This is the severest form. There is severe skeletal disease present at birth and the mortality is greater than 50%.
2. The childhood type. This is a self-limiting disease of moderate severity appearing after 6 months of age.
3. The adult type. This is characterized by the appearance of osteoporosis and bone fragility in early adult life.

A fourth clinical type may exist (Bixler *et al.*, 1974). It is characterized by low serum alkaline phosphatase activity, premature loss of deciduous incisors, and absence of bone lesions. This disorder is much milder than the foregoing types and the serum enzyme levels, although reduced, are not so low.

The anterior teeth may be shed spontaneously or become mobile after relatively minor trauma. There is an absence of severe periodontal inflammation. The teeth most frequently lost are incisors. Occasionally, the dentition may appear to manifest hypereruption and be loose in the alveolus without the evidence of either classical chronic gingivitis or periodontitis (Baer, Brown and Hamner, 1964; Kjellman *et al.*, 1973). Cementum may be completely absent as in Casson's (1969) two cases. When present, the cementum is often very thin or present only in islands.

The degree of cementum aplasia is related to the severity of the overall disease itself (Bruckner, Rickles and Porter, 1962). Even those teeth not exfoliated in affected persons do not have normal amounts of cementum (Beumer *et al.*, 1973). It has also been shown that the periodontal ligament fibres may lack an attachment to the cementum and may even run parallel to the root surface (Listgarten and Houpt, 1969). When cementum is absent, the periodontal ligament fibres approach, but are not attached to, the dentine.

The basic anomaly appears to lie in the matrix.

Fraser and Yendt (1955) showed that the cartilage of rachitic rats would calcify in the serum of patients with hypophosphatasia. However, cartilage from the patients themselves would not calcify in serum from unaffected subjects.

It has been suggested that because serum alkaline phosphatase activity represents a mixture of isoenzymes from bone, liver, and intestine, variation in the isoenzymes themselves may help to explain the spectrum of clinical disease (Scriver and Cameron, 1969; Aminoff, Austrins and Zolfaghari, 1971). Bixler *et al.* (1974) noted electrophoretic variation in the enzymes from one of their families and the report by Hosenfeld and Hosenfeld (1973) also described isoenzyme electrophoretic variation in this disease complex.

A simple autosomal recessive mode of inheritance has been demonstrated for the various types of hypophosphatasia that show markedly decreased serum alkaline phosphatase activity, increased urinary excretion of phosphoethanolamine, rachitic-like bone diseases, and premature loss of deciduous incisors. Thus the genetic patterns appear the same for the infantile, childhood, and adult types. This does not mean, however, that there is not heterogeneity within this grouping, and most workers believe there is more than a single type of hypophosphatasia. Indirect support for this comes from the observation that the heterozygous gene carriers in some families have a serum alkaline phosphatase activity intermediate between that of the affected and the normal (Glimcher and Krane, 1962). However, numerous other families have not shown this result. A similar problem has been observed when testing heterozygotes for phosphoethanolamine excretion (Harris and Robson, 1959). A tentative interpretation of these results has been non-penetrance, but it seems more likely that there is more than one disease entity in the entire group, all with a recessive mode of inheritance (Poland *et al.*, 1972).

There may also be a dominantly inherited form of hypophosphatasia (Bixler, 1976). Affected individuals have no bone disease, but a lowered serum alkaline phosphatase (not so severe as in the recessive form), and show premature incisor loss. Bixler (1976) reported no example of non-penetrance, and the clinical picture was remarkably consistent. The presence of two genetic forms of hypophosphatasia, one recessive and the other dominant, makes it clear that at least two genes are involved in this disease complex, and the variability in clinical phenotype of the recessive form suggests additional genes, allelic or otherwise.

Skin diseases

HYPERKERATOSIS PALMOPLANTARIS AND PERIODONTOCLASIA IN CHILDHOOD (PAPILLON—LEFÈVRE SYNDROME)

This syndrome is characterized by hyperkeratosis of the palms and soles with premature destruction of the periodontal ligament of deciduous and permanent teeth, resulting in their early loss (Gorlin, Sedano and Anderson, 1964; Carvel, 1969). Following normal eruption of deciduous teeth, the gingivae become red and swollen and bleed easily. At about the same time, the palmar and plantar hyperkeratosis usually begins to appear. With the full eruption of the second deciduous molars, destruction of the periodontal ligament is noted. Deep periodontal pockets are formed which exude pus on pressure and marked halitosis may be noted. The teeth become mobile and radiographs show marked destruction of the supporting alveolar bone. By 4 to 5 years of age, the teeth are exfoliated, often in a sequence similar to that in which they erupted. The gingival inflammation resolves with the loss of the deciduous teeth. A similar process begins with the commencement of eruption of permanent teeth, although the symptoms may be more marked. By about 15 years of age, all permanent teeth except the third molars usually have been shed. When all permanent teeth are lost, the gingival tissue resumes its normal appearance (Carvel, 1969; Sedano et al., 1977).

Gorlin, Sedano and Anderson (1964) consider this condition to be an autosomal recessive trait and have estimated the frequency of the condition to be approximately 1 : 1,000,000. Between 1924, when first described, and 1969 there were fifty-three case reports (Carvel, 1969).

There are several syndromes characterized by palmoplantar hyperkeratosis but the Papillon—Lefèvre is the only one with such rampant precocious periodontal destruction. Histologically, the periodontal ligament is destroyed and replaced by chronic granulation tissue. There is considerable osteoclastic activity in the ligament. The cementum along most of the root surface is very thin except in the apical area where some cellular cementum may be present (Martinez Lalis, Lopez Otero and Carranza, 1965). Using disc electrophoresis, Shoshan, Finkelstein and Rosenzweig (1970) compared collagen from clincally healthy gingiva and clinically inflamed gingiva of otherwise healthy young people with that of a 14-year-old patient with Papillon—Lefèvre syndrome. They postulated that the periodontal involvement may result from a functional imbalance of collagenolytic activity in the periodontal ligament.

REFERENCES

AEBI, H. E. & WYSS, S. R. (1978) Acatalasemia. In: *The metabolic basis of inherited disease,* J. B. STANBURY, I. B. WYNGARDEN and D. S. FREDRICKSON (eds.) (4th ed.), pp. 1792–1807. New York, McGraw-Hill.

AMINOFF, D., AUSTRINS, M. & ZOLFAGHARI, S. P. (1971) Plasma alkaline phosphatase isozymes: isolation and characterization of isozymes. *Biochem. Biophys. Acta* **242,** 108–122.

BAER, P. N. (1971) The case for periodontosis as a clinical entity. *J. Periodont.* **42,** 516–520.

BAER, P. N., BROWN, N. C. & HAMNER, J. E. (1964) Hypophosphatasia: report of two cases with dental findings. *Periodontics* **2,** 209–215.

BAER, P. N. & GAMBLE, J. W. (1966) Autogenous dental transplants as a method of treating the osseous defect in periodontosis. *Oral Surg.* **22,** 405–410.

BAER, P. N. & LIEBERMAN, J. E. (1959) Observations on some genetic characteristics of the periodontium in three strains of inbred mice. *Oral Surg.* **12,** 820–829.

BARABAS, G. M. (1969) The Ehlers—Danlos Syndrome. Abnormalities of the enamel, dentine, cementum and the dental pulp: an histological examination of 13 teeth from 6 patients. *Br. dent. J.* **126,** 509–515.

BARROS, L. & WITKOP, C. J. (1963) Oral and genetic study of Chileans. 1960. III. Periodontal disease and nutritional factors. *Archs. oral Biol.* **8,** 195–206.

BENJAMIN, S. D. & BAER, P. N. (1967) Familial patterns of advanced alveolar bone loss in adolescence (periodontosis). *Periodontics* **5,** 82–88.

BERRY, A. C. (1978) Anthropological and family studies on minor variants of the dental crown. In: *Development, function and evolution of teeth,* P. M. BUTLER & K. A. JOSEY (eds.), pp. 81–96. London, Academic Press.

BEUMER, J., TROWBRIDGE, H. O., SILVERMAN, S. & EISENBERG, E. (1973) Childhood hypophosphatasia and the premature loss of teeth. *Oral Surg.* **35**, 631–640.

BISSADA, N. F. & ABDELMALEK, R. G. (1973) Incidence of cervical enamel projections and its relationship to furcation involvement in Egyptian skulls. *J. Periodont.* **44**, 583–585.

BIXLER, D. (1976) Heritable disorders affecting cementum and the periodontal structure. In: *Oral facial genetics*, R. E. STEWART & G. H. PRESCOTT (eds.), pp. 262–287. St. Louis, Mosby.

BIXLER, D., POLAND, C. P., BRANDT, I. K. & NICHOLAS, N. J. (1974) Autosomal dominant hypophosphatasia without skeletal disease. American Society of Human Genetics, 26th Annual Meeting, Portland, Ore., 1974.

BORRING-MØLLER, G. & FRANDSEN, A. (1978) Autologous tooth transplantation to replace molars lost in patients with juvenile periodontitis. *J. Clin. Periodont.* **5**, 152–158.

BOYDE, A. & JONES, S. J. (1972) Scanning electron microscopic studies of the formation of mineralized tissues. In: *Developmental aspects of oral biology*, H. C. SLAVKIN & L. A. BAVETTA (eds.), pp. 261–263. New York, Academic Press.

BROOK, A. H. & WINTER, G. B. (1970) Double teeth. A retrospective study of 'geminated' and 'fused' teeth in children. *Brit. dent. J.* **129**, 123–130.

BROWN, R. H. (1978) A longitudinal study of periodontal disease in Down's syndrome. *N. Z. dent. J.* **74**, 137–144.

BRUCKNER, R. J., RICKLES, N. H. & PORTER, D. R. (1962) Hypophosphatasia with premature shedding of teeth and aplasia of cementum. *Oral Surg.* **15**, 1351–1359.

BUDTZ-JORGENSEN, E., ELLEGAARD, J., ELLEGAARD, B., JORGENSEN, F. & KELSTRUP, J. (1978) Cell-mediated immunity in juvenile periodontitis and levamisole treatment. *Scand. J. dent. Res.* **86**, 124–129.

BUTLER, J. H. (1969) A familial pattern of juvenile periodontitis (periodontosis). *J. Periodont.* **40**, 115–118.

CARMICHAEL, A. F. (1965) The distribution of ABO blood groups in cases of periodontal disease. *Dent. Mag.* (Lond.) **82**, 255–257.

CARVEL, R. I. (1969) Palmo-plantar hyperkeratosis and premature periodontal destruction. *J. Oral Med.* **24**, 73–82.

CASSON, M. (1969) Oral manifestations of primary hypophosphatasia. *Br. dent. J.* **127**, 561–566.

CAWSON, R. A. (1962) The oral changes in gargoylism. *Proc. R. Soc. Med.* **55**, 1066–1077.

CHUNG, C. S., RUNCK, D. W., NISWANDER, J. D., BILBEN, S. E. & KAU, M. C. W. (1970) Genetic and epidemiologic studies of oral characteristics in Hawaii's school children. I. Caries and periodontal disease. *J. dent. Res.* **49**, 1374–1385.

CIANCIOLA, L., GENCO, R. J., PATTERS, M. R., McKENNA, I. & VAN OSS, C. J. (1977) Defective polymorphonuclear leukocyte function in a human periodontal disease. *Nature* **265**, 445–447.

CLARK, R. A., PAGE, R. C. & WILDE, G. (1977) Defective neutrophil chemotaxis in juvenile periodontitis. *Infect. Immun.* **18**, 694–700.

COHEN, D. W. & GOLDMAN, H. M. (1960) Clinical obser-

vations on the modification of human oral tissue metabolism by local intraoral factors. *Ann. N.Y. Acad. Sci.* **85**, 68–95.

COHEN, M. M. (1960) Periodontal disturbances in the mentally subnormal child. *Dent. Clin. N. Amer.* 483–489.

COHEN, M. M., WINER, R. A., SCHWARTZ, S. & SHKLAR, G. (1961) Oral aspects of mongolism. Part I. Periodontal disease in mongolism. *Oral Surg.* **14**, 92–107.

CULLINAN, M. P., SACHS, G., WOLF, E. & SEYMOUR, G. J. (1980) The distribution of HLA-A and B antigens in patients and their families with periodontosis. *J. periodont. Res.* **15**, 177–184.

CUTRESS, T. W. (1971) Periodontal disease and oral hygiene in trisomy 21. *Archs. oral Biol.* **16**, 1345–1355.

CUTRESS, T. W., BROWN, R. H. & GUY, E. (1970) Occurrence of some bacterial species in dental plaque of trisomic 21 (mongoloid), other mentally retarded and normal subjects. *N. Z. dent. J.* **66**, 40–45.

DELGADO, W. A. & CALDERON, R. (1979) Acatalasia in two Peruvian siblings. *Oral Path.* **8**, 358–368.

DI BIASE, D. D. (1971) The effects of variations in tooth morphology and position on eruption. *Dent. Practnr.* **22**, 95–108.

DI BIASE, D. D. (1976) Dental abnormalities affecting eruption. In: *The eruption and occlusion of teeth*, D. F. G. POOLE & M. V. STACK (eds.). Colston Papers No. 27. pp. 156–168. London, Butterworths.

DOW, R. S. (1951) A preliminary study of periodontoclasia in mongolian children at Polk State School. *Amer. J. ment. Defic.* **55**, 535–538.

DUCKWORTH, R. (1962) Abnormal attachment of labial mucosa in maleruption of teeth. *Brit. dent. J.* **113**, 312–314.

EVERETT, F. G. & KRAMER, G. M. (1972) The distolingual groove in the maxillary lateral incisor: a periodontal hazard. *J. Periodont.* **43**, 352–361.

FOUREL, J. (1972) Periodontosis: a periodontal syndrome. *J. Periodont.* **43**, 240–255.

FRANDSEN, A. (1978) Personal communication cited by Saxen (1980).

FRASER, D. (1957) Hypophosphatasia. *Amer. J. Med.* **22**, 730–746.

FRASER, D. & YENDT, E. R. (1955) Metabolic abnormalities in hypophosphatasia. *Amer. J. Dis. Child.* **90**, 552–554.

FRIEDMAN, S. A., FARBER, P. A. & SALKIN, L. M. (1976) Histopathology of juvenile periodontitis. I. Surface morphology of inflammatory cells. *J. dent. Res.* **55**, B259 (abs.).

GLIMCHER, M. J. & KRANE, S. M. (1962) Studies of the interactions of collagen and phosphate. I. The nature of inorganic and organophosphate binding. In: *Radioisotopes and bone*, P. LACROIX & A. M. BUDY (eds.), pp. 393–418. Oxford, Blackwell.

GOODMAN, R. M. & GORLIN, R. J. (1977) *Atlas of the face in genetic disorders*, pp. 17–18. St. Louis, Mosby.

GORLIN, R. J. (1976) In: *Oral facial genetics*, R. E. STEWART & G. H. PRESCOTT (eds.), pp. 338–384. St. Louis, Mosby.

GORLIN, R. J., PINDBORG, J. J. & COHEN, M. M. (1976) *Syndromes of the head and neck*. McGraw-Hill, New York.

GORLIN, R. J., SEDANO, H. & ANDERSON, V. E. (1964) The syndrome of palmar-plantar hyperkeratosis and premature periodontal destruction of the teeth. *J. Pediatr.* **65**, 895–908.

GORLIN, R. J., STALLARD, R. E. & SHAPIRO, B. L. (1967) Genetics and periodontal disease. *J. Periodont.* **38**, 5–10.

HAMNER, J. E., WITKOP, C. J. & METRO, P. S. (1964) Taurodontism, report of a case. *Oral Surg.* **18**, 409–418.

HARRIS, H. & ROBSON, E. B. (1959) A genetical study of ethanolamine phosphate excretion in hypophosphatasia. *Ann. Human Genet.* **23**, 421–441.

HOLT, R. D. (1976) *The prevalence of root anomalies in children.* M.Sc. dissertation, Univ. London.

HOLT, R. D. & BROOK, A. H. (1979) Taurodontism: a criterion for diagnosis and its prevalence in mandibular first molars in a sample of 1,115 British school children. *J. Int. Assoc. Dent. Child.* **10**, 41–47.

HOSENFELD, D. & HOSENFELD, A. (1973) Qualitative and quantitative examinations of the isoenzymes of serum alkaline phosphatase in hypophosphatasia. *Klin. Paediatr.* **185**, 437–443.

HOWARD, R. D. (1966) The unerupted incisor. *Trans. Br. Soc. Study Orthod.* 30–40.

JACOBSON, L., SVÄRDSTRÖM, G. & DANIELSSON, D. (1978) Post juvenile periodontitis. Immunological screening of 30 patients. *Swed. dent. J.* **2**, 209–212.

JOHNSON, N. P. & YOUNG, M. A. (1963) Periodontal disease in mongols. *J. Periodont.* **34**, 41–47.

JOHNSTON, W. P. (1969) Treatment of palatally impacted canine teeth. *Amer. J. Orthodont.* **56**, 589–596.

JORGENSON, R. J., LEVIN, L. S., HUTCHERSON, S. T. & SALINAS, C. F. (1975) Periodontosis in sibs. *Oral Surg.* **39**, 396–402.

KASLICK, R. S., WEST, T. L. & CHASENS, A. I. (1980) Association between ABO blood groups, HL-A antigens and periodontal diseases in young adults: a follow-up study. *J. Periodont.* **51**, 339–342.

KASLICK, R. S., WEST, T. L., CHASENS, A. I., TERASAKI, P. I., LAZZARA, R. & WEINBERG, S. (1975) Association between HL-A2 antigen and various periodontal diseases in young adults. *J. dent. Res.* **54**, 424.

KEITH, A. (1913) Problems relating to the teeth of the earlier forms of prehistoric man. *Proc. R. Soc. Med.* **6**, 103–119.

KERR, D. A. (1961) The cementum: its role in periodontal health and disease. *J. Periodont.* **32**, 183–189.

KIRKHAM, L. B. (1977) Periodontosis – general discussion and report of familial cases. *J. Wisconsin dent. Assoc.* **53**, 347–349.

KISLING, E. & KREBS, G. (1963) Periodontal conditions in adult patients with mongolism (Down's syndrome). *Acta odont. Scand.* **21**, 391–405.

KJELLMAN, M., OLDFELT, V., NORDENRAM, A. & OLOW-NORDENRAM, M. (1973) Five cases of hypophosphatasia with dental findings. *Int. J. Oral Surg.* **2**, 152–158.

LAVINE, W. S., MADERAZO, E. G., STOLMAN, J., WARD, P. A., COGEN, R. B., GREENBLATT, I. & ROBERTSON, P. B. (1979) Impaired neutrophil chemotaxis in patients with juvenile and rapidly progressing periodontitis. *J. periodont. Res.* **14**, 10–19.

LEE, K. W., LEE, E. C. & POON, K. Y. (1968) Palato-gingival grooves in maxillary incisors. *Br. dent. J.* **124**, 14–18.

LEGUM, C. P., SCHORR, S. & BERMAN, E. R. (1976) The genetic mucopolysaccharidoses and mucolipidoses: review and comment. *Adv. Pediatr.* **22**, 305–347.

LEHNER, T., WILTON, J. M. A., IVANYI, L. & MANSON, J. D. (1974) Immunological aspects of juvenile periodontitis (periodontosis). *J. periodont. Res.* **9**, 261–272.

LEIB, A. M., BERDON, J. K. & SABES, W. R. (1967) Furcation involvements correlated with enamel projections from the cementoenamel junction. *J. Periodont.* **38**, 330–334.

LILJENBERG, B. & LINDHE, J. (1980) Juvenile periodontitis. Some microbiological, histopathological and clinical characteristics. *J. Clin. Periodont.* **7**, 48–61.

LISTGARTEN, M. A. & HOUPT, M. (1969) Ultrastructural features of the rooth surface of deciduous teeth in patients with hypophosphatasia. *J. periodont. Res.* Suppl. 4, 34–35.

MALENA, D. E. (1972) ABO phenotypes and periodontal disease. *J. dent. Res.* **51**, 1504.

MANSON, J. D. (1977) Juvenile periodontitis (periodontosis). *Int. dent. J.* **27**, 114–118.

MANSON, J. D. & LEHNER, T. (1974) Clinical features of juvenile periodontitis (periodontosis). *J. Periodont.* **45**, 636–640.

MARTINEZ LALIS, R. R., LOPEZ OTERO, R. & CARRANZA, F. A. (1965) A case of Papillon–Lefèvre syndrome. *Periodontics* **3**, 292–295.

MASTERS, D. H. & HOSKINS, S. W. (1964) Projections of cervical enamel into molar furcations. *J. Periodont.* **35**, 49–53.

McMILLAN, R. S. & KASHGARIAN, M. (1961) Relation of human abnormalities of structure and function to abnormalities of the dentition. II. Mongolism. *J. Amer. dent. Assoc.* **63**, 368–373.

MELNICK, M., SHIELDS, E. D. & BIXLER, D. (1976) Periodontosis: a phenotypic and genetic analysis. *Oral Surg.* **42**, 32–41.

MÜHLEMANN, H. R. (1972) Karies und Parodontopathien beim Menschen in genetischen Sicht. *Schweiz. Monatschr. Zahnheilk.* **82**, 942–959.

NISENGARD, R. J., MYERS, D. & NEWMAN, M. G. (1977) Human antibody titres to periodontosis – associated microbiota. *J. dent. Res.* **56**, A73 (abs.).

NISWANDER, J. D. (1975) Genetics of common dental disorders. In: *Dent. Clin. N. Amer.* **19**, 197–206.

OEHLERS, F. A. C. (1958) The radicular variety of dens invaginatus. *Oral Surg.* **11**, 1251–1260.

PETERSON, R. J. & MARSH, C. L. (1979) The relationship of Alpha-antitrypsin to inflammatory periodontal disease. *J. Periodont.* **50**, 31–35.

POLAND, C. P., EVERSOLE, L. R., BIXLER, D. & CHRISTIAN, J. C. (1972) Histochemical observations of hypophosphatasia. *J. dent. Res.* **51**, 333–338.

POLEVITZKY, K. (1929) Blood types in pyorrhea alveolaris. *J. dent. Res.* **9**, 285 (abs.).

PRADHAN, A. C., CHAWLA, T. N., SAMUEL, K. C. & PRADHAN, S. (1971) The relationship between periodontal disease and blood groups and secretor status. *J. periodont. Res.* **6**, 294–300.

RAO, S. S. & TEWANI, S. V. (1968) Prevalence of periodontosis among Indians. *J. Periodont.* **39**, 27–34.

REINHOLDT, J., BAY, I. & SVEJGAARD, A. (1977) Association between HLA-antigens and periodontal disease. *J. dent. Res.* **56**, 1216–1263.

REISEL, J. H. (1971) Clinical osteoporosis and periodontal disease. *Ned. Tijdschr. Tandheelkd.* **78**, 132–135.

ROBERTSON, P. B. & COOPER, M. D. (1974) Oral manifestations of IgA deficiency. *Adv. Exp. Med. Biol.* **45**, 497–503.

ROBERTSON, P. B., MACKLER, B. F., WRIGHT, T. E. & LEVY, B. M. (1980) Periodontal status of patients with abnormalities of the immune system. Observations over a 2-year period. *J. Periodont.* **51**, 70–73.

RUSHTON, M. A. (1957) Hereditary or idiopathic hyperplasia of the gums. *Dent. Practit.* **7**, 136–146.

SAUK, J. J. (1980) Defects of the teeth and tooth-bearing structures. In: *Textbook of pediatric dentistry,* R. L. BRAHAM & M. E. MORRIS (eds.), pp. 57–83. Baltimore, Williams and Wilkins.

SAXEN, L. (1980) Juvenile periodontitis: a review. *J. Clin. Periodont.* **7**, 1–19.

SCRIVER, C. R. & CAMERON, D. (1969) Pseudohypophosphatasia. *N. Engl. J. Med.* **281**, 604–606.

SEDANO, H. O., SAUK, G. G. & GORLIN, R. J. (1977) *Oral manifestations of inherited disorders,* pp. 168, 191 and 194–195. Boston, Butterworths.

SHILOAH, J. & KOPCZYK, R. A. (1979) Developmental variations of tooth morphology and periodontal disease. *J. Amer. dent. Assoc.* **99**, 627–630.

SHOSHAN, S., FINKELSTEIN, S. & ROSENZWEIG, K. A. (1970) Disc electrophoretic pattern of gingival collagen isolated from a patient with palmoplantar hyperkeratosis. *J. periodont. Res.* **5**, 255–258.

SOBEL, A. E., STRAZZULLA, M., SHERMAN, B. S., ELKAN, B., MORGENSTERN, S. W., MARIUS, N. & MEISEL, A. (1958) Vitamin A absorption and other blood composition studies in mongolism. *Amer. J. ment. Defic.* **62**, 642–655.

SUSSMAN, H. I. & BAER, P. N. (1978) Three generations of periodontosis: Case report. *Ann. Dent.* **37**, 8–11.

SWALLOW, J. N. (1964) Dental disease in children with Down's syndrome. *J. ment. Defic. Res.* **8**, 102–118.

SZNAJDER, N., CARRARO, J. J., OTERO, E. & CARRANZA, F. A. (1968) Clinical periodontal findings in trisomy 21 (Mongolism). *J. periodont. Res.* **3**, 1–5.

TAKAHARA, S. (1952) Progressive oral gangrene probably due to lack of catalase in the blood (acatalasemia). Report of nine cases. *Lancet* **2**, 1101–1104.

TOLLEFSEN, T., SALTVEDT, E. & KOPPANG, H. S. (1978) The effect of immunosuppressive agents on periodontal disease in man. *J. periodont. Res.* **13**, 240–250.

TSUNEMITSU, A., HONJO, K., KANI, M. & MATSUMURA, T. (1964) Citric acid metabolism in periodontosis. *Archs. oral Biol.* **9**, 83–86.

VAN SWOL, R. L., GROSS, A., SETTERSTROM, J. A. & D'ALESSANDRO, S. M. (1980) Concentrations of immunoglobulins in granulation tissue from pockets of periodontosis and periodontitis patients. *J. Periodont.* **51**, 20–24.

WITKOP, C. J. (1975) Hereditary defects of dentin. *Dent. Clin. N. Amer.* **19** (1), 25–45.

WITKOP, C. J., MacLEAN, C. J. & SCHMIDT, P. J. (1966) Medical and dental findings in the Brandywine isolate. *Ala. J. Med. Sci.* **3**, 382–403.

ZIMMERMAN, B. R. & BAKER, W. A. (1960) Effect of geographic location and race on gingival disease in children. *J. Amer. dent. Assoc.* **51**, 542–547.

Chapter 14

TRAUMA AND THE PERIODONTAL LIGAMENT
H. N. Newman and J. D. Strahan

INTRODUCTION

To date, there has been no systematic review of the effects of trauma to the periodontal ligament. Periodontologists have been concerned mainly with trauma to the lateral portion of the ligament; endodontists have been interested mostly in periapical changes induced by their procedures. There are also few documented instances of experimental physical and chemical injury to the periodontal ligament. Information on changes as they relate to human periodontal ligament is scarce, particularly for occlusal traumatism. No one seems to have produced in experimental animals an occlusal traumatism like that which occurs in man in the presence of dental plaque.

This review has been written with these limitations in mind. As the range of responses is limited, it seemed logical to consider the subject matter under the headings of types of traumatic factor rather than resultant damage. The first section considers the effects of occlusal trauma, including excessive orthodontic forces, and surgical trauma, including replants and implants. The second section is concerned with the sequelae of endodontic injury. The final section collates information on the more abstruse forms of physical and chemical injury to which periodontal ligaments have been subjected.

We have not discussed damage resulting from a variety of iatrogenic procedures, for example from the subgingival placement of orthodontic bands and elastics, gingival retraction cords, copper rings, impression materials, restorations with subgingival overhanging margins, or from the use of a range of periodontal surgical procedures (including pericision) since these affect almost exclusively the gingival ligament.

From the studies reported it will be shown that the periodontal ligament has a considerable potential for repair, often following comparatively severe injury. The role of occlusal trauma in chronic inflammatory periodontal disease has been less well defined. It seems that complete resolution will occur in the absence of infective matter (i.e. plaque) and that occlusal trauma is a factor in progressive ligament destruction only when combined with plaque. Regarding periapical responses to injury, it seems that chemically induced damage using clinically suitable endodontic materials is often transient, and that overinstrumentation is a more significant clinical cause of periapical ligament injury.

OCCLUSAL TRAUMA

Parafunction

Early work concerning the influence of parafunction on the human periodontal ligament was summarized in the statement that functionless teeth show poorly developed ligament, consisting merely of loose connective tissue almost devoid of fibre bundles, whereas ligaments subjected to excessive, abnormal function undergo hypertrophy (Kronfeld, 1931). Coolidge (1938) noted that jaws in which many teeth were missing furnished the most frequent evidence of trauma (in the periodontal ligaments of the remaining teeth). He listed these injuries as haemorrhage, thrombosis and hyalinization of the ligament. In instances of severe damage, he observed tissue necrosis. He claimed that the likelihood of necrosis was increased by excessive pressure and that less severe forces resulted in hyalinization of the affected portion of the ligament, with loss of fibroblast nuclei. He also noted instances of repair following removal of the trauma. Early conclusions such as these were based on extrapolations from jaw biopsies. Most investigators since have tried to relate ligament changes to the type of trauma. However, in none of the studies does the periodontal ligament appear to have been subjected to stresses typical of occlusal traumatism which clinically is related to an unusually rapid rate of ligament destruction. Attempts to correlate occlusal traumatism and chronic periodontitis using human autopsy and biopsy material are inconclusive (Waerhaug, 1979).

One of the early methods of applying stress was to place a wedge (e.g. a piece of rubber dam) between two teeth (Macapanpan and Weinmann, 1954). This caused a widening of the ligament on the tension side and a narrowing on the pressure side within 3 days. After 3 days, young fibroblasts differentiated in the stretched portion of ligament near the alveolar crest. Leukocytes seemed to enter the ligament at this site. Capillary damage and small areas of haemorrhage were observed. Macapanpan and Weinmann (1954) were among many in observing that traumatism of the ligament will not by itself produce the lesion of chronic inflammatory periodontal disease. Further studies (Macapanpan, Meyer and Weinmann, 1954)

revealed that the rate of mitotic activity of periodontal fibroblasts was directly proportional to the increase in width of the ligament due to tension, becoming greatest between 24 and 36 hours from the time of insertion of the rubber dam, and reducing to zero by 48 hours. They concluded that fibroblast proliferation is part of the process by which the damaged fibre bundles of abruptly enlarged periodontal spaces are repaired.

Bhaskar and Orban (1955) produced traumatism with premature contact from high crowns placed on monkey premolar teeth. After 3 days there was necrosis of periodontal fibres on the pressure side and widening of the periodontal space and vascular thrombosis on the tension side. Both features became more pronounced after 3 weeks. Following removal of the high contacts, repair occurred within 3 to 6 months. Neither gingival changes nor pocket formation were observed. Similar features were observed by Glickman and Weiss (1955). In addition, they noted that loss of principal fibres was most marked adjacent to bone on the pressure side, where the tissue was more vascular and cellular than normal, many of the cells being osteoclasts. The tension side contained densely packed fibre bundles, many fibroblasts and dilated blood vessels.

Wentz, Jarabak and Orban (1958) fitted rhesus monkeys with high gold crowns and an appliance to produce jiggling forces. In both 3- and 6-month specimens, the periodontal space was elongated apically and was 3 times its original lateral width. However, neither gingivitis nor periodontitis was present. Pressure (132 days) without jiggling led to depression of the tooth in its socket, altered orientation of transseptal fibres and persistence of any necrotic areas. Such changes resolved if the pressure was removed. Glickman and Smulow (1962, 1968) suggested that excessive force was necessary to damage the ligament on the tension side. On the pressure side of their specimens, the periodontal fibres underwent moderate compression, disorientation, realignment and degeneration and there was engorgement of blood vessels. Eventually, most periodontal fibres became realigned parallel to root and bone. The compressed ligament becomes either acellular or shows pyknotic nuclei (Picton, 1976; Polson, Meitner and Zander, 1976 a and b). Leukocytes penetrate between the injured periodontal fibres. In areas subjected to severe pressure, the ligament necroses (Glickman and Smulow, 1962, 1968). Picton (1976) suggested that this was due to prolonged ischaemia followed by autolysis.

Crumley (1964) carried out a rubber dam-type traumatism study on rats. He observed orientation of the fibre bundles on the tension side in the direction of stress between bone and cementum but poor organization of fibres in areas subjected to pressure. Using labelling with tritiated proline, he showed that most cell activity in the stressed ligament was initially osteoblastic, the periodontal fibre bundles exhibiting only slight labelling. In 1- and 3-day specimens the Sharpey's fibres in bone were relatively heavily labelled. The coronal third of the ligament adjacent to cementum showed little labelling, unlike the corresponding apical third. Crumley indicated that this may be due to cementum forming mainly on the apical third. He found no concentration of labelling at any time in the central zone of the periodontal ligament. Silver grains in the ligament were mostly over the cells, mainly fibroblasts (but including vascular endothelium), 30 minutes after ^{3}H-proline administration. Later, a small but significant number of grains was extracellular and at 4 hours there was moderately heavy labelling of loose perivascular connective tissue. There was no dense labelling in any areas of ligament exposed to pressure. At the earliest (30 minutes) and latest (72 hours) time intervals, the proportion of extracellular grains was highest in the zone of ligament adjacent to bone. Crumley (1964) concluded that fibroblast activity was responsible for fibre production in the periodontal ligament, and that extracellular labelling in the ligament after tritiated proline administration was due to the presence of a collagen-bound derivative of the labelled proline. It should be remembered that proline-labelling is not specific for collagen.

In a histologic and autoradiographic study of periodontal healing following wedging (compressive) interdental injury in mice, Solt and Glickman (1968) observed after 4 days compressive necrosis of alveolar crest and transseptal fibres and a moderate level of inflammation around the necrotic zone. Using tritiated proline, they claimed that in the injured tissue there was a decrease in collagen formation in transseptal and crestal ligaments. By 8 days, there was an increase in ligament cellularity and reorientation of transseptal and crestal fibres. New collagen formation was greatest between 4 and 8 days. By 2 weeks, there was only moderate inflammation and transseptal and alveolar crest fibres were organized into bundles. By 3 weeks, the test and control ligaments were indistinguishable histologically. There was a corresponding increase in collagen formation interdentally and interradicularly in the periodontal ligaments of teeth opposing those subjected to injury, although they appeared histologically normal. Similarly, the usual pressure and tension side changes may take place in distant teeth due to trauma from occlusion (Nascimento and Sallum, 1975).

Few workers have investigated the biophysics of occlusal traumatism. Palcanis (1973) applied excessive occlusal loads for 48 hours to dog canines. He showed that the histological changes described by others resulted from microcirculatory injury due to pressure. Less severe hyperfunction, as from the placing of slightly high amalgams, leads to an increase in the gingival vascular network, but only rarely to similar changes in the periodontal ligament (Koivumaa and Lassila, 1971). Occlusal trauma causes an increase in resting intra-ligament pressure (Palcanis, 1973; Walker, Ng and Burke, 1978).

There has always been difficulty in correlating histological changes with the clinical features of occlusal traumatism. Mobility of teeth may not correlate with radiographic signs such as widening of the periodontal space (Posselt and Maunsbach, 1957; Mühlemann and Herzog, 1961). Glickman and Smulow (1962, 1969) attempted to correlate occlusal traumatism with the pattern of tissue destruction in chronic inflammatory periodontal disease, using high gold crowns in rhesus monkeys. Their work suggested that excessive forces (particularly pressure) could determine the path of tissue damage. These and other studies using human biopsy and autopsy material have led to the conclusion that trauma from occlusion and gingival inflammation were co-destructive factors responsible for the production of vertical patterns of ligament and alveolar bone destruction (Glickman, 1963; Glickman and Smulow, 1965, 1967). Similar studies in monkeys also showed that periodontal pockets advance more rapidly in the presence of excessive occlusal loads (Waerhaug and Hansen, 1966) (Fig. 1). However, there is contradictory evidence, in that histological examination of

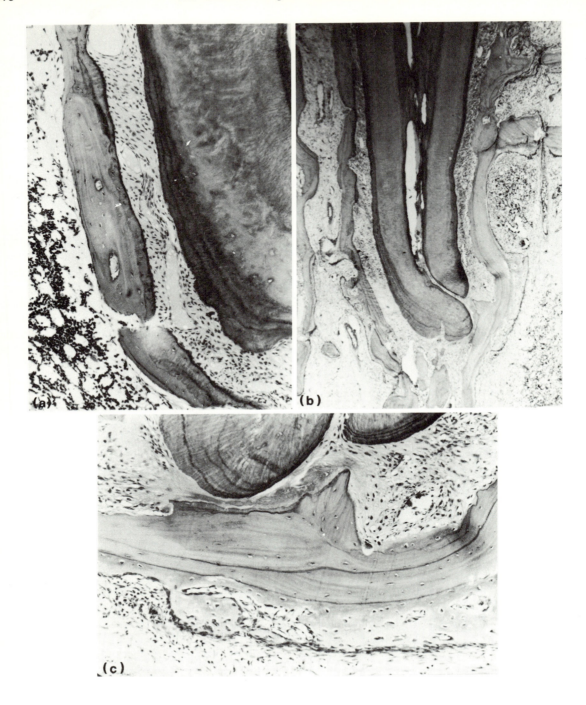

FIG. 1. Effects of trauma on primate (Squirrel monkey) periodontal ligament. (a) Control. ×40. (b) Periodontal ligament after 2 weeks of subjection to mesiodistal jiggling forces. Note increases in width of ligament on left (tension) side. ×40. (c) Specimen as in (b). Note acellularity and narrowing of ligament in pressure area at root apex. ×160. (d) Specimen as in (b). Tension side. The ligament is wider and less cellular than normal. ×160. (e) After 10 weeks of mesiodistal jiggling forces. Reversion to more normal appearance, but increased width of ligament still apparent. ×160. (f) Specimen as in (e). Pressure side. Note more normal cellularity of still narrow ligament. ×160.

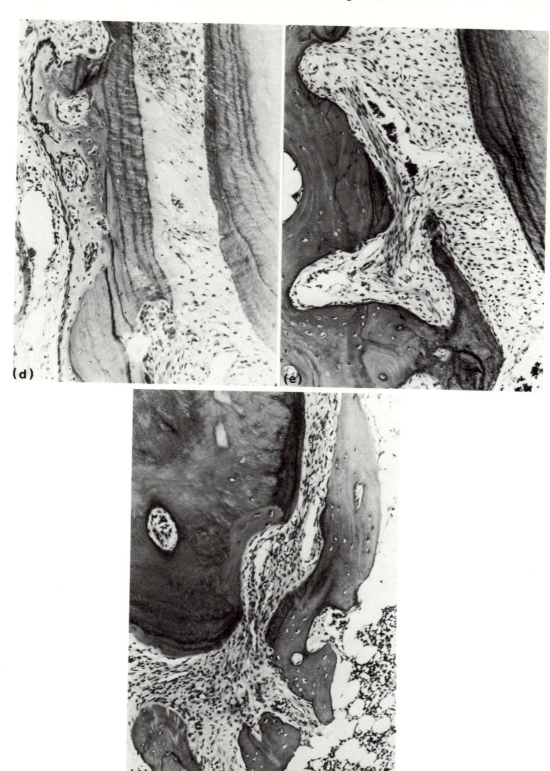

human periodontal ligaments subjected to occlusal hyperfunction as assessed from autopsy material showed minimal change (Koivumaa and Lassila, 1971).

Experimental hypermobility of (dog) teeth has been achieved with a cap splint which displaced the tooth and a spring mechanism tending to return the tooth to its original position. Over 13 days, this caused a widening of the periodontal ligament and the types of bone defect associated by earlier workers with occlusal traumatism (Svanberg and Lindhe, 1973). Similar jiggling-type forces produced prolonged hypermobility if the forces were maintained. In addition, Svanberg and Lindhe (1974) and Svanberg (1974) observed increasing width and vascularity of the alveolar crest periodontal ligament on the pressure side. Trauma from occlusion neither induced gingivitis nor influenced the level or extent of established gingivitis. However, around dogs' teeth with surgically created bony pockets allowed to accumulate plaque, jiggling forces produced more rapid increase in pocket depth, although gingivitis and plaque levels were similar on test and control sides (Lindhe and Svanberg, 1974). Dogs with healthy periodontal tissues adapted to the altered occlusion within 6 months of the start of the experiment, whereas those animals with experimental periodontitis still showed ligament abnormalities after this time, including increased vascular leakage, leucocyte migration and osteoclastic activity.

Polson (1974), using a circumdental ligature technique to produce a progressive periodontitis in squirrel monkeys, found no evidence for occlusal trauma as a co-destructive factor in chronic inflammatory periodontal disease. Nor could others (Lindhe and Ericsson, 1976; Ericsson and Lindhe, 1977) find any evidence that jiggling-type occlusal trauma and the resulting tooth hypermobility detrimentally affect healing following periodontal surgery (in dogs), providing plaque control is maintained. Similarly, pocketing was a likely (though not invariable) sequel to 'conversion' of a supragingival into a subgingival plaque by orthodontic means. When normal orthodontic forces were applied to plaque-free teeth, the tilting movement did not result in the formation of infrabony pockets (Ericsson et al., 1977). Ericsson, Thilander and Lindhe (1978) showed that in the absence of plaque orthodontic forces moving individual teeth do not (at least in the dog) induce gingivitis.

Nor were such forces, in the presence of plaque, capable of converting a gingivitis into a destructive and progressive periodontitis. In dogs with a progressive periodontitis, however, repeated jiggling mediated an enhanced rate of ligament and bone destruction (Nyman, Lindhe and Ericsson, 1979). However, jiggling forces produced by alternate siting of wedges caused no increased bone loss unless in the presence of a pre-existing periodontitis. Jiggling trauma in the presence of periodontitis did not affect the loss of ligament attachment (Polson, Meitner and Zander, 1976 a, b; Polson, 1977). It is concluded from the relatively sparse literature that occlusal traumatism may be a factor in progressive destruction of the periodontal ligament, but only in the presence of active chronic periodontitis. One may note also the finding of a severe case of juvenile periodontitis following orthodontic treatment in one individual (Deli and Picarelli, 1977). Occlusal traumatism does not initiate loss of ligament attachment. Accelerated loss of attachment occurred in the dog but not in the monkey model. Bone regeneration (in monkeys) occurs if inflammation is controlled, even though traumatism persists (Polson, 1980). Unfortunately, human studies are rare, and the dog and monkey experiments cited may bear little relation to human occlusal traumatism.

Excessive orthodontic forces

The response of the periodontal ligament to axial and horizontal stress has been considered already in Chapter 8. Discussion here concerns only excessive orthodontic forces applied mainly for experimental purposes. Excessive force produced by intermaxillary elastics in rats (Waldo and Rothblatt, 1954) increased the width and vascularity of the periodontal ligament. As with occlusal traumatism, pressure areas showed regions of vasoconstriction by 24 hours. Tension areas showed a widened periodontal space and slight vasodilation. The responses were maximal by 3 days. On the pressure side of the ligament there was haemorrhage and crushing and eventually resorption of periodontal fibres. This study also confirmed the observation that bodily movements of teeth produce most damage since they cut off the blood supply on the pressure side (Moyers, 1950). Bien (1967) posed the question — why do orthodontic forces move teeth while chewing forces which are much greater do not drive a tooth into a skull? He concluded that rate rather than magnitude of force was related to ligament injury. He did not make conclusions about the significance of the direction of force or of its duration.

The level of force capable of producing damage is low. Gianelly (1969) showed that forces exceeding 50 g reduced the vascular flow in (dog) periodontal ligament, but many vessels remained patent. Forces of 150 g almost completely occluded vessels at the alveolar crest. A force of 75 g applied for 7 days did not significantly impair the structural integrity of the ligament. A 125 g force applied for 7 days produced a distorted fibre apparatus, many of the periodontal fibres becoming aligned parallel to the long axis of the affected tooth. The 75 g and 125 g forces compressed the ligament and its blood vessels. This fits with Miura's (1973) finding that pressures of approximately 80 g/cm^2 decrease the blood flow to the ligament and at the same time compress its thickness to two-thirds of its original lateral dimension.

Orthodontic forces can delay healing of the periodontal ligament following root canal treatment and apicectomy (Baranowskyj, 1969). Singer, Furstman and Bernick (1967) suggested that fewer areas of hyalinization occurred, and were delayed and less intense, in (rat) periodontal ligament subjected to orthodontic loads if the animals had previously received 100 ppm fluoride in their diet, though the mechanism was not clarified.

Root fractures

In most of the numerous reports of injuries to teeth, there is little or no mention of the effects of such injuries on the periodontal ligament (Andreasen and Hjörting-Hansen, 1966). The ligament is mentioned usually as a possible source of repair tissue between apical and coronal portions of a fractured root (e.g. Pindborg, 1955; Arwill, 1962). Bevelander (1942) examined tissue reactions in experimental tooth root fracture in dogs. Adjacent to the fracture

site, a mild inflammatory reaction was observed. The periodontal ligament formed a fibrous union between root fragments in most cases. Where lateral displacement of the fragments had occurred, there was complementary alveolar resorption to allow for the maintenance of a normal width of periodontal space. Uniform width of ligament seems to be established after about 6 months. However, Blackwood (1959) still noted changes in orientation of periodontal fibres and many dilated vascular channels after about 6 months. Torn cementum appears to be repaired by bone, cementum or an unidentified calcified tissue (Claus and Orban, 1953). In rats, enlarged periodontal spaces were observed adjacent to fracture sites (Dreyer and Blum, 1967). The fibres were less dense and organized. There was a downgrowth of crevicular epithelium associated with traumatic detachment of underlying periodontal fibres so that pockets of depths varying as far as the rooth apex formed.

In root fractures, the ligament around the apical fragment shows histologic changes indicative of loss of normal function. It becomes uniformly thinner, its collagen fibres are less dense and arranged mostly parallel to the root surface (Kronfeld, 1936). Its thickness ranges from 0.03 to 0.13 mm, which is within the limits for periodontal ligaments of embedded teeth and teeth without antagonists. By contrast, the ligament around the coronal fragment was about 0.3 mm wide, within the range typical of ligaments subjected to heavy masticatory forces and showed fibres aligned normally. Pindborg (1955) studied intra-alveolar fractures of upper central incisors and concluded that root-fracture repair tissue was organized from both pulp and periodontal ligament. He also reported the proliferation in the region of the fracture line of epithelial rests of Malassez.

SURGICAL TRAUMA

The response of the human periodontal ligament to surgical trauma from clinical periodontics is poorly documented, except for the extraction of teeth. The main reason is that most procedures aimed at eliminating periodontal pockets encroach minimally on healthy ligament. In any event, in most instances of chronic inflammatory periodontal disease, the ligament is intact and free from inflammation apical to the coronal transseptal fibres (see Chapter 13). Therefore, correct periodontal surgery should not result in injury to any but a small proportion of supracrestal fibres. Even in the case of pericision one is cutting only the extra-alveolar fibres, which re-form in their new position without severe consequences locally or to the deeper ligament, providing plaque control is adequate (Strahan and Mills, 1970). Therefore, the remarks that follow derive mainly from experimental studies.

Morris (1953) studied periodontal re-attachment following surgical detachment around periodontally sound human anterior teeth due for extraction for prosthetic reasons. Connective tissue healing took place in all surgical pockets against dentine or cementum. Ligament fibres were aligned parallel to the root in all except the oldest (106 day) specimen, in which Sharpey's fibres were present. There was apparently no attachment to the dentine of non-vital teeth (Morris, 1957).

Burkland, Heeley and Irving (1976) carried out a histological study of regeneration of the completely disrupted periodontal ligament in the rat. The maxillary first molar was elevated and replaced immediately with the torn periodontal ligament in the original socket. After 2 days, the ligament was inflamed, necrotic and without orientated fibres. After 5 days, some collagen fibres had united to bone and cementum. The oriented fibres were more developed cervically and less so apically. Oxytalan fibres were more abundant than in normal periodontal ligaments. By 10 days, scattered areas of inflammation were still present. The transseptal and principal fibres had regained their normal orientation and were only slightly less abundant than in normal ligaments. The apical ligament now showed greater regeneration of collagen than the lateral areas. Oxytalan fibres were still more abundant than in control specimens. At 15 days, orientation of the still sparse collagen fibres appeared normal but at 20 days oxytalan fibres were still more abundant than normal. By 30 days, some animals showed degeneration and hyalinization of part of the ligament. In others, the ligament was thinner than normal. After 50 days, the disrupted ligament was still not fully repaired, being discontinuous over areas of root resorption. It was concluded that the repair process was not maintained because

of the persistence of necrotic matter leading to root resorption. Hair impaction and inflammation were absent, and bacterial contamination was present only initially. In a similar study of ligament healing adjacent to (monkey) extraction sockets, Chase and Revesz (1944) found that transseptal fibres formed and connected the teeth on either side of the socket after 5 weeks.

Hurst (1972) reasoned that oxytalan fibres may be needed in the initial healing process to hold the tooth stable until collagen fibres mature. He also noted that some mobility may be necessary for proper collagen fibre regeneration after initial attachment since, of a number of splinted teeth, the only specimen which did not ankylose was that from which the splint had been dislodged accidentally after 6 weeks. Occlusal trauma may destabilize the healing process. Glickman et al. (1966) applied a traumatic splint to the mandibular anterior teeth of dogs which then received mucogingival surgery. Surgery in this study consisted either of a flap reflected from the gingival margin to the fornix of the vestibule or of an apically repositioned flap. Ligament widening was observed in both groups. Collagen fibre bundles appeared well formed, and blood vessels were increased in number and appeared dilated. There were irregular areas of bone resorption covered with new bone into which new periodontal fibres were inserted. The alveolar crest fibres were shorter and more nearly perpendicular to the tooth than in hypofunctional teeth.

Pietrokovski (1967) investigated roots fractured during extraction of (rat) teeth and left in situ. After 1 week the periodontal ligament near the wound surface had lost its regular structure, and the main components of the periodontal space were blood capillaries, lymphocytes and neutrophils. There was widening of the ligament between the apical foramen and the bony fundus. After 4 weeks, the periodontal space around the root remnant was enlarged and occupied by obliquely orientated collagen fibres and many fibroblasts. Exfoliative movement of the root took place within the healing socket.

In a similar study, Johansen (1970) observed the incorporation of tritiated thymidine into the epithelial cell rests up to 6 days after attempted extraction. He suggested that the experimental injury and subsequent inflammatory response provided the stimulus for epithelial cell rest proliferation. In the case of root fracture with retention of both portions, repair seems also to depend upon the activity of the periodontal ligament, with its invagination into the fracture site, and infiltration into the same site of chronic inflammatory cells (Michanowicz, Michanowicz and Abou-Rass, 1971).

Melcher (1967 a, b) studied the effects of mechanical injury with a saline-cooled bur on rat incisor periodontal ligament. At 4 days, the disorganized ligament contained many active fibroblasts with a high cytoplasm—nucleus ratio. A well-organized cellular connective tissue formed within 1 week of injury. At 6 weeks, the ligament was wider than normal.

The same group studied the response of (mouse molar) periodontal ligament to similar bur-induced injury, which exposed but did not extirpate the ligament through a hole in alveolar bone (Gould, Melcher and Brunette, 1977, 1980). The wound site was isolated by mylar film from the overlying connective tissue. It was found that most dividing progenitor cells in the wounded ligament were close to blood vessels but external to the basement lamina of the latter (Gould, Melcher and Brunette, 1977).

Labelling by autoradiography was apparent in some cells even 30 hours after injury, although most of the affected ligament was necrotic at this time (Gould, Melcher and Brunette, 1980). Reorganization was marked by 5 days. The labelled cells were shown to be moving away from blood vessels to repopulate the reorganizing ligament. Repopulation was delayed by 800 r caesium irradiation. Labelled cells taking part in repair while mainly fibroblasts included endothelial cells, osteoblasts and cementoblasts. They concluded that there is in (mouse molar) periodontal ligament a population of progenitor cells located within 5 mm of blood vessels, the number of these cells remaining relatively stable during the healing of a ligament wound.

Replantation and transplantation

There has been much debate as to the advantages of the presence of an intact periodontal ligament on the tooth to be replanted. Perhaps the best results are obtained using unerupted teeth with only partially formed roots, as in the replacement by third molars of first molars compromised by periodontosis (Borring-Møller and Frandsen, 1978).

In a study of the changes following removal of periodontal tissues from dogs' teeth Yoshida (1976) found that within the first few days the wound sites became filled with granulation tissue containing undifferentiated mesenchyme cells that proliferated from the periodontal ligament of adjoining teeth, periosteum and endosteum. Seven to 9 days after the operation, cementoblasts were arranged on the prepared dentine surface. After 2 weeks, collagen fibre bundles were attached perpendicular to the cavity walls. After 3 weeks, new ligament had formed between the original cementum and newly formed bone. At 4 weeks, the ligament was wide, highly cellular, vascular but poorly organized.

For teeth with complete roots, the best results follow endodontics, washing and avoiding delay prior to replacement with minimal interference with residual periodontal ligament (Hammer, 1955).

If replantation is to have any chance of success, it is essential to maintain the viability of the periodontal ligament (Hunter, 1778; Sherman, 1968). Two important points are to avoid dehydration of the ligament and loss of viability of its cell rests (Löe and Waerhaug, 1961). Söder *et al.* (1977) observed that after 2 hours at 20% relative humidity and 25°C no periodontal ligament cells were viable on tissue culture.

The main problem is the prevention of external resorption and ankylosis (Barbakow, Austin and Cleaton-Jones, 1977). In the investigation of Simons, Jensen and Kimura (1975), six human tooth roots examined whether 22 or 30 months after replantation all showed external resorption. There were acute and chronic inflammatory cells in the ligament. Resorbed cementum and dentine were bordered by non-inflamed fibrous connective tissue. Most roots had scattered areas of relatively normal ligament attached to unresorbed root surfaces. Similar results were obtained by Andreasen and Hjörting-Hansen (1966). Another study involved implantation of (monkey) roots in bone and in contact with replaced flaps. No new ligament formed on those portions of roots which had been exposed to plaque, and then planed thoroughly prior to implantation. In areas where the ligament had been preserved a fibrous re-attachment occurred between the root and adjacent gingival tissue (derived from the flaps) (Nyman *et al.,* 1980).

In further studies using animals it has been possible to follow the sequence of events more closely. Nasjleti, Castelli and Blankenship (1975) observed that 1 day after replantation there was only blood clot at the wound site, consisting of fibrin, erythrocytes and many neutrophils. Granulation tissue was present at 3 days. It occupied most of the periodontal space by 14 days when it was still oedematous and contained many fibroblasts, and macrophages and epithelial rests, the latter especially in the cervical third of the space. Three-week specimens compared with untreated specimens showed increased cellularity and a tendency towards orientation of the new ligament collagen fibres. Nasjleti *et al.* (1975) found that root resorption could be avoided by storage of teeth prior to replantation at +4°C for up to 1 year. Storage at −10°C resulted in moderate inflammation with neutrophil and lymphocyte infiltration of the ligament, followed by a failure of the ligament to organize properly, and root resorption and ankylosis. Eventually these teeth were exfoliated. Even those preserved at +4°C may not show resolution in the long term, ligament fibres often failing to regain or retain functional orientation, and partial or complete ankylosis may supervene (Caffesse, Nasjleti and Castelli, 1977).

In a study using Syrian hamsters Costich *et al.* (1958) observed normal fibroblast orientation around molar teeth 3 months after replantation. Ankylosis occurred around half of the teeth; bone resorption in relation to all but one specimen. Transplantation of teeth from young to adult animals was relatively unsuccessful, most cases forming a poor attachment, although ankylosis did not occur (Hoek, Costich and Hayward, 1958).

Castelli *et al.* (1980) investigated the vascular response of (monkey) incisor periodontal ligament after replantation of teeth. Apical and cervical vessels regained their patency after 4 days, the middle third vessels after 7 days because of better sources of supply to the former. At 4 days the vascular network was disordered, blood vessels intermingling with reparative cells and disrupted collagen fibres. This, the authors suggest, allowed a maximum contact area at the blood vessel/ground substance interface

for nutrient supply. Areas of hyaline degeneration in the middle third of the ligament at this time were associated with a scarcity of reparative cells. By 7 days the hyperaemic reaction was accompanied by proliferation of fibroblasts and endothelial cells. At 15 days, focal spots of increased vascular density were observed in areas undergoing reparative remodelling, and areas adjacent to cementum resorption. In areas where pre-ankylotic bony trabeculae were forming the vasculature appeared less pronounced. Three months after replantation the periodontal vascular network had regained its normal appearance.

Andreasen *et al.* (1978) studied the effects of tissue culture on teeth scheduled for replantation. Tooth crowns were cleaned before extraction, irrigated with phosphate-buffered saline after extraction, and placed in tissue culture medium either immediately or after drying at room temperature and humidity for 1 hour. Teeth were replanted after 5, 7 or 14 days in culture medium. Normal ligament formed only in those specimens where no drying had been permitted. Some of the dried specimens showed inflammation due to resorption of necrotic remnants of ligament and extensive root resorption, and only a few areas of normal ligament persisted. Separation lines in the ligaments of replanted (monkey) teeth can disappear within 2 weeks of immediate replantation (Andreasen, 1980).

In another study, using monkeys, the periodontal ligament was removed by scraping and the root surface decalcified before replantation (Nordenram, Bang and Anneroth, 1973). The inflammatory response varied from mild to intense, the latter especially periapically. About half the teeth became ankylosed.

As to rate of repair of ligament this, as stated above, depends on the degree of preservation of existing ligament. Sharpey's fibres (in dogs) have been observed between 4 to 6 weeks after replantation (Hammer, 1955). If the ligament has been removed, the area between cementum and bone becomes filled after 4 days with poorly formed young connective tissue which will form a new ligament after 2 or 3 months. Unfortunately, all such cases eventually undergo ankylosis (Hammer, 1955; Löe and Waerhaug, 1961). Ankylosis has been observed in such specimens as early as 30 days after replantation. It may be concluded that the prognosis for a replanted tooth depends on the viability of its periodontal ligament.

Implants

Because they are intended to occupy or traverse the original periodontal space, this section considers only those implants designed to fit extraction sockets (the least successful of all implants) and diodontic implants which extend through the root canal into the alveolar bone.

Epithelialization is an almost invariable result. In the case of porcelain 'roots', Dewey and Zugsmith (1933) observed a highly vascularized granulation tissue surrounded by a connective tissue layer of variable thickness. Epithelialization occurred only in favourable circumstances, namely, following relatively atraumatic extraction. Polymethylmetha-crylate implants appear to be retained in sockets by a dense collagenous tissue, the fibres being aligned parallel to the surface of the implant (Hodosh, Povar and Shklar, 1965).

DIODONTIC/ENDODONTIC IMPLANTS

A variety of pins have been used in an attempt to stabilize teeth with minimal alveolar bone support (particularly those requiring endodontic treatment). These traverse the apical periodontal ligament and penetrate the alveolar bone. The best tolerated material seems to be the metal alloy vitallium. Histo-logic evaluation revealed little if any adverse reaction to the implant itself (Fig. 2), any slight chronic inflammatory reaction having been attributed to the presence of root canal sealer, AH26 being more irritant than Diaket (Franks and Abrams, 1969; Scopp et al., 1971; Seltzer et al., 1976). A dense, thin connective tissue layer forms around the metal, its constituent fibres being aligned parallel to the surface of the pin (Franks and Abrams, 1969; Seltzer et al., 1973). Some fibres also form perpendicular to the implant (Scopp et al., 1971). Some lymphocytes and polymorphs are interspersed around the implant. Occasionally, macrophages are present. Corrosion of the metal and ankylosis have been observed, not necessarily in the same specimens (Seltzer et al.,

1973). There can be considerable variation in the dimensions of the implant 'ligament'. No evidence had been found to indicate that the soft tissue around an implant of this type functions in any way like a natural periodontal ligament (Picton et al., 1974).

ENDODONTIC INJURY

Mechanical

Early studies of injury to the periapical periodontal ligament lacked experimental detail, but revealed considerable recovery properties on the part of this portion of the ligament. For example, following unspecified experimental trauma to dog teeth, Sippy (1928) found complete repair. Similarly, while root amputation of cat teeth led to ankylosis, functional stimulation resulted in renewal of normal ligament structure (Bauer, 1923). This, and similar work using dogs (Sippy, 1927), showed that loss of pulp vitality need not interfere with periodontal function. More recently Stahl (1960) has observed (in rat teeth) no periapical changes 3 hours after pulp and ligament exposure. At 6 hours there was increased vascularity and cellularity of the periapical ligament, and some evidence of argyrophilic fibre formation and fuchsi-nophilia, indicating reticulin and ground substance formation. Between 1 and 3 days, neutrophils (PMN) became abundant and capillaries and argyrophilic fibres proliferated. This process continued until 6 days from injury. Many disoriented fibroblasts appeared. Granulation tissue was most abundant by 10 days. After 2 weeks, it was being replaced slowly by organizing connective tissue which appears to wall off inflammatory cells at the apical foramen. Hyaluronic acid and collagen increased in amount with collagen formation. By 44 days, the periapical tissue was composed mainly of organized collagen bundles. Cysts sometimes appeared by 30 days. Epithelial cell rest proliferation was observed in five of twenty specimens. Stahl (1960) noted that peri-apical tissue organized more rapidly and showed more extensive collagen formation than comparably injured gingiva, perhaps because the former was more protected from the oral environment. Similar events

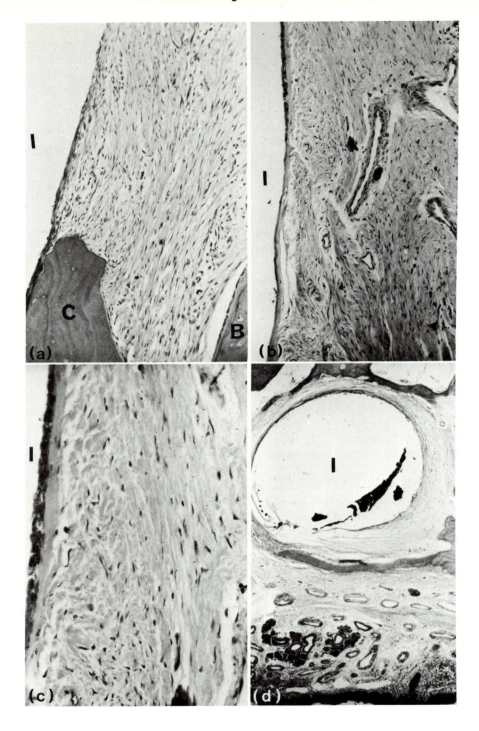

follow pulpectomy and root canal filling. As will be made clear, however, the chemical composition of filling materials can modify periapical healing. In general, competent endodontic treatment results in successful periapical healing, with true or pseudo-encapsulation of any filling material projecting from the apex (Kukidome, 1959; Fukunaga, 1960). Complete regeneration may take a year or more (Hiatt, 1959) and take the form of a relatively avascular fibrous tissue of repair rather than of a regenerated ligament (Penick, 1961).

Pulpal injury itself can lead to periapical changes. The placing of amalgam in direct contact with exposed rat pulps caused less periapical destruction if the restoration were not a cause of premature contact, indicating an exacerbating role for occlusal traumatism in periapical injury (Stahl, Miller and Goldsmith, 1958). Winter and Kramer (1965) observed that experimental pulpal injury (to kitten deciduous molars) led to acute periapical inflammation followed by granuloma formation. In a similar (rat) study, Stahl, Tonna and Weiss (1969) observed an initial reduction in labelling of periapical ligament fibroblasts by tritiated thymidine. After 24 hours, there was an increase in labelling of fibroblasts, osteoblasts and cementoblasts, which by 4 days had spread to the adjacent ligament. The rate of proliferation diminished by 20 days, at which time a well-circumscribed granuloma had formed. At the same time, periapical vessels proliferated (Strömberg, 1971).

Pulpectomy without further instrumentation (in humans and rhesus monkeys) leads to acute and chronic inflammatory changes periapically. Curiously, these seem as likely to resolve as to undergo suppuration, even if the canal is not filled (Sinai et al., 1967). There is no tendency for inflammation to spread from exposed pulps to the furcation rather than periapically. Previous contrary conclusions were based upon the use of kittens rather than primates

(*Macaca irus*) as experimental animals (Winter and Kramer, 1965, 1972).

Seltzer and co-workers (1968, 1973) compared the effects of endodontic instrumentation short of and beyond root apices. Immediately following under instrumentation in rhesus monkey teeth, a slight polymorphonuclear infiltrate was observed periapically. In humans 2 weeks after treatment, dilated vessels, oedema, haemorrhage and granulation tissue were present periapically. In one case, epithelial cell rest proliferation occurred. Four to 6 weeks later, the response varied from mild inflammation to resolution or granuloma formation. After 90 days, apical granulomas were the commonest finding. Dilation of apical ligament blood vessels was observed at 4 days. After 11 days (Seltzer et al., 1969), compression of the ligament by dentine chips was observed, with the accumulation of neutrophils and red blood cells around the latter. After about 4 weeks, chronic inflammation supervened and it took between 6 months and 1 year for repair or further breakdown to occur. The least periapical damage resulted when root canals were underinstrumented (Seltzer et al., 1969; Bhaskar and Rappoport, 1971; Davis, Joseph and Buchner, 1971). Seltzer's group and others (Penick, 1961; Andreasen and Rud, 1972a) noted that the tissue of repair was usually a thickened fibrous layer which, by producing the appearance on radiographs of a widened periodontal space, could give a false impression of continuing disease.

Seltzer et al. (1968, 1973) noted that overinstrumentation caused profuse periapical haemorrhage and the dissemination of dentine particles beyond the apical foramina. The periodontal ligament became oedematous and an intense mainly neutrophil inflammatory infiltrate formed. After 5—6 weeks, the periapical ligament underwent granuloma or occasionally abscess formation. After 180 days, some

FIG. 2. Periodontal responses to cobalt chromium (Vitallium) diodontic implants in monkeys (*Macaca irus*). Maxillary incisor region. Stained haematoxylin and eosin. (a) Apex of tooth. Implant space (I) on left. 4 months *in situ*. Fibres attached to cementum merge with the fibrous capsule surrounding the implant. The fibrous tissue is more dense immediately adjacent to the implant and extends between implant and cementum (C). Longitudinal section. B = bone. ×72. (b) Near apex of implant. 18 months *in situ*. Implant space on left. Note amorphous layer adjacent to condensed fibrous layer adjoining implant. Epithelium—ligand cavities are mucous glands close to normal. Longitudinal section. ×72. (c) Higher magnification of B. Shows detail of implant 'capsule' from left, densely stained, amorphous disordered and orientated collagen layers. ×240. (d) Near apex of implant. 40 months *in situ*. Floor of nares at bottom of micrograph. In the transverse plane of this section, the 'capsule' fibres can be seen to extend circumferentially around the implant. ×36.

epithelial rest proliferation generally was apparent (Fig. 3).

Periapical abscess formation need not impede completion of root formation. In a study of developing monkey (*Macaca irus*) incisors after pulpectomy or pulpotomy, all showed completed root formation, in spite of prior abscesses (the root canals were sealed only with cotton pellets and amalgam) (Torneck

and Smith, 1970). Teeth which had been 'irritated' by caries and restorations prior to endodontic treatment exhibited root canal narrowing but no significant periapical inflammation after endodontics, provided the root canals had been underinstrumented (Seltzer *et al.*, 1968).

Root perforation appears to cause inflammation even if the defect is filled immediately. After approxi-

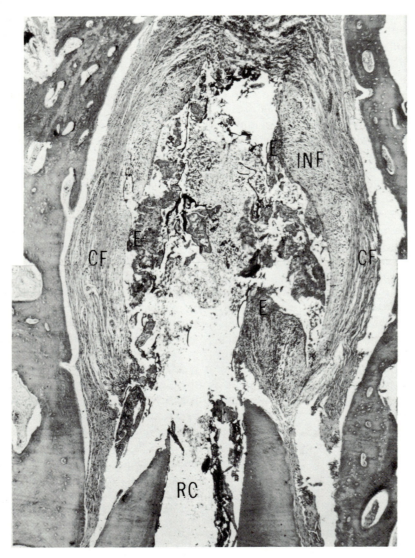

FIG. 3. Following instrumentation beyond the root apex, the root canal (RC) has been overfilled. Stratified squamous epithelium (E) has proliferated around the filling (5 months after treatment). Chronic inflammation (INF) is evident. The lesion is surrounded by collagen fibres (CF). ×59.

mal or bifurcation perforation of dogs' teeth with a machine-driven reamer, followed by pulpectomy and immediate filling under aseptic conditions, the ligament at the site of injury suffered acute and, after 6 weeks, chronic inflammatory changes. These were least when the defect was filled immediately, with chloroform-rosin and gutta-percha cones, and greatest when left open to contamination, even if restored subsequently (Lantz and Persson, 1967). Seltzer, Sinai and August (1970) studied the periodontal effects of root perforation before and during endodontic procedures, experimenting with varying intervals between perforation and closure. They found inflammation to be most severe when perforations were not closed, either immediately or at all, and concluded that the prognosis was doubtful in all cases but better if the defect were closed immediately. A more promising prognosis for perforated roots derived from a similar study using dogs (Lantz and Persson, 1970). In this instance, however, the perforation was made after aseptic pulpectomy, and root canal filling with chloroform rosin and gutta-percha cones. The result was mild chronic inflammation with the appearance of scattered lymphocytes and plasma cells. Inflammation was more marked when amalgam was substituted for gutta-percha. This would seem to be because of leakage around amalgam. A well-organized fibrous capsule formed around gutta-percha but only sparse collagen fibres around amalgam. If the perforations were sealed with zinc phosphate cement, there was a similar mild chronic inflammatory reaction in the periapical ligament (Lantz and Persson, 1970). In a study using rats, Andreasen and Skougaard (1972) showed comparable temporary inflammatory changes around the sites of perforation in vital teeth. In these specimens, early ankylosis was followed after only 3 weeks by re-establishment of an intact periodontal ligament (Fig. 4).

Chemical

There have been many investigations determining the effects of the wide range of materials used in endodontics on short- and long-term healing of periapical tissues. The periapical ligament response seems to depend both on the texture of the filling material and on its chemical composition. When hard and compact the material tends to become encapsulated, although a zone of loose connective tissue containing many macrophages frequently forms between the 'capsule' and the filling material. When less compact, the material is resorbed more rapidly. Resorbable pastes (e.g. iodoform) whilst being rapidly resorbed produce an intense polymorph-rich infiltrate and necrosis of the surrounding ligament due to obliteration of the local blood supply (Muruzábal, Erausquin and Devoto, 1966). In contrast to the persistent inflammation produced by zinc oxide–eugenol root canal filling, other studies suggest that iodoform pastes only rarely produce necrosis (Erausquin and Muruzábal, 1969a; Holland *et al.*, 1971).

Various pastes and resins have been used as root-canal fillers. With Diaket (a polyvinyl resin, with bismuth phosphate and an antiseptic, dihydroxy-dichlorodiphenyl-methane) and AH-26 (a compound of silver, bismuth oxide, titanium oxide, hexamethylene tetramine and bisphenol diglycidyl ether) moderate periapical inflammatory infiltration was observed whether roots were under- or overfilled. Overfilled material compressed the periodontal ligament producing the appearance of a pseudo-capsule. By 15 days, the overfilled material was separated from the surrounding tissue by a fibrous layer outside a zone of macrophages, foreign-body giant cells and stellate fibroblasts. After 30 days, only the overfilled sites showed persistent inflammation. The pseudo-capsule also persisted except at the periphery of the filling material where it had been replaced by new fibrous tissue. Diaket overfill was surrounded by a fibrous capsule with a loose structure, containing macrophages and giant cells, the cytoplasm of which was loaded with particles of Diaket when in direct contact. AH-26 overfill disintegrated, and many phagocytes were found among the particles. The overfilled mass often was surrounded by a poorly organized fibrous capsule. By 60 days, the AH-26 overfill showed little change, and had not been completely removed at 90 days (Muruzábal and Erausquin, 1966). This study was extended to include Riebler resin (basically a phenol-formaldehyde resin (Erausquin and Muruzábal, 1969a). Again, the response seemed to depend primarily on the level to which the root was filled.

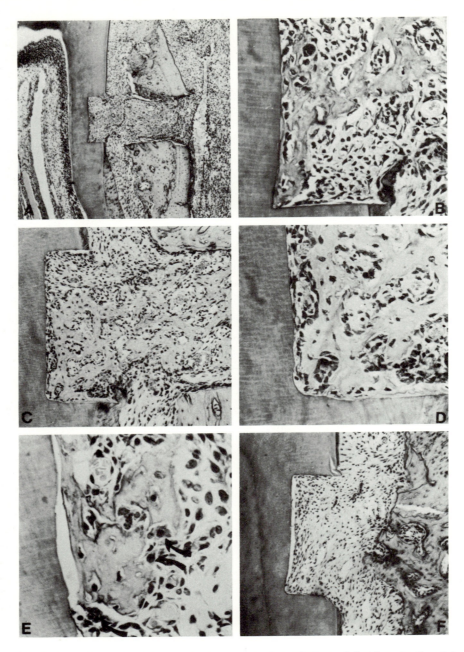

FIG. 4. Lateral periodontal ligament injury. Sequence of events following experimental perforation of (rat) periodontal ligament is depicted in photomicrographs A–F. A. Deposition of immature bone upon surface of exposed dentine after 7 days. ×38. B. Higher magnification of A. ×330. C. Extensive ankylosis covering almost all exposed dentine after 7 days. ×132. D. Higher magnification of C. ×330. E. Removal of ankylosis area by osteoclastic resorption (arrows). Observation period: 10 days. ×330. F. Re-establishment of a new periodontal ligament 3 weeks after injury. ×132.

Overfilling produced either necrosis of the apical periodontal ligament, or neutrophil and macrophage, and later giant cell infiltration. This was followed by encapsulation, or occasionally abscess or granuloma formation. This response was typical of the industrial epoxy resins and of root-canal cements containing resins, the latter producing a slight but persistent neutrophil infiltrate replaced eventually by macrophages and giant cells (Erausquin *et al.*, 1966; Erausquin and Muruzábal, 1969b). Chloroform rosin and gutta-percha led to acute inflammation even when used to fill perforations immediately after the defects had been created (Lantz and Persson, 1967).

Hydron, poly-2-hydroxyethyl methacrylate, a gel which polymerizes in the presence of water, has recently been tested for its endodontic potential. This agent was found to produce little or no periapical reaction, although histiocytes took up the barium salt filler (Benkel *et al.*, 1976; Kronman *et al.*, 1977).

Silicone rubber used as a root-canal filling produced periapical fibrotic encapsulation with slight inflammation. There was some phagocytosis of the material by giant cells, but it was not broken down. There was no evidence of a severe foreign-body reaction in any of the specimens examined (Kasman and Goldman, 1977).

The results using root-canal cements are highly variable. Phosphate cement has been associated with progressive periodontal destruction when used to fill root perforations (Lantz and Persson, 1967). Zinc oxide–eugenol produced a larger zone of necrosis than N2 or Kerr cements, particularly if the cement was mixed with tissue debris due to instrumentation. However, all such lesions were eventually encapsulated (Erausquin and Muruzábal, 1968). Rowe (1967) used various combinations of zinc oxide, eugenol, barium sulphate, olive oil, glycyrrhetinnic acid, 2% cortisone acetate, paraformaldehyde, calcium hydroxide, Kri paste (iodoform paste containing a blend of parachlorphenol, camphor and menthol), an unidentified resorbable material, Grossman's root-canal sealer (zinc oxide, staybelite resin, bismuth subcarbonate, barium sulphate, eugenol and almond oil), Ledermix cement (zinc oxide, calcium hydroxide, triamcinolone acetonide, demethylchlortetracycline hydrochloride) and paste (water-soluble cream, triamcinolone acetonide, demethylchlortetracycline-cal-

cium) and N2 (paraformaldehyde, an anti-inflammatory agent called hydroxydimethyl octodien, zinc oxide, barium sulphate and oil of cloves). Results obtained 2 weeks after pulpectomy of cat teeth and extension of fillings at least to apical thirds were similar, irrespective of the material used. All but one of fifty-eight teeth showed considerable periapical inflammation, the main inflammatory cells being polymorphs, with some plasma cells and lymphocytes. Using zinc oxide–eugenol, inflammation was still present after 16 weeks. The addition of barium sulphate and olive oil resulted in less inflammation. No improvement was obtained by the addition of glycyrrhetinnic acid. When the latter was replaced by 2% cortisone acetate, marked inflammation occurred. Paraform and glycyrrhetinnic acid with zinc oxide and eugenol produced minimal inflammation. Calcium hydroxide with distilled water produced the most severe reaction with abscess formation. None of the proprietary pastes prevented inflammation.

It should be emphasized that these reactions are usually transient, whether periapically or in relation to lateral canals (Rud and Andreasen, 1972) and do not warrant the rejection of those materials which produce only a mild inflammation for a brief period (Barker and Lockett, 1972 a, b). For example, N2 (in dogs' teeth) showed very little periapical disturbance 3 months after placement (Barker and Lockett, 1972b).

Erausquin and Muruzábal (1968) compared the effects of filling short of, to, and beyond the root apices of rat molars, using zinc oxide–eugenol, Grossman's, N2 and Kerr root-canal cements. They found that overfilling produced infarction of the periapical periodontal ligament due to destruction, compression or thrombosis of the apical vessels, regardless of the cement used. Necrosis was most extensive with zinc oxide–eugenol, although necrotic tissue was replaced within 4 days. Mild inflammation resulted whether the filling extended to or slightly beyond the apex. More severe inflammation occurred if the overfilled mass was not compact. Tightly packed cements resorbed very slowly. Resorption was carried out partly by foreign-body giant cells which appeared on the surface of the overfilled material. N2 temporarily tended to fragment with the release of granules of titanium dioxide that were phagocytosed rapidly by macrophages. Polymorphs tended to disappear 2 weeks after filling, and encapsulation of excess filling material occurred usually by 90 days. In two cases of overfill with Grossman's cement and one with zinc oxide—eugenol, bone was deposited directly on the cementum.

Similar results were obtained when acrylic polymer was added to these various root-canal cements, the position of the cement in relation to the apex being of apparently greater consequence than its chemical composition (Erausquin and Muruzábal, 1968).

Erausquin (1970) tested root-canal filling materials containing zinc, titanium, lead and aluminium oxides. Propylene glycol, polyethylene glycol, petrolatum-lanolin and silicone cream were used as excipients. Zinc and lead oxides produced a moderate inflammatory infiltrate 1 week after placement. This was still slightly in evidence 90 days post-operatively. Over-filled material was surrounded by fibrous tissue. Titanium dioxide produced a dense polymorph infiltrate containing many macrophages loaded with the oxide. Granulomas and apical abscesses were frequent sequels. The reaction was more severe if petrolatum-lanolin was used as the excipient. Aluminium oxide stimulated production of a marked infiltrate with subsequent encapsulation. Zinc and lead oxides which had no tendency to disperse underwent encapsulation. Titanium and aluminium oxides tended to disperse, and this exacerbated the inflammatory response.

One of the least offensive root-canal fillings seems to be calcium hydroxide, notwithstanding Rowe's (1967) early results. In studies of periapical response to root-canal treatment of incompletely formed dog teeth, this agent was used with distilled water or as the proprietary paste Calxyl (calcium hydroxide, sodium bicarbonate and sodium, potassium and calcium chlorides) (Binnie and Rowe, 1973, 1974). Some canals were filled with Grossman's root-canal sealer, which produced mild but occasionally severe inflammation not observed following the use of either calcium hydroxide preparation (Fig. 5). Mild transient inflammation did occur soon after placement (Binnie and Rowe, 1973; Holland *et al.*, 1977).

Citrome and Hever (1979) compared a calcium

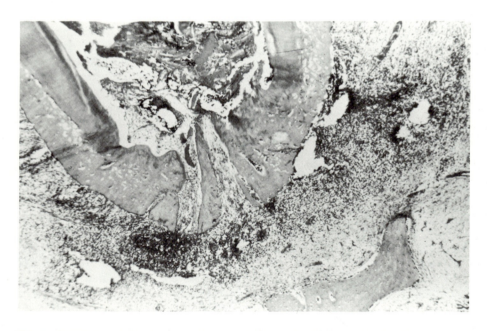

FIG. 5. Chemical endodontic injury to periapical periodontal ligament of pulpless immature (dog) teeth. Severe inflammatory reaction 4 weeks after root-canal filling with Grossman's root-canal sealer. Root formation appears complete but apical cementum is necrotic and there is extensive inflammation of the associated periodontal ligament and periapical bone resorption. ×23.

hydroxide—saline paste and a collagen—calcium phosphate gel as root-canal filling materials. The gel produced severe inflammation, in the form of acute abscesses followed by granulomas or cysts. Little inflammation followed the use of the calcium hydroxide—saline preparation. Calcium hydroxide used with or without iodoform produced good healing in dog teeth with open apices (Holland *et al.*, 1971).

Polycarboxylates were tested as root-canal cements by Seltzer *et al.* (1976). They found them to be no better than other cements, nor were there particular advantages to be gained by using them in combination with other materials, including tin hydroxide, stannous fluoride, calcium hydroxide or calcium fluoride in various concentrations. In most cases, the cements were forced into the periapical ligament producing the typical overfill reaction (Fig. 6). This invalidates this study as a test of the materials themselves.

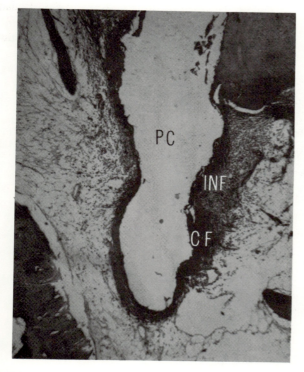

FIG. 6. Periapical periodontal ligament response to overfilling with polycarboxylate cement plus 10% calcium fluoride. 165 days after vital pulpectomy and root filling. Excess cement (PC) is surrounded by collagen fibres (CF). A small amount of inflammation (INF) persists. ×66.

The use of corticosteroid-containing root-canal preparations was investigated by Barker and Lockett (1972c). They reported that prolonged contact of Ledermix paste with (dog) periapical tissues had no harmful consequences. Cortril, which contains hydrocortisone in a water-miscible base, caused severe periapical inflammation, including abscess formation. This was attributed to the effects of the base, although it had been shown previously (Rowe, 1967) that the use of cortisone in a root-canal cement was itself associated with marked periapical inflammation. Cortisone administered systemically is known to impair fibroblast metabolism and collagen synthesis (Dreizen, Levy and Bernick, 1971) (see Chapter 18). Erausquin (1972) filled root canals with corticoid-containing materials and found only a minimal inflammatory reaction periapically if radicular pulp and dentine chips were compressed beforehand to form an apical plug between the cement and the ligament. After local application of prednisolone following pulpectomy, Strömberg (1972) observed periapical vascular proliferation in a group of dogs which had undergone partial pulpectomy. In a similar total pulpectomy group, a comparable increase in vascularity occurred by the third instead of the tenth day. Otherwise, no differences between the two groups were noted.

Regarding the effects of amalgam, reimplantation of rhesus monkey teeth which had been extracted, root filled and an amalgam restoration placed midway along the root was followed by severe inflammation. Omitting the ligament effects produced by this severe trauma, inflammation appeared to be more severe and prolonged in relation to the restoration (Nasjleti, Castelli and Caffesse, 1977).

Erausquin and Devoto (1970) investigated the potential of different root-canal cements to produce ankylosis. They found this rarely followed the use of zinc oxide—eugenol or Grossman's root-canal sealer. Formaldehyde-containing derivatives caused frequent ankylosis. However, trioxymethylene powder (a constituent of N2) rarely produced ankylosis unless combined with a corticoid. If the root canal was filled (with trioxymethylene-containing N2) but the vital pulp not removed, there was periapical inflammation but no ankylosis. After pulpectomy the same N2 paste produced acute periapical inflammation followed by ankylosis or granuloma formation (Langeland, 1974) (Fig. 7). Ankylosis was less frequent and extensive when the root canal was underfilled. The addition of acrylic to the paste resulted in the production of only slight inflammation and moderate fibrosis (Bordoni and Erausquin, 1970).

Erausquin and Devoto (1970) noted that where healing started in the healthy ligament, following periapical instrumentation, there was functional rehabilitation of the tissues. Where regeneration began in the alveolar bone marrow, they observed ankylosis as a sequel. Either the newly formed fibrous tissue which had replaced necrotic ligament underwent trabecular bone formation, or the necrotic ligament calcified.

None of the root-canal cements tested by Binnie and Rowe (1973) nor various zinc and magnesium salts with water, glutaraldehyde or eugenol caused epithelial cell rest proliferation. It was concluded that the presence of rests was a characteristic of the individual animal rather than a response to a particular filling material (Binnie and Rowe, 1974). Epithelial rests also proliferate following mechanical injury, e.g. following attempted tooth extraction (Johansen, 1970).

Attention has been drawn above to the variability in response of the periapical periodontal ligament to a variety of endodontic procedures and filling materials, and to the short-term delay in healing in most instances. Healing shows a similar variability. The ligament may regenerate or ankylosis may occur with or without persistent mild inflammation. Fibrous scar tissue may form adjacent to healthy ligament or an ankylosis, in the presence of varying grades of inflammation. Moderate or severe inflammation may persist in the absence of tissue repair. These conclusions were drawn from a study of seventy cases of human endodontic surgery 1–14 years after the original endodontic therapy, including amalgam or gutta-percha and retrograde or orthograde filling (Andreasen and Rud, 1972c). Andreasen (1973) observed that lateral ligament inflammation was more inclined to persist following pulp necrosis in younger (rats') teeth due to the greater permeability of younger dentine permitting more ready spread of necrotic pulp products.

Only isolated studies have been reported concerning the effects of drugs and poisons on the periodontal ligament. Most of these derive from endodontic studies and will be reviewed here.

The acute secondary agranulocytosis resulting

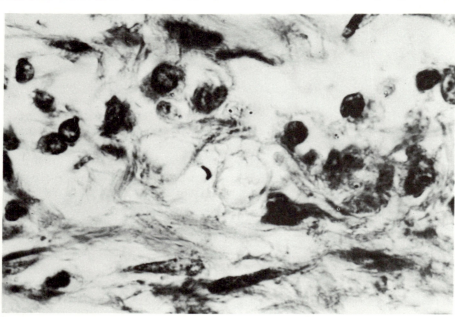

FIG. 7. Periapical periodontal ligament after N2 overfilling. Lymphocytes and macrophages with granular N2 inclusions. ×700.

from arsphenamine treatment has been associated with extensive haemorrhage and ultimately necrosis of the periodontal ligament, due to the activity of anaerobic organisms in periodontal pockets (Bauer, 1946). Similarly, arsenical pulp devitalizers were observed to cause acute periapical inflammation if pushed through the apex (Glasser, 1957). 20 ppm arsenic supplements to the diet of rats led to a slightly increased severity of chronic periodontitis (Shaw, 1973).

Attalla (1968) observed that beechwood creosote, an antiseptic used to clean root canals, caused a severe periapical reaction with abscess formation in 60% of specimens in a test using dogs. Similar treatment with chloramine, however, produced no significant reaction.

Butyl-2-cyanoacrylate was applied in one study to exposed rat molar pulps. After 1 week there had been no extension of (minimal) pulpal inflammation to the periodontal ligament. Marked periapical inflammation with microabscess formation occurred in those specimens exposed to cavity liner varnish. However, widening of the apical periodontal space was evident in the cyanoacrylate-treated cases after 7 weeks (Wade, 1969).

When cold cure acrylic was placed in root surface cavities in extracted monkey teeth, subsequently replanted after 4 minutes outside the mouth, inflammation and fibre disorientation were more marked and prolonged in relation to the ligament apposed to the resin, and fibres which did form remained parallel to the restoration surface (Nasjleti, Castelli and Keller, 1972).

Accidental injection of sodium hypochlorite beyond the root apex has been reported on one occasion as producing an acute periapical reaction spreading to involve the face (Becker, Cohen and Borer, 1974). Routine canal irrigation with 1% NaOCl or with 1% NaOCl followed by 2% iodine potassium iodide produced insignificant and transient periapical inflammation (Lamers, van Mullem and Simon, 1980). There are few reported non-endodontic cases of chemical damage to the periodontal ligament. The local application of carbolic acid to (rat) interdental papilla resulted in loss of alveolar crest ligament fibres after 3 days. These regenerated 4 days later, but there was still diminished birefringence of the fibres after 30 days. The fibre changes were accompanied by a round cell infiltrate (Tonna and Stahl, 1967).

Ogle and Ciancio (1971) showed that a protracted exposure to anticholinergic agents was associated with a more severe periodontal response to plaque, perhaps due to reduction in salivary flow.

The addition of either strontium or beryllium to rat diets led to ankylosis in the periodontal ligament (Gravina. Cabrini and Carranza, 1970). There is one reported case of generalized widened periodontal spaces due to mercury poisoning following weekly injections of mersalyl (Zamet, 1967). There is also a report of tooth exfoliation following cytotoxic therapy with Bleomycin and CCNU for a case of Hodgkin's disease, possibly due to post-herpes zoster damage to the ligament (Vickery and Midda, 1976).

PHYSICAL AGENTS

Radiation

Leist (1926) and Zerosi (1938, 1940) observed degenerative changes in the ligaments of young dogs, with hyperaemia, exudation, a reduced number of principal fibres and reduced cellularity due to thrombosis and vascular degeneration. By contrast, radium sulphate administered through the alveolar bone of young rabbits led to fibrous hypertrophy and the development of cysts from epithelial rests (Rosenthal, 1937).

Shapiro, Brat and Ershoff (1960) found that whole body irradiation of 1200 r induced (in mice) severe periodontal destruction within 100 days. Two cases of 2000 r radiation damage to child dentitions were recorded in which the periodontal ligament was widened (Fronman and Ratzkowski, 1966).

A study using kittens revealed a decrease in ligament width with loss of normal insertion of fibres following two doses of 1000 r each 1 week apart. Ankylosis occurred in nearly half the animals (Winter and Kramer, 1965). Frandsen (1965) noted extensive periodontal destruction (in rats) related to ulceration spreading from the overlying mucosa, if the tooth and supporting tissues were irradiated. Whole body irradiation (1000 r) resulted only in decreased cellularity of the ligament 2—58 days after irradiation. Frandsen

(1963) in a further study of local roentgen irradiation, to the molar regions of rats, found no difference between dosages of 1725 r and 2400 r. No extensive destruction originated in the ligament, which showed only oedema or degeneration of some fibres. A dose of 1000 r to the head produced decreased cellularity of the ligament. A dose of 2000 r or 3000 r led to death before ligament involvement had occurred although there had been gingival epitheliolysis. Mayo *et al.* (1962) observed that a threshold of 700 r total body irradiation was necessary to produce lesions in Syrian hamsters. In rats, 1020 r from 200 kV radiation was found to produce decreased ligament vascularity, only occasional small sclerotic blood vessels being present. There was also a reduced number of fibroblasts, which were smaller, rounded and more deeply staining than normal. Cementoblasts were also scarcer. A similar radiation dose from cobalt 60 produced very slight alterations, the ligament generally possessing normal vascularity and cellularity although there was a slight decrease in the density of collagen fibre distribution. Doubling the dose of standard radiation of 2040 r exacerbated the ligament changes seen with half the dosage, whereas a 2040 r dose of cobalt 60 radiation produced little change. Meyer, Shklar and Turner (1962) concluded that cobalt 60 radiation was much less damaging than standard high-voltage radiation. However, Zach *et al.* (1973) observed ligament inflammation whether high voltage or cobalt 60 irradiation was used. They administered fractionated doses of 333 r thrice weekly over 6 weeks (total 600 r) to thirty-four adult rhesus monkeys, at a rate of 35 rads per minute.

Diet texture may modify the response to radiation. While no changes were observed in mice fed a routine diet, soft food consumption resulted in disorganization of the periodontal ligament, especially along the apical third of the root, with hyalinization and fragmentation of collagen fibres and nuclear pyknosis of fibroblasts. Both groups had received 200 r whole body X-irradiation repeated once weekly until 1200 r had been given (Mayo *et al.*, 1962; Ershoff *et al.*, 1967). While the authors did not explain their findings, it is known that typical chronic inflammatory periodontal disease advances only in animals consuming diet of soft texture, due to the lack of prevention of plaque accumulation at the site of onset (Egelberg, 1965; Newman, 1974).

Laser radiation has been found to produce periodontal degenerative and inflammatory changes, attributable to the heat produced by the beam (Taylor, Shklar and Roeber, 1965).

Temperature

When rats were maintained between 0–2°C, for periods of up to 2 weeks, the periodontal ligament appeared more granular than fibrillar (Shklar and Glickman, 1959). Fibroblasts were reduced in number and irregular in distribution, size and shape. Their nuclei became small, spherical rather than elliptical, and deeply staining. There were reduced numbers of cementoblasts and osteoblasts. By 4 weeks, the collagen fibres looked normal, but there were still fewer fibroblasts. By 4 months, no significant differences were noted between control and experimental animals. The initial changes were attributed to adrenal stress, although no clear mechanism was put forward.

In a further study of rats exposed to the same temperatures for up to 18 months, Shklar (1966) observed a decreased cellularity and a separation and irregularity of collagen bundles in the ligament. There were many dilated and engorged capillaries. He attributed the changes on this occasion to loss of normal function following prolonged exposure of the animals to stress. At the other extreme, mice subjected to temperatures of 42°C and 90% relative humidity for 10 minutes suffered an initial depression of ligament fibroblast labelling by tritiated thymidine. Subsequent peak labelling values at 4–8 or 24–48 hours were double those for control tissues. Thereafter, labelling values returned to those of the control animals (McKibben and Pechersky, 1972).

A local application of high temperature to the ligament was obtained by insertion after pulpectomy of an electrosurgery tip 2.5 mm apical to the cement—enamel junction of squirrel monkey teeth (Atrizadeh, Kennedy and Zander, 1971). Necrosis occurred 3–7 days later in the ligament near where the broach had been inserted. Fibroblasts, cementoblasts and osteoblasts were destroyed and there was a reduction in staining of ligament fibres. At the periphery of the necrotic area, fibroblasts and blood vessels proliferated 2 weeks after injury. The vascular and cellular responses were more marked apically than coronally. Many osteoclasts were seen. Granulation tissue formation and widening of ligament space due to bone resorption proceeded. However, between 3 and 6 months ankylosis occurred, the ligament became less cellular than normal, and many collagen fibres were aligned parallel to the root surface. Similar findings were obtained by Line, Polson and Zander (1974).

ACKNOWLEDGEMENT

We thank Mr. F. J. Harty, Clinical Senior Lecturer in Conservative Dentistry at the Eastman Dental Hospital for his helpful comments on the endodontics section.

REFERENCES

ANDREASEN, J. O. (1973) Effect of pulpal necrosis upon periodontal healing after surgical injury in rats. *Int. J. oral Surg.* **2**, 62–68.

ANDREASEN, J. O. (1980) A time-related study of periodontal healing and root resorption activity after replantation of mature permanent incisors in monkeys. *Swed. dent. J.* **4**, 101–110.

ANDREASEN, J. O. & HJÖRTING-HANSEN, E. (1966) Replantation of teeth, II. Histological study of 22 replanted anterior teeth in humans. *Acta odont. Scand.* **24**, 287–300.

ANDREASEN, J. O., REINHOLDT, J., RÜS, I., DYBDAHL, R., SÖDER, P.-Ö. & OTTERSKOG, P. (1978) Periodontal and pulpal healing of monkey incisors preserved in tissue culture before replantation. *Int. J. oral. Surg.* **7**, 104–112.

ANDREASEN, J. O. & RUD, J. (1972a) Correlations between histology and radiography in the assessment of healing after endodontic surgery. *Int. J. oral Surg.* **I**, 161–173.

ANDREASEN, J. O. & RUD, J. (1972b) A histobacteriologic study of dental and periapical structures after endodontic surgery. *Int. J. oral Surg.* **I**, 272–281.

ANDREASEN, J. O. & RUD, J. (1972c) Modes of healing histologically after endodontic surgery in 20 cases. *Int. J. oral Surg.* **I**, 148–160.

ANDREASEN, J. O. & SKOUGAARD, M. R. (1972) Reversibility of surgically induced dental ankylosis in rats. *Int. J. oral Surg.* **I**, 98–102.

ARWILL, T. (1962) Histopathologic studies of traumatized teeth. *Odont. Tidskr.* **70**, 91–117.

ATRIZADEH, F., KENNEDY, J. & ZANDER, H. (1971) Ankylosis following thermal injury. *J. periodont. Res.* **6**, 159–167.

ATTALLA, M. N. (1968) Effect of beechwood creosote and chloramine on periapical tissue of dogs. *J. Canad. dent. Assoc.* **34**, 190–195.

BARANOWSKYJ, G. R. T. (1969) A histologic investigation of tissue response to an orthodontic intrusive force on a dog maxillary incisor with endodontic treatment and root resection. *Amer. J. Orthodont.* **56**, 623–624.

BARBAKOW, F. H., AUSTIN, J. C. & CLEATON-JONES, P. E. (1977) Experimental replantation of root-canal-filled and untreated teeth in the vervet monkey. *J. Endod.* **3**, 89–93.

BARKER, B. C. W. & LOCKETT, B. C. (1972a) Reaction of dog tissue to immediate root filling with zinc oxide cement and gutta percha. *Austral. dent. J.* **17**, 1–8.

BARKER, B. C. W. & LOCKETT, B. C. (1972b) Periapical response to N2 and other paraformaldehyde compounds confined within or extruded beyond the apices of dog root canals. *Dent. Practit.* **22**, 370–379.

BARKER, B. C. W. & LOCKETT, B. C. (1972c) Reaction of dog pulp and periapical tissue to two glucocorticosteroid preparations. *Oral Surg.* **33**, 249–262.

BAUER, W. (1923) The histology of the periapical region after amputation. *Dent. Cosmos.* **65**, 1145.

BAUER, W. H. (1946) The supporting tissues of the tooth in acute secondary agranulocytosis (arsphenamin neutropenia). *J. dent. Res.* **25**, 501–508.

BECKER, G. L., COHEN, S. & BORER, R. (1974) The sequelae of accidentally injecting sodium hypochlorite beyond the root apex. *Oral Surg.* **38**, 633–638.

BENKEL, B. H., RISING, D. W., GOLDMAN, L. B., ROSEN, H., GOLDMAN, M. & KRONMAN, J. H. (1976) Use of hydrophilic plastic as a root canal filling material. *J. Endod.* **2**, 196–202.

BEVELANDER, G. (1942) Tissue reactions in experimental tooth fracture. *J. dent. Res.* **21**, 481–487.

BHASKAR, S. N. & ORBAN, B. (1955) Experimental occlusal trauma. *J. Periodont.* **26**, 270–284.

BHASKAR, S. N. & RAPPOPORT, H. M. (1971) Histologic evaluation of endodontic procedures in dogs. *Oral Surg.* **31**, 526–535.

BIEN, S. M. (1967) Difficulties and failures in tooth movement – biophysical responses to mechanotherapy. *Trans. Eur. Orthod. Soc.* **43**, 55–67.

BINNIE, W. H. & ROWE, A. H. R. (1973) A histological study of the periapical tissues of incompletely formed pulpless teeth filled with calcium hydroxide. *J. dent. Res.* **52**, 1110–1116.

BINNIE, W. H. & ROWE, A. H. R. (1974) The incidence of epithelial rests, proliferations and apical periodontal cysts following root canal treatment in young dogs. *Br. dent. J.* **137**, 56–60.

BLACKWOOD, H. J. J. (1959) Tissue repair in intra-alveolar root fractures. *Oral Surg.* **12**, 360–370.

BORDONI, N. & ERAUSQUIN, J. (1970) Periapical tissue reaction to root canal filling with a paste containing 7 per cent trioxymethylene. *Oral Surg.* **29**, 907–914.

BORRING-MØLLER, G. & FRANDSEN, A. (1978) Autologous tooth transplantation to replace molars lost in patients with juvenile periodontitis. *J. Clin. Periodont.* **5**, 152–158.

BURKLAND, G. A., HEELEY, J. D. & IRVING, J. T. (1976) A histological study of regeneration of the completely disrupted periodontal ligament in the rat. *Archs. oral Biol.* 21, 349–354.

CAFFESSE, R. G., NASJLETI, C. E. & CASTELLI, W. A. (1977) Long term results after intentional tooth reimplantation in monkeys. *Oral Surg.* 44, 666–678.

CASTELLI, W. A., NASJLETI, C. E., CAFFESSE, R. G. & DIAZ-PEREZ, R. (1980) Vascular response of the periodontal membrane after replantation of teeth. *Oral Surg.* 50, 390–397.

CHASE, S. W. & REVESZ, J. (1944) Re-establishment of transseptal fibres following extraction. *J. dent. Res.* 23, 333–336.

CITROME, G. P. & HEVER, M. A. (1979) A comparative study of tooth apexification in the dog. *J. Endod.* 5, 290–297.

CLAUS, E. C. & ORBAN, B. (1953) Fractured vital teeth. *Oral Surg.* 6, 605–613.

COOLIDGE, E. D. (1938) Traumatic and functional injuries occurring in the supporting tissues of human teeth. *J. Amer. dent. Assoc.* 25, 343–357.

COSTICH, E. R., HOEK, R. B. & HAYWARD, J. R. (1958) Replantation of molar teeth in the Syrian hamster. *J. dent. Res.* 37, abs. 851, p. 36.

CRUMLEY, P. J. (1964) Collagen formation in the normal and stressed periodontium. *Periodontics* 2, 53–61.

DAVIS, M. S., JOSEPH, S. W. & BUCHNER, J. F. (1971) Periapical and intracanal healing following incomplete root canal fillings in dogs. *Oral Surg.* 31, 662–675.

DELI, R. & PICARELLI, A. (1977) A case of juvenile periodontitis particularly severe due to orthodontic treatment. *Riv. Ital. Stomatol.* 46, 12–17.

DEWEY, K. W. & ZUGSMITH, R. (1933) An experimental study of tissue reactions about porcelain roots. *J. dent. Res.* 13, 459–472.

DREIZEN, S., LEVY, B. M. & BERNICK, S. (1971) Studies on the biology of the periodontium of marmosets. X. Cortisone induced periodontal and skeletal changes in adult cotton top marmosets. *J. Periodont.* 42, 217–224.

DREYER, C. J. & BLUM, L. (1967) Effect of root fracture on the epithelial attachment. *J. dent. Assoc. S.A.* 22, 103–105.

EGELBERG, J. (1965) Local effect of diet on plaque formation and development of gingivitis in dogs. I. Effects of hard and soft diets. *Odont. Revy* 16, 31–41.

ERAUSQUIN, J. (1970) Periapical tissue reaction to root canal fillings with zinc, titanium, lead, and aluminium oxides. *Oral Surg.* 30, 545–554.

ERAUSQUIN, J. (1972) Periapical tissue response to the apical plug in root canal treatment. *J. dent. Res.* 51, 483–487.

ERAUSQUIN, J. & DEVOTO, F. C. H. (1970) Alveolodental ankylosis induced by root canal treatment in rat molars. *Oral Surg.* 30, 105–116.

ERAUSQUIN, J. & MURUZÁBAL, M. (1968) A tissue reaction to root canal cements in the rat molar. *Oral Surg.* 26, 360–373.

ERAUSQUIN, J. & MURUZÁBAL, M. (1969a) Tissue reaction to root canal fillings with absorbable pastes. *Oral Surg.* 28, 567–578.

ERAUSQUIN, J. & MURUZÁBAL, M. (1969b) Tissue reaction to root canal fillings with plastic cements. *Oral Surg.* 29, 91–101.

ERAUSQUIN, J., MURUZÁBAL, M., DEVOTO, F. C. H. & RIKLES, A. (1966) Necrosis of the periodontal ligament in root canal overfillings. *J. dent. Res.* 45, 1084–1092.

ERICSSON, I. & LINDHE, J. (1977) Lack of effect of trauma from occlusion on the recurrence of experimental periodontitis. *J. Clin. Periodont.* 4, 115–127.

ERICSSON, I., THILANDER, B. & LINDHE, J. (1978) Periodontal conditions after orthodontic tooth movements in the dog. *Angle Orthodont.* 48, 210–218.

ERICSSON, I., THILANDER, B., LINDHE, J. & OKAMOTO, H. (1977) The effect of orthodontic tilting movements on the periodontal tissues of infected and non-infected dentitions in dogs. *J. Clin. Periodont.* 4, 278–293.

ERSHOFF, B. H., BAJWA, G. S., SHAPIRO, M. & BERNICK, S. (1967) Comparative effects of a purified diet and natural food stock rations on the periodontium of mice exposed to multiple sublethal doses of total body X-irradiation. *J. dent. Res.* 46, 1051–1057.

FRANDSEN, A. M. (1962) Periodontal tissue changes induced in young rats by roentgen irradiation of the molar regions of the head. *Acta odont. Scand.* 20, 393–410.

FRANDSEN, A. M. (1963) Experimental investigations of socket healing and periodontal disease in rats. Effects of vitamin A deficiency. *Acta odont. Scand.* 21, suppl. 37.

FRANKS, A. L. & ABRAMS, A. M. (1969) Histologic evaluation of endodontic implants. *J. Amer. dent. Assoc.* 78, 520–524.

FRONMAN, S. & RATZKOWSKI, E. (1966) Two cases of radiation damage to the growing dentition and their supporting structures in children. *Dent. Practit.* 16, 344–348.

FUKUNAGA, K. (1960) Healing of periapical tissues in human teeth after pulp extirpation and root canal filling. *D. Abs.* 5, 595.

GIANELLY, A. A. (1969) Force-induced changes in the vascularity of the periodontal ligament. *Amer. J. Orthodont.* 55, 5–11.

GLASSER, M. M. (1957) Acute periapical necrosis from arsenical pulp devitalizer. *Oral Surg.* 10, 216–217.

GLICKMAN, I. (1963) Inflammation and trauma from occlusion, co-destructive factors in chronic inflammatory periodontal disease. *J. Periodont.* 34, 5–10.

GLICKMAN, I. & SMULOW, J. B. (1962) Alterations in the pathway of gingival inflammation into the underlying tissues induced by excessive occlusal forces. *J. Periodont.* 33, 7–13.

GLICKMAN, I. & SMULOW, J. B. (1965) Effect of excessive occlusal forces upon the pathway of gingival inflammation in humans. *J. Periodont.* 36, 141–147.

GLICKMAN, I. & SMULOW, J. B. (1967) Further observations on the effects of trauma from occlusion in humans. *J. Periodont.* 38, 280–293.

GLICKMAN, I. & SMULOW, J. B. (1968) Adaptive alterations in the periodontium of the rhesus monkey in chronic trauma from occlusion. *J. Periodont.* 39, 101–105.

GLICKMAN, I. & SMULOW, J. B. (1969) The combined effects of inflammation and trauma from occlusion in periodontitis. *Int. dent. J.* 19, 393–407.

GLICKMAN, I., SMULOW, J. B., VOGEL, G. & PASSA-MONTI, G. (1966) The effect of occlusal forces on healing following mucogingival surgery. *J. Periodont.* 37, 319–325.

GLICKMAN, I. & WEISS, I. (1955) Role of trauma from occlusion in initiation of periodontal pocket formation in experimental animals. *J. Periodont.* 26, 14–20.

GOULD, T. R. L., MELCHER, A. H. & BRUNETTE, D. M. (1977) Location of progenitor cells in periodontal ligament stimulated by wounding. *Anat. Rec.* 188, 133–141.

GOULD, T. R. L., MELCHER, A. H. & BRUNETTE, D. M. (1980) Migration and division of progenitor cell populations in periodontal ligament after wounding. *J. periodont. Res.* 15, 20–42.

GRAVINA, O., CABRINI, R. L. & CARRANZA, F. A. (1970) Effect of a strontium-containing diet on periodontal tissues of rat molars. *J. Periodont.* 41, 174–177.

HAMMER, H. (1955) Replantation and implantation of teeth. *Int. dent. J.* 5, 439–457.

HIATT, W. H. (1959) Regeneration of the periodontium after endodontic therapy and flap operation. *Oral Surg.* 12, 1471–1477.

HODOSH, M., POVAR, M. & SHKLAR, G. (1965) Periodontal tissue acceptance of plastic tooth implants in primates. *J. Amer. dent. Assoc.* 70, 362–371.

HOEK, R. B., COSTICH, E. R. & HAYWARD, J. R. (1958) Homogenous transplantation of hamster second molars from young to adult animals. *J. dent. Res.* 37, abs. 84, p. 36.

HOLLAND, R., DE MELLO, W., NERY, M. J., BERNABE, P. F. E. & DE SOUZA, V. (1977) Reaction of human periapical tissue to pulp extirpation and immediate root canal filling with calcium hydroxide. *J. Endod.* 3, 63–67.

HOLLAND, R., DE SOUZA, V., TAGLIAVINI, R. L. & MILANEZI, L. A. (1971) Healing process of teeth with open apices: histological study. *Bull. Tokyo dent. Coll.* 12, 333–338.

HUNTER, J. (1778) *The natural history of the human teeth: Explaining their structure, use, formation, growth and diseases*, pp. 127–128 Part I; pp. 94–112 Part II. London, Johnson.

HURST, R. V. V. (1972) Regeneration of periodontal and transseptal fibres after autografts in *Rhesus* monkeys: a qualitative approach. *J. dent. Res.* 51, 1183–1192.

JOHANSEN, J. R. (1970) Incorporation of tritiated thymidine by the epithelial rests of Malassez after attempted extraction of rat molars. *Acta odont. Scand.* 28, 463–470.

KASMAN, F. G. & GOLDMAN, M. (1977) Tissue response to silicone rubber when used as a root canal filling. *Oral Surg.* 43, 607–614.

KOIVUMAA, K. K. & LASSILA, V. (1971) Angiographical investigation of the influence of occlusal hyper- and hypofunction on the periodontium in rat. *Suom. Hammaslääk Toim.* 67, 102–122.

KRONFELD, R. (1931) Histologic study of the influence of function on the human periodontal membrane. *J. Amer. dent. Assoc.* 18, 1242–1274.

KRONFELD, R. (1936) A case of tooth fracture with special emphasis on tissue repair and adaptation following traumatic injury. *J. dent. Res.* 15, 429–446.

KRONMAN, J. H., GOLDMAN, M., LIN, P. S., GOLDMAN, L. B. & KLIMENT, C. (1977) Evaluation of intracytoplasmic particles in histiocytes after endodontic therapy with a hydrophilic plastic. *J. dent. Res.* 56, 795–801.

KUKIDOME, K. (1959) Histopathological study on healing of periapical tissues after infected root canal treatment of human teeth. *D. Abs.* 4, 44–45.

LAMERS, A. C., VAN MULLEM, P. J. & SIMON, M. (1980) Tissue reactions to sodium hypochlorite and iodine potassium iodide under clinical conditions in monkey teeth. *J. Endod.* 6, 788–792.

LANGELAND, K. (1974) Root canal sealants and pastes. *Dent. Clin. N. Amer.* 18, 309–327.

LANTZ, B. & PERSSON, P.-A. (1967) Periodontal tissue reactions after root perforations in dogs' teeth. A histologic study. *Odont. Tidskr.* 75, 209–220.

LANTZ, B. & PERSSON, P.-A. (1970) Periodontal tissue reactions after surgical treatment of root perforations in dogs' teeth. A histologic study. *Odont. Revy* 21, 51–62.

LEIST, M. (1926) Experimentelle Untersuchungen über die Einwirkung der Röntgenstrahlen und des Radiums auf die zweite Dentition. *Z. Stomat.* 24, 452–460.

LINDHE, J. & ERICSSON, I. (1976) The influence of trauma from occlusion on reduced but healthy periodontal tissues in dogs. *J. Clin. Periodont.* 3, 110–122.

LINDHE, J. & SVANBERG, G. (1964) Influence of trauma from occlusion on progression of experimental periodontitis in the beagle dog. *J. Clin. Periodont.* 1, 3–14.

LINE, S. E., POLSON, A. M. & ZANDER, H. A. (1974) Relationship between periodontal injury, selective cell repopulation and ankylosis. *J. Periodont.* 45, 725–730.

LÖE, H. & WAERHAUG, J. (1961) Experimental replantation of teeth in dogs and monkeys. *Archs. oral Biol.* 3, 176–184.

MACAPANPAN, L. C., MEYER, J. & WEINMANN, J. P. (1954) Mitotic activity of fibroblasts after damage to the periodontal membrane of rat molars. *J. Periodont.* 25, 105–112.

MACAPANPAN, L. C. & WEINMANN, J. P. (1954) The influence of injury to the periodontal membrane on the spread of gingival inflammation. *J. dent. Res.* 33, 263–272.

MAYO, J., CARRANZA, F. A., EPPER, C. E. & CABRINI, R. L. (1962) The effect of total irradiation on the oral tissues of the Syrian hamster. *Oral Surg.* 15, 739–745.

McKIBBEN, D. H. & PECHERSKY, J. L. (1972) Effect of thermal stress on cell proliferation of the submandibular gland and periodontal ligament of CH^{-3} male mice. *Archs. oral Biol.* 17, 291–298.

MELCHER, A. H. (1967a) Wound repair in the periodontium of the rat incisor. *Archs. oral Biol.* 12, 1645–1647.

MELCHER, A. H. (1967b) Remodelling of the periodontal ligament during eruption of the rat incisor. *Archs. oral Biol.* 12, 1649–1651.

MEYER, I., SHKLAR, G. & TURNER, J. (1962) A comparison of the effects of 200 kV radiation and cobalt-60 radiation on the jaws and dental structure of the white rat. A preliminary report. *Oral Surg.* 15, 1098–1108.

MICHANOWICZ, A. E., MICHANOWICZ, J. P. & ABOU-RASS, M. (1971) Cementogenic repair of root fractures. *J. Amer. dent. Assoc.* **82**, 569–579.

MIURA, F. (1973) Effect of orthodontic force on blood circulation in periodontal membrane. *Trans. 3rd Int. Orthod. Congr. London.* abs. 63, p. 21.

MORRIS, M. L. (1953) The reattachment of human periodontal tissues following surgical detachment: a clinical and histological study. *J. Periodont.* **24**, 270–278.

MORRIS, M. L. (1957) Healing of human periodontal tissues following surgical detachment from non-vital teeth. *J. Periodont.* **28**, 222–238.

MOYERS, R. E. (1950) The periodontal membrane in orthodontics. *J. Amer. dent. Assoc.* **40**, 22–27.

MÜHLEMANN, H. R. & HERZOG, H. (1961) Tooth mobility and microscopic tissue changes produced by experimental occlusal trauma. *Helv. odont. Acta* **5**, 33–39.

MURUZÁBAL, M. & ERAUSQUIN, J. (1966) Response of periapical tissues in the rat molar to root canal fillings with Diaket and AH-26. *Oral Surg.* **21**, 786–804.

MURUZÁBAL, M., ERAUSQUIN, J. & DEVOTO, F. C. H. (1966) A study of periapical overfilling in root canal treatment in the molar of rat. *Archs. oral Biol.* **11**, 373–383.

NASCIMENTO, A. & SALLUM, A. W. (1975) Periodontal changes in distant teeth due to trauma from occlusion. *J. periodont. Res.* **10**, 44–48.

NASJLETI, C. E., CASTELLI, W. A. & BLANKENSHIP, J. R. (1975) The storage of teeth before reimplantation in monkeys. *Oral Surg.* **39**, 20–29.

NASJLETI, C. E., CASTELLI, W. A. & CAFFESSE, R. G. (1977) Effects of amalgam restorations on the periodontal membrane in monkeys. *J. dent. Res.* **56**, 1127–1131.

NASJLETI, C. E., CASTELLI, W. A. & KELLER, B. E. (1972) Effects of acrylic restorations on the periodontium of monkeys. *J. dent. Res.* **51**, 1328–1382.

NEWMAN, H. N. (1974) Diet, attrition, plaque and dental disease. *Br. dent. J.* **136**, 491–497.

NORDENRAM, A., BANG, G. & ANNEROTH, G. (1973) A histopathologic study of replanted teeth with superficially demineralised root surfaces in Java monkeys. *Scand. J. dent. Res.* **81**, 294–302.

NYMAN, S., KARRING, T., LINDHE, J. & PLANTÉN, S. (1980) Healing following implantation of periodontitis-affected roots into gingival connective tissue. *J. Clin. Periodont.* **7**, 394–401.

NYMAN, S., LINDHE, J. & ERICSSON, I. (1979) The effect of progressive tooth mobility on destructive periodontitis in the dog. *J. Clin. Periodont.* **5**, 213–215.

OGLE, R. E. & CIANCIO, S. G. (1971) The effect of anticholinergic agents on the periodontium. *J. Periodont.* **42**, 280–282.

PALCANIS, K. G. (1973) Effect of occlusal trauma on interstitial pressure in the periodontal ligament. *J. dent. Res.* **52**, 903–910.

PENICK, E. C. (1961) Periapical repair by dense fibrous connective tissue following conservative endodontic therapy. *Oral Surg.* **14**, 239–242.

PICTON, D. C. A. (1976) Experimental evidence on the role of abnormal contacts in the aetiology of periodontal disease. In: *Mastication,* D. J. ANDERSON & B. MATTHEWS (eds.), pp. 251–258. Bristol, Wright.

PICTON, D. C. A., JOHNS, R. B., WILLS, D. J. & DAVIES, W. I. R. (1974) The relationship between the mechanisms of tooth and implant support. In: *Oral Sci. Rev.* **5**, A. H. MELCHER & G. A. ZARB (eds.), pp. 3–22. Copenhagen, Munksgaard.

PIETROKOVSKI, J. (1967) Extraction wound healing after tooth fracture in rats. *J. dent. Res.* **46**, 233–240.

PINDBORG, J. J. (1955) Clinical, radiographic and histological aspects of intraalveolar fractures of upper central incisors. *Acta odont. Scand.* **13**, 41–71.

POLSON, A. M. (1974) Trauma and progression of marginal periodontitis in squirrel monkeys. II. Mechanical. *J. periodont. Res.* **9**, 108–113.

POLSON, A. M. (1977) Interactions between periodontal trauma and marginal periodontitis. *Int. dent. J.* **27**, 107–113.

POLSON, A. M. (1980) Interrelationship of inflammation and tooth mobility (trauma) in pathogenesis of periodontal disease. *J. Clin. Periodont.* **71**, 351–360.

POLSON, A. M., MEITNER, S. W. & ZANDER, H. A. (1976a) Trauma and progression of marginal periodontitis in squirrel monkeys. III. Adaptation to repetitive injury. *J. periodont. Res.* **11**, 279–289.

POLSON, A. M., MEITNER, S. W. & ZANDER, H. A. (1976b) Trauma and progression of marginal periodontitis in squirrel monkeys. IV. Trauma and inflammation. *J. periodont. Res.* **11**, 290–298.

POSSELT, U. & MAUNSBACH, O. (1957) Clinical and roentgenographic studies of trauma from occlusion. *J. Periodont.* **28**, 192–196.

ROSENTHAL, M. (1937) Experimental radium poisoning. II. Changes in teeth of rabbits produced by oral administration of radium sulphate. *Amer. J. Med. Sci.* **193**, 495–501.

ROWE, A. H. R. (1967) Effect of root filling materials on the periapical tissues. *Br. dent. J.* **122**, 98–102.

RUD, J. & ANDREASEN, J. O. (1972) Operative procedures in periapical surgery with contemporaneous root filling. *Int. J. Oral Surg.* **1**, 297–310.

SCOPP, I. W., DICTROW, R. L., LICHTENSTEIN, B. & BLECHMAN, H. (1971) Cellular response to endodontic endosseous implants. *J. Periodont.* **42**, 717–720.

SELTZER, S., GREEN, D. B., DE LA GUARDIA, R., MAGGIO, J. & BARNETT, A. (1973) Vitallium endodontic implants: a scanning electron microscope, electron microprobe and histologic study. *Oral Surg.* **35**, 828–860.

SELTZER, S., MAGGIO, J., WOLLARD, R. R., BROUGH, S. O. & BARNETT, A. (1976) Tissue reactions to polycarboxylate cements. *J. Endod.* **2**, 208–214.

SELTZER, S., MAGGIO, J., WOLLARD, R. R. & GREEN, D. (1976) Titanium endodontic implants: a scanning electron microscope, electron microprobe, and histologic investigation. *J. Endod.* **2**, 267–276.

SELTZER, S., SINAI, I. & AUGUST, D. (1970) Periodontal effects of root perforations before and during endodontic procedures. *J. dent. Res.* **49**, 332–339.

SELTZER, S., SOLTANOFF, W., SINAI, I., GOLDENBERG, A. & BENDER, I. B. (1968) Biologic aspects of endodontics. Part III. Periapical tissue reactions to root canal instrumentation. *Oral Surg.* **26**, 534–546, 694–705.

SELTZER, S., SOLTANOFF, W., SINAI, I. & SMITH, J. (1969) Biologic aspects of endodontics. IV. Periapical tissue reactions to root-filled teeth whose canals had been instrumented short of their apices. *Oral Surg.* **28**, 724–738.

SHAPIRO, M., BRAT, V. & ERSHOFF, B. H. (1960) Periodontal changes following multiple sublethal doses of X-irradiation in the mouse. *J. dent. Res.* **39**, abs. 46, p. 668.

SHAW, J. H. (1973) Relation of arsenic supplements to dental caries and the periodontal syndrome in experimental rodents. *J. dent. Res.* **52**, 494–497.

SHERMAN, P. (1968) Intentional replantation of teeth in dogs and monkeys. *J. dent. Res.* **47**, 1066–1071.

SHKLAR, G. (1966) Periodontal disease in experimental animals subjected to chronic cold stress. *J. Periodont.* **37**, 377–383.

SHKLAR, G. & GLICKMAN, I. (1959) The effect of cold as a stressor agent upon the periodontium of albino rats. *Oral Surg.* **12**, 1311–1320.

SIMONS, J. H. S., JENSEN, J. L. & KIMURA, J. T. (1975) Histologic observations of endodontically treated replanted roots. *J. Endod.* **1**, 178–180.

SINAI, I., SELTZER, S., SOLTANOFF, W., GOLDENBERG, A. & BENDER, I. B. (1967) Biologic aspects of endodontics. Part II. Periapical tissue reactions to pulp extirpation. *Oral Surg.* **23**, 664–679.

SINGER, J., FURSTMAN, L. & BERNICK, S. (1967) A histologic study of the effect of fluoride on tooth movement in the rat. *Amer. J. Orthodont.* **53**, 296–308.

SIPPY, B. O. (1927) Regeneration of tissues following experimental injury of the tooth roots. *Dent. Cosmos.* **69**, 771–780.

SIPPY, B. O. (1928) Regeneration of bone, peridental membrane, and cementum, following experimental injury in dogs. *J. dent. Res.* **8**, abs. 3, p. 9.

SÖDER, P.-Ø., OTERSKOG, P., ANDREASEN, J. O. & MODÉER, T. (1977) Effect of drying on viability of periodontal membrane. *Scand. J. dent. Res.* **95**, 164–168.

SOLT, C. W. & GLICKMAN, I. (1968) A histologic and radiographic study of healing following wedging interdental injury in mice. *J. Periodont.* **39**, 249–254.

STAHL, S. S. (1960) Response of the periodontium, pulp and salivary glands to gingival and tooth injury in young adult male rats. I. Periodontal tissues. II. Pulp and periapical tissues. *Oral Surg.* **13**, 613–626; 734–742.

STAHL, S. S., MILLER, S. C. & GOLDSMITH, E. D. (1958) The influence of occlusal trauma and protein deprivation on the response of periapical tissues following pulpal exposures in rats. *Oral Surg.* **11**, 536–540.

STAHL, S. S., TONNA, E. A. & WEISS, R. (1969) Autoradiographic evaluation of periapical responses to pulpal injury. II. Mature rats. *Oral Surg.* **29**, 270–274.

STRAHAN, J. D. & MILLS, J. R. E. (1970) A preliminary report on the severing of gingival fibres following rotation of teeth. *Dent. Practnr.* **21**, 101–102.

STRÖMBERG, T. (1971) The apical blood vessel topography, with special reference to pulpectomy. A microangiographic and histologic study in dogs. *Odont. Revy* **22**, 163–177.

STRÖMBERG, T. (1972) The effect of pulpectomy and root canal filling in the same treatment, with special reference to local prednisolone therapy. A microangiographic and histologic study in dogs. *Odont. Revy* **23**, 221–230.

SVANBERG, G. (1974) Influence of trauma from occlusion on the periodontium of dogs with normal or inflamed gingivae. *Odont. Revy* **25**, 165–178.

SVANBERG, G. & LINDHE, J. (1973) Experimental hypertooth-mobility in the dog. *Odont. Revy* **24**, 269–282.

SVANBERG, G. & LINDHE, J. (1974) Vascular reactions in the periodontal ligament incident to trauma from occlusion. *J. Clin. Periodont.* **1**, 58–67.

TAYLOR, R., SHKLAR, G. & ROEBER, F. (1965) The effects of laser radiation on teeth, dental pulp and oral mucosa of experimental animals. *Oral Surg.* **19**, 786–795.

TONNA, E. A. & STAHL, S. S. (1967) A polarized light microscopic study of rat periodontal ligament following surgical and chemical gingival trauma. *Helv. odont. Acta* **11**, 90–105.

TORNECK, C. S. & SMITH, J. (1970) Biologic effects of endodontic procedures on developing incisor teeth. I. Effect of partial and total pulp removal. *Oral Surg.* **30**, 258–266.

VICKERY, I. M. & MIDDA, M. (1976) Dental complications of cytotoxic therapy in Hodgkin's disease – a case report. *Br. J. Oral Surg.* **13**, 282–288.

WADE, G. W. (1969) Pulpal and periapical tissue response to butyl 2-cyanoacrylate. *Oral Surg.* **28**, 226–234.

WAERHAUG, J. (1979) The angular bone defect and its relationship to trauma from occlusion and downgrowth of subgingival plaque. *J. Clin. Periodont.* **6**, 61–82.

WAERHAUG, J. & HANSEN, E. R. (1966) Periodontal changes incident to prolonged occlusal overload in monkeys. *Acta odont. Scand.* **24**, 91–105.

WALDO, C. M. & ROTHBLATT, J. M. (1954) Histologic response to tooth movement in the laboratory rat. *J. dent. Res.* **33**, 481–486.

WALKER, T. W., NG, G. C. & BURKE, P. S. (1978) Fluid pressures in the periodontal ligament of the mandibular canine tooth in dogs. *Archs. oral Biol.* **23**, 753–765.

WENTZ, F. M., JARABAK, J. & ORBAN, B. (1958) Experimental occlusal trauma imitating cuspal interferences. *J. Periodont.* **29**, 117–127.

WINTER, G. B. & KRAMER, I. R. H. (1965) Changes in periodontal membrane and bone following experimental injury in deciduous molar teeth in kittens. *Archs. oral Biol.* **10**, 279–289.

WINTER, G. B. & KRAMER, I. R. H. (1972) Changes in periodontal membrane, bone and permanent teeth following experimental pulpal injury in deciduous molar teeth of monkeys (*Macaca irus*). *Archs. oral Biol.* **17**, 1771–1779.

YOSHIDA, M. (1976) An experimental study on regeneration

of cementum, periodontal ligament and alveolar bone in the intradentinal cavities in dogs. *Shikwa Gakuho* **76**, 1197–1222.

ZACH, L., COHEN, G., SCOPP, I. & KAPLAN, G. (1973) Experimental radio osteonecrosis in rhesus macaque jaws; therapeutic irradiation dose effect on dental extraction wound healing. *Amer. J. Phys. Anthropol.* **38**, 325–330.

ZAMET, J. S. (1967) Report of a case of mercurial periodontitis. *J. Periodont.* **38**, 255–258.

ZEROSI, C. (1938) Experimentelle Untersuchungen über Reaktionen und histopathologische Veränderungen, welche durch Röntgen- und Radiumsbestrahlungen in dentalen und periodontalen Gewebe verursacht werden. *Zahnärtzl. Rdsch.* **47**, 265–272.

ZEROSI, C. (1940) Experimentelle Forschungen über die histologischen Reaktionen und Veränderungen der dentalen und periodontalen Gewebe infolge von Röntgen- und Radiumbestrahlung. *Z. Stomat.* **38**, 278–304; 322–339.

Chapter 15

INFECTION AND THE PERIODONTAL LIGAMENT

H. N. Newman

INTRODUCTION

To many periodontologists, the term 'periodontal disease' is synonymous with chronic inflammatory periodontal disease. Even when the inflammatory aspects due to infection are considered more fully, it is common to find a lack of coordination between studies of changes in periapical and lateral portions of the periodontal ligament. This chapter considers features of both lateral and periapical periodontal ligament consequent upon acute and chronic infection. Discussion of more esoteric oral infections is limited to the sparse information available concerning periodontal ligament involvement by these conditions. Changes due to trauma-induced inflammation are considered in Chapter 14. Gingival changes are omitted, except where they relate to the transitional stages between gingivitis and periodontitis. As will become apparent from this review, surprisingly little is known about the pathology of the ligament in infectious inflammatory periodontal diseases as compared with our knowledge of gingival changes in the same diseases.

LATERAL PERIODONTITIS

Chronic inflammatory periodontal disease

The general features of this, the most widespread human disease, resemble those of other long-term chronic inflammatory diseases affecting connective tissue (Page and Schroeder, 1976). The lack of research on the periodontal ligament changes in this disease is surprising, when one considers that these are responsible for the majority of teeth lost in adult life. At the present time, it is not clear what factors determine the transition from gingivitis to periodontitis or the rate of progression of the latter. Furthermore, mechanisms of periodontal ligament destruction have to be deduced from studies of changes in gingival connective tissue, for most of the research has concentrated on the early stages of the disease.

Chronic inflammatory periodontal disease is neither linear nor continuous in its progression. Periods of quiescence, and even of acute exacerbation with abscess formation, occur (Page and Schroeder, 1976).

Nor can we yet distinguish between established lesions which will remain stable and those which will advance rapidly.

The change from gingivitis to periodontitis may be said to occur when the alveolar crest collagen fibres are replaced by inflammatory exudate (Goldman, 1957 a, b; Heijl, Rifkin and Zander, 1976). How soon after the onset of chronic gingivitis periodontal ligament changes occur has not been determined in man. One experiment, in dogs fed a soft diet, suggests that significant loss of fibre attachment takes place after about 6 months in relation to molars, and after approximately 8 months in relation to premolars and incisors (Lindhe, Hamp and Löe, 1973).

Tissue damage proceeds from the gingival connective tissue until the transseptal fibres are involved. The main body of the ligament shows little inflammatory change throughout the disease process (Warwick James and Counsell, 1927; Wade, 1965). The principal alteration is progressive destruction spreading apically from its coronal periphery. The alveolar bone seems to show more dramatic changes than the periodontal ligament (Warwick James and Counsell, 1927). The ligament fibres initially lose their attachment to bone and then to cementum (Figs. 1—3). If occlusal trauma be a complication (see Chapter 14), the ligament may be involved before the bone (Macapanpan and Weinmann, 1954).

The first part of the periodontal ligament to be involved is its interdental portion (Melcher, 1962). Resorption of interdental bone results in contact being established between contiguous ligament fibres previously inserted into the intervening bone. In this way the destroyed transseptal fibres are replaced, a state of affairs which persists throughout the disease process (Fig. 4). Some of the fibres extend not simply between adjacent tooth surfaces at the same level, but from the depths of bony craters across the residual alveolar crest into the adjacent tooth cementum. This persistent transseptal fibre layer is usually densely fibrous, and infiltrated by small numbers of chronic inflammatory cells, and is thought to assist in walling off noxious matters from the deeper tissues (Garant, 1976). With the progression of the disease in

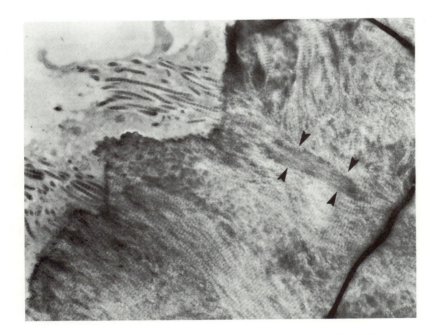

FIG. 1. Transmission electron micrograph. Extensive destruction of the fibre attachment to cementum. Only a few collagen fibrils remain attached to the hard tissue. The matrix fibrils, which mostly are arranged in the plane of the section, exhibit the cross banding of collagen. In one area, however, the cross-banding is absent (between the arrows). Section decalcified on the grid by phosphotungstic acid. ×14,000.

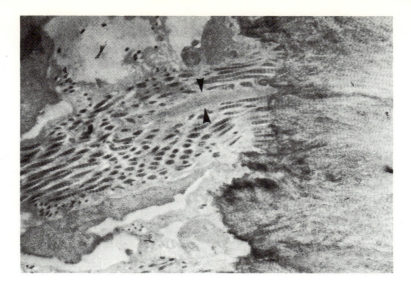

FIG. 2. Transmission electron micrograph. Area similar to that illustrated in Fig. 1. A bundle of fine, non-banded filaments is located within a collagen fibre (between the arrows). Cross-banding is present in the embedded portion of the filamentous structure. Section decalcified on the grid by phosphotungstic acid. ×14,000.

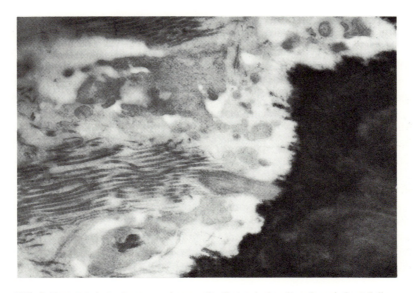

FIG. 3. Transmission electron micrograph. Extensively altered periodontal ligament. Only a bundle of filaments remains attached to the cementum in this area. This bundle appears to be continuous with the bundle of collagen fibrils. The periodicity of collagen is faintly visible in the embedded portion of this and other matrix fibrils. ×14,000.

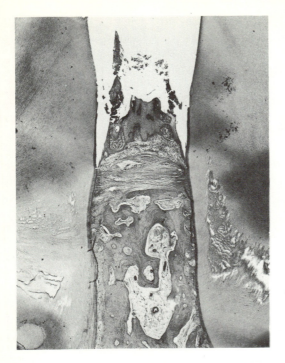

FIG. 4. Light micrograph. Note intact transseptal fibres walling off inflamed tissue from the alveolar bone. Interdental area /67 stained peracetic acid—aldehyde fuchsin—Halmi. × 11.

clearly requires further clarification, as do so many aspects of the disease. The zone of completely and partially destroyed ligament fibres at the periphery of the advancing lesion is another feature which persists throughout the disease (Saglie, Johansen and Flötra, 1975). Another characteristic which, with the preceding, suggests that the periodontal tissues retreat in good order is the usually almost intact epithelial lining of the periodontal pocket, which suggests an apparent equilibrium between cell division and desquamation (Ruben, Goldman and Schulman, 1970). This equilibrium may be upset by an increase in noxious stimuli of plaque or host origin, leading to ulceration at the base of the pocket. Then the adjacent epithelium shows increased mitotic activity and hyperplasia, and penetration of the disrupted corium by extending rete pegs. It seems clear that only an intact original transseptal fibre system prevents the epithelium from extending apically (Goldman, 1951).

VASCULAR AND INFLAMMATORY CELL CHANGES

Warwick James and Counsell (1927) observed that in the initial stages of inflammation the periodontal ligament vessels were enlarged, so that the ligament appeared hyperaemic. Later the vessels showed constriction and were surrounded by loose connective tissue. In the crestal region, infiltration by inflammatory cells was noted where small arteries traversed the coronal part of the ligament from bone to gingiva. Regarding vascular changes in the deeper ligament, there is an increase in both number and size of blood vessels in the inflamed (marmoset) ligament, most of which pass through the lamina dura (Fig. 5) (Page *et al.* 1972) and join ligament and supracrestal vessels (Kennedy, 1974). In spontaneous 7-week periodontitis in rats fed a high sucrose diet, Garant and Cho (1979b) observed several features consistent with endothelial proliferation, namely increased endothelial cell processes, penetration of the basal lamina by these processes and increased prominence of granular endoplasmic reticulum and Golgi complex.

Increased vascularity has been related to the accumulation of an inflammatory infiltrate (Kennedy, 1974) which seems to form in tissue planes in the transseptal fibre region between fibre bundles and in

gnotobiotic rats, osteoclasts accumulate in the remains of the transseptal fibres, sometimes in dense groups (Irving, Socransky and Heeley, 1974). Eventually this fibrous zone extends around the tooth, the bands of fibrous tissue being separated by zones of inflammatory cells (Weinmann, 1941; Fullmer, 1961; Ruben, Goldman and Schulman, 1970). Fullmer (1961) observed that the initial degradation of periodontal ligament collagen occurred in regions apart from the inflammatory focus.

Periodontal ligament changes appear generally some distance ahead of the advancing plaque, due to a lack of bacterial invasion and the probable diffusion of acellular toxic matter into the tissues (Newman, 1976). Also, the distance from the base of the periodontal pocket to the alveolar crest seems to remain constant throughout the disease (Stanley, 1955). This may be due to the production in the inflammatory focus of 'diffusible compounds' which inhibit enzyme reactions in the ligament (Paunio and Mäkinen, 1969). This

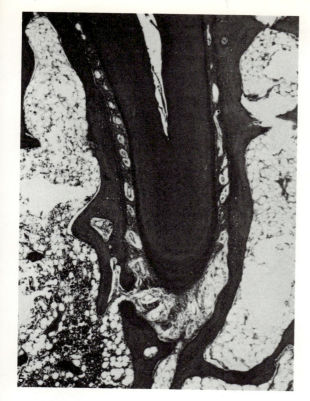

FIG. 5. Light micrograph. Periodontal ligament of first premolar illustrating the presence of numerous large blood vessels. Stained haematoxylin and eosin. ×57.

ligament lymphatics (Melcher, 1962). The latter are also inflamed and contain lymphocytes and plasma cells (Bernick and Grant, 1978). Granulocytes and macrophages account for most of the increased tissue cell content, there being an accompanying decrease in the number of fibroblasts in this location (Adams, Zander and Polson, 1979).

CONNECTIVE TISSUE CHANGES

Page and Schroeder (1976) have summarized the main features of the advanced lesion of chronic periodontitis as comprising an acute exudative vasculitis and chronic fibrotic inflammation, the chronic infiltrate consisting of plasma cells, lymphocytes and macrophages. They found clusters of plasma cells between the remains of collagen fibre bundles and around blood vessels. Many plasma cells were degenerating. The

perivascular proliferation of plasma cells extended from the gingival connective tissue to the ligament. Proliferation of the epithelial attachment apically is followed by only a slight cellular, mainly plasma cell, infiltration of the deeper connective tissue (Orban and Weinmann, 1942; Goldman, 1957 a, b). On the bony aspect of the ligament, osteoclasts are the most obvious cells. Garant (1976) also observed binucleated cells with fibroblasts or osteoblast-like cytoplasm and small mononuclear cells, all rich in acid phosphatase activity like osteoclasts, next to the bone surface.

Throughout the disease process, as mentioned previously, the collagen fibre bundles remain intact, except at the cervical periphery of the ligament. Deep to this the main changes seem to be a disruption of the perivascular connective tissue (Warwick James and Counsell, 1927), which is replaced largely by ground substance, PAS-positive mucopolysaccharide (Stahl, Sandler and Suben, 1958; Toto, Pollock and Gargiulo, 1964). Acidic mucopolysaccharide and reticulin fibres seem to be more abundant in inflamed tissue close to alveolar bone, and in areas of ground substance infiltrated by leukocytes (Stahl, Sandler and Suben, 1958; Quintarelli, 1960).

The local perivascular changes are followed by degeneration of the principal fibres of the ligament, with localized widening of the periodontal space due to adjacent alveolar bone resorption. Capillaries proliferate with the development of loose connective tissue (Orban and Weinmann, 1942). The fibre bundles acquire an open-weave appearance, due possibly to fluid accumulation within and around them, prior to their disintegration (Melcher, 1962).

There seems to have been little study of non-collagenous fibres in the inflamed ligament. There are varying opinions as to the fate of oxytalan fibres. Fullmer (1962) believed they were broken down, similarly to collagen, at some distance from the inflammatory focus. Kohl and Zander (1962) observed that oxytalan resisted denaturation better than collagen.

At an ultrastructural level, the first deviation from normal ligament collagen structure appears as a relaxation of packing of fibrils within each collagen fibre. Some fibrils appear swollen and non-banded fibrils are interposed parallel to the remaining collagen fibres (Selvig, 1966). Other fibrils have a beaded appearance, with a periodicity of beading similar to that of collagen cross-banding. Breakdown of the fibres is characterized by separation followed by a longitudinal splitting of component fibrils. These changes are followed by loss in orientation of the fibres and fibrils (Figs. 1—3) (Selvig, 1966, 1968). These ultra-structural changes are supported by a biochemical study which indicates that periodontal ligament from periodontitis patients is both more soluble and more unstable than that from healthy teeth (Paunio, 1965), due apparently to deficiencies in inter- rather than intra-molecular links (Paunio, Mäkinen and Paunio, 1970). As well as showing less collagen cross-linking than in healthy tissue, the diseased ligament also possesses increased fibroblast activity (Paunio, 1969 a, b).

There is little evidence as to changes with inflammation in the types of collagen in the ligament. There is an indication that fibroblasts from individuals with chronic periodontitis synthesize a type I collagen of altered composition, $\alpha 1$ (I)3, which is not synthesized by cells from normal gingiva (Page et al., 1979), but produce no type III molecules.

It has been estimated from a biochemical study that approximately 20% of the diseased collagen is abnormal (Narayanan and Page, 1976). The diseased ligament shows increased galactosamine: glucosamine and chondroitin sulphate: hyaluronic acid ratios. There is a need for further research into changes with inflammation in this most important component of the ligament as well as the fluid so relevant to its properties (see Chapter 6). Water-soluble proteins increase in amount but do not seem to alter in composition (Paunio, 1969 a, b). One report suggests that elastic fibres occur in the ligament only in advanced disease with little overt inflammation (Popov, 1965).

Some enzyme changes have been noted in the chronically inflamed ligament, though their significance is not clear. In hamster periodontitis there are reductions in fibroblast succinic dehydrogenase, and in di- and tri-phosphopyridine nucleotide diaphorase. There was a decrease in succinic dehydrogenase, and increase in triphosphopyridine nucleotide diaphorase activity in periodontal pocket epithelium (Carlson, 1964). This study is too isolated to permit any useful conclusions although the fibroblast changes suggest decreased metabolic activity in diseased ligament.

The most important sequel of chronic inflammatory periodontal disease is the loss of teeth by exfoliation or extraction. Clearly the loss of supporting tissue and the maintenance of unchanged occlusal load would, as in the case of deciduous root resorption, result eventually in exfoliation. It is also a common clinical finding that patients resort to softer foods when faced with the discomfort of chewing their usual diet with loose teeth. There has been little scientific study of how chronic inflammatory periodontal disease affects the mobility of teeth. The effects of occlusal trauma both alone and in conjunction with infectious inflammation have attracted more attention (see Chapter 14). Picton (1962) observed no increase in mobility with the development of gingivitis over a 1-month period, but increased mobility in relation to teeth affected by early periodontitis with slight horizontal bone loss (Mühlemann, 1954).

MECHANISMS OF LIGAMENT DESTRUCTION

It seems likely that collagen breakdown in chronic periodontitis is a multifactorial process and that mechanisms may differ at various stages of the disease (Soames and Davies, 1977). The mechanisms proposed include elements of the immune response and alterations in fibroblast activities and from the discussion which follows, it will be seen that these may be inter-related.

Schultz-Haudt and Aas (1960) suggested that collagen loss in chronic inflammatory periodontal disease was primarily the result of disorganization of fibre bundles, and secondarily due to the reduced ability of ligament fibroblasts to form collagen precursors. Lymphocytes have been observed in close contact with degenerating gingival fibroblasts (Schroeder and Page, 1972). This led to the suggestion that cytotoxic activity of these lymphocytes was at least partly responsible for fibroblast lysis and for a resultant reduced rate of collagen synthesis in humans (Page and Schroeder, 1976). Damage to fibroblasts may be produced by plaque-derived substances bound to the cells, by the cytotoxic action of lymphotoxin or by immune complex formation on the fibroblast surface with consequent complement activation (Horton, Oppenheim and Mergenhagen, 1973; Schluger, Yuodelis and Page, 1977). There may be an important species difference regarding this phenomenon since in rats a rapid and severe loss of periodontal tissues can occur without any apparent cytotoxic changes in the normal cells of the ligament or in those of the inflammatory infiltrate (Garant, 1976). Garant (1976) also observed close contacts between lymphocytes (and small macrophages) and fibroblasts, but could find no cytoplasmic alterations within such fibroblasts. A similar species difference may explain the contradictory finding in marmosets of increased collagen synthesis in the immediate proximity of periodontal pocket epithelium (Skougaard and Levy, 1971). It seems likely that reduced fibroblast activity occurs in the human periodontal ligament, since one of the first signs of inflammatory involvement is an increase in fibroblast and osteoblast glycogen content (Michel and Frank, 1970). This storage polymer also occurs between collagen fibrils, apparently due to cell rupture (Fig. 6). Michel and Frank (1970) reasoned that glycogen accumulated because it was not being used routinely for energy. They concluded that the phenomenon indicated an upset in fibroblast metabolism induced by inflammation. A similar conclusion was reached by Rippin (1978). On the basis of similarities between rat molar and human periodontal ligament regarding structure, function and biochemistry, unlike the extreme situation observed by Garant

(1976), he labelled rat molar periodontal ligament with tritiated proline and observed a reduced rate of collagen synthesis in the inflamed ligament, in terms of reduced uptake of the tracer. He also suggested that there was no evidence of a major collagenolytic plaque or host factor, and concluded that reduced rate of collagen formation was the most likely reason for loss of ligament collagen in chronic inflammatory periodontal disease.

There is evidence to suggest that collagenolysis is an important factor in the disease. Morphometric study suggests, at least in early gingivitis, that collagen loss is too rapid to be explained by a decrease in the rate of collagen synthesis by damaged fibroblasts (Page and Schroeder, 1976). Collagen fibrils have been observed in human fibroblasts from tissue affected by apical or juvenile periodontitis (Figs. 7 and 8) (Eley and Harrison, 1975; Garant, 1976; Garant and Cho, 1979 a, b) and in beagle dog fibroblasts and macrophages from lesions of early chronic gingivitis (Soames and Davies, 1977). There is also evidence that both macrophages and fibroblasts can phagocytose and resorb collagen fibres (Parakkal, 1969). Soames and Davies (1977) noted that the presence of collagen within cytoplasmic vacuoles did not constitute proof

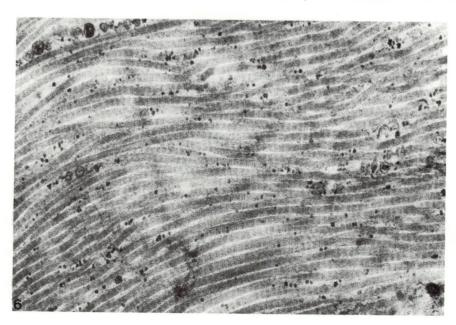

FIG. 6. Transmission electron micrograph. Bundle of collagen fibres of the periodontal ligament. Between the fibrils are glycogen granules. ×9700.

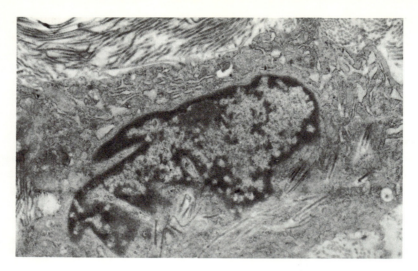

FIG. 7. Transmission electron micrograph. A fibroblast is seen containing intracellular banded collagen fibrils and rough endoplasmic reticulum, and is surrounded
by collagen fibrils. Section of periodontal ligament from /6̄. ×8000.

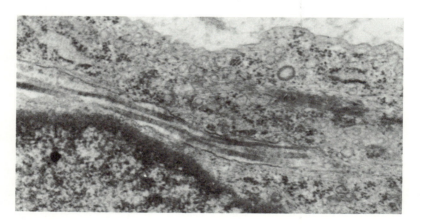

FIG. 8. Transmission electron micrograph. Banded collagen fibrils are seen in an
elongated membrane-bound vacuole adjacent to the nucleus, and above in a less
clearly defined elongated vacuole. The plasma membrane is seen at the top of the
photograph. Section of part of a fibroblast in periodontal ligament from 6/. ×38,000.

of phagocytosis. However, from their observations of
the frequency of occurrence of intracellular fibrils,
the varied orientation of fibrils within cytoplasmic
vacuoles in the same cell and the demonstration of
acid hydrolase-containing bodies of similar morphology to fibril-containing vacuoles, they concluded that
phagocytosis of collagen did occur, at least in early
gingivitis. A similar line of reasoning and conclusion
followed from Garant's (1976) work. On the basis

of this evidence, there seems no reason why a similar
situation should not exist in the inflamed periodontal
ligament. There are several supporting reports from the
concept of physiologic phagocytosis and intracellular
collagenolysis of the periodontal soft connective
tissues (Ten Cate, 1972; Ten Cate and Deporter, 1975).

In a study of rapidly (7 weeks) developing gingivitis
and periodontitis in rats fed a high sucrose diet,
Garant and Cho (1979a) observed cytopathic altera-

tion of fibroblasts limited mostly to areas adjacent to epithelium. They also noted that altered fibroblasts in this location were not usually in contact with lymphocytes, and questioned whether the deterioration of fibroblasts in gingivitis was always lymphocyte mediated. In the infiltrated dense connective tissue of advanced lesions (Garant and Cho, 1979b) they did observe a lymphocyte–fibroblast interaction, but found no changes in macrophages, endothelial cells or pericytes. They also found clusters of fibroblasts rich in intracellular collagen fibrils in the dense connective tissue of advanced lesions, and large and apparently active fibroblasts in older lesions, which they suggested represented a fibrotic or wound healing response. Although the periodontal lesions described by Garant and Cho developed rapidly, they provide further evidence for lymphocyte–fibroblast interaction and fibroblast collagenolysis as mechanisms of ligament breakdown in chronic inflammatory periodontal disease.

There is some evidence that extracellular collagenolysis occurs during periodontitis. The ground substance seems to be affected first, since ligament hyaluronidase activity has been found to increase prior to that of collagenase (Paunio, 1969b). Extracellular collagenases may derive from plaque bacteria, neutrophils, macrophages and fibroblasts. While bacterial collagenase may affect the rate of production or the activity of endogenous collagenase, the latter is apparently the exclusive form of the enzyme associated with the affected tissues (Fullmer, Baer and Driscoll, 1969).

Lysosomal enzymes other than collagenase may have an important role in periodontal ligament destruction. This is indicated by the more rapid periodontal destruction noted in mink affected by Chediak–Higashi syndrome, in which the hereditary defect is an abundance of lysosome-like granules in leucocytes, mainly polymorphs, but including lymphocytes (Gustafson, 1969). Lysosomes from macrophages may also release enzymes which help to break down ligament connective tissue (Hamp and Folke, 1968; Paunio and Mäkinen, 1969). It may be noted that in one study increases and decreases in the numbers of granulocytes and macrophages in (monkey) transseptal fibres correlated respectively with initiation and slowing down of ligament destruction. This was related to the known capacity of these cells for causing cell damage, collagen degradation and bone resorption

(Adams, Zander and Polson, 1979). At the same time these workers pointed out that the granulocytes might serve the more important function of limiting antigens to the tissue adjacent to the gingival crevice.

THE INFLAMMATORY/IMMUNE RESPONSE

Mention has been made of possible relationships between the inflammatory/immune response and ligament destruction. Although there is as yet little evidence that the relationships occur *in vivo*, certain factors seem relevant, and will be described. Most, if not all, of the cellular and acellular components of an inflammatory/immune response to plaque microorganisms and their products accumulate in the soft periodontal tissues. They include neutrophils, plasma cells, T- and B-lymphocytes, macrophages, immunoglobulins and complement components. It has been suggested that the severity or rate of advance of the lesion is increased by activation of the host response, perhaps by uncontrolled production of lymphokines, prostaglandins and hydrolytic enzymes (for review see Schluger, Yuodelis and Page, 1977). Alternatively or concomitantly, the same could result from increases in the levels of gram-negative anaerobes in the dento-gingival plaque (Grigsby and Sabiston, 1976). Some research indicates a linear relationship between peripheral blood lymphocyte transformation, an excellent indicator of the intensity of host response, and the severity of periodontitis, except in severe periodontitis (Ivanyi and Lehner, 1970, 1971; Ivanyi, Wilton and Lehner, 1972; Horton, Leikin and Oppenheim, 1972). However, there is one dissenting study (Kiger, Wright and Creamer, 1974). The greatest stimulation of peripheral blood lymphocytes seems to occur when the lesion has extended to the ligament (Patters *et al.*, 1976). This postulated relationship between lymphocyte response and tissue damage is supported by work suggesting that positive lymphocyte transformation, cytotoxicity and migration inhibition tests indicate cell-mediated immune responses consistent with damage to periodontal tissues (Ivanyi and Lehner, 1970, 1971; Ivanyi, Wilton and Lehner, 1972; Horton, Leikin and Oppenheim, 1972). Lest one be led to consider the possibility of chronic inflammatory periodontal disease being an auto-immune process, one should remember that the disease is chronic, lasting many years in most patients, and that the periodontal soft tissues and alveolar bone retreat in good order ahead of the advancing front of the lesion, as described in an earlier section. Also, as in many non-specific chronic infectious inflammatory conditions, the central lesion is effectively walled off from deeper healthy tissue by zones of chronic inflammatory cells and fibrous tissue. There is additional evidence that in most patients the inflammatory/immune response tends to be self-limiting as the disease advances. This relates to the observation that the stimulation index of lymphocyte transformation by ultrasonicates of several plaque organisms is decreased significantly in cases of severe chronic periodontitis, due, it is postulated, to the presence of inhibitory or the absence of stimulatory factors in serum (Ivanyi *et al.*, 1972). Lymphocyte transformation appears to be comparable in normal patients and in those with severe periodontitis (Ivanyi and Lehner, 1971).

A further problem concerns the role of the individual components of the host response in the small amount of tissue loss that takes place. It seems that both T- and B-lymphocytes contribute to fibroblast damage through lymphokine production, although there is no direct evidence for this (Mackler *et al.*, 1974) or for any other proposed mechanism, for that matter. The main inflammatory cell in the advanced lesion is the plasma cell. This may relate to the role of B-lymphocytes in the production of relevant lymphokines, for example, osteoclast activating factor (Page and Schroeder, 1976). Regarding the comparative importance of T- and B-lymphocytes, there is evidence that the established human lesion is dominated by B-lymphocytes (Walker, 1977) and that the T-cell role, while including other features of cell-mediated immunity, may be mainly one of helper activity (Seymour and Greenspan, 1979).

Mast cells have been associated with regions of collagen breakdown, so they, too, could be involved in ligament destruction (Barnett, 1974). Mast-cell heparin can stimulate collagenase production and activity (Sakamoto, Goldhaber and Glimcher, 1973). Mast-cell neutral proteases may digest both collagen and non-collagenous ligament proteins after initial cleavage by collagenase (Page and Schroeder, 1976).

As mentioned previously, macrophages by virtue of their enzymic activity, particularly lysosomal and including collagenase, may have a part in tissue breakdown. In addition activated macrophages can form prostaglandins which are thought to inhibit lymphocyte transformation. This might be a further mechanism inhibiting the host response in advanced periodontitis (Morley, 1974; Schluger, Yuodelis and Page, 1977). Prostaglandins seem capable of producing different effects, from collagen synthesis (Raisz and Koolemans-Beynen, 1974) to fibrotic ligament changes (Blumenkrantz and Söndergaard, 1972). Schluger, Yuodelis and Page (1977) have suggested that prostaglandins may suppress the immune response, but inhibit fibroblast mitosis, and the synthesis and turnover of both collagen and non-collagenous proteins. However, one experiment suggests that prostaglandins, particularly PGE_1, may increase ligament collagen resorption without affecting many fibroblasts (Rao, Moe and Heersche, 1978).

Because of the lack of any firm experimental evidence the precise role of the humoral response during periodontitis can only be surmised. One possibility is that immune complex formation could activate complement resulting in C3b stimulation of hydrolytic enzyme (including collagenase) secretion by macrophages (Berglund, 1971; Schluger, Yuodelis and Page, 1977). Fibroblast lysis may result from complement activation at its surface by immune complex formation between specific antibody and plaque antigens or from the activation by immune complex of killer lymphocytes (K-cells) (Brandtzaeg, 1966).

There has been little study of the possibility of genetic predisposition to rapid ligament destruction, although an inverse relationship does seem to exist between this and the frequency of HL-A2 antigen occurrence in patients, suggesting that the genes controlling susceptibility to microbial agents from plaque may be linked to the HL-A locus (Terasaki *et al.*, 1975).

Periodontosis

This condition involves rapid destruction of the periodontal ligament in young people. Hence the designation juvenile periodontitis by some workers (Lehner *et al.*, 1974). Typically, the disease is restricted initially to first molars and incisors, although, if left unchecked, it may involve the entire dentition. (Genetic aspects of this disease are considered in Chapter 13.)

The alveolar attachment of the periodontal ligament fibres is lost initially (Baer *et al.*, 1963). This is followed by a widening of the periodontal 'space' due to bone resorption. The principal fibres are eventually replaced by a loose and disorientated collagen network, though they are still recognizable until the more advanced stages of the disease (Baer *et al.*, 1963). Remaining ligament fibres run parallel to the root surface (Baer *et al.*, 1963; Kaslick and Chasens, 1968 a, b). The picture is one of rapid alveolar fibre destruction and apical proliferation of epithelial attachment (Fig. 9) (Bouyssou and Fourel, 1973). Ligament vessels are numerous and markedly dilated, although there is minimal inflammation (Wade, 1965; Fourel, 1972). There may (Orban and Weinmann, 1942) or may not (Fourel, 1972) be proliferation of the rests

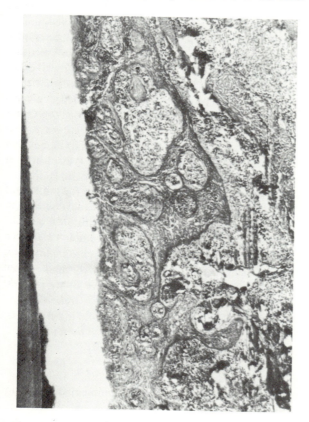

FIG. 9. Light micrograph. Section from periodontosis periodontal ligament (10½-year-old boy). Extensive inflammatory infiltrate and epithelial proliferation. ×21.

of Malassez. There are variable but usually small numbers of plasma cells, with fewer polymorphs (Fourel, 1972).

In spite of a lack of proven aetiological factors in periodontosis genetic factors are suspected, although no genetic defect of collagen synthesis or metabolism has yet been demonstrated. There is now no doubt that plaque is involved, its distribution being similar on teeth affected by periodontitis and periodontosis, although much thinner on the latter (Waerhaug, 1976, 1977). The flora associated with periodontosis increases in numbers of various gram-negative rods found in lesser amounts in periodontitis-associated plaque (Newman *et al.*, 1976; Slots, 1976). Deficient neutrophil function as regards chemotaxis and phagocytosis has been demonstrated in patients with this disease (Cianciola *et al.*, 1977; Clark, Page and Wilde, 1977). It has been shown that polymorphs limit subgingival plaque growth (Attström and Schroeder, 1979) and that there is a poor response by polymorphs to gram-negative rods such as *Capnocytophaga* thought to be important in periodontosis (Lindhe and Socransky, 1979). A combination of this type of organism, with defective polymorph function as described, provides a reasonable hypothesis for the aetiology of periodontosis. There also seems to be an impaired lymphocyte response in this condition (Lehner *et al.*, 1974). Van Swol (1973) described a patient with both sarcoidosis and periodontosis. He suggested that the two diseases might have something immunological in common, although he did not admit coincidence as the more likely possibility.

Lateral periodontal abscess

There has been little research into periodontal ligament changes in this condition. Its aetiology has been attributed, without good evidence, to sudden alterations in ecology in the bacterial population of periodontal pockets, produced, for example, by scaling or probing, especially where there are deep infrabony defects or involvement of the furcations of multirooted teeth (Pritchard, 1953; McFall, 1964; Miyasato, 1975). Acute changes are therefore superimposed generally on tissues already chronically inflamed. The histopathology resembles in many respects that of the periapical abscess (see succeeding section on suppurative apical periodontitis), with an abundance of polymorphs being the main feature. Chronic change results in reversion to a predominance of plasma cells and lymphocytes, with peripheral fibrosis (Stahl, 1973).

APICAL PERIODONTITIS

Non-suppurative apical periodontitis

The acute form of this lesion usually follows physical trauma or chemical irritation, but may be infective in origin. There are the typical changes associated with acute inflammation, including hyperaemia, oedema, neutrophil infiltration and some widening of the periodontal space (Darling, 1970). The chronic variety is often a sequel to the acute form with a change to a chronic inflammatory cell infiltrate comprising mainly plasma cells and macrophages. There is moderate vasodilation and new capillary formation, together with fibroblast activity. This results in the formation of a granuloma which gradually increases in volume, with associated bone resorption, and a fibrous tissue layer and new bone may be found at the periphery of the lesion (Wade, 1965; Darling, 1970). The granuloma itself consists mainly of chronic inflammatory granulation tissue composed mainly of numerous plasma cells, lymphocytes, a few polymorphs, proliferating fibroblasts and a varying density of collagen bundles (Figs. 10 and 12) (Gardner, 1962a). It varies macroscopically from one which is firm and adherent to the root apex to a soft or haemorrhagic granuloma easily damaged during tooth extraction. This variation relates to differences in the density and degree of order of connective tissue fibres in the lesion (Lyons et al., 1970). The fibrous tissue of the lesion is continuous at its periphery with the healthy periodontal ligament (Leuin, 1957). On a histological basis, Yanagisawa (1980) has divided periapical granulomas into four types: exudative, granulomatous, granulo-fibrous and fibrous. Cases of more than 1 year's duration showed much fibrosis.

Elimination or reduction in the severity of irritation can allow the lesion to proceed to complete repair. Ankylosis of tooth to bone can occur (Wade, 1965; Darling, 1970). There may be a widening of the perio-

dontal space, with breaks in continuity of the lamina dura, associated with granuloma formation (Narita, 1956). Root resorption, osteosclerosis or hypercementosis can occur, but usually only in long-standing cases (Darling, 1970).

Epithelial cell rests occur in the lesion and one (monkey) study suggests that the rests are larger, but not more numerous, than in normal tissues, and can eventually occupy most of a granuloma (Valderhaug, 1974). Detailed study shows that the epithelial cells in apical lesions are polygonal, adhering to each other by fewer desmosomes than in normal squamous epithelium. The cells have irregular nuclei, prominent nucleoli and much euchromatin. There is a decrease in the nuclear:cytoplasmic ratio. Some contain lipid droplets. The cells also contain scattered polyribosomes and dilated rough endoplasmic reticulum. Their cytoplasm contains bundles of tonofilaments and keratohyalin granules, scattered mitochondria, a well-developed Golgi apparatus and occasional membrane whorls or residual myelin bodies. Micropinocytotic vesicles and large vacuoles are also present, but phagosomes are rare (Ten Cate, 1972b; Summers and Papadimitriou, 1975). It has been suggested that the stimulus causing proliferation of the epithelial cells is a local change in pH or CO_2 tension (Grupe, Ten Cate and Zander, 1967).

The epithelial (and capillary endothelial) basement membranes in these lesions are strongly PAS-positive, the intensity of staining increasing with subacute or acute inflammatory change (Diniotou et al., 1975). This is indicative of connective tissue breakdown and an increase in the amount of ground substance mucopolysaccharide (Obručnik and Meduna, 1959). Diniotou et al. (1975) suggested that chronic inflammatory changes in apical granulomas were marked by a gradual disappearance of connective tissue mucopolysaccharides, and the replacement of reticulin by collagen. Oxytalan fibres have been found in periapical granulomas, although the significance of their presence has not been explained (Fullmer, 1960).

Lack of pain from the lesion has been associated with lack of nerve endings (Gardner, 1962a), although nerve endings are present in small numbers in at least half of chronic inflammatory periapical lesions (Bynum and Flieder, 1960).

Periapical lesions contain several fat residues of tissue degeneration. These include glycerides, free

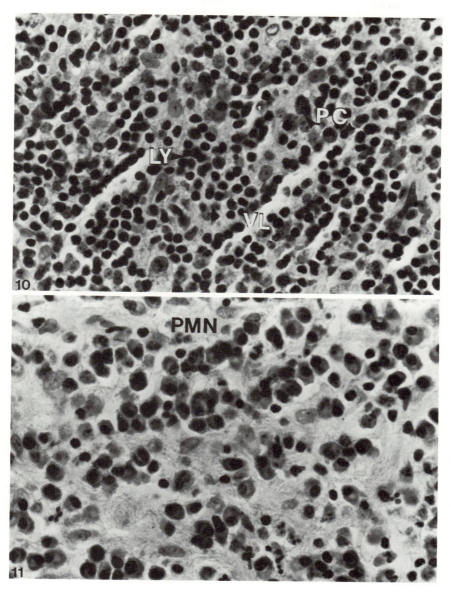

FIGS. 10 and 11. Light micrographs. Chronically inflamed periapical tissue composed of numerous inflammatory cells in loose connective tissue stroma. Prominent features of lesion in Fig. 10 include abundant lymphocytes (LY) and mature plasma cells (PC) as well as numerous immature blood vessels (vessel lumen, VL). In other specimens (Fig. 11) numerous plasma cells and scattered polymorphonuclear leucocytes (PMN) are observed. Stained haematoxylin and eosin. ×350.

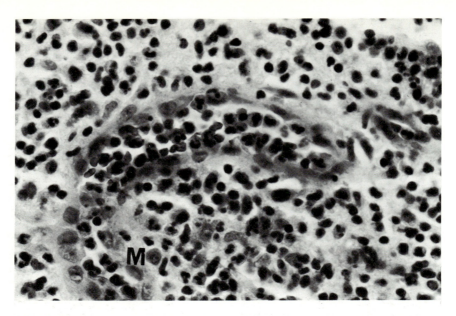

FIG. 12. Light micrograph. Neutrophil lesion. PMN may be prominent inflammatory cells and in such cases are often observed penetrating vessel walls. A few macrophages (M) and numerous PMN are scattered through connective tissue stroma. Stained haematoxylin and eosin. ×350.

and esterified cholesterol and phospholipids (Bozzo, Valdrighi and Vizioli, 1972). Cholesterol clefts are common, the crystals themselves having been removed, of course, during routine tissue processing. The clefts are surrounded by foreign-body giant cells, Russell bodies and haemosiderin pigment (Gardner, 1962a; Leonard, Lunin and Provenza, 1974). Cholesterol and other fat residues may result from fatty degeneration of cells (Gardner, 1962a). Cholesterol also forms in blood clots which congest the many capillaries in the inflamed tissue. The disintegrating red thrombi may release their lipids to form the characteristic spindle-shaped aggregates of cholesterol crystals which are enveloped by the endothelial walls of small vessels (Browne, 1971; Arwill and Heyden, 1973). Foam cells occur adjacent to the zone of fibrosis (Yanagisawa, 1980).

The capillaries in apical lesions are hard to discern, but may be distinguished by their high ATP-ase activity. Pericytes of the inflamed capillary endothelium show increased lysosomal function, and may form eventually foreign-body giant cells with tissue-degrading properties leading to resorption of components of the apical lesion (Browne, 1971; Arwill and Heyden, 1973).

Immunoglobulin-producing cells are common in periapical lesions (Figs. 13 and 14) (Morse, Lasater and White, 1975; Morton, Clagett and Yavorsky, 1977). Of the plasma cells, those containing IgG are most numerous. Some cells contain IgA, but few IgM. A recent study of periapical granulomas indicated that IgG, IgA, IgM and IgE cells represented 70, 14, 4 and 10% respectively of the immunoglobulin-containing cells observed (Pulver, Taubman and Smith, 1978). Many lymphocytes, including T-cells (Farber, 1975), occur in the typical granuloma, and complement components, mainly C3, are also present (Kuntz *et al.*, 1977). Granulomas having marked lymphocyte infiltration are found more frequently in cases which had endodontic treatment. In contrast, a mainly plasma cell infiltrate was more frequent in untreated cases with open pulp chambers, as was epithelial proliferation. Mast cells in exudative and granulomatous zones may release histamine, increasing vascular permeability. In the fibrous zone, mast cells may contribute to breakdown and formation of collagen and ground substance (Yanagisawa, 1980).

There is no clear evidence that immune complexes contribute to the inflammatory events or subsequent

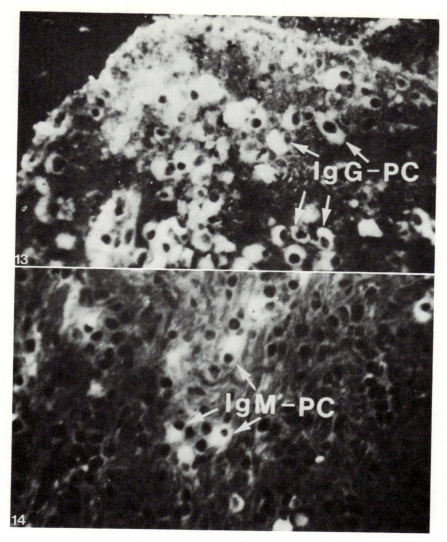

FIGS. 13 and 14. Light micrographs. Immunofluorescence photomicrographs of unfixed periapical tissues stained with fluoresceinated anti-human IgG and IgM respectively. As in Fig. 13, abundant IgG-containing plasma cells (IgG-PC) are present in most instances. To a lesser extent, IgM plasma cells (IgM-PC) were also observed (Fig. 14). ×280.

bone loss of periapical periodontitis (Morton, Clagett and Yavorsky, 1977). Bacteria occur rarely in inflamed periapical tissue (Block *et al.*, 1976; Langeland, Block and Grossman, 1977). Abundant mast cells were found in apical granulomas in one study (Mathiesen, 1973). In general, there appears to be too little information available to comment usefully on the significance of these demonstrated components of the host response in periapical lesions, except to suggest that as in lateral periodontitis, they serve to counter infection. However, it appears that immune complexes and IgE-mediated reactions may play a role in periapical pathosis (Yanagisawa, 1980).

Suppurative apical periodontitis

These lesions have been reviewed by Gardner (1962a)

and Darling (1970), though there is a lack of literature on the topic. The periapical suppurative lesions are composed of a focus of infection around the apical foramen which, with necrosis and the accumulation of polymorphs, results in pus formation. The acute central necrotic area is surrounded by a dense polymorph infiltrate and some chronic inflammatory cells. This zone is encompassed by inflammatory granulation tissue and then by an area of fibrosis, the latter being more abundant in chronic lesions. External to the fibrotic zone is a region of hyperaemia, oedema and bone resorption, producing widening of the periodontal space. The chronic lesion contains lymphocytes, plasma cells, some neutrophils and bacteria and serous pus. The cavity in both acute and chronic forms centres on the root apex foramen, a lateral canal, or the furcation area of a multi-rooted tooth. In the chronic lesion, the central zone is surrounded by inflammatory granulation tissue infiltrated with chronic inflammatory and giant cells, with a peripheral fibrous capsule between this and the alveolar bone. Pus may accumulate in the adjacent bone marrow spaces as well as the periapical periodontal space (Gardner, 1962b).

RARE INFECTIONS OF THE PERIODONTAL LIGAMENT

Actinomycosis

Periodontal lesions are usually secondary to cervicofacial actinomycosis. The rare ligament lesions often contain epithelial rests which may form cysts. Chronic abscess formation is a more usual sequel. This displays a central zone of bacterial filaments surrounded by lymphocytes, polymorphs, endothelioid and giant cells, and a peripheral thick fibrous layer (Figs. 15 and 16) (Wade, 1965; August and Levy, 1973; Samanta, Malik and Aikat, 1975; Krolls, Westbrook and Hess, 1977). The lesion may spread to involve the jaw or present gingivally as an enlarging painless nodule which softens, usually after several months, and breaks down, discharging yellow pus containing typical sulphur granules (Wade, 1965). Periapical actinomycosis has been reported also with demonstrable actinomycetes in the periapical region sur-

rounded by polymorphs and other inflammatory cells (August and Levy, 1973; Samanta, Malik and Aikat, 1975; Krolls, Westbrook and Hess, 1977).

Acute necrotizing ulcerative gingivitis

Spread to involve the periodontal ligament is uncommon, but extensive destruction of the ligament can occur (Hornstein and Gorlin, 1970). In such instances there is loss of crestal bone, and the ligament is affected by marked vasodilation and thrombosis, resulting in a localized ischaemic necrosis. An intense acute inflammatory infiltrate may spread to the marrow spaces, and the transseptal fibres are then usually disrupted (Cohen, 1965; Wade, 1965). Among the possible mechanisms underlying the pathogenesis of this condition is an excessive cell-mediated immune response to one of the associated organisms, fusiform bacilli (Nisengard, 1977). Lehner (1969) found significantly depressed IgG and raised IgM concentrations within 1 to 4 days of onset of clinical symptoms, followed by rises in levels of IgG and IgM during the first month of onset. Complement levels appeared to be normal. He suggested that these changes could be effected by a relative hypogammaglobulinaemia of the IgG class or by the (unspecified) activity of gram-negative endotoxin-producing organisms.

Tuberculosis

The oral lesion is usually a crateriform painless ulcer with a caseated base which may rarely extend to the ligament and cause tooth loss. If extension occurs, the lesion presents as an endosteal granuloma with a chronic sinus which often persists after local treatment (Wade, 1965). One individual with acute disseminated miliary tuberculosis was found to have very loose teeth with numerous yellowish, pinhead-sized tubercles on the affected gingival margins. The roots of extracted teeth were covered by soft, adherent granulomatous tissue containing many tubercles (Grant and Bernick, 1972). Cases have been reported of apical granulomas containing closely packed tubercles with epithelioid and giant cells, but little caseation (Bradnum, 1961). In general, periodontal

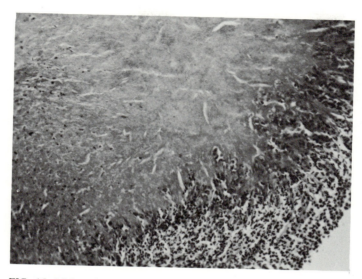

FIG. 15. Light micrograph. Periodontal actinomycotic abscess. Periodic acid Schiff stain demonstrates a granule of one of the colonies of the actinomyces organisms surrounded by polymorphonuclear leucocytes. ×325.

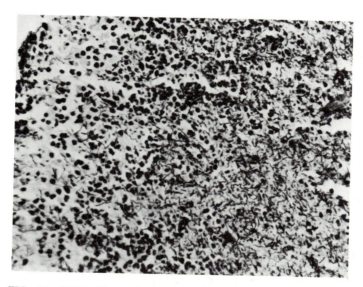

FIG. 16. Light micrograph. Periodontal actinomycotic abscess. The Brown and Brenn staining technique demonstrates the actinomyces organisms among numerous inflammatory cells. ×420.

lesions are secondary to pulmonary tuberculosis (Jian, 1956).

Leprosy

Gingival ulceration in lepromatous leprosy may spread to cause severe periodontal destruction, affecting particularly the maxillary incisors (Epker and Via, 1969; Reichart, Ananatasan and Reznik, 1976). There seem to be no reports of tuberculoid leprosy affecting the periodontal ligament. The lepromatous lesion typically causes widening of both lamina dura and periodontal space. Histologically, the ligament changes differ little from non-specific chronic inflammation. Occasionally, scanty acid-fast fragmented, granular bacilli, representing the degenerate forms of once viable *Myobacterium leprae*, occur in relation to macrophages (Fig. 17) (Reichart, Ananatasan and Reznik, 1976).

Aspergillosis

A single case of aspergillosis of the nasal cavity, caused by a strain of the filamentous fungus *Aspergillus*, and arising probably from a maxillary incisor periapical

abscess, has been reported in a patient debilitated by acute myelogenous leukaemia (Fields, 1977).

Glanders

This disease of horses is caused by the gram-negative bacillus *Loefflerella mallei*. Human glanders, occurring usually in those working with affected animals, may on rare occasions produce destructive crateriform gingival ulcers extending in even rarer instances to alveolar bone, leading to dental exfoliation. The lesion develops quickly into an ulcer which enlarges by marginal breakdown or confluence of adjacent ulcers, and discharges a yellowish, blood-streaked oily fluid (Hornstein and Gorlin, 1970).

Leishmaniasis

Protozoa of the genus *Leishmania,* closely related to the trypanosomes, may cause disease in man. On extremely rare occasions leishmaniasis may involve the periodontal ligament, endarteritis accelerating the process of destruction. This occurs only in the serious mucocutaneous form of the disease, in which the lesions are reported as firm, partly ulcerative, partly

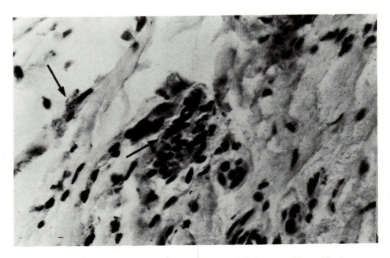

FIG. 17. Light micrograph. Portion of periodontal ligament affected by leprosy. Small fragments of *Mycobacterium leprae.* ×215.

polypoid, severely mutilating, chronic and progressive (Hornstein and Gorlin, 1970). Detailed ligament histopathology is lacking.

Histoplasmosis

A single case of histoplasmosis as periapical pathology has been documented (Pisanty, 1979). The fungus was identified in a periapical granuloma in relation to a symptomless upper first molar, for which vitality tests had been inconclusive. There had been no periodontal pockets around the affected tooth. Histologically, large numbers of fungus-laden phagocytes were present. These contained many minute yeast-like bodies with prominent round nuclei surrounded by a clear zone and a distinct peripheral capsule, compatible with the appearance of *Histoplasma capsulatum*. Pisanty (1979) suggested that the organism had gained entry to the tissue during previous extraction of an adjoining tooth. The patient had no systemic involvement and the intradermal histoplasmin skin test and chest radiography were negative.

CONCLUSIONS

Surprisingly little attention has been given to changes in the periodontal ligament in the infectious inflammatory periodontal diseases, whether rare or common. Concerning the most widespread of these periodontal diseases, there is still inadequate information concerning mechanisms of ligament degradation, although there are suggestions that defective cellular host response factors, especially polymorphonuclear, and a range of gram-negative rods in plaque may accelerate the rate of tissue loss. This would point to the elaboration by live organisms or the passive release by dead or dying bacteria of factors of which some are more noxious than others to the ligament. One of the most important features requiring clarification is the mechanism whereby gingivitis spreads to involve the deeper tissues, and how this change occurs at different times and rates in different patients. There needs to be more effort to establish the mechanisms of collagen loss, and more detail is required of the changes which occur in both the collagen fibre structure and the

ground substance. Is collagen loss effected directly by plaque enzymes or other factors or by host tissue factors alone? The general details of the host response remain confusing at the present time. There exists in the literature a level of hypothesis concerning the role of the inflammatory/immune reaction to plaque out of proportion to the experimental and observational evidence. It is to be hoped that future research will clarify the situation *in vivo*. This should involve the subjection of periodontal tissue to a variety of putative protective or destructive factors in order to assess the effects of these singly and in combination on the rate of development and progression of chronic inflammatory periodontal disease.

REFERENCES

ADAMS, R. A., ZANDER, H. A. & POLSON, A. M. (1979) Cell populations in the transseptal fibre region before, during and after experimental periodontitis in squirrel monkeys. *J. Periodont.* **50**, 7–12.

ARWILL, T. & HEYDEN, G. (1973) Histochemical studies on cholesterol formation in odontogenic cysts and granulomas. *Scand. J. dent. Res.* **81**, 406–410.

ATTSTRÖM, R. & SCHROEDER, H. E. (1979) Effect of experimental neutropenia on initial gingivitis in dogs. *Scand. J. dent. Res.* **87**, 7–23.

AUGUST, O. S. & LEVY, B. A. (1973) Periapical actinomycosis. *Oral Surg.* **36**, 585–588.

BAER, P. N., STANLEY, H. R., BROWN, K., SMITH, L., GAMBLE, J. & SWERDLOW, H. (1963) Advanced periodontal disease in an adolescent (periodontosis). *J. Periodont.* **34**, 533–539.

BARNETT, M. L. (1974) The fine structure of human connective tissue mast cells in periodontal disease. *J. Periodont. Res.* **9**, 84–91.

BERGLUND, S. E. (1971) Immunoglobulins in human gingiva with specificity for oral bacteria. *J. periodont.* **42**, 546–551.

BERNICK, S. & GRANT, D. A. (1978) Lymphatic vessels of healthy and inflamed gingiva. *J. dent. Res.* **57**, 810–817.

BLOCK, R. M., BUSHELL, A., RODRIGUES, H. & LANGELAND, K. (1976) A histopathologic, histobacteriologic and radiographic study of periapical endodontic surgical specimens. *Oral Surg.* **42**, 656–678.

BLUMENKRANTZ, N. & SÖNDERGAARD, J. (1972) Effect of prostaglandins on biosynthesis of collagen. *Nature* (New Biol.) **239**, 246.

BOUYSSOU, M. & FOUREL, J. (1973) La parodontite aiguë juvenile et le syndrome de Papillon-Lefèvre. Problème clinique, pathologique et étiologique. *Acta Stomatol. Belgica* **70**, 71–113.

BOZZO, L., VALDRIGHI, L. & VIZIOLI, M. R. (1972) Lipid components of human dental periapical lesions. Histochemical and histophysical observations. *Oral Surg.* **34**, 166–171.

BRADNUM, P. (1961) Tuberculous sinus of face associated with an abscessed lower third molar. *Dent. Practnr.* **12**, 127–128.

BRANDTZAEG, P. (1966) Local factors of resistance in the gingival area. *J. periodont. Res.* **1**, 19–42.

BROWNE, R. M. (1971) The origin of cholesterol in odontogenic cysts in man. *Archs. oral Biol.* **16**, 107–114.

BYNUM, J. W. & FLIEDER, D. E. (1960) Demonstration of nerve tissue in periapical inflammatory lesions. *J. dent. Res.* **39**, 737 (abs.).

CARLSON, D. R. (1964) Histochemistry of oxidative enzymes in hamster periodontal disease. *J. dent. Res.* **43**, 846 (abs.).

CIANCIOLA, L. J., GENCO, R. J., PATTERS, M. R., McKENNA, J. & VAN OSS, C. J. (1977) Defective polymorphonuclear leukocyte function in a human periodontal disease. *Nature* **265**, 445–447.

CLARK, R. A., PAGE, R. C. & WILDE, G. (1977) Defective neutrophil chemotaxis in juvenile periodontitis. *Infect. Immunol.* **18**, 694–700.

COHEN, D. W. (1965) Pathology of periodontal disease. In: *Oral pathology*, R. W. TIECKE (ed.), pp. 131–167. New York, McGraw-Hill.

DARLING, A. I. (1970) Periapical inflammation of the teeth. In: *Thoma's oral pathology*, Vol. I, R. J. GORLIN & H. M. GOLDMAN (eds.), pp. 335–358. St. Louis, C. V. Mosby.

DINIOTOU, M., CROISIER, N., POMPIDOU, A., MARE, B., MUGNIER, A. & SCHRAMM, B. (1975) Contribution à l'étude histopathologique des granulomes apexiens. *Bull. Group Eur. Rech. Sc. Stomat. et Odont.* **18**, 25–35.

ELEY, B. M. & HARRISON, J. D. (1975) Intracellular collagen fibrils in the periodontal ligament of man. *J. periodont. Res.* **10**, 168–170.

EPKER, B. N. & VIA, W. F. (1969) Oral and perioral manifestations of leprosy. Report of a case. *Oral Surg.* **28**, 342–347.

FARBER, P. A. (1975) Scanning electron microscopy of cells from periapical lesions. *J. Endod.* **1**, 291–294.

FIELDS, B. N. (1977) Case 36-1977. Case records of the Massachusetts General Hospital. *New England J. Med.* **297**, 546–551.

FOUREL, J. (1972) Periodontosis: a periodontal syndrome. *J. Periodont.* **43**, 240–255.

FULLMER, H. M. (1960) Observations on the development of oxytalan fibres in dental granulomas and radicular cysts. *Arch. Path.* **70**, 59–67.

FULLMER, H. M. (1961) A histochemical study of periodontal disease in the maxillary alveolar processes of 135 autopsies. *J. Periodont.* **32**, 206–218.

FULLMER, H. M. (1962) A critique of normal connective tissues of the periodontium and some alterations with periodontal disease. *J. dent. Res.* **41**, 223–229 and 229–234.

FULLMER, H. M., BAER, P. & DRISCOLL, E. (1969) Correlation of collagenase production to periodontal disease. *J. periodont. Res.* **4**, suppl. 4, 30–31.

GARANT, P. R. (1976) An electron microscopic study of the periodontal tissues of germfree rats and rats monoinfected with *Actinomyces naeslundii*. *J. periodont. Res.* (Suppl.) **11**, 3–79.

GARANT, P. R. & CHO, M. I. (1979a) Histopathogenesis of spontaneous periodontal disease in conventional rats. I. Histometric and histologic study. *J. periodont. Res.* **14**, 297–309.

GARANT, P. R. & CHO, M. I. (1979b) Histopathogenesis of spontaneous periodontal disease in conventional rats. II. Ultrastructural features of the inflamed subepithelial connective tissue. *J. periodont. Res.* **14**, 310–322.

GARDNER, A. F. (1962a) A survey of periapical pathology. Part 1. *Dent. Digest* **68**, 162–167.

GARDNER, A. F. (1962b) A survey of periapical pathology. Part 2. *Dent. Digest* **68**, 223–227.

GOLDMAN, H. M. (1951) The topography and role of the gingival fibres. *J. Periodont.* **30**, 331–336.

GOLDMAN, H. M. (1957a) The behaviour of transseptal fibres in periodontal disease. *J. dent. Res.* **36**, 249–259.

GOLDMAN, H. M. (1957b) Extension of exudate into supporting structures of teeth in marginal periodontitis. *J. Periodont.* **28**, 175–183.

GRANT, D. & BERNICK, S. (1972) The periodontium of ageing humans. *J. Periodont.* **43**, 660–667.

GRIGSBY, W. R. & SABISTON, C. B. (1976) The periodontal disease process. *J. oral Path.* **5**, 175–188.

GRUPE, H. E., TEN CATE, A. R. & ZANDER, H. A. (1967) A histochemical and radiobiological study of *in vitro* and *in vivo* human epithelial cell rest proliferation. *Archs. oral Biol.* **12**, 1321–1329.

GUSTAFSON, G. T. (1969) Increased susceptibility to periodontitis in mink affected by a lysosomal disease. *J. periodont. Res.* **4**, 259–267.

HAMP, S-E. & FOLKE, L. E. A. (1968) The lysosomes and their possible role in periodontal disease. *Odont. Tidskr.* **76**, 353–375.

HEIJL, L., RIFKIN, B. R. & ZANDER, H. A. (1976) Conversion of chronic gingivitis to periodontitis in squirrel monkeys. *J. Periodont.* **47**, 710–716.

HORNSTEIN, O. P. & GORLIN, R. J. (1970) Infectious oral diseases. In: *Thoma's oral pathology*, Vol. 2, R. J. GORLIN & H. M. GOLDMAN (eds.), pp. 708–774. St. Louis, C. V. Mosby.

HORTON, J. E., LEIKIN, S. & OPPENHEIM, J. J. (1972) Human lympho-proliferative reaction to saliva and dental plaque-deposits: an *in vitro* correlation with periodontal disease. *J. Periodont.* **43**, 522–527.

HORTON, J. E., OPPENHEIM, J. J. & MERGENHAGEN, S. E. (1973) Elaboration of lymphotoxin by cultured human peripheral blood leucocytes stimulated with dental-plaque deposits. *Clin. Exp. Immunol.* **13**, 383–393.

IRVING, J. T., SOCRANSKY, S. S. & HEELEY, J. D. (1974) Histological changes in experimental periodontal disease in gnotobiotic rats and conventional hamsters. *J. periodont. Res.* **9**, 73–80.

IVANYI, L. & LEHNER, T. (1970) Stimulation of lymphocyte transformation by bacterial antigens in patients with periodontal disease. *Archs. oral Biol.* **15**, 1089–1096.

IVANYI, L. & LEHNER, T. (1971) Lymphocyte transformation by sonicates of dental plaque in human periodontal disease. *Archs. oral Biol.* **16**, 1117–1121.

IVANYI, L., WILTON, J. M. A. & LEHNER, T. (1972) Cell-mediated immunity in periodontal disease: cytotoxicity, migration inhibition and lymphocyte transformation studies. *Immunology* **22**, 141–145.

JIAN, W. (1956) Parodontolyses et tuberculose. *Parodontol. Zürich* 10, 66–69.

KASLICK, R. S. & CHASENS, A. I. (1968a) Periodontosis with periodontitis: A study involving young adult males. Part I. Review of the literature and incidence in a military population. *Oral Surg.* 25, 305–326.

KASLICK, R. S. & CHASENS, A. I. (1968b) Periodontosis with periodontitis: a study involving young adult males. Part II. Clinical, medical and histopathologic studies. *Oral Surg.* 25, 327–350.

KENNEDY, J. E. (1974) Effect of inflammation on collateral circulation of the gingiva. *J. periodont. Res.* 9, 147–152.

KIGER, R. D., WRIGHT, W. H. & CREAMER, H. R. (1974) The significance of lymphocyte transformation responses to various microbial strains. *J. Periodont.* 45, 780–785.

KOHL, J. & ZANDER, H. A. (1962) Fibres conjonctives 'oxytalan' dans le tissu gingival interdentaire. *Paradontologie* 16, 23–30.

KROLLS, S. O., WESTBROOK, S. D. & HESS, D. S. (1977) Actinomycosis as periapical pathology. Case report. *J. Oral Med.* 32, 41–43.

KUNTZ, D. S., GENCO, R. J., GUTTUSO, J. & NATIELLA, J. R. (1977) Localization of immunoglobulins and the third component of complement in dental periapical lesions. *J. Endod.* 3, 68–73.

LANGELAND, K., BLOCK, R. M. & GROSSMAN, L. I. (1977) A histopathologic and histobacteriologic study of 35 periapical endodontic surgical specimens. *J. Endod.* 3, 8–23.

LEHNER, T. (1969) Immunoglobulin abnormalities in ulcerative gingivitis. *Br. dent. J.* 127, 165–169.

LEHNER, T., WILTON, J. M. A., IVANYI, L. & MANSON, J. D. (1974) Immunological aspects of juvenile periodontitis (periodontosis). *J. periodont. Res.* 9, 261–272.

LEONARD, E. P., LUNIN, M. & PROVENZA, D. V. (1974) On the occurrence and morphology of Russell bodies in the dental granuloma. An evaluation of seventy-nine specimens. *Oral Surg.* 38, 584–590.

LEUIN, I. S. (1957) Infections and tumors arising in and from the periapical tissues. *Oral Surg.* 10, 1291–1301.

LINDHE, J., HAMP, S-E., & LÖE, H. (1973) Experimental periodontitis in the beagle dog. *J. periodont. Res.* 8, 1–10.

LINDHE, J. & SOCRANSKY, S. S. (1979) Chemotaxis and vascular permeability produced by human periodontopathic bacteria. *J. periodont. Res.* 14, 138–146.

LYONS, D. C., YAZDI, I., NONPARAST, B. & MIRIOHI, M. (1970) The histopathologic variations of the chronic dental granuloma. *J. Oral Med.* 25, 46–50.

MACAPANPAN, L. C. & WEINMANN, J. P. (1954) The influence of injury to the periodontal membrane on the spread of gingival inflammation. *J. dent. Res.* 33, 263–272.

MACKLER, B. F., ALTMAN, L. C., WAHL, S., ROSENSTREICH, D. L., OPPENHEIM, J. J. & MERGENHAGEN, S. E. (1974) Blastogenesis and lymphokine synthesis by T and B lymphocytes from patients with periodontal disease. *Infect. Immunol.* 10, 844–850.

MATHIESEN, A. (1973) Preservation and demonstration of mast cells in human apical granulomas and radicular cysts. *Scand. J. dent. Res.* 81, 218–229.

McFALL, W. T. (1964) Periodontal abscess. *J. N. Carolina D. Soc.* 47, 34–36.

MELCHER, A. H. (1962) Pathogenesis of chronic gingivitis. I. The spread of the inflammatory process. *Dent. Practit.* 13, 2–7.

MICHEL, G. & FRANK, R. M. (1970) Surcharge glycogénique des cellules ligamentaires et osseuses au cours des parodontolyses. *Parodontologie* 24, 3–9.

MIYASOTO, M. C. (1975) The periodontal abscess. *Perio. Abstr.* 23, 53–59.

MORLEY, J. (1974) Prostaglandins and lymphokines in arthritis. *Prostaglandins* 8, 315–326.

MORSE, D. R., LASATER, D. R. & WHITE, D. (1975) Presence of immunoglobulin-producing cells in periapical lesions. *J. Endod.* 1, 338–343.

MORTON, T. B., CLAGETT, J. A. & YAVORSKY, J. D. (1977) Role of immune complexes in human periapical periodontitis. *J. Endod.* 3, 261–268.

MÜHLEMANN, H. R. (1954) Tooth mobility. The measuring method. Initial and secondary tooth mobility. *J. Periodont.* 25, 22–29.

NARAYANAN, A. S. & PAGE, R. C. (1976) Biochemical characterization of collagens synthesized by fibroblasts derived from normal and diseased human gingiva. *J. Biol. Chem.* 251, 5464–5471.

NARITA, T. (1956) Histopathologic study on natural healing in chronic periapical periodontitis. *Bull. oral Path. Tokyo* 1, 163–185.

NEWMAN, H. N. (1976) The apical border of plaque in chronic inflammatory periodontal disease. *Brit. dent. J.* 141, 105–113.

NEWMAN, M. G., SOCRANSKY, S. S., SAVITT, E. D., PROPAS, D. A. & CRAWFORD, A. (1976) Studies of the microbiology of periodontosis. *J. Periodont.* 47, 373–379.

NISENGARD, R. J. (1977) The role of immunology in periodontal disease. *J. Periodont.* 48, 505–516.

OBRUČNIK, M. & MEDUNA, J. (1959) Histological and histochemical characteristics of apical granulomas. *Českoslov. Stomat.* 59, 317–328.

ORBAN, B. & WEINMANN, J. P. (1942) Diffuse atrophy of the alveolar bone (periodontosis). *J. Periodont.* 13, 31–45.

PAGE, R. C., KO, S. D., HASSELL, T. M. & NARAYANAN, A. S. (1979) The role of fibroblast subpopulations in the connective tissue alterations of gingival and periodontal diseases. *J. periodont. Res.* 14, 266.

PAGE, R. C. & SCHROEDER, H. E. (1976) Pathogenesis of inflammatory periodontal disease. A summary of current work. *Lab. Invest.* 34, 235–249.

PAGE, R. C., SIMPSON, D. M., AMMONS, W. F. & SHECHTMAN, L. R. (1972) Host tissue response in chronic periodontal disease. III. Clinical, histopathologic and ultrastructural features of advanced disease in a colony-maintained marmoset. *J. periodont. Res.* 7, 283–296.

PARAKKAL, P. F. (1969) Involvement of macrophages in collagen resorption. *J. Cell Biol.* 41, 345–354.

PATTERS, M. R., GENCO, R. J., REED, M. J. & MASHIMO, P. A. (1976) Blastogenic response of human lymphocytes to oral bacterial antigens: comparison of individuals with periodontal disease to normal and edentulous subjects. *Infect. Immunol.* 14, 1213–1220.

PAUNIO, K. (1965) Studies on the connective tissue components in the periodontal membrane. *Odont. Tidskr.* **73**, 613–614 (abs.).

PAUNIO, K. (1969a) The age change of acid mucopolysaccharides in the periodontal membrane of man. *J. periodont. Res.* **4**, suppl. 4, 32–33.

PAUNIO, K. (1969b) Periodontal connective tissue. Biochemical studies of disease in man. *Suomen Hammas. Toim.* **65**, 249–290.

PAUNIO, K. & MÄKINEN, K. (1969) Studies on hydrolytic enzyme activity in the connective tissue of the human periodontal ligament. Observations apart from areas of inflammation. *Acta odont. Scand.* **27**, 153–171.

PAUNIO, K. U., MÄKINEN, K. K. & PAUNIO, I. K. (1970) The stability of extracted collagen molecules from human periodontal membrane. *Acta odont. Scand.* **28**, 959–966.

PICTON, D. C. A. (1962) A study of normal tooth mobility and the changes with periodontal disease. *D. Practit.* **12**, 167–173.

PISANTY, S. (1979) Histoplasmosis as periapical pathology. *J. oral Med.* **34**, 116–118.

POPOV, C.-P. (1965) Sur la présence et la signification des fibres élastiques dans le paradentium. *Rev. Stomatol.* (Paris) **66**, 553–556.

PRITCHARD, J. F. (1953) Management of the periodontal abscess. *Oral Surg.* **6**, 474–482.

PULVER, W. H., TAUBMAN, M. A. & SMITH, D. J. (1978) Immune components in human dental periapical lesions. *Archs. oral Biol.* **23**, 535–543.

QUINTARELLI, G. (1960) Histochemistry of the gingiva. IV. Preliminary investigations on the mucopolysaccharides of connective tissue. *Archs. oral Biol.* **2**, 277–284.

RAISZ, L. G. & KOOLEMANS-BEYNEN, A. R. (1974) Inhibition of bone collagen synthesis by prostaglandin E_2 in organ culture. *Prostaglandins* **10**, 377–385.

RAO, L. G., MOE, H. K. & HEERSCHE, J. N. M. (1978) *In vitro* culture of porcine periodontal ligament cells: response of fibroblast-like and epithelial-like cells to prostaglandin E_1, parathyroid hormone and calcitonin and separation of a pure population of fibroblast-like cells. *Archs. oral Biol.* **23**, 957–964.

REICHART, P., ANANATASAN, T. & REZNIK, G. (1976) Gingiva and periodontium in lepromatous leprosy. A clinical, radiological and microscopical study. *J. Periodont.* **47**, 455–460.

RIPPIN, J. W. (1978) Collagen turnover in the periodontal ligament under normal and altered functional forces. II. Adult rat molars. *J. periodont. Res.* **13**, 149–154.

RUBEN, M. P., GOLDMAN, H. M. & SCHULMAN, S. M. (1970) Diseases of the periodontium. In: *Thoma's oral pathology,* Vol. I, R. J. GORLIN & H. M. GOLDMAN (eds.), pp. 394–444. St. Louis, C. V. Mosby.

SAGLIE, R., JOHANSEN, J. R. & FLÖTRA, L. (1975) The zone of completely and partially destroyed periodontal fibres in pathological pockets. *J. Clin. Periodont.* **2**, 198–202.

SAKAMOTO, S., GOLDHABER, P. & GLIMCHER, M. J. (1973) Mouse bone collagenase: the effect of heparin on the amount of enzyme released in tissue culture and on the activity of the enzyme. *Calc. Tiss. Res.* **12**, 247–258.

SAMANTA, A., MALIK, C. P. & AIKAT, B. K. (1975) Periapical actinomycosis. *Oral Surg.* **39**, 458–462.

SCHLUGER, S., YUODELIS, R. A. & PAGE, R. C. (1977) Pathogenic mechanisms. In: *Periodontal disease.* Philadelphia, Lea & Febiger.

SCHROEDER, H. E. & PAGE, R. (1972) Lymphocyte fibroblast interaction in the pathogenesis of inflammatory gingival disease. *Experimentia* **28**, 1228–1230.

SCHULTZ-HAUDT, S. D. & AAS, E. (1960) Observations on the status of collagen in human gingiva. *Archs. oral Biol.* **2**, 131–142.

SELVIG, K. A. (1966) Ultrastructural changes in cementum and adjacent connective tissue in periodontal disease. *Acta odont. Scand.* **24**, 459–500.

SELVIG, K. A. (1968) Nonbanded fibrils of collagenous nature in human periodontal connective tissue. *J. periodont. Res.* **3**, 169–179.

SEYMOUR, G. J. & GREENSPAN, J. S. (1979) The phenotypic characterization of lymphocyte subpopulations in established human periodontal disease. *J. periodont. Res.* **14**, 39–46.

SKOUGAARD, M. R. & LEVY, B. M. (1971) Collagen metabolism in periodontal membrane of the marmoset. Influence of periodontal disease. *Scand. J. Dent. Res.* **79**, 518–572.

SLOTS, J. (1976) The predominant cultivable organisms in juvenile periodontitis. *Scand. J. Dent. Res.* **84**, 1–10.

SOAMES, J. V. & DAVIES, R. M. (1977) Intracellular collagen fibrils in early gingivitis in the beagle dog. *J. periodont. Res.* **12**, 378–386.

STAHL, S. S. (1973) Marginal lesions. In: *Periodontal therapy,* 5th ed., H. M. GOLDMAN & D. W. COHEN (eds.), pp. 94–142. St. Louis, C. V. Mosby.

STAHL, S. S., SANDLER, H. C. & SUBEN, E. (1958) Histochemical changes in inflammatory periodontal disease. *J. Periodont.* **29**, 183–191.

STANLEY, H. R. (1955) The cyclic phenomenon of periodontitis. *Oral Surg.* **8**, 598–610.

SUMMERS, L. & PAPADIMITRIOU, J. (1975) The nature of epithelial proliferation in apical granulomas. *J. oral Path.* **4**, 324–329.

TEN CATE, A. R. (1972a) Morphological studies of fibrocytes in connective tissue undergoing rapid remodelling. *J. Anat.* **112**, 401–414.

TEN CATE, A. R. (1972b) The epithelial cell rests of Malassez and the genesis of the dental cyst. *Oral Surg.* **34**, 956–964.

TEN CATE, A. R. & DEPORTER, D. A. (1975) The degradative role of the fibroblast in the remodelling and turnover of collagen in soft connective tissue. *Anat. Rec.* **182**, 1–14.

TERASAKI, P. I., KASLICK, R. S., WEST, T. L. & CHASENS, A. I. (1975) Low HL-A2 frequency and periodontitis. *Tissue Antigens* **5**, 286–288.

TOTO, P. D., POLLOCK, R. J. & GARGIULO, A. W. (1964) Pathogenesis of periodontitis. *Periodontics* **2**, 197–201.

VALDERHAUG, J. (1974) Epithelial cells in the periodontal membrane of teeth with and without periapical inflammation. *Int. J. oral Surg.* **3**, 7–16.

VAN SWOL, R. L. (1973) Periodontosis in a patient with previously diagnosed sarcoidosis. *J. Periodont.* **44**, 697–704.

WADE, A. B. (1965) *Basic periodontology.* John Wright, Bristol.

WAERHAUG, J. (1976) Subgingival plaque and loss of attachment in periodontosis as observed in autopsy material. *J. Periodont.* **47**, 636–642.

WAERHAUG, J. (1977) Subgingival plaque and loss of attachment in periodontosis as evaluated on extracted teeth. *J. Periodont.* **48**, 125–130.

WALKER, D. M. (1977) Lymphocytes and macrophages in the gingiva. In: *The borderland between caries and periodontal disease,* T. LEHNER (ed.), pp. 185–198. London, Academic Press.

WARWICK JAMES, W. & COUNSELL, A. (1927) A histo-

logical investigation into so-called pyorrhoea alveolaris. *Brit. dent. J.* **48**, 1237–1252.

WEINMANN, J. P. (1941) Progress of gingival inflammation into the supporting structure of the teeth. *J. Periodont.* **12**, 71–82.

YANAGISAWA, S. (1980) Pathologic study of periapical lesions. 1. Periapical granulomas: Clinical, histopathologic and immunohistopathologic studies. *J. oral Path.* **9**, 288–300.

Chapter 16

NEOPLASTIC INVOLVEMENT OF THE PERIODONTAL LIGAMENT

A. K. Adatia

INTRODUCTION

Neoplasia of the periodontal ligament is rare. However, involvement of the periodontal ligament leading to looseness of teeth is often the earliest manifestation of neoplastic disease of the jaws (Burkitt, 1958; Cohen, 1958; Adatia, 1966; Bertelli, Costa and Miziara, 1970; Oikarinen, Calonius and Sainio, 1975). The variety of its cellular elements predisposes the periodontal ligament to almost any of the neoplasms which are commonly found in the jaws. Thus, the cell rests of Malassez could give rise to epithelial tumours, the connective tissue elements to fibroblastic lesions, osseous elements to osteomas, osteogenic sarcomas and giant cell tumours, cemental cells to cementomas, and the cells of the undifferentiated mesenchyme and lymphoreticular system to a variety of lymphoreticular neoplasms. The purpose of this chapter is to discuss the place of periodontal ligament and its constituent elements in the natural history of jaw neoplasia. Most of the information which follows is essentially a record of the neoplastic lesions which can occur in the periodontal ligament. It is, of course, beyond the scope of this chapter to give details of their general histopathology which can be readily obtained elsewhere. Furthermore, because of their rarity and the lack of experimental models, as yet most studies have simply been case reports.

LOCALIZED LESIONS

Benign neoplasms

Most localized neoplasms affecting the periodontal ligament are benign, e.g. cementoma, fibroma, and osteoma. All of these are thought to arise from their respective cellular elements in the ligament. When such lesions are small and associated with loss of lamina dura around affected teeth, it is tempting to assume that the condition arose in the periodontal ligament. However, such an assumption might be incorrect without supporting histological evidence.

A number of benign, fibro-osseous and cementoid lesions of the jaw have been shown to occur in the periodontal ligament. These include ossifying fibroma, cementifying fibroma, cemento-ossifying fibroma, cementoblastoma, gigantiform cementoma and periapical cemental and fibrous dysplasias (Hamner, Scofield and Cornyn, 1968; Pindborg,

Kramer and Torloni, 1971; Waldron and Giansanti, 1973; Punniamoorthy, 1980). A cementoma is formed by enlargement and fusion of droplets of cementum to produce a dense, acellular cementum mass in a sparse, avascular, loose connective tissue stroma. Various combinations of identifiable cementum and bone are found in periapical cementomas, cementifying and ossifying fibromas, and periapical fibrous and cemental dysplasias. Cementifying fibromas consist of fibrous and fibroblastic tissue interspersed by tiny cementicles; they can also contain irregularly distributed cementoid. A cementoma is considered as a variant with scanty stroma (Khanna, Khanna and Varanasi, 1979). The cementoblastoma (Fig. 1) attached to the roots of affected teeth consists of cementum-like material containing many reversal lines, and minimal intervening soft tissue. There is a discrete connective tissue layer, derived probably from the periodontal ligament between the lesion and the surrounding alveolar bone. Periapical cemental dysplasia resembles cementifying or ossifying fibroma, but shows marked osteoblastic and osteoclastic activity, lack of inflammatory cells, and benign connective tissue stroma (Regezi, Kerr and Courtney, 1978). Of forty-three well-documented cases in sixty-five records of benign fibro-osseous lesions of the jaws studied by Waldron and Giansanti (1973), all appeared to arise from cells of the periodontal ligament and were restricted to the tooth-bearing region of the jaws.

Benign osteoblastoma, a rare tumour characterized by the formation of osteoid and bone, can involve the ligament causing looseness and migration of teeth. The lesion consists of many bony trabeculae lined with osteoblasts in a vascular, loosely arranged fibrillar stroma. Clinical findings, history and radiographs help to differentiate it from osteosarcoma (Sidhu, Parkash and Khanani, 1980).

Odontogenic fibromyxoma may also derive from the ligament. This lesion is composed of relatively loose fibrous tissue, the matrix of which contains few fibres within an abundant palely staining (H and E) ground substance. The cells appear spindle-shaped or stellate (Schneider and Weisinger, 1975) though their overall morphology in three dimensions has yet to be determined.

There are few reports of other myxomatous jaw tumours involving periodontal ligament (Kangur and Dahlin, 1975).

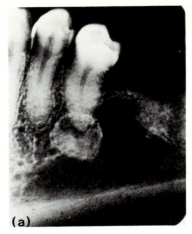

(a)

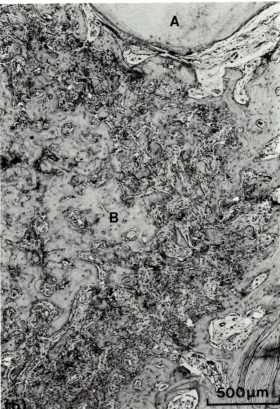

FIG. 1. (a) Radiograph of left mandibular second premolar with a vital pulp in a 30-year-old female, who complained of ill-defined pain in that region. Loss of lamina dura in the affected area and the consistency and disposition of the radioopacity near the apex suggest a cementoblastoma. (b) Photomicrograph of the excised lesion. (A) root apex; (B) lesional tissue. Haematoxylin and eosin. ×40.

A ligament origin for peripheral odontogenic fibroma is indicated by its content of oxytalan fibres (Wright and Jennings, 1979), structures which exist mainly though not exclusively in the ligament (Hamner and Fullmer, 1966). There is a report of periodontal ligament involvement in adenomatoid odontogenic tumour (Berghagen, Bergström and Valerius-Olsson, 1973).

Neurofibroma has been reported as developing from periapical neural elements in a tooth socket. Toth *et al.* (1975) found such a lesion in the socket of a maxillary first molar where there had been acute periapical inflammation. They suggested that the tumour had developed from neural elements within the alveolar defect. Smith and Smith (1979) describe a similar condition in a patient with neurofibromatosis, multiple lesions appearing as epulides 3 weeks after multiple extractions. An instance of neurilemmoma of the jaws, originating between lower incisors and invading the associated periapical periodontal ligament, has been reported by Rengaswamy (1978).

Plasma cell granuloma is a benign lesion occurring almost exclusively in periodontal tissues but affecting mainly gingiva. It is composed chiefly of plasma cells arranged diffusely, as solid sheets or in lobules (Bhaskar, Levin and Frisch, 1968). Because of its benign clinical behaviour it is now considered a non-neoplastic lesion.

Melanotic neuroectodermal tumour of infancy has been reported around a mobile upper central incisor in a 4-month-old boy. It appeared to have originated in alveolar bone. This tumour may superficially resemble retino-, neuro- and medulloblastomas (Barfield and Pleasants, 1976). It is believed to arise from neural crest cells (Lucas, 1976).

Locally invasive lesions

Although ameloblastomas are locally invasive tumours, in most cases they present as localized lesions (Fig. 2) (Small and Waldron, 1955; Singleton, 1970). On the other hand, tumours such as adenomatoid odontogenic tumour (adenoameloblastoma), ameloblastic fibroma and calcifying odontogenic tumour do not usually recur following conservative surgery (Ackerman and Rosai, 1974; Lucas, 1976). There is general

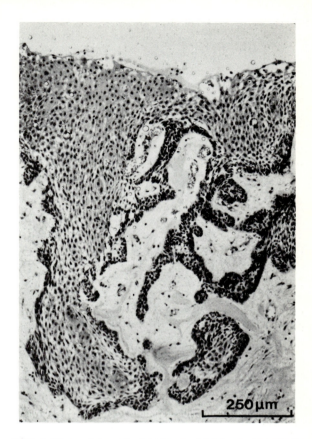

FIG. 2. Photomicrograph showing ameloblastoma apparently arising from the epithelial lining of an odontogenic cyst. Haematoxylin and eosin. ×98.

agreement that odontogenic epithelial residues are implicated in the histogenesis of both ameloblastoma (Fig. 2) and the calcifying odontogenic tumour (Pindborg, 1958; Kramer, 1963; Abrams and Howell, 1967; Seward and Duckworth, 1967; Vap, Dahlin and Turlington, 1970; Lucas, 1976). The neoplastic potential of epithelial residues in the periodontal ligament remains obscure. In their report of eighty-four cases of ameloblastoma arising in the walls of odontogenic cysts, Shteyer, Lustmann and Lewin-Epstein (1978) record seven instances of periodontal cyst origin.

DISSEMINATING LESIONS

Malignant neoplastic lesions in the jaws can be

divided broadly into primary neoplasms in the jaws or metastatic lesions.

Primary neoplasms

Primary carcinoma of the mandible (Fig. 3) is rare (Ackerman and Rosai, 1974; Lucas, 1976; Coonar, 1979; McGowan, 1980). In the maxilla, primary carcinoma is associated mainly with carcinoma of the antrum. The epithelial cell rests in the periodontal ligament feature prominently in the histogenesis of primary carcinoma in the jaws (Shear, 1969; McGowan, 1980). Carcinomatous change occurring in radicular, lateral periodontal and follicular cysts has been reported by several authors (Martensson, 1955; Hankey and Pedler, 1957; Bradfield and Broadway, 1958; Kay and Kramer, 1962; Ward and Cohen, 1963; Baker et al., 1979). Primary gingival carcinoma can lead to loosening of teeth after periodontal ligament involvement. It may present at this stage as a poorly defined, irregular, periodontal radiolucency so that it can be confused with a routine periodontal pocket. Coonar (1979) reported a case of carcinoma in the upper incisor region which became apparent 10 months after the teeth were extracted on the basis of a diagnosis of chronic periodontitis.

Osteosarcoma is one of the few malignant neoplasms clearly associated with definitive periodontal ligament changes. Primary jaw osteosarcoma often presents radiographically as a symmetrical widening of the periodontal space about one or more teeth (Garrington et al., 1967; Gardner and Mills, 1976; Schofield and Johnson, 1977). The altered ligament features cementicles both attached to cementum and free within the tumour-affected tissue. The lesion tissue consists mainly of a malignant fibrous stroma, the original principal fibre bundles of the ligament being destroyed. Malignant osteoid is also present (Gardner and Mills, 1976).

Chondrosarcoma does not appear to produce a similar widening of periodontal space, although it destroys lamina dura, as observed in a case of maxillary clear cell chondrosarcoma occurring between the roots of a lateral incisor and canine (Shootweg, 1980).

Primary malignant haemangioendothelioma can involve the periodontal ligament (Wesley, Mintz and Wertheimer, 1975), as can benign haemangioma (Sznajder et al., 1973). Other rare instances of ligament involvement by primary malignant neoplasms include non-Burkitt's malignant lymphoma (Cook, 1961), fibrohistocytoma, presenting as apparently 'necrotic' areas around the roots of teeth (Jee, Domboski and Milobsky, 1978), and leiomyosarcoma. The latter was diagnosed at autopsy in an extraction socket in the maxilla (Takagi and Ishikawa, 1972).

Metastatic neoplasms

Jaw metastases are relatively uncommon (Figs. 4—13). Since, however, they may present as loss of lamina dura and loosening of teeth, they could be confused with simple periodontitis. Their serious import obviously necessitates a rapid diagnosis as the primary lesion may be treatable. Among malignant neoplasms reported as having metastasized to the jaws and involving the periodontal ligament are carcinomas including lung carcinoma (Cherry and Glass, 1977), pancreatic carcinoma (Schofield, 1974), colonic adenocarcinoma (Levy and Smith, 1974; Lopez and Lobos, 1976), malignant melanoma (Fig. 4) (Mosby, Sugg and Hiatt, 1973), rhabdomyosarcoma (Khanna, Khanna and Varanasi, 1979), leukaemia (Fig. 5) (Bender, 1944; Stern and Cole, 1973; Michaud et al., 1977), retinoblastoma (Zegarelli, 1976), chorioepithelioma (Bakeen, Hiyarat and Al-Ubaidy, 1976; Sato et al., 1978), Hodgkin's disease (Forman and Wesson, 1970), non-Hodgkin's lymphoma (Mittelman and Kaban, 1976) and hepatocellular carcinoma (Yacabucci, Mainous and Kramer, 1972) and reticulum cell sarcoma (Fig. 6).

Leukaemia, manifesting clinically with demonstrable jaw involvement, has characteristic features, namely, the young age of the patient, alveolar swelling, lip paraesthesia, pain, looseness of teeth and peripheral lymph node enlargement. There may be loss of lamina dura, widening of periodontal space and furcation involvement, all due to infiltration by leukaemia cells (Fig. 5) (Bender, 1944; Curtis, 1971; Stern and Cole, 1973; Michaud et al., 1977; Ruprecht and Arora, 1978). Remission of leukaemia by chemotherapy may be associated with re-establishment of lamina dura (Fig. 5).

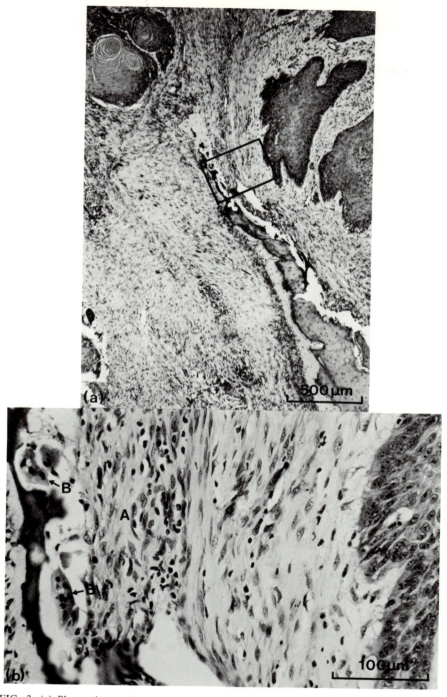

FIG. 3. (a) Photomicrograph of primary squamous cell carcinoma in the mandible. Haematoxylin and eosin. ×40. (b) High-power view of the area in the square in (a) to show the
advancing edge of the tumour (A) and the osteoclasts (B) associated with the resorption of
bone. Haematoxylin and eosin. ×250.

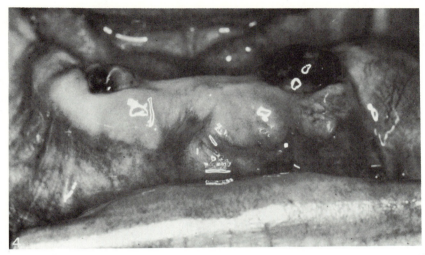

FIG. 4. Metastatic melanoma in the sockets of the mandibular canines in a 60-year-old woman. The right canine was removed 11 weeks previously, and the left canine 4 weeks later. The wounds had healed normally until the appearance of the tumour. The patient had undergone surgery 2 years earlier for malignant melanoma of the rectum.

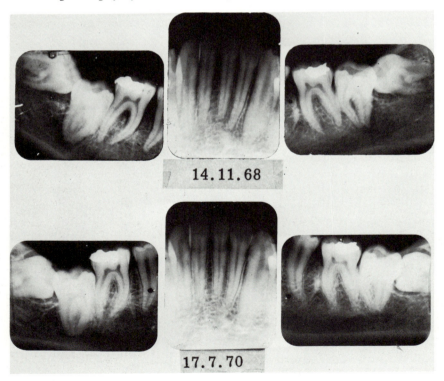

FIG. 5. Periapical radiographs of the mandibular teeth of 18-year-old male, who complained of incisor pain and lower lip paraesthesia. Loss of or break in the lamina dura around most of the teeth and periapical radiolucency affecting the second molars is evident in the radiographs taken on 14.11.68. Examination of the sternal marrow suggested acute myelogenous leukaemia. Note the reconstitution of the alveolar trabeculae and lamina dura evident in the radiographs taken 21 months following chemotherapy.

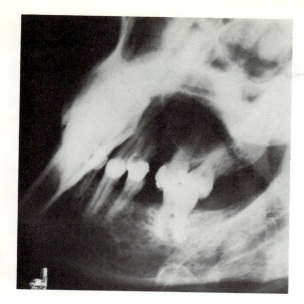

FIG. 6. Radiograph of a 32-year-old man with reticulum cell sarcoma of the left mandible.

Burkitt's lymphoma is unusual in having a predilection for the jaws (see Chapter 9). Loosening of teeth due to loss of lamina dura and destruction of periodontal ligament (Fig. 7) may be its first clinical feature in the jaw (Burkitt, 1958; Adatia, 1966).

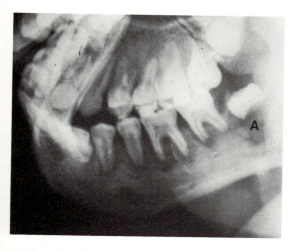

FIG. 7. As in this case of Burkitt's lymphoma, mobility of teeth and radiographic appearance in cases of neoplasia may resemble that seen in chronic inflammatory periodontal disease.

In Burkitt's lymphoma, ligament invasion appears to occur by tumour cells spreading between the collagen fibres (Figs. 8, 9 and 10). Although teeth may be dislodged as the tumour grows, the periodontal ligament may retain its attachment to cementum and bone or gingiva until a late stage. Successful chemotherapy leads to rapid regression of the tumour and a remarkable restoration of tooth position and development (Fig. 11) (Adatia, 1968, 1970). This suggests that odontogenic tissue survives attack by both the tumour and the cytotoxic chemotherapy, and that the periodontal ligament can regenerate

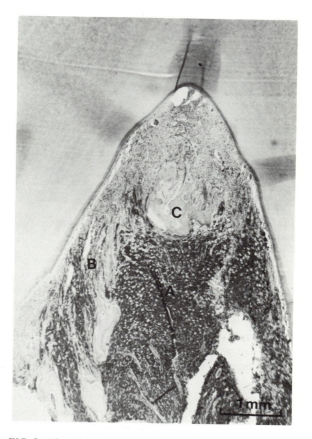

FIG. 8. Photomicrograph showing Burkitt's lymphoma invading the interradicular region of a mandibular second deciduous molar. The tumour appears to have replaced most of the alveolar bone (A) and is spreading between the fibres of the periodontal ligament (B). Woven bone (C) seen in the bifurcation may be a manifestation of normal response to occlusal displacement of the tooth by the tumour. Haematoxylin and eosin. ×16.

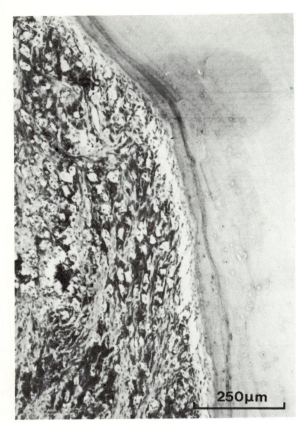

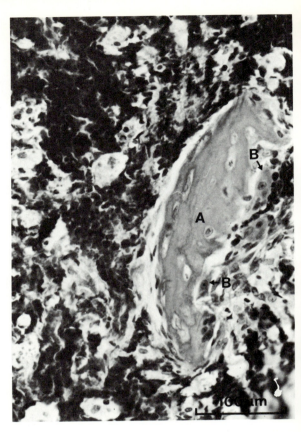

FIG. 9. High-power view of Burkitt's lymphoma in the perio-dontal ligament. Haematoxylin and eosin. ×98.

FIG. 10. Spicule of bone (A), surrounded by Burkitt's lymphoma in the mandible, is being resorbed by osteoclasts (B). Haematoxylin and eosin. ×256.

(Fig. 12). Lamina dura and periodontal ligament begin to be re-established within 4 weeks of therapy (Fig. 13). Within this periodontal ligament are fibres which may have survived tumour and treatment and others derived from the activity of fibroblasts which develop from surviving undifferentiated mesenchyme. Persistence of the epithelial root sheath may help by preventing ankylosis (see Chapter 12). Recent experiments in rats injected with therapeutic doses of cyclophosphamide (Adatia and Berkovitz, in press) have shown that the periodontal ligament does not form until a layer of dentine has been deposited (Fig. 14). Repair and regeneration phenomena in the periodontal ligaments of treated Burkitt's lymphoma patients may also be due in part to the persistence of epithelial rests (Fig. 12).

PATHOGENESIS OF PERIODONTAL NEOPLASIA

As yet, there is no explanation for the malignant change which can occur in the epithelial residues in the periodontal ligament, or for the high incidence of jaw lesions in Burkitt's lymphoma and some cases of leukaemia. Three possibilities can be considered. Malignant neoplasms may arise in the jaws, they may be metastatic tumours of clonal origin, or they may be one of several tumours occurring simultaneously in different parts of the body.

Shafer, Hine and Levy (1974) have argued that a carcinoma becoming manifest in a socket following extraction of a loose tooth may have originated in the gingival epithelium. Gingival cuff (Ten Cate

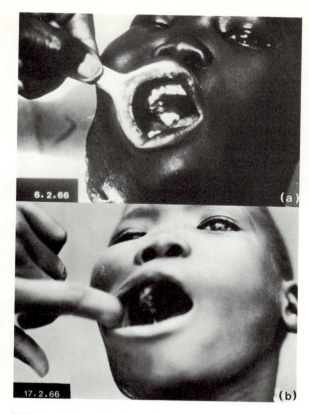

FIG. 11. (a) Gross displacement of the right maxillary first permanent molar due to Burkitt's lymphoma. (b) Photograph of the same patient taken 2 weeks later demonstrates the precision in the return of the affected tooth to its position in the jaw upon regression of the tumour following cyclophosphamide therapy.

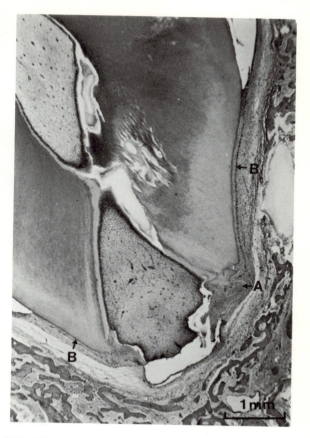

FIG. 12. Photomicrograph of the maxillary permanent canine of a 6-year-old girl 80 days after regression of massive maxillary Burkitt's lymphoma which had caused gross displacement of the teeth. (A) Bulge in the root. (B) Residual odontogenic epithelium in the periodontal ligament. Haematoxylin and eosin. ×16.

1975) and epithelial cell rests in the ligament (Spouge, 1980) are the two possible sources of epithelial proliferation. Ten Cate (1975) has shown that the epithelium of the gingival cuff is an actively proliferating tissue. Main (1970) showed that infection of odontogenic epithelium *in vitro* by polyoma virus could give rise to cells resembling those found in ameloblastoma. Stanley, Dawe and Law (1964) showed that mice inoculated with polyoma virus at birth developed tumours from gingival epithelium, which resembled ameloblastoma; similar tumours were also present in the periodontal ligament. It is thus possible to speculate that benign proliferative activity of epithelium in gingival cuff and periodontal ligament may undergo neoplastic change if an oncogenic factor is present at a susceptible stage in the life cycle of the affected cell. There is much evidence to suggest that Epstein—Barr (EB) virus may act as an oncogenic agent in patients who have become susceptible to its neoplastic propensity by previous infection, e.g. malaria (Burkitt, 1969; Epstein and Achong, 1973, 1979; Wright, 1973). Burkitt's lymphoma provides an instance of such a sequence of events affecting a different target cell. Proliferation of epithelial cells in the follicle of an unerupted tooth surrounded by Burkitt's lymphoma has been seen (in one case) (Fig. 15).

It has been argued that the frequency of jaw lesions in Burkitt's lymphoma is related not so much to the presence of teeth, but to odontogenesis (Adatia,

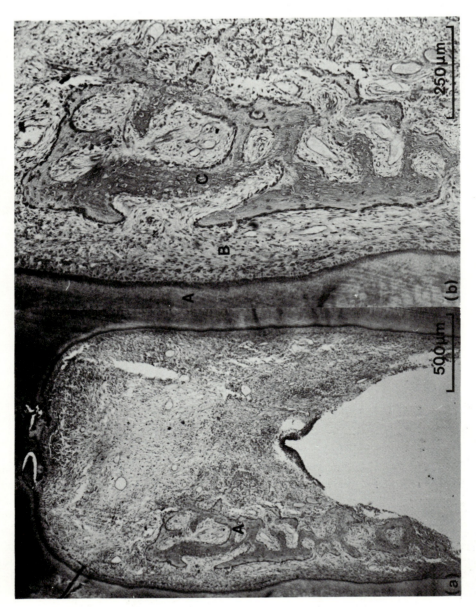

FIG. 13. (a) Photomicrograph of inter-radicular region of a first maxillary molar 4 weeks following chemotherapy (Endoxan) for Burkitt's lymphoma in the maxilla. Woven bone demonstrating regeneration of the lamina dura (A) is evident. Haematoxylin and eosin. ×42. (b) Detail of new bone and the associated periodontal ligament from (a). (A) Tooth root. (B) Periodontal ligament. (C) Bone. ×96.

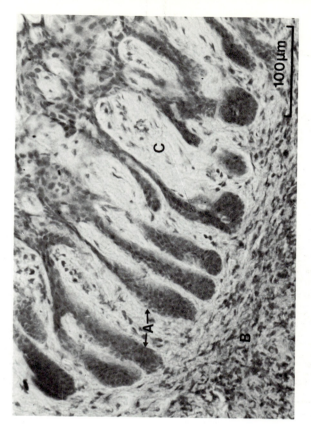

FIG. 15. Epithelial proliferation (A) in the follicle of a premolar involved in Burkitt's lymphoma (B). Note the tumour-free zone (C) adjacent to the epithelial strands, reminiscent of the inductive influence of the ondotogenic epithelium. Haematoxylin and eosin. ×256.

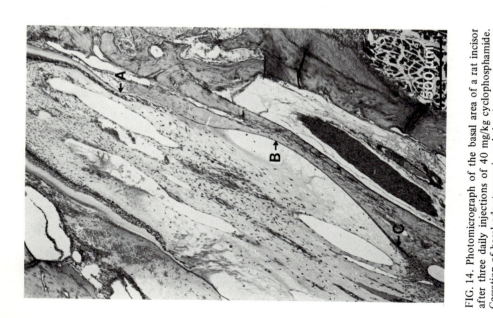

FIG. 14. Photomicrograph of the basal area of a rat incisor after three daily injections of 40 mg/kg cyclophosphamide. Cessation of basal odontogenesis and the absence of dentine, cementum and the fibres of the periodontal ligament are evident below the dentine (A) formed before the injection of the cytotoxic drug. Note the continuity of the epithelial root sheath (B) with the basal odontogenic epithelium (C). Haematoxylin and eosin. ×42.

1978). It is possible that, during odontogenesis, jaws offer either a greater concentration of target tissue, or particularly suitable conditions for colonization by the circulating tumour cells. According to Epstein and Achong (1973), EB virus is present in large quantity in saliva in infected persons and healthy carriers. MacGregor (1936) showed that the lymphatic drainage from the gingival sulcus is through the periodontal ligament, and that the lymphatic vessels pass through bone before reaching the submandibular lymph nodes. This could create a high concentration of the carcinogenic agent in the jaws at a time of marked proliferative activity by susceptible cells.

Paucity of red marrow in the adult jaw may explain the rarity of metastatic tumours commonly occurring late in life. However, jaws have not been investigated sufficiently in all cases to account for the apparent difference in incidence of the various malignant neoplasms (Cohen, 1958). This is unfortunate, for jaws are easily accessible and can be studied with relative precision both clinically and radiologically. Initial radiographic changes may precede even the early clinical signs and give a better indication for early histological examination. Radiological examination of large bones does not always succeed in demonstrating detectable changes, even when infiltration by neoplastic cells is present histologically (Vieta, Friedell and Craver, 1942). Loss of lamina dura would require far less osteolytic change than may be needed for demonstrable radiolucency in a vertebra or in a long bone. Moreover, being easily accessible, any change demonstrated radiologically can be confirmed relatively easily by biopsy.

Available evidence suggests that jaw screening could arguably form part of the protocol for every case of malignant neoplasia, whether jaws are involved or not. There are several reasons for persuading overselves to take such a step. It needs to be recognized that jaws contain a large share of embryonic elements which persist post-natally (Cohen, 1976). It needs to be appreciated also that pathologic processes affecting these elements may give a clue to the nature of such processes in other regions. A system of clinical examination recommended recently (Adatia, 1978), particularly for cases of neoplastic disorders which frequently disseminate to the skeleton, may suggest an association of jaw lesions with particular pathological entities. At the same time, experiments may elucidate the nature of the neoplastic propensities of these elements. This knowledge should enhance greatly co-operation between dental and other scientists engaged in cancer research.

REFERENCES

ABRAMS, A. M. & HOWELL, F. V. (1967) Calcifying epithelial odontogenic tumours: report of four cases. *J. Amer. dent. Assoc.* **74**, 1231–1240.

ACKERMAN, L. V. & ROSAI, J. (1974) *Surgical pathology* (5th ed.). St. Louis, Mosby.

ADATIA, A. K. (1966) Burkitt's tumour in the jaws. *Br. dent. J.* **120**, 315–326.

ADATIA, A. K. (1968) Response of the dental elements to chemotherapy of Burkitt's tumour. *Int. dent. J.* **18**, 646–654.

ADATIA, A. K. (1970) Dental aspects. In: *Burkitt's lymphoma*, D. P. BURKITT and D. H. WRIGHT (eds.), pp. 34–42. Edinburgh, Livingstone.

ADATIA, A. K. (1978) Significance of jaw lesions in Burkitt's lymphoma. *Br. dent. J.* **145**, 263–266.

ADATIA, A. K. & BERKOVITZ, B. K. B. (in press) The effects of cyclophosphamide on eruption of the continuously growing mandibular incisor of the rat. *Archs. oral Biol.*

BAKEEN, G., HIYARAT, A. M. & AL-UBAIDY, S. S. (1976) Chorio-epithelioma presenting as a bleeding gingival mass. *Oral Surg.* **41**, 467–471.

BAKER, R. D., D'ONOFRIO, E. D., CORIO, R. L., CRAWFORD, B. E. & TERRY, B. C. (1979) Squamous-cell carcinoma arising in a lateral periodontal cyst. *Oral Surg.* **47**, 495–499.

BARFIELD, G. H. & PLEASANTS, J. E. (1976) Melanotic neuroectodermal tumour of infancy. *J. oral Surg.* **34**, 839–841.

BENDER, I. B. (1944) Bone changes in leucemia. *Oral Surg.* **30**, 556–563.

BERGHAGEN, N., BERGSTRÖM, J. & VALERIUS-OLSSON, H. (1973) Adenomatoid odontogenic tumour. Periodontal aspects on diagnosis and treatment. *Sven. Tandlak. Tidskr.* **66**, 467–474.

BERTELLI, A. DE P., COSTA, F. Q. & MIZIARA, J. E. A. (1970) Metastatic tumors of the mandible. *Oral Surg.* **30**, 21–28.

BHASKAR, S. N., LEVIN, M. P. & FRISCH, J. (1968) Plasma cell granuloma of periodontal tissues. Report of 45 cases. *Periodontics* **6**, 272–276.

BRADFIELD, W. J. D. & BROADWAY, E. S. (1958) Malignant change in a dentigerous cyst. *Br. J. Surg.* **45**, 657–659.

BURKITT, D. (1958) A sarcoma involving the jaws in African children. *Br. J. Surg.* **46**, 218–223.

BURKITT, D. P. (1969) Etiology of Burkitt's lymphoma — an alternative hypothesis to a vectored virus. *J. Nat. Cancer Inst.* **42**, 19–28.

CHERRY, C. Q. & GLASS, R. T. (1977) Large-cell carcinoma

metastatic to the jaw. Report of a case. *Oral Surg.* 44, 358–361.

COHEN, B. (1958) Secondary tumours of the mandible. *Ann. R. Coll. Surg. Eng.* 23, 118–130.

COHEN, B. (1976) The enigma of vestigial tissues. *Ann. R. Coll. Surg. Eng.* 58, 104–114.

COOK, H. P. (1961) Oral lymphomas. *Oral Surg.* 14, 690–704.

COONAR, H. S. (1979) Primary intra-osseous carcinoma of maxilla. *Br. dent. J.* 147, 47–48.

CURTIS, A. B. (1971) Childhood leukaemias: Osseous changes in jaws on panoramic dental radiographs. *J. Amer. dent. Assn,* 83, 844–847.

EPSTEIN, M. A. & ACHONG, B. G. (1973) Various forms of Epstein–Barr virus infection in man: established facts and a general concept. *Lancet* 2, 836–839.

EPSTEIN, M. A. & ACHONG, B. G. (1979) The relationship of the virus to Burkitt's lymphoma. In: *The Epstein–Barr virus,* M. A. EPSTEIN & B. G. ACHONG (eds.), pp. 321–337. Heidelberg, Springer-Verlag.

FORMAN, G. H. & WESSON, C. M. (1969–70) Hodgkin's disease of the mandible. *Br. J. oral Surg.* 7, 146–152.

GARDNER, D. G. & MILLS, D. M. (1976) The widened periodontal ligament of osteosarcoma of the jaws. *Oral Surg.* 41, 652–656.

GARRINGTON, G. E., SCOFIELD, H. H., CORNYN, J. & HOOKER, S. P. (1967) Osteosarcoma of the jaws. Analysis of 56 cases. *Cancer* 20, 377–391.

HAMNER, J. E. & FULLMER, H. M. (1966) Oxytalan fibres in benign fibro-osseous jaw lesions. *Arch. Path.* 82, 35–39.

HAMNER, J. E., SCOFIELD, H. H. & CORNYN, J. (1968) Benign fibro-osseous jaw lesions of periodontal membrane. *Cancer* 22, 861–878.

HANKEY, G. T. & PEDLER, J. A. (1957) Primary squamous-cell carcinoma of mandible arising from epithelial lining of dental cyst. *Proc. R. Soc. Med.* 50, 680–681.

JEE, A., DOMBOSKI, M. & MILOBSKY, S. A. (1978) Malignant fibro-histocytoma of the maxilla presenting with endodontically involved teeth. *Oral Surg.* 45, 464–469.

KANGUR, T. T. & DAHLIN, D. C. (1975) Myxomatous tumours of the jaws. *J. oral Surg.* 33, 523–528.

KAY, L. W. & KRAMER, I. R. H. (1962) Squamous-cell carcinoma arising in a dental cyst. *Oral Surg.* 15, 970–979.

KHANNA, S., KHANNA, N. N. & VARANASI, M. S. (1979) Primary tumours of the jaws in children. *J. oral Surg.* 37, 800–804.

KRAMER, I. R. H. (1963) Ameloblastoma: a clinicopathological appraisal. *Br. J. oral Surg.* 1, 13–28.

LEVY, B. & SMITH, W. K. (1974) A jaw metastasis from the colon. *Oral Surg.* 38, 769–772.

LOPEZ, N. & LOBOS, N. (1976) Metastatic adenocarcinoma of gingiva. Report of a case. *J. Periodont.* 47, 358–360.

LUCAS, R. B. (1976) *Pathology of tumours of the oral tissues.* Edinburgh, Churchill Livingstone.

McGOWAN, R. H. (1980) Primary intra-alveolar carcinoma. A difficult diagnosis. *Br. J. oral Surg.* 18, 259–265.

MacGREGOR, A. (1936) An experimental investigation of the lymphatic system of the teeth and jaws. *Proc. R. Soc. Med.* 29, 1237–1272.

MAIN, J. H. P. (1970) Transformation of odontogenic epithelium by polyoma virus *in vitro. J. dent. Res.* 48, 738–744.

MARTENSSON, G. (1955) Cysts and carcinoma of the jaws. *Oral Surg.* 8, 673–681.

MICHAUD, M., BAEHNER, R. L., BIXLER, D. & KAFRAWY, A. H. (1977) Oral manifestations of acute leukaemia in children. *J. Amer. dent. Assoc.* 95, 1145–1150.

MITTELMAN, D. & KABAN, L. B. (1976) Recurrent non-Hodgkin's lymphoma presenting with gingival enlargement. Report of a case. *Oral Surg.* 42, 792–800.

MOSBY, E. L., SUGG, W. E. & HIATT, W. R. (1973) Gingival and pharyngeal metastasis from a malignant melanoma. Report of a case. *Oral Surg.* 36, 6–10.

OIKARINEN, V. J., CALONIUS, P. E. B. & SAINIO, P. (1975) Metastatic tumours to the oral region. I. An analysis of cases in the literature. *Proc. Finn. dent. Soc.* 71, 58–67.

PINDBORG, J. J. (1958) A calcifying epithelial odontogenic tumour. *Cancer* 11, 838–843.

PINDBORG, J. J., KRAMER, I. R. H. & TORLONI, H. (1971) *Histological typing of odontogenic tumours, jaw cysts and allied lesions. International Classification of Tumours No. 5,* pp. 31–34. Geneva, W.H.O.

PUNNIAMOORTHY, A. (1980) Gigantiform cementoma: review of the literature and a case report. *Br. J. oral Surg.* 18, 221–229.

REGEZI, J. A., KERR, D. A. & COURTNEY, R. M. (1978) Odontogenic tumours: analysis of 706 cases. *J. oral Surg.* 36, 771–778.

RENGASWAMY, V. (1978) Central neurilemmoma of the jaws. Review of literature and case report. *Int. J. oral Surg.* 7, 300–304.

RUPRECHT, A. & ARORA, B. K. (1978) Involvement of the mandible in leukaemia. *Dentomaxillofac. Radiol.* 7, 27–34.

SATO, M., NISHIO, J., YOSHIDA, H., MAEDA, N., URADE, M., MIYAZAKI, T., YAMAMOTO, Y. & HAYASHI, S. (1978) Metastatic choriocarcinoma involving the gingiva. *Int. J. oral Surg.* 7, 192–196.

SCHNEIDER, L. C. & WEISINGER, E. (1975) Odontogenic fibromyxoma arising from the periodontal ligament. *J. Periodont.* 46, 493–497.

SCHOFIELD, I. D. F. & JOHNSON, R. H. (1977) Osteosarcoma: An example of the thickened periodontal ligament space. *J. Periodont.* 48, 487–491.

SCHOFIELD, J. J. (1974) Oral metastatic deposit from carcinoma of the head of the pancreas. A case report. *Br. dent. J.* 137, 355–356.

SEWARD, G. R. & DUCKWORTH, R. (1967) A review of the pathology of the calcifying odontogenic cysts and tumours. *Dent. Practnr.* 18, 83–98.

SHAFER, W. G., HINE, M. K. & LEVY, B. M. (1974) *A textbook of oral pathology* (3rd ed.). Philadelphia, Saunders.

SHEAR, M. (1969) Primary intra-alveolar epidermoid carcinoma of the jaw. *J. Pathol.* 97, 645–651.

SHOOTWEG, P. J. (1980) Clear-cell chondrosarcoma of the maxilla. *Oral Surg.* 50, 233–237.

SHTEYER, A., LUSTMANN, J. & LEWIN-EPSTEIN, J. (1978) The mural ameloblastoma: a review of the literature. *J. oral Surg.* 36, 866–872.

SIDHU, S. S., PARKASH, H. & KHANANI, N. (1980) Benign osteoblastoma of the mandible. *J. Dentistry* 8, 254–256.

SINGLETON, J. McL. (1970) Malignant ameloblastoma. *Br. J. oral Surg.* **8**, 154–158.

SMALL, I. A. & WALDRON, C. A. (1955) Ameloblastoma of the jaw. *Oral Surg.* **8**, 281–297.

SMITH, G. C. & SMITH, R. J. (1979) Multiple neurofibromatosis (von Recklinghausen's disease). Case report. *Aust. dent. J.* **24**, 253–255.

SPOUGE, J. D. (1980) A new look at the rests of Malassez: a review of their embryological origin, anatomy, and possible role in periodontal health and disease. *J. Periodont.* **51**, 437–444.

STANLEY, H. R., DAWE, C. J. & LAW, L. W. (1964) Oral tumours induced by polyoma in mice. *Oral Surg.* **17**, 547–558.

STERN, M. H. & COLE, W. L. (1973) Radiographic changes in the mandible associated with leukemic cell infiltration in a case of acute myelogenous leukemia. *Oral Surg.* **36**, 343–348.

SZNAJDER, N., DOMINGUEZ, F. V., CARRARO, J. J. & LIS, G. (1973) Hemorrhagic hemangioma of gingiva: a report of a case. *J. Periodont.* **44**, 579–582.

TAKAGI, M. & ISHIKAWA, G. (1972) An autopsy case of leiomyosarcoma of the maxilla. *J. oral Pathol.* **1**, 125–132.

TEN CATE, A. R. (1975) The dento-gingival junction. An interpretation of the literature. *J. Periodont.* **46**, 475–477.

TOTH, B. B., LONG, W. H. & PLEASANTS, J. E. (1975) Central pacinian neurofibroma of the maxilla. *Oral Surg.* **39**, 630–634.

VAP, D. R., DAHLIN, D. C. & TURLINGTON, E. G. (1970) Pindborg tumour: the so-called calcifying epithelial odontogenic tumours. *Cancer* **25**, 629–636.

VIETA, J. O., FRIEDELL, H. L. & CRAVER, L. F. (1942) A survey of Hodgkin's disease and lymphosarcoma in bone. *Radiology* **39**, 1–14.

WALDRON, C. A. & GIANSANTI, J. S. (1973) Benign fibro-osseous lesions of the jaws: a clinical–radiologic–histologic review of sixty-five cases. II. Benign fibro-osseous lesions of periodontal ligament origin. *Oral Surg.* **35**, 340–350.

WARD, T. G. & COHEN, B. (1963) Squamous carcinoma in a mandibular cyst. *Br. J. oral Surg.* **1**, 8–12.

WESLEY, R. K., MINTZ, S. M. & WERTHEIMER, F. W. (1975) Primary malignant hemangioendothelioma of the gingiva. Report of a case and review of the literature. *Oral Surg.* **39**, 103–112.

WRIGHT, B. A. & JENNINGS, E. H. (1979) Oxytalan fibres in peripheral odontogenic fibromas. A histochemical study of eighteen cases. *Oral Surg.* **48**, 451–453.

WRIGHT, D. H. (1973) Lymphoreticular neoplasms In: *Tumours in a tropical country. A survey of Uganda 1964–1968,* A. C. TEMPLETON (ed.), pp. 270–291. London, Heinemann.

YACABUCCI, J. E., MAINOUS, E. G. & KRAMER, H. S. (1972) Hepatocellular carcinoma, diagnosed following metastasis to the mandible. Report of a case. *Oral Surg.* **33**, 888–893.

ZEGARELLI, D. J. (1976) Primary and metastic intraoral carcinoma. *N. Y. State dent. J.* **42**, 478–481.

Chapter 17

PERIODONTAL LIGAMENT FEATURES IN BLOOD AND LYMPHORETICULAR DISORDERS
R. M. Browne

INTRODUCTION

As in any vascular tissue, a significant proportion of the volume of the periodontal ligament is made up of its blood vessels and their contained blood, so that large numbers of red and white blood cells are continually circulating through it. As a consequence, any abnormality of these cells may lead to disturbance of periodontal function. In many instances such effects are functional rather than morphological and thus no overt changes are demonstrable. But in a number of disorders the periodontal ligament may exhibit clinical and/or microscopical changes. Although the periodontal ligament may be directly involved by the abnormal blood cells circulating through it, or by changes in the scattered lymphocytes and histiocytes normally present in the interstitial connective tissue, it is likely that most of the changes occur secondarily to two other events.

Firstly, in modern man the incidence of gingivitis is very high, indicating that in most individuals there is some degree of irritation by plaque micro-organisms. Since leucocytic infiltration into the gingiva is an essential component of the defence response to these micro-organisms, defective leucocytic response, a consequence either of deficient numbers of cells or of abnormalities in their function, may lead to an accelerated rate of spread of the natural progression of gingivitis into periodontitis.

Secondly, the periodontal ligaments of the teeth are surrounded by alveolar bone and its marrow spaces. The marrow spaces of the jaws contain scattered lymphocytes and histiocytes and in certain parts, especially in children, erythropoietic tissue. The periodontal ligament may thus be affected by abnormalities of these cells which arise primarily in the marrow spaces of the alveolar bone.

As might be expected, the most important changes accompany abnormalities of the leucocytes.

ANAEMIA

Anaemia is the state in which there is an inadequate quantity of circulating haemoglobin. The anaemias fall into two major groups, those consequent upon a deficiency of some factor essential for the development and/or maturation of the erythrocytes and those consequent upon an excessive loss or breakdown of the erythrocytes once they have been formed. In both groups the oral mucosa may exhibit pallor, due to the lowered concentration of circulating haemoglobin. In addition, there are other striking features, particularly in the lingual mucosa, which may be present in the deficiency anaemias (Ferguson, 1975). For example, iron, cyanocobalamin and folic acid, in addition to being essential for the formation of erythrocytes, are important constituents of enzymes and co-enzymes involved in general cellular metabolism. Thus, other cell systems which exhibit marked cell turnover, such as the oral epithelium, are also directly affected (Jones, 1973).

On the other hand, there is no evidence that the anaemia of iron deficiency has any direct effect upon the periodontal ligament. In a study of 752 patients with periodontal disease, no correlation was obtained between the haematocrit, haemoglobin concentration or erythrocyte count and the level of disease (Lainson, Brady and Fraleigh, 1968). A similar lack of correlation has also been observed in rats (Deutsch, Dreizen and Stahl, 1969). However, there does not appear to have been any attempt to correlate serum iron levels with periodontal disease, although it is known that the lymphocytes from sideropenic patients exhibit deficient immune responses (Joynson et al., 1972). In man there is no clear evidence that the megaloblastic anaemias of vitamin B_{12} or folic acid deficiency have any direct effect upon the periodontal tissues, although there are reports that gingivitis and periodontitis are features of folate deficiency in man (Day et al., 1938) and other primates (Dreizen, Levy and Bernick, 1970; Siddons, 1974).

Mild anaemia is a variable feature of ascorbic acid, riboflavin and pyridoxine deficiency in man (Ferguson, 1975). Swollen haemorrhagic gums together with accelerated progression of established periodontal disease leading to destruction of the periodontal ligament and loosening of the teeth are also common features of ascorbic acid deficiency, scurvy (Dreizen, 1971; Hodges et al., 1971; Schluger, Yuodelis and Page, 1977). However, there is no evidence that the anaemia is of significance in these changes. It is more likely that it is the defective

hydroxylation and thus cross linking of secreted tropocollagen molecules, which is dependent upon the presence of ascorbic acid, that leads to them. Such defective collagen metabolism results in weakening of the walls of capillaries (Priest, 1970) and other small vessels and the inadequate maintenance of the fibres of the periodontal ligament (Dreizen, Levy & Bernick, 1969). However, there is evidence that plaque must be present for the periodontal changes to occur, so that avitaminosis C may lead also to an altered host response to local irritation (Wolbach and Bessy, 1942; Glickman, 1948, 1964; El-Ashiry, Ringsdorf and Cheraskin, 1964; O'Leary et al., 1969; Schluger et al., 1977).

Since it is primarily the direct effect of the deficient factor upon the oral tissues rather than the anaemia itself which causes the important changes in the deficiency anaemias, it would be anticipated that none would occur in anaemias that arise from an excessive rate of destruction of the erythrocytes, the haemolytic anaemias and haemoglobinopathies. There is indeed no association between this group of anaemias and lesions of the periodontal ligament. However, there are characteristic changes in the alveolar bone in some of the haemoglobinopathies, notably in sickle cell disease and to a lesser extent in thalassemia.

Sickle cell disease is characterized by the presence of haemoglobin S in the erythrocytes. In haemoglobin S, valine is substituted for glutamic acid in the β-chain of the molecule and this leads to a rigidity and distortion of the shape of the erythrocyte to form the characteristic sickle appearance (Catena, 1975). The disorder is transmitted as a non-sex linked dominant and is of variable expressivity according to whether the subject is heterozygous or homozygous and to the penetrance of the gene. The heterozygous form, or sickle cell trait, is the more common and affects 8—11% of American Negroes (Catena, 1975). Anaemia, which affects particularly the homozygotes, results from haemolytic episodes brought on by such factors as hypoxia and infection. As a result of the anaemia there is erythroplasia of bone marrow which results in generalized osteoporosis, including the alveolar bone. Indeed osteoporosis can be detected here before in other bones (Robinson and Sarnat, 1952), probably due to the greater definition obtained on intra-oral radiographs rather than to any predilection for this site.

In the jaws there is a generalized osteoporosis with fewer, but sharply defined trabeculae, which show a characteristic 'step-ladder' pattern in the alveolar bone, the trabeculae arising from a distinct lamina dura which remains intact (Robinson and Sarnat, 1952; Morris and Stahl, 1954; Prowler and Smith, 1965; Massucco, 1966; Catena, 1975). All reports stress that the periodontal ligament space remains normal. In addition irregular osteosclerotic areas may be present (Prowler and Smith, 1965; Catena, 1975), probably indicative of past focal infarcts which have repaired by bone sclerosis. The changes are more obvious and more prevalent in homozygotes than those with sickle-cell trait (Prowler and Smith, 1965). In addition to the bone changes, abnormalities of tooth structure may also occur (Soni, 1966).

Similar bone changes have also been reported in homozygous haemoglobin C disease (Halstead, 1970). In haemoglobin C, lysine is substituted for glutamic acid in the β-chain of the molecule. This disorder is much less common, the heterozygous form affecting only approximately 2% of American Negroes (Smith and Conley, 1953).

In thalassemia (Cooley's anaemia) osteoporosis may also affect the alveolar bone although it is not an outstanding feature (Catena, 1975). In thalassemia, which affects predominantly the races living around the Mediterranean Sea, the defect lies in the rate of globin synthesis in the β-chain of the haemoglobin molecule. It is transmitted as an autosomal recessive.

POLYCYTHAEMIA

Polycythaemia is an abnormal increase in the erythrocyte mass in the circulation, usually as a consequence of an increased number of cells, but may occur as a result of haemoconcentration. It can be primary (polycythaemia vera) or secondary to some other condition such as renal carcinoma. Occasionally patients with polycythaemia have gingival bleeding which is probably a consequence of thrombocytosis (Ferguson, 1975). Thrombocytosis, an increase in the number of circulating platelets, may accompany polycythaemia and leukaemia, and results in defective thromboplastin generation.

DEFECTIVE HAEMOSTASIS

Defective haemostasis can arise in three basic ways: from abnormalities of the coagulation factors involved in the clotting mechanism, from defective platelet function, and from impaired support of the blood vessels. Defective platelet function may be a consequence of reduced numbers (thrombocytopenia), increased numbers (thrombocytosis), or of abnormalities in their metabolism (thrombocytosthenia). These latter disorders, and impaired support of blood vessels as occurs in avitaminosis C, are discussed elsewhere.

Defective haemostasis arising as a consequence of abnormalities of coagulation factors, haemophilia, is due to deficiencies of factors VIII, IX, and XI. Eighty per cent are due to deficiencies of factor VIII (anti-haemophilic globulin), 15% of factor IX (Christmas factor, plasma thromboplastin component) and 1–2% of factor XI (plasma thromboplastin antecedent) and are called haemophilia A, B and C respectively (Green, 1974; Grossman, 1975). In addition, in von Willebrand's disease there is a deficiency of factor VIII (Nilsson *et al.*, 1957) as well as defective platelet function (Hellem, 1960).

The major oral problem in such patients is the risk of post-surgical haemorrhage. The extent of the deficiency varies very much from patient to patient and from time to time in the same patient, and hence the clinical manifestations are variable. In classical haemophilia, haemophilia A, levels of anti-haemophilic globulin at 25% or less of normal are likely to lead to prolonged haemorrhage after dental extractions: levels at 5% or less may lead to spontaneous haemorrhage (Green, 1974), including gingival haemorrhage. In addition to the factors VIII, IX and XI, spontaneous gingival haemorrhage has also been reported in factor X (Stuart–Prower factor) deficiency (Bhoweer, Shirwatkar and Desai, 1977).

THROMBOCYTOPENIA

A reduction in the numbers of circulating platelets, thrombocytopenia, results in a prolongation of the bleeding time together with defective clot retraction. The outstanding clinical sign is the presence of numerous petechial haemorrhages, a purpuric rash on the skin, but which can also involve the oral mucosa. Most commonly thrombocytopenic purpura is secondary to drug toxicity, and can occur at any age; less commonly it arises as idiopathic thrombocytopenic purpura which usually occurs in young adults. This form of the disease is believed to be an auto-immune condition and is accompanied by the presence of anti-platelet antibodies in the plasma which leads to their agglutination (Harrington, Minnich and Arimura, 1956) and subsequent lysis in the spleen (McKelvy, Satinover and Sanders, 1976). The platelet/anti-platelet complexes can also lead to complement activation in the tissues (Yeager, 1975) and thus to destruction of the peripheral blood vessels. Such changes can occur in the gingiva where the capillaries may exhibit extensive serofibrinous perivascular exudation (McKelvy et al., 1976). As a consequence there may be gingival haemorrhage (Laskin, 1974; Yeager, 1975) and/or swelling (McKelvy et al., 1976).

There is a third, rare form of thrombocytopenia, thrombotic thrombocytopenic purpura, which is accompanied by thrombosis of the terminal arterioles and capillaries (Moschcowitz, 1925). It most commonly affects adolescents and young adults and runs a rapidly fatal course (Amorosi and Ultmann, 1966; Hill and Cooper, 1968). Although there are no significant oral features clinically, it has been demonstrated that the gingival vessels exhibit the same changes as elsewhere and provide an invaluable site for biopsy for confirmation of the diagnosis (Schwartz, Rosenberg and Cooperberg, 1972; Goldenfarb and Finch, 1973; Fox, Gordon and Williams, 1977). The arterioles and capillaries contain hyaline thrombi which occlude their lumens and there is endothelial proliferation. The aetiology of this form of the disease is unknown, but drug sensitivity and auto-immunity may both be factors (Fox et al., 1977).

Defective platelet function (thrombocytosthenia), such as occurs in uraemia (Merril and Peterson, 1970) and in Glanzmann's thrombasthenia, may also lead to gingival bleeding (Nixon, Keys and Brown, 1975). In the latter condition there are normal numbers of platelets, but they fail to aggregate normally in response to adenosine diphosphate and collagen, thus leading to defective clot retraction. Adenosine diphosphate activation of platelet thrombo-

plastic factor is also inhibited in uraemia. No periodontal ligament changes have been reported.

LEUCOPENIA

Leucopenia is regarded as being present when the white cell count drops below 3000/c mm and agranulocytosis when there is a virtual absence of granulocytes from the blood.

Most cases of agranulocytosis are a consequence of drug toxicity (Mishkin, Akers and Darby, 1976), are acute and are rapidly fatal due to overwhelming infection, most commonly by Gram-negative organisms. In addition to the cytotoxic and immunosuppressive agents given for the treatment of malignant disease and immune disorders, the drugs most commonly associated with agranulocytosis are the aminopyrines, phenothiazines, barbiturates, arsenicals, sulphonamides, thiouracils, gold and anti-malarials (Pretty et al., 1965; Cohen, 1977). Although ulceration of the oral mucosa, including the gingiva, is a frequent occurrence, the periodontal ligament is rarely involved, probably because of the short clinical course of the disorder. For example, it has been demonstrated in dogs that severe leucopenia induced either with nitrogen mustard (Attström and Egelberg, 1971a) or anti-neutrophil serum (Attström and Egelberg, 1971b) over periods of 4 days results in no change in the gingival index (Rylander, Attström and Lindhe, 1975; Attström and Schroeder, 1979).

Agranulocytosis may also occur as part of the complete cessation of haematopoiesis that occurs in aplastic anaemia. Again, although mucosal ulceration is a usual feature, involvement of the periodontal ligament as part of the overall necrotizing stomatitis is rare (Stamps, 1974; Lerman and Grodin, 1977).

Sometimes a more chronic course may ensue, in which case there may be extensive gingival ulceration resembling the lesions of acute ulcerative gingivitis, together with exposure of necrotic alveolar bone, destruction of the periodontal ligament and increased mobility of the affected teeth (Swenson, Redish and Manne, 1965).

Involvement of the periodontal ligament is a more important feature of the rare conditions of congenital neutropenia and cyclical neutropenia. In these conditions which affect the polymorphonuclear leucocytes and not the other forms of granulocyte, there is a persistent or cyclical absence or reduction of the cells to very low levels in the circulation.

In congenital neutropenia there is persistent neutropenia with a differential count usually below 5% and often a relative lymphocytosis, monocytosis and eosinophilia. Approximately 70% of these patients die in the first 3 years of life (Mishkin et al., 1976), but some survive into adolescence. In these, severe periodontitis is a characteristic feature with extensive destruction of the alveolar bone and periodontal ligament, and rapid loosening and premature loss of both the deciduous and permanent dentition (Levine, 1959; Cutting and Lang, 1964; Andrews et al., 1965; Davey and Konchak, 1969; Gates, 1969; Kyle and Linman, 1970; Miller, Oski and Harris, 1971; Awbrey and Hibbard, 1973; Lampert and Fesseler, 1975; Vann and Oldenburg, 1976; Mishkin et al., 1976; Reichart and Dornow, 1978). This rapid periodontal destruction occurs despite rigorous oral hygiene and is presumably a consequence of uninhibited irritation of the tissues by the plaque micro-organisms due to deficient phagocytosis. In support of this is the observation that despite the neutropenia, extraction sockets heal normally (Andrews et al., 1965; Mishkin et al., 1976). Further, necrotizing periodontitis has been demonstrated in rats in whom granulocytopenia was induced for 30–60 days with either methyl folic acid (Franklin et al., 1947; Pindborg, 1949) or neoarsphenamine (Bauer, 1946).

The condition occurs in a variety of forms some of which are transmitted as an autosomal recessive (Kostman, 1956; Andrews, McClellan and Scott, 1960; MacGillwray et al., 1964; Matsaniotis et al., 1966) and others as a dominant (Cutting and Lang, 1964), although most cases have no familial pattern. In some it has been demonstrated that there is a failure of the normal granulocyte maturation in the bone marrow to progress beyond the myelocyte or metamyelocyte stage (Cutting and Lang, 1964; Gates, 1969; Mishkin et al., 1976), whereas in others there are normal numbers of mature neutrophils in the marrow but these do not enter the circulation or respond well to chemical or inflammatory stimuli in the other tissues (Miller et al., 1971). In the latter case the neutrophils exhibit normal phagocytosis but respond weakly to chemotactic stimuli. In some

forms of the disease monocyte activity is enhanced, presumably to compensate for the lack of neutrophils (Biggar et al., 1974; Kay et al., 1976).

In cyclical neutropenia the neutrophils disappear from or are markedly reduced in the peripheral blood every 21 days (Reimann and de Baradinis, 1949). The cell count increases again after 5–8 days but rarely attains a count greater than 50% of normal. During the periods of neutropenia there is a complete suppression of neutrophil leucopoiesis or a maturation arrest at the promyelocyte stage in the bone marrow. Despite the periods of neutropenia these patients usually remain in good health, although they are subject to recurrent infections.

The most common oral symptom is recurrent oral ulceration, crops of ulcers coinciding with the periods of neutropenia (Cohen and Morris, 1961). In some patients there are reports of advanced periodontal disease with bifurcation and trifurcation involvement and marked increase in tooth mobility (Page and Good, 1957; Gorlin and Chaudhry, 1960; Cohen and Morris, 1961; Telsey et al., 1962; Wade and Stafford, 1963; Cohen, 1965; Binon and Dykema, 1974). Since such cases are usually diagnosed in the first decade, rapidly progressing periodontal disease may be an early diagnostic feature of the condition. In general, neither the extent of the periodontitis nor the number of patients exhibiting this feature is as great as in congenital neutropenia, presumably because the neutropenia occurs for only short periods.

CHEDIAK–HIGASHI SYNDROME

Chediak–Higashi syndrome (Chediak, 1952; Higashi, 1954) is a genetically transmitted disease which is characterized by partial oculo-cutaneous albinism, photophobia, nystagmus, recurrent pyogenic infections and abnormally large granules in all the granulocytic cells of the body (Kritzler et al., 1964; Blume and Wolff, 1972). It is transmitted as an autosomal recessive, and has not been reported in negroes. In addition to man it affects mink (Leader, Padgett and Gorham, 1963), cattle and mice (Padgett et al., 1964). In man death usually occurs before the age of 20 either from recurrent infections or from an accelerated, lymphoma-like stage of the disease in which there is widespread lympho-/histiocytic infiltration, pancytopenia, thrombocytopenia, lymphadenopathy and hepatosplenomegaly (Kritzler *et al.*, 1964). It is not clear whether this stage of the disease is reactive (Padgett *et al.*, 1967; Blume and Wolff, 1972) or neoplastic (Dent *et al.*, 1966).

Abnormal, large granules are present within the polymorphonuclear leucocytes, eosinophils, basophils and their precursors, and under the electron microscope have been demonstrated to be lysosomally derived (White, 1966). There is defective chemotactic attraction (Clark and Kimball, 1971) and although bacterial ingestion is unaffected there is defective degranulation and intracellular killing, not dependent upon diminished peroxidase activity. In addition there is granulocytopenia, possibly a result of intramedullary breakdown of the abnormal cells (Blume *et al.*, 1968).

Associated with the decreased numbers of circulating granulocytes which are abnormal, patients exhibit severe gingivitis and advanced periodontitis leading to marked mobility and loss of teeth, even before the end of the first decade (Weary and Bender, 1967; Gillig and Caldwell, 1970; Blume and Wolff, 1972; Tempel *et al.*, 1972; Hamilton and Giansanti, 1974). It is generally believed that this accelerated tissue destruction is a consequence of defective protection by the abnormal leucocytes allowing unhindered periodontal breakdown by the plaque micro-organisms (Lavine, Page and Padgett, 1976) rather than increased tissue destruction by the abnormal cells. It has been demonstrated that leucocytes from patients with Chediak—Higashi syndrome exhibit no cytotoxic effect upon HeLa cells in tissue culture (Taubman, Cogen and Lepow, 1974).

The periodontal tissues are infiltrated densely by lymphocytes and plasma cells, in some areas closely packed into 'abscesses' (Gustaffson, 1969) and relatively few polymorphonuclear leucocytes. Radiographically there is extensive bone loss around the affected teeth, often with a 'moth-eaten' appearance (Lavine *et al.*, 1976). In addition to periodontitis there may be gingival haemorrhage (Blume and Wolff, 1972), mucosal ulceration and glossitis (Gillig and Caldwell, 1970).

CHRONIC GRANULOMATOUS DISEASE

This disease, which is thought to be genetically transmitted, is characterized by the inability of the circulating leucocytes to kill certain micro-organisms after ingestion. As a consequence, multiple purulent granulomas develop in the lymph nodes, spleen, liver, skin and lungs, and the child seldom survives to adolescence (Berendes, Bridges and Good, 1957; Johnston and Baehner, 1971). The defective intracellular killing is associated with a failure to synthesize hydrogen peroxide which is apparently essential for this activity. Many bacteria themselves synthesize hydrogen peroxide sufficient to maintain the intracellular killing activity of the leucocytes, but many in addition contain catalase which degrades hydrogen peroxide (Good and Fisher, 1971). It is such catalase positive micro-organisms which cause the infections in chronic granulomatous disease, examples of which are *Candida albicans,* staphylococci, *Escherichia coli* and *Nocardia.*

The oral changes include stomatitis and oral ulceration (Johnston and Baehner, 1971; Wolf and Ebel, 1978). In addition, if survival beyond childhood occurs, a severe gingivitis, with bright red coloration of the affected tissue, including the alveolar mucosa, may be present (Wolf and Ebel, 1978). Since there is marked improvement of the lesions with plaque control, it is probable that they arise as a consequence of the reduced host response to the plaque micro-organisms.

INFECTIOUS MONONUCLEOSIS

Infectious mononucleosis (glandular fever) is a systemic lymphoproliferative disease which is characterized by the presence of large numbers of atypical mononuclear cells in the peripheral blood. It occurs almost exclusively in adolescents and young adults (Hoagland, 1960; Dunnet, 1963) among whom it is believed that kissing is an important mode of transmission (Cassingham, 1971), and is most common in the spring and autumn. Most commonly there is a febrile illness with ulcero-membranous pharyngitis and generalized lymphadenopathy involving variable numbers of lymph nodes, but almost invariably those in the posterior triangle of the neck (Banks, 1967).

The most striking oral feature is a palatal enanthematous eruption (Shiver, Berg and Frenkel, 1956; Caird and Holt, 1958; Courant and Sobkov, 1969). Less commonly there may be an ulcero-membranous gingivitis which resembles acute ulcerative gingivitis (Contratto, 1944; Fraser-Moodie, 1959; Banks, 1967; Valentine, 1971), sometimes associated with partially erupted lower third molars, where it resembles pericoronitis (Fraser-Moodie, 1959; Banks, 1967). It is not clear whether the periodontal ligament is involved under these circumstances.

The striking finding in infectious mononucleosis is the presence of heterophil antibodies in the serum, which cause the lysis of sheep red blood cells (Paul and Bunnell, 1932). The association between the presence of these antibodies and infection with Epstein—Barr virus was first demonstrated in 1968 (Henle, Henle and Diehl, 1968; Niederman *et al.* 1968) and it is now widely accepted that this is the most frequent causative virus (Evans, 1974). The incubation period is uncertain, estimates varying from a few days to several weeks (Hoagland, 1964; Valentine, 1971). However, there are some patients with all the clinical features of infectious mononucleosis but who do not have heterophil antibodies in their serum, and there is evidence that whereas some of these may also be a consequence of infection with Epstein—Barr virus (Evans, Niederman and McCollum, 1968; Klemola *et al.,* 1970), approximately 50% are associated with cytomegalovirus infection (Klemola and Kaariainen, 1965; Klemola *et al.,* 1970; Jordan *et al.,* 1973) and occasionally with other unknown agents (Evans, 1972; Jordan, 1975).

LEUKAEMIA

Leukaemia is characterized by the neoplastic proliferation of leucocyte precursor cells within the haemopoietic tissues leading to replacement of the normal haemopoietic constituents and usually to accumulation of large numbers of cells in the peripheral blood. According to the type of leucocyte involved, lymphocytic, myelocytic and monocytic

forms are recognized, although rare variants, involving eosinophils and basophils, have been reported. It occurs in acute and chronic forms, the former being more common in children and adolescents and the latter in adults.

Oral lesions have been observed in 55—80% of cases with acute leukaemia and 15—49% with chronic leukaemia (Sinrod, 1957; Duffy and Driscoll, 1958; Lynch and Ship, 1967b; Bodey, 1971). There is, however, little doubt that many oral lesions in leukaemics are the consequence of the treatment of the disease rather than of the disease itself. The oral lesions have accordingly been classified into primary, secondary and tertiary (Segelman and Doku, 1977). Primary lesions arise from infiltration of the tissues by the leukaemic cells. Secondary lesions are a consequence of the myelophthisic effects of the leukaemic infiltrate in the bone marrow leading to granulocytopenia and thrombocytopenia. Tertiary lesions are due to the myelo-/immuno-suppressive and cytotoxic effects of the drugs used in the treatment of the disease. Some drugs, such as methotrexate and methyl GAG, are more commonly associated with oral lesions than others (Bodey, 1971). It is not surprising, therefore, that there is considerable variation in the reported incidence of oral lesions in leukaemia. Indeed, the incidence of oral lesions as presenting symptoms in acute leukaemia is substantially lower than the above figures, being only 20—38% (Roath, Israels and Wilkinson, 1964; Lynch and Ship, 1967a; Curtis, 1971).

Involvement of the periodontal tissues in leukaemia is not uncommon. Hyperplastic gingivitis, ulceration, necrosis with pseudo-membrane formation and haemorrhage are the most frequent changes (Figs. 1 and 2) (Segelman and Doku, 1977). Hyperplastic gingivitis has been observed in 15—53% of all cases of leukaemia (Kaufman and Lowenstein, 1940; Duffy and Driscoll, 1958; Boggs, Wintrobe and Cartwright, 1962). As with the oral lesions, the incidence of hyperplastic gingivitis as a presenting feature is substantially less, varying from 10—33% (Southam *et al.,* 1951; Lynch and Ship, 1967a), being twice as common in acute as in chronic leukaemia (Lynch and Ship, 1967a). The incidence is also lower in acute leukaemia in children, varying from 1—10% (Curtis, 1971; Michaud *et al.,* 1977).

The lower incidence in children is probably a

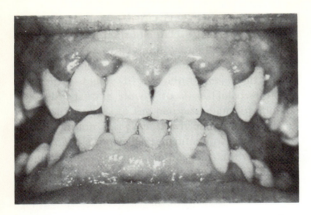

FIG. 1. Acute leukaemia. There is a hyperplastic gingivitis with enlargement of the interdental papillae, some of which are haemorrhagic.

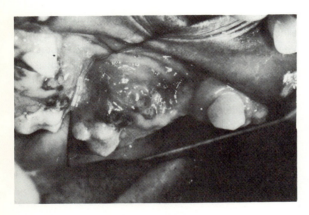

FIG. 2. Acute leukaemia. There is a haemorrhagic ulcero-necrotic swelling of the maxillary ridge, involving the periodontal tissues of the molar tooth.

consequence of the varying incidence of oral lesions in the different forms of leukaemia. According to Sinrod (1957), Lynch and Ship (1967a) and Shafer, Hine and Levy (1974), oral lesions occur in 20—53% of cases of acute lymphatic leukaemia, 40—47% acute myelogenous leukaemia and 80—91% acute monocytic leukaemia. There is much evidence that hyperplastic gingivitis occurs most commonly in acute monocytic leukaemia (Shaw, 1978) although figures for the incidence are again somewhat variable, ranging from 34 to 100% (Hubler and Netherton, 1947; Sinn and Dick, 1956; Berkheiser, 1957; Boggs et al., 1962; Michaud et al., 1977) and least commonly in acute lymphocytic leukaemia, figures varying from

0 to 4.7% (Boggs et al., 1962; Curtis, 1971; Michaud et al., 1977). A complete absence of gingival inflammation was noted in 56% of children with acute lymphocytic leukaemia (White, 1970). Since acute lymphocytic leukaemia is the commonest leukaemia of childhood, it is not suprising that hyperplastic gingivitis is uncommon in childhood leukaemia.

Evidence for involvement of the periodontal ligament is, on the other hand, largely circumstantial and not well documented. There are a number of clinical reports in which reference is made to the presence of generalized bone loss (Keene, Hussman and Bruner, 1972; Presant, Safdar and Cherrick, 1973; Segelman and Doku, 1977), increased mobility of teeth (McCarthy and Karcher, 1946; Stern and Cole, 1973; Michaud et al., 1977; Pogrel, 1978) and protrusion of teeth (Mallett et al., 1947; Taliano and Wakefield, 1966; Smillie and Cowman, 1969). Since most of these occurred in adults, the extent to which the periodontal changes were a consequence of a pre-existing chronic periodontitis and not due to leukaemic infiltration is not clear. However, more definitive evidence is derived from radiological studies, particularly in children where bone changes as a consequence of chronic periodontitis are unlikely. Curtis (1971) studied the oral radiographs of 214 children with leukaemia and observed bone changes in 87 (41%). There was a significant difference between children with active disease (62%) and those in remission (5%), and between patients with acute lymphocytic leukaemia (65%) and acute myelogenous leukaemia (47%). The most characteristic changes were a loss of the lamina dura around erupted teeth, with widening of the periodontal ligament space, and loss of the crypt outline around unerupted teeth. Similar changes have been mentioned in other case reports (Bender, 1944; Sinrod, 1957; Taliano and Wakefield, 1966; Stern and Cole, 1973; Michaud et al., 1977).

In children the changes are most commonly observed around the last developing molar tooth (Curtis, 1971) and involve the periapical part of the periodontium rather than the crestal part. The involvement of the periapical part of the periodontal ligament prior to the crestal part in leukaemia is confirmed from histological studies in both AKR (Carranza and Cabrini, 1965) and CFW mice (Flanagan et al., 1970). In both these studies no infiltration of the gingiva was present. It has been suggested (Curtis, 1971) therefore that the primary event is infiltration of the marrow spaces by the leukaemic cells which spread to involve the lamina dura and periodontal ligament of the involved teeth (Fig. 3). Since haemopoietic bone marrow persists longest in the posterior and molar regions of the jaws in children, this might

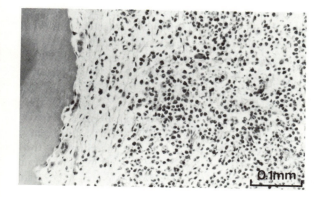

FIG. 3. Acute myelogenous leukaemia. The periodontal ligament is infiltrated by leukaemic cells which exhibit pleomorphism. The collagen fibres have been destroyed and there is active odontoclastic resorption of the root surface. H & E. ×134.

account for the more frequent involvement of the molar teeth (Curtis, 1971; Jones, 1975) in the early stages of leukaemia. Infiltration of the pulp has also been reported both in humans (Sinrod, 1957; Duffy and Driscoll, 1958; Smillie and Cowman, 1969) and in mice (Carranza and Cabrini, 1965; Flanagan *et al.,* 1970). As far as can be determined such infiltration usually occurs only in the pulps of incompletely formed or continuously forming teeth, both of which have open apices.

The pathogenesis of the destructive changes in the periodontal tissues in leukaemia is unclear. The relative frequency of gingival changes, including hyperplasia, haemorrhage and ulcero-necrosis, are considered a consequence of the high incidence of pre-existing chronic gingivitis. Several authors have emphasized that the gingival changes are less marked or even suppressed if excellent oral hygiene measures are maintained (Sinrod, 1957; McGowan, Gorman and Otridge, 1970; Segelman and Doku, 1977; Pogrel, 1978; Carranza, 1979). Gingival biopsy reveals a dense infiltrate of the gingiva with leukaemic

cells, the infiltrate characteristically being separated from the gingival epithelium by a narrow band of normal connective tissue (Sinrod, 1957; Lucas, 1976a). Leukaemic cells have been variously reported as exhibiting defective immune responses (Dupuy *et al.,* 1971), and also impaired phagocytosis (Lehrer *et al.,* 1972). Thus in sites where, prior to the disease, inflammation already existed, such as in the gingiva in chronic gingivitis, greater numbers of cells would be attracted.

There is no information on the mechanism of tissue destruction once the leukaemic cells have arrived in the tissues. However, several authors have observed blood vessels occluded by dense aggregates of leukaemic cells (Fig. 4) (Burkett, 1940; Sinrod, 1957;

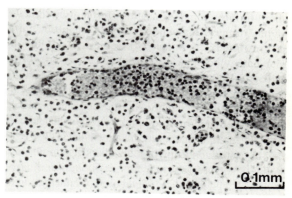

FIG. 4. Acute myelogenous leukaemia. A venule from the inter-radicular region of a lower molar, partially occluded by aggregates of leukaemic cells. H & E. ×134.

Bodey, 1971; Segelman and Doku, 1977) and that this may lead to necrosis of the gingiva and periodontal ligament. Intra-vascular leucocyte thrombi and aggregates are a particular feature of myelogenous leukaemia (McKee and Collins, 1974) and occur in sites other than the periodontal ligament with increasing frequency proportional to the circulating leucocyte count. Although no such study has been made of the periodontal ligament, the incidence of leukaemic cell infiltration of non-ulcerated labial mucosa in acute myelogenous leukaemia shows a similar relationship to the circulating leucocyte count (Basu and Pollock, unpublished). However, the circulating level of leucocytes is only one of probably many factors, since radiological changes in alveolar bone have been reported in preleukaemia when the circulating leucocytes are still within normal limits (Deasy et al., 1976). Whether bone resorption is a consequence of a direct effect of the release of lysosomal enzymes from the leukaemic cells or of stimulation of osteoclasts is uncertain. In studies of leukaemia in mice, particular note was made of the paucity of osteoclasts in histological examination of the alveolar bone, despite the marked destruction of the lamina dura and adjacent bone (Carranza and Cabrini, 1965). On the other hand, marked odontoclastic activity can occur in the periodontal ligament in acute leukaemia (Fig. 3).

Another factor of possible significance is the change in the oral flora in leukaemic patients. Leukaemic patients are particularly susceptible to infections (Hersh et al., 1965) as a consequence partly of their defective immune responses, and partly of the myelo-suppression, immuno-suppression and cytotoxicity which are side effects of the chemo-therapeutic treatment of the disease (Dreizen, Bodey and Brown, 1974). In the course of the disease, particularly during periods of remission in patients with acute myelogenous leukaemia, patients are granulocytopenic for approximately 50% of the time (Bodey et al., 1966) and it is during such periods that they are particularly prone to infection. The infections are caused predominantly by opportunist organisms, in particular the Gram-negative bacilli and Candida species (Dreizen et al., 1974). In the oral cavity Escherichia coli, Klebsiella and Pseudomonas are commonly cultured from patients with leukaemia (Bodey, 1971; Brown, Dreizen and Bodey, 1973) whereas they are rare in the mouths of healthy patients. The reason for this change in the oral flora is unclear, although it should be noted that there is a reduction in the level of parotid secretory IgA in patients with acute myelogenous leukaemia (Brown et al., 1973; Basu, Pollock and Gordon, 1978) and acute lymphoblastic leukaemia (Schiliro et al., 1977).

In addition to the above micro-organisms, infections of the oral mucosa associated with Candida albicans (Bodey, 1971; McGowan, Gorman and Otridge, 1970; Segelman and Doku, 1977; Michaud et al., 1977) are not uncommon. In one study candida were recovered from the mouths of 93% of patients (Segelman and Doku, 1977). Less commonly acute

ulcerative gingivitis has been reported (Michaud et al., 1977; Segelman and Doku, 1977).

The frequency of involvement of the periodontal ligament is, therefore, uncertain. However, changes occur in children, probably as a result of secondary invasion from the marrow spaces, and in adults as a consequence of spread of tumour cells attracted into the periodontal tissues previously altered by chronic periodontal disease. Whether this difference between children and adults is a consequence of the different incidence of the various forms of leukaemia in the two groups or of the different prevalence of pre-existing inflammatory changes, or of other factors, is unclear.

MALIGNANT LYMPHOMAS

Malignant lymphomas are neoplastic lesions of the cells of the lymphoreticular system and occur predominantly in the lymph nodes of the body. The cervico-facial lymph nodes are commonly involved although, since the spread of tumour cells to involve other groups of lymph nodes is often rapid, indeed the neoplasm may be multicentric in origin, other groups of nodes are usually also affected. In approximately 10% of cases (Rosenberg et al., 1961), the tumour is first noted in the head and neck region.

They are subdivided into two main groups, the non-Hodgkin's lymphomas and Hodgkin's disease. Extranodal lesions in malignant lymphomas occur either from progression of a tumour previously confined to the lymph nodes or less commonly as a primary neoplasm. In the former it is usually other lymphoreticular organs such as the spleen, or the lymphoid tissue of Waldeyer's ring, the gastro-intestinal tract and bone marrow which are involved. In the latter, a primary lymphoma may occur in almost any tissue of the body, including the oral mucosa and jaws. There is a form of lymphoma, Burkitt's lymphoma, in which involvement of the jaw is a particular characteristic (Burkitt, 1958) (see Chapter 16).

Non-Hodgkin's lymphomas

Non-Hodgkin's lymphomas are traditionally classified according to their cytological and histological features, and the most widely accepted classification is that of Rappaport (1966, 1977), in which five categories are recognized: lymphocytic, well differentiated; lymphocytic, poorly differentiated; mixed lymphocytic/histiocytic; histiocytic; undifferentiated. There are a number of more recent classifications of the nodal lesions in non-Hodgkin's lymphomas, based upon their relationship to the T and B systems of lymphocytes and the cellular changes that normally accompany lymphocyte transformation (Lukes and Collins, 1974, 1975, 1977; Gerard-Marchant *et al.,* 1974; Dorfman, 1974; Bennett *et al.,* 1974; Lennert, Stein and Kaiserling, 1975; Mathe *et al.,* 1976). Such studies indicate that the majority of nodal non-Hodgkin's lymphomas, including those classified as histiocytic, are derived from B-cells, and although they provide a better understanding of the pathogenesis of these lesions, their value in assessing the clinical behaviour and thus of formulating appropriate treatment regimes is as yet unproven. The inter-relationships of the various classifications with emphasis on nodal lymphomas in the head and neck is fully discussed elsewhere (Schnitzer and Weaver, 1979). No similar studies have been made of the extranodal lesions affecting the mouth and jaws.

Poorly differentiated lymphocytic, mixed lymphocytic–histiocytic, and histiocytic lymphomas can occur in both a nodular and diffuse form (Wong *et al.,* 1975). In the nodular form, which is more frequently found in the first two types, follicle-like groupings of tumour cells are present. Such lymphomas usually have a better prognosis, although a proportion of them probably undergo transition to a more diffuse form. This change, which may take many years, is accompanied by a worsening of the prognosis (Rappaport, Winter and Hicks, 1956; Schnitzer, Loesel and Reed, 1970).

Extranodal lesions in non-Hodgkin's lymphomas are common, occurring in approximately 60% of cases (Peters, Hasselback and Brown, 1968; McNelis and Pai, 1969; Johnson *et al.,* 1974). Fuller *et al.* (1975) reported 58% of stage I and II non-Hodgkin's lymphomas with primary extranodal presentation and 61% of these occurred in the head and neck. In this region, Waldeyer's ring forms the commonest site (Wong *et al.,* 1975), the gingivae, floor of mouth, vestibular sulcus and cheek accounting for approximately 8%. Males are affected nearly twice as com-

monly as females, the tumours becoming increasingly common with age. Most patients are over 50, the peak incidence being in the seventh decade.

Apart from Burkitt's lymphoma most reports have described lymphomas in the mouth and jaws as either reticulum cell sarcoma or lymphosarcoma. Both may arise either within the mucous membrane overlying the alveolus or as a primary tumour within the marrow spaces, the periodontal ligament becoming secondarily involved. In the maxilla, the tumour may arise in the antrum, which is the commonest site of origin of lymphomas involving this bone (Steg, Dahlin and Gores, 1959). Nodular forms of the tumour are rare in extranodal sites in the head and neck (Wong *et al.,* 1975; McNelis and Pai, 1969).

The most common complaint is of a painful swelling (Steg *et al.,* 1959), which may involve the bone of the maxilla and mandible or be restricted to the gingivae (Silverman, 1955; Orsos, 1958; Harvey and Thomson, 1966; Calderwood, 1967; Mittelman and Kaban, 1976). In dentate jaws mobility of the teeth is an outstanding feature (Seldin, Seldin and Rakower, 1954; Gerry and Williams, 1955; Kennedy, 1957; Cook, 1961; Chaudhry and Vickers, 1962; Tillman, 1965; Keusch, Poole and King, 1966; Binnie, Bret Day and Lynn, 1971; Mittelman and Kaban, 1976) due to destruction of the periodontal ligament and alveolar bone. Thus the radiological features associated with such lesions are predominantly those of poorly defined areas of osteolysis

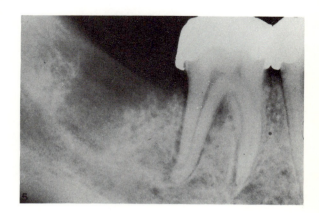

FIG. 5. Radiograph of diffuse lymphocytic lymphoma. There is irregular diffuse bone loss with loss of the lamina dura and widening of the periodontal ligament space on the distal root of the molar.

(Fig. 5) (Seldin *et al.,* 1954; Gerry and Williams, 1955; Steg *et al.,* 1959; Cook, 1961; Blake and Beck, 1963; Gould and Main, 1969; Binnie *et al.,* 1971) although in one report there is specific reference to the loss of the lamina dura and to the appearance of floating teeth (Blake and Beck, 1963).

The occurrence of primary intra-osseous lymphomas in bone was first established by Parker and Jackson (1949) and it is likely that in the jaws involvement of the periodontal ligament is secondary to that of the bone marrow spaces.

When the periodontal ligament is involved it is infiltrated by dense sheets of lymphocytic cells resulting in destruction of the fibre bundles and the adjacent alveolar bone (Fig. 6). According to the

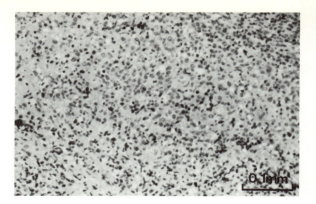

FIG. 7. Diffuse mixed lymphocytic/histiocytic lymphoma. The tumour is composed of a dense infiltrate of large and small lymphoid and histiocytoid cells. H & E. ×134.

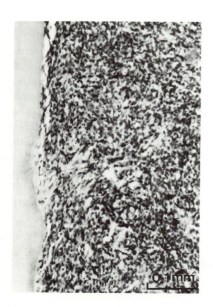

FIG. 6. Diffuse lymphocytic lymphoma. The fibres of the periodontal ligament have been destroyed and replaced by a dense infiltrate of small and large lymphoid cells. H & E. ×134.

stage of differentiation of the neoplastic cells, they will vary in appearance from small lymphocytes with darkly staining nuclei, through larger, less-well-differentiated cells with vesicular nuclei and poorly defined cytoplasm (Fig. 7), to larger cells which may closely resemble histiocytes. Resorption of the roots of the teeth has been reported (Blake and Beck, 1963; Keusch *et al.,* 1966). Preliminary

studies with immunoperoxidase techniques indicate that the tumour cells exhibit a monoclonality with regard to the distribution of both immunoglobulins and kappa and lambda short chains, similar to that exhibited by non-Hodgkin's lymphomas in lymph nodes (Matthews and Basu, in press).

There is a particular form of malignant lymphoma in which extranodal lesions are frequent and which commonly affects the jaws in children living in the central part of Africa and in New Guinea. This tumour was first described by Burkitt (1958) and is now known eponymously. In these endemic regions of the world, Burkitt's tumour affects the jaws in 50–60% of cases, although other bones are only rarely involved (Burkitt, 1958, 1964; Burkitt and Davies, 1961; Edington, McLean and Okubadejo, 1964; Davies, 1964; Adatia, 1968 a and b; Wright, 1971).

Its cytological appearance is distinctive, being composed of sheets of undifferentiated lympho-blastic cells of remarkably uniform appearance each .with a round to oval nucleus containing coarsely shaped chromatin and one to four prominent nucleoli. Their cytoplasm is vacuolated and strongly pyronino-philic (WHO Bulletin, 1969) due to the large numbers of ribosomes. Scattered among these malignant cells are varying numbers of large macrophages which are reactive rather than neoplastic in type and whose cytoplasm frequently contains substantial quantities of nuclear debris. Their scattered distribution among the tumour cells forms a characteristic 'starry-sky' pattern. Recent studies indicate that the tumour cells have the characteristics of B-lymphocytes and are probably derived from germinal follicles (Schnitzer and Weaver, 1979).

In Africa the tumour is rare in children under 2 and over 15 years of age (Burkitt, 1958) and the peak involvement of the jaws is at 3 years (Kramer, 1965; Adatia, 1968b). Involvement of the jaws becomes decreasingly common as the age of the patient increases. This association probably explains the less frequent involvement of the jaws in Burkitt's lymphoma occurring in non-endemic areas, where only 15% have jaw involvement (Adatia, 1968b) since the average age of these patients is rather greater (Schnitzer and Weaver, 1979). In any event involvement of the jaws is uncommon after the age of 15.

The maxilla is involved approximately twice as commonly as the mandible (Burkitt, 1964; Adatia, 1968b) and the tumour usually first affects the molar regions. More than one quadrant is commonly affected, simultaneous involvement of all four being the most frequent form of multiple presentation (Adatia, 1968b). Radiological studies suggest that more than one jaw is involved in 83% of patients. Loosening of the primary molars is the earliest sign and usually precedes the onset of swelling. There is rapid dissemination of the tumour cells through the posterior parts of the jaws so that varied radiological changes may be seen including scattered foci of radiolucency which may coalesce forming larger areas (Adatia, 1968b) loss of the lamina dura (Adatia, 1966, 1968b), focal enlargement of the periodontal ligament space (Adatia, 1970) and enlargement of the crypts around unerupted teeth (Adatia, 1966). There is rapidly progressive infiltration of the tumour cells among the fibres of the periodontal ligament and dental follicle, resulting in their displacement and destruction. Active osteoclastic resorption accounts for the breakdown of the alveolar bone. Subsequently the entire attachment between the tooth and bone is disrupted and the tooth may be displaced out of the remains of its socket, thus forming a radiological image of floating teeth.

The pulp is also frequently infiltrated by tumour cells penetrating through the incompletely closed apex of developing teeth. Outwards displacement of the epithelial diaphragm may occur, leading to the formation of hook-like deformities in the roots of those teeth where dentinogenesis continues (Adatia, 1968b, 1973).

The genome for Epstein–Barr virus is present in the tumour cells of 97% of African patients (Ziegler, 1977) although this close association is not a feature of cases reported in non-endemic areas (Pagano, Huang and Levine, 1973; Judson, Henle and Henle, 1977). The significance of this association in the pathogenesis of Burkitt's lymphoma remains uncertain. The aetiology of the other forms of non-Hodgkin's lymphoma affecting the jaws is unknown, although it has been demonstrated that implantation of a known carcinogen, dimethylbenzanthrocene, into extraction sockets in hamsters results in lymphoma formation (Mesrobian and Shklar, 1971).

Hodgkin's disease

Hodgkin's disease is the commonest form of malignant lymphoma and is a multicentric condition that affects the lymph nodes and many other tissues, in particular the spleen and liver. The cervical lymph nodes are commonly involved and the presenting symptom in approximately 50% of cases (Forman and Wesson, 1970). As in the non-Hodgkin's lymphomas, males are affected approximately twice as frequently as females. It occurs particularly in adolescents and young adults and beyond the age of 50.

Bone involvement is not commonly reported, being observed radiologically in from 8 to 15% of cases (Steiner, 1943; Tiwari, 1973). However, much greater involvement has been reported in histological studies of autopsy material, Steiner (1943) finding tumour foci in 78.6% affecting mostly the vertebrae, pelvis, sternum and ribs. Tumour deposits in the jaws are rare being found in only 0–0.86% of cases (Steiner, 1943; Jackson and Parker, 1945; Fuscilla and Hannam, 1961; Tiwari, 1973). It is not surprising, therefore, that there are few clinical reports of lesions involving the mouth and jaws. In three of the four cases with involvement of the periodontal ligament (Ames, 1958; Meyer, Roswit and Unger, 1959; Forman and Wesson, 1970; Tiwari, 1973), the lesion arose in the mandibular molar region in patients who were under treatment for the disease. In the fourth case the maxilla was primarily involved. The typical radiological changes were the presence of a diffuse irregular radiolucency in relation to the roots of the involved teeth, together with loss of the lamina dura. Clinically, tenderness and looseness of the teeth were a feature.

Histologically, the nodal lesions of Hodgkin's disease are characterized by the presence of Reed—Sternberg cells which are believed to be derived from reticulum cells. Reed—Sternberg cells have large vesicular nuclei with prominent acidophilic nucleoli and classically are binucleate, the nuclei being arranged in a mirror image pattern, although mononuclear and multinucleate forms occur. In addition, there are varying numbers of lymphocytes, plasma cells, eosinophils and polymorphonuclear leucocytes. The lesions are classified into four distinct types, namely lymphocyte dependent, nodular sclerosing, mixed cellularity, and lymphocyte depleted, according to the proportions of the constituent cells (Lukes and Butler, 1966). Such a classification is of clinical importance since the prognosis is substantially better in the two former types than in the latter two. The paucity of data on the extra-nodal lesions involving the jaws does not allow any conclusion as to whether a similar classification can be applied to these lesions.

Herpes zoster is common in patients with Hodgkin's disease, occurring in approximately 15% of patients (Wilson, Marsa and Johnson, 1972; Goffinet, Glatstein and Merigan, 1972). It is generally considered that Hodgkin's disease is a neoplasm of T-lymphocytes and is accompanied by defects of cell-mediated immunity. It is likely that these defects contribute to the increased incidence of zoster infections. However, the precise relationship between the two is unclear since the changes in immune responsiveness occur early in the disease although zoster infections are usually late complications (Cassazza, Duvall and Carbone, 1966; Goffinet *et al.,* 1972). As a rare complication of herpes zoster infections of the trigeminal nerve in Hodgkin's disease, necrosis of the alveolar process and periodontal ligament may occur leading to loosening and exfoliation of the teeth (Delaire *et al.,* 1964; Chenitz, 1976; Vickery and Midda, 1976).

MALIGNANT GRANULOMA AND WEGENER'S GRANULOMATOSIS

Malignant granuloma classically arises within the nose, usually in the midline, but the oral tissues may become secondarily affected. It is a destructive, granulomatous lesion which causes progressive necrosis of the midline of the face, usually culminating in rapid death (Batsakis, 1979). Very occasionally the oral lesion may be the first sign (Garrett and Ludman, 1965; Hamilton, Sherrer and Schwartz, 1965; Butler and Thompson, 1972), in which case pain associated with the maxillary teeth is the commonest symptom. Irregular bone loss related to the teeth, with loss of the lamina dura, may be present radiographically.

The lesion is characterized by a diffuse granulomatous infiltrate of lymphocytes and histiocytes accompanied by varying amounts of necrosis and fibrosis (Fig. 8). The cellular infiltrate is usually

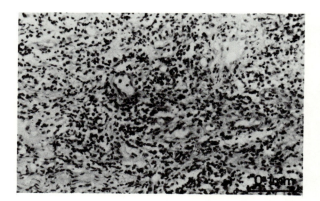

FIG. 8. Malignant granuloma of the maxilla. There is a mixed lympho-/histiocytic infiltrate, together with scattered polymorphonuclear leucocytes and some fibrosis. H & E. ×134.

well differentiated, showing none of the cellular features of malignant neoplasms. Vasculitis may be present. A more disseminated type of the disease is recognized (Friedman, 1964) although such variants may represent a form of Wegener's granulomatosis (Wegener, 1936). This condition is characterized by a triad of features: necrotizing granulomatous lesions of the upper and lower respiratory passages, generalized focal necrotizing vasculitis of arteries and veins, usually affecting the lungs, and glomerulitis with necrosis and thrombosis of the capillary loops, often accompanied by capsular adhesion (Godman and Churg, 1954). As with the malignant granuloma, the oral tissues may be involved, oral ulceration being the most common feature (Walton, 1958; Reed *et al.,* 1963; Scott and Finch, 1972a). Gingivitis may also occur and some cases exhibit an unusual form of granulomatous gingivitis in the early stages, which may be pathognomonic (Morgan and O'Neil, 1956; Reed *et al.,* 1963; Cawson, 1965; Kakehashi *et al.,* 1965; Brooke, 1969; Scott and Finch, 1972a; Edwards and Buckerfield, 1978). The gingiva is erythematous and granular, the changes spreading beyond the mucogingival junction, and, although they may be localized in the early stages, usually becoming segmental or panoral in distribution. Areas of irregular bone loss, with destruction of the lamina dura and periodontal ligament of the affected teeth, are often present. In Wegener's granulomatosis there is a polymorphic infiltrate of inflammatory cells with numerous polymorphonuclear leucocytes, lymphocytes and macrophages, some of them being multinucleate of both the foreign body and Langhan's type (Fig. 9). Tissue eosinophilia is frequently a pro-

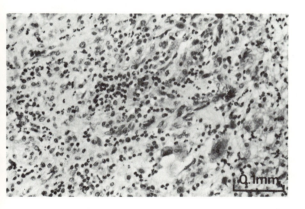

FIG. 9. Wegener's granulomatosis. A gingival biopsy containing a polymorphic infiltrate of polymorphonuclear leucocytes, lymphocytes, eosinophils and histiocytes, some of them multinucleate. H & E. ×134.

minent feature. Vasculitis with fibrinoid necrosis is not a significant finding in the periodontal lesions.

The aetiology and pathogenesis of both disorders are unknown, although hypersensitivity (Edwards and Buckerfield, 1978) and selective immunodeficiency (Shillitoe *et al.,* 1974) may be factors.

PLASMACYTOMA AND MULTIPLE MYELOMA

Plasma cell tumours uncommonly affect the jaws and when they do it is usually as a manifestation of multiple myelomatosis. Deposits of myeloma in the jaws most frequently arise in patients with established disease (Sherman, 1951), although occasionally the jaw lesions may be the first manifestations (Wolff and Nolan, 1944; Meloy, Gunter and Sampson, 1945; Calman, 1952; Ewing and Foote, 1952; Silverman and Shklar, 1962; Lewin and Cataldo, 1967). The reason for this probably arises from the observation that the tumour has a predilection for bones containing active haematopoietic marrow, and since multiple myelomatosis is uncommon before the sixth decade it is not surprising that the jaws are only infrequently involved, the mandible more often than the maxilla (Bruce and Quentin-Royer, 1953). However, it has been pointed out that deposits of myeloma can often be demonstrated histologically in bones in the absence of radiological changes (Linarzi, 1951) and it is likely that the jaws are involved more frequently than is generally reported (Bruce and Quentin-Royer, 1953; Cataldo and Meyer, 1966; Willis, 1967). It is suggested that myelomatosis is a multifocal disease rather than a single neoplasm that metastasizes (Christopherson and Miller, 1950) and therefore also sometimes occurs as a solitary tumour or plasmacytoma (Stout and Kenney, 1949; Christopherson and Miller, 1950; Ewing and Foote, 1952). However, it is possible that if most solitary lesions are followed up long enough, disseminated lesions will eventually appear (Lucas, 1976b).

Solitary tumours may arise within the bones of the jaws, most commonly in the mandible (Spitzer and Price, 1948; Christopherson and Miller, 1950; Ewing and Foote, 1952; Lane, 1952; Hinds, Pleasants and Bell, 1956; Whitlock and Hughes, 1960), or in the overlying soft tissues (Stout and Kenney, 1949; Ewing and Foote, 1952). In the latter sites, particularly when there is involvement of the gingiva, it may be difficult to distinguish between a solitary plasma cell neoplasm and dense infiltrations of plasma cells which are believed to be reactive in nature. Plasma cell infiltration is a feature of chronic periodontal disease, particularly in progressive chronic periodontitis and chronic hyperplastic gingivitis, although some authorities consider that when such infiltrates are prominent, they represent a specific disease process that has variably been called plasmacytosis (Poswillo, 1967; Ginwalla, Bhoweer and D'Silva, 1977) or plasma cell granuloma of the gingiva (Bhaskar, Levin and Frisch, 1968; Warson and Preis, 1969; Acevedo and Buhler, 1977). However, insufficient is known about these conditions at present to determine if they are distinct diseases or merely extreme variants of the chronic inflammatory process.

Whether the tumours are multiple or solitary, infiltration of the periodontal ligament may occur by spread of tumour cells from the medullary spaces of the mandible and maxilla or from the overlying soft tissues. Although pain is the most common complaint, looseness of the teeth may, therefore, be an early feature (Meloy *et al.,* 1945; Calman, 1952; Bruce and Quentin-Royer, 1953; Whitlock and Hughes, 1960; Orlean and Blewitt, 1965; Nally, 1968; Wood, 1975). When there is infiltration of the periodontal ligament there is usually radiographic evidence of irregular destruction of the lamina dura around the involved teeth (Calman, 1952; Bruce and Quentin-Royer, 1953; Whitlock and Hughes, 1960; Orlean and Blewitt, 1965; Nally, 1968; Wood, 1975), together with solitary or multiple 'punched-out' areas of radiolucency of variable size which may become confluent. Occasionally there may be single or multiple gingival swellings (Stout and Kenney, 1949; Bruce and Quentin-Royer, 1953; Smith, 1957; Orlean and Blewitt, 1965). In multiple myelomatosis there is often widespread replacement of the normal haematopoietic marrow tissue by tumour cells which may result in thrombocytopenia, and post-extraction haemorrhage (Ramon *et al.,* 1965) or delayed healing (Meloy *et al.,* 1945; Spitzer and Price, 1948; Hinds *et al.,* 1956) may occur.

When the periodontal ligament is involved in plasma cell tumours its structure is progressively destroyed by the dense infiltrate of plasma cells (Fig. 10). They may exhibit some pleomorphism and binucleate and occasionally multinucleate forms may be present. The tumour has a scant stroma of reticulin fibres within which deposition of amyloid sometimes occurs. Occasionally active resorption of the tooth root may be present.

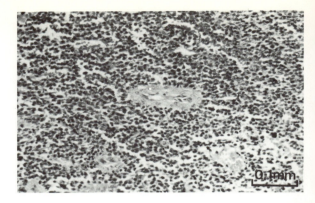

FIG. 10. Multiple myelomatosis. The tissue of the mandible is infiltrated by a dense mass of plasmacytoid cells. There is total destruction of the normal tissue components, only the blood vessels remaining. H & E. × 134.

With multiple tumours abnormal, monoclonal immunoglobulin paraproteins can be demonstrated in the serum and Bence–Jones protein in the urine, although these are not usually present in solitary tumours. In addition amyloidosis may arise as a complication of multiple myelomatosis in 7–15% of cases (Gold, 1961) and deposits of amyloid may occur in the oral mucosa, particularly in the tongue (Cahn, 1957; Tillman, 1957). Although such deposits can also rarely be demonstrated in the gingiva (Calkins and Cohen, 1960) in multiple myelomatosis, there is no evidence of involvement of the periodontal ligament.

Deposition of amyloid in the gingiva in primary and secondary amyloidosis (Symmers, 1956) is probably more common than in myelomatosis, although the frequency has varied greatly in different reports from 0 to 78% (Selikoff and Robizek, 1947; Gorlin and Gottsegen, 1949; Symmers, 1956; Cooke, 1958; Calkins and Cohen, 1960; Trieger, Cohen and Calkins, 1960; Lovett, Cross and van Allen, 1965; Pettersson and Wegelius, 1972; van der Waal, Fehmers and Kraal, 1973). In the early stages the deposits occur only in the walls of the small blood vessels and sinusoids and at the basement membrane of the gingival epithelium and do not therefore cause any clinical signs. There are no reports of deposits in the walls of the blood vessels of the periodontal ligament in man, although they have been demonstrated experimentally in mice 22 weeks following the subcutaneous injection of casein (Miller and Clark,

1968). Further there is a report of a primary form of the disease in two siblings, aged 7 and 12, in whom in addition to gingival hyperplasia, there was loosening of some of the teeth, although there was no histological examination of the periodontal ligament (Hornova and Dluhosova, 1968).

HISTIOCYTOSIS X

The histiocytoses comprise a group of disorders of unknown aetiology which are characterized by the presence of solitary or multiple destructive histiocytic lesions. The histiocytes often contain large quantities of lipid and in some disorders, the lipid histiocytoses, the nature of the lipid has been identified, such as in Niemann—Pick disease (sphingomyelin) and Gaucher disease (cerebroside). In others, the so-called non-lipid histiocytoses, the nature of the lipid is uncertain. It is these latter which may particularly affect the periodontal tissues.

Three particular forms of the non-lipid histiocytoses have been identified. Letterer—Siwe disease is the acute disseminated form in which almost any tissue of the body may be affected. This eponym was first proposed by Abt and Denenholz (1936) after the original descriptions of the disease (Letterer, 1924; Siwe, 1933). If not present at birth, it is usually manifest during the first 6 months of life and rapidly fatal. Hand—Schüller—Christian disease, named eponymously after the original descriptions (Hand, 1893; Schüller, 1915; Christian, 1919), is the chronic disseminated form of the disease and affects particularly the skeleton and certain viscera, notably the lungs, liver and spleen. The original descriptions drew attention to a triad of features, namely exophthalmos, diabetes insipidus and multiple skeletal lesions, although this triad is probably present in only 10% of cases. The disease is usually diagnosed in the first decade of life and is fatal in from 30 to 70%. Eosinophilic granuloma (Lichtenstein and Jaffe, 1940) is the localized form of the disease, usually affecting only one bone. It is usually diagnosed in adolescents and adults before the age of 30, and is only rarely fatal. It is widely believed that these three disorders are variants of the same disease process and as such there are many examples which do not fit clearly into one category or the other. As a

consequence the term histiocytosis X (Lichtenstein, 1953, 1964) is used to cover the entire range of these diseases.

Oral lesions are common in histiocytosis X, having been variably reported from 21% to 77% (Sleeper, 1951; Blevins *et al.*, 1959; Sedano *et al.*, 1969; Lucaya, 1971; Sigala *et al.*, 1972). Of greater importance is the fact that the oral lesions are the presenting symptoms in 10—28% of cases (Blevins *et al.*, 1959; Sedano *et al.*, 1969; Lucaya, 1971; Sigala *et al.*, 1972). In Letterer—Siwe disease and Hand—Schüller—Christian disease the most common change is the presence of ulcero-necrotic enlargement of the gingiva, together with looseness of the teeth (Blevins *et al.*, 1959; Johnson and Mohnac, 1967; Sedano *et al.*, 1969; Sigala *et al.*, 1972; Scott and Finch, 1972b). These changes most commonly occur in the mandible and usually first affect the molar teeth and subsequently spread to involve the anterior teeth. The ulcero-necrotic lesions lead to marked halitosis. The bone loss may progress rapidly and lead to premature loss of the primary and permanent teeth.

Radiographically there is advanced bone loss around the affected teeth, with loss of the lamina dura (Winther, Fejerskov and Philipsen, 1972) and often marked areas of radiolucency. The destruction of alveolar bone may be so complete that the teeth, particularly in the molar regions, have the appearance of floating in the alveolus (Keusch, Poole and King, 1966; Fasulo and Vangaasbeek, 1966; Boggs and McMahon, 1968; Schofield and Gardner, 1971; Betts and McNeish, 1972; Uthman, 1974). Several authors have emphasized that the histiocytoses are an important cause of advanced periodontal disease in children (Kaufman, 1951; Holst, Husted and Pindborg, 1953; Blevins *et al.*, 1959; Meranus *et al.*, 1968; Schofield and Gardner, 1971). In addition, cyst-like osteolytic lesions may be present.

In eosinophilic granuloma, osteolytic lesions of the jaws are the more common presentation. Not uncommonly these are associated with the apical regions of the teeth, thus simulating both clinically and radiologically a periapical granuloma, abscess or cyst and may in the first instance be treated as such (Whitehead, 1972; Carraro *et al.*, 1972). However, the lesions will recur and spread to involve adjacent teeth or other parts of the jaw.

In all forms of histiocytosis X the periodontal ligament of the involved teeth is extensively infiltrated and destroyed by the dense histiocytic infiltrate. In Letterer–Siwe disease and Hand–Schüller–Christian disease the infiltrate consists of large numbers of histiocytes (Fig. 11) which contain

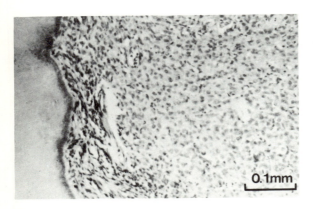

FIG. 11. Hand–Schüller–Christian disease. The periodontal ligament has been infiltrated by large histiocytic cells, together with scattered lymphocytes and eosinophils. Residual collagen fibres persist in the lower part of the field. H & E. ×134.

varying numbers of fat droplets (Georgiewa *et al.,* 1965; Ritter, 1966; Markert, 1967) and may assume such large proportions to give the cells the appearance of foam cells, particularly in Hand–Schüller–Christian disease. Varying numbers of eosinophils are present. As the lesion progresses there may be some fibrosis. Occasionally resorption of the cementum of the tooth root occurs (Carraro, de Sereday and Sznajder, 1967).

In eosinophilic granuloma, the cellular infiltrate is more mixed and contains variable proportions of histiocytes, lymphocytes and eosinophils, although the latter usually predominate (Fig. 12). The eosinophils typically are formed into focal groups, the centres of which are often necrotic. The focal areas of necrosis may become confluent and form a predominant feature of the lesion. As the lesion progresses, there is increasing fibrosis and the characteristic cellular infiltrate may become decreasingly conspicuous.

The aetiology of histiocytosis X is unknown, and although it is generally believed that Letterer–Siwe

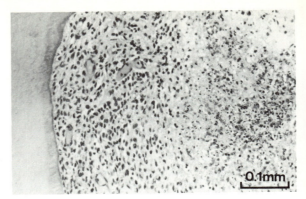

FIG. 12. Eosinophilic granuloma. The periodontal ligament is infiltrated with eosinophils, histiocytes and lymphocytes and its normal structure has been destroyed. To the right there is a focal group of eosinophils, which is necrotic. H & E. ×134.

disease and Hand–Schüller–Christian disease are neoplastic forms, and eosinophilic granuloma a reactive form, the evidence for this is slight.

REFERENCES

ABT, A. F. & DENENHOLZ, E. J. (1936) Letterer–Siwe's disease. *Amer. J. Dis. Child.* **51**, 499–522.

ACEVEDO, A. & BUHLER, J. E. (1977) Plasma cell granuloma of the gingiva. *Oral Surg.* **43**, 196–200.

ADATIA, A. K. (1966) Burkitt's tumour in the jaws. *Br. dent. J.* **120**, 315–326.

ADATIA, A. K. (1968a) Response of the dental elements to chemotherapy of Burkitt's tumour. *Int. dent. J.* **18**, 646–654.

ADATIA, A. K. (1968b) Dental tissues and Burkitt's tumour. *Oral Surg.* **25**, 221–234.

ADATIA, A. K. (1970) Dental aspects. In: *Burkitt's lymphoma,* D. P. BURKITT & D. H. WRIGHT (eds.), p. 36. Edinburgh, Livingstone.

ADATIA, A. K. (1973) Dental changes in Burkitt's lymphoma. *Pathol. Microbiol.* **39**, 196–203.

AMES, M. I. (1958) Oral manifestations of Hodgkin's disease. *Oral Surg.* **11**, 155–157.

AMOROSI, E. L. & ULTMANN, J. E. (1966) Thrombotic thrombocytopenic purpura: report of 16 cases and review of the literature. *Medicine* **45**, 139–159.

ANDREWS, J. P., McCLELLAN, J. T. & SCOTT, C. H. (1960) Lethal congenital neutropenia with eosinophilia occurring in two siblings. *Amer. J. Med.* **29**, 358–362.

ANDREWS, R. G., BENJAMIN, S., SHORE, N. & CANTER, S. (1965) Chronic benign neutropenia of childhood with associated oral manifestations. *Oral Surg.* **20**, 719–725.

ATTSTRÖM, R. & EGELBERG, J. (1971a) Effect of experimental leucopenia on chronic gingival inflammation in dogs. I. Induction of leucopenia by nitrogen mustard. *J. periodont. Res.* 6, 194–199.

ATTSTRÖM, R. & EGELBERG, J. (1971b) Effect of experimental leucopenia on chronic gingival inflammation in dogs. II. Induction of leucopenia by heterologous anti-neutrophil serum. *J. periodont. Res.* 6, 200–210.

ATTSTRÖM, R. & SCHROEDER, H. E. (1979) Effect of experimental neutropenia on initial gingivitis in dogs. *Scand. J. dent. Res.* 87, 7–23.

AWBREY, J. J. & HIBBARD, E. D. (1973) Congenital agranulocytosis. *Oral Surg.* 35, 526–530.

BANKS, P. (1967) Infectious mononucleosis: a problem of differential diagnosis to the oral surgeon. *Br. J. oral Surg.* 4, 227–234.

BASU, M. K., POLLOCK, A. & GORDON, P. A. (1978) Serum and salivary immunoglobulin in acute myelogenous leukaemia. *Proc. 17th Cong. Int. Soc. Haematol.*, p. 792. Paris. II.

BATSAKIS, J. G. (1979) Tumours of the head and neck. *Clinical and pathological considerations* (2nd ed.), pp. 492–500. Baltimore, Williams & Wilkins.

BAUER, W. (1946) The supporting tissues of the tooth in acute secondary agranulocytosis (arsphenamin neutropenia). *J. dent. Res.* 25, 501–508.

BENDER, I. B. (1944) Bone changes in leukaemia. *Amer. J. Orthod.* 30, 556–563.

BENNETT, M. H., FARRER-BROWN, G., HENRY, K. & JELIFFE, A. M. (1974) Classification of non-Hodgkin's lymphomas. *Lancet* 2, 405–406.

BERENDES, H., BRIDGES, R. A. & GOOD, R. A. (1957) A fatal granulomatosis of childhood: the clinical study of a new syndrome. *Minn. Med.* 40, 309–312.

BERKHEISER, S. W. (1957) Studies on the comparative morphology of monocytic leukaemia, granulocytic leukaemia and reticulum-cell sarcoma. *Cancer* 10, 606–616.

BETTS, P. R. & McNEISH, A. S. (1972) Oral manifestations of Letterer–Siwe disease. *Archs. Dis. Child.* 47, 463–464.

BHASKAR, S. N., LEVIN, M. P. & FRISCH, J. (1968) Plasma cell granuloma of periodontal tissues: report of 45 cases. *Periodontics* 6, 272–276.

BHOWEER, A. L., SHIRWATKAR, L. G. & DESAI, A. J. (1977) Possible congenital deficiency of factor X (Stuart-Prower): a case report. *Ann. Dent.* 36, 1–7.

BIGGAR, W. D., HOLMES, B., PAGE, A. R., DEINARD, A. S., L'ESPERANCE, P. & GOOD, R. A. (1974) Metabolic and functional studies of monocytes in congenital neutropenia. *Br. J. Haematol.* 28, 233–243.

BINNIE, W. H., BRET DAY, R. C. & LYNN, A. H. (1971) Lymphosarcoma presenting with oral symptoms. *Br. dent. J.* 130, 235–238.

BINON, P. P. & DYKEMA, R. W. (1974) Rehabilitative management of cyclic neutropenia. *J. Prosthet. Dent.* 31, 52–60.

BLAKE, M. N. & BECK, L. (1963) Reticulum cell sarcoma: report of a case. *J. oral Surg.* 21, 165–168.

BLEVINS, C., DAHLIN, D. C., LOVESTEDT, S. A. & KENNEDY, R. L. J. (1959) Oral and dental manifestations of histiocytosis X. *Oral Surg.* 12, 473–483.

BLUME, R. S., BENNETT, J. M., YANKEE, R. A. & WOLFF, S. M. (1968) Defective granulocyte regulation in the Chediak–Higashi syndrome. *New Engl. J. Med.* 279, 1009–1015.

BLUME, R. S. & WOLFF, S. M. (1972) The Chediak–Higashi Syndrome: Studies in four patients and a review of the literature. *Medicine* 51, 245–280.

BODEY, G. P. (1971) Oral complications of the myeloproliferative diseases. *Postgrad. Med.* 49, 115–121.

BODEY, G. P., BUCKLEY, M., SATHE, Y. S. & FREIREICH, E. J. (1966) Quantitative relationships between circulating leukocytes and infection in patients with acute leukaemia. *Ann. Intern. Med.* 64, 328–340.

BOGGS, D. C. & McMAHON, L. J. (1968) Hand–Schüller–Christian disease presenting as gingivitis. *Oral Surg.* 26, 261–264.

BOGGS, D. R., WINTROBE, M. M. & CARTWRIGHT, G. E. (1962) The acute leukaemias. *Medicine* 41, 163–225.

BROOKE, R. I. (1969) Wegener's granulomatosis involving the gingivae. *Br. dent. J.* 127, 34–36.

BROWN, L. R., DREIZEN, S. & BODEY, G. P. (1973) Effect of immuno-suppression on the human oral flora. Comparative immunology of the oral cavity. *DHEW Publication No. (NIH)* 73–428, 204–220.

BRUCE, K. W. & QUENTIN-ROYER, R. (1953) Multiple myeloma occurring in the jaws. *Oral Surg.* 6, 729–744.

BURKETT, L. W. (1940) Histopathologic explanation for oral lesions in acute leukaemia. *Amer. J. Orthod.* 30, 516–523.

BURKITT, D. (1958) A sarcoma involving jaws in African children. *Br. J. Surg.* 46, 218–224.

BURKITT, D. (1964) A lymphoma syndrome dependent upon the environment. Part I. Clinical aspects. In: *Symposium on Lymphomatous Tumours in Africa,* 1963. F. C. ROULET (ed.), p. 80. Basel, Karger.

BURKITT, D. & DAVIES, J. N. P. (1961) Lymphoma syndrome in Uganda and tropical Africa. *Med. Press.* 245, 367–369.

BUTLER, D. J. & THOMPSON, H. (1972) Malignant granuloma. *Br. J. oral Surg.* 9, 208–221.

CAHN, L. (1957) Oral amyloid as a complication of myelomatosis. *Oral Surg.* 10, 735–742.

CAIRD, F. I. & HOLT, P. R. (1958) The enanthema of glandular fever. *Br. Med. J.* 1, 85–87.

CALDERWOOD, R. G. (1967) Primary reticulum cell sarcoma of gingiva. *Oral Surg.* 24, 71–77.

CALKINS, E. & COHEN, A. S. (1960) Diagnosis of amyloidosis. *Bull. Haem. Dis.* 10, 215–218.

CALMAN, H. I. (1952) Multiple myeloma. Report of a case first observed in the maxilla. *Oral Surg.* 5, 1302–1311.

CARRANZA, F. A. (1979) *Glickman's clinical periodontology* (5th ed.), pp. 529–530. Philadelphia, Saunders.

CARRANZA, F. A. (1979) *Glickman's clinical periodontology* (5th ed.), pp. 529–530. Philadelphia, Saunders. 374–379.

CARRARO, J. J., DE SEREDAY, M. & SZNAJDER, N. (1967) Oral manifestations of histiocytosis X. *J. Periodont.* 38, 521–525.

CARRARO, J. J., SZNAJDER, N., BARROS, R. & LALIS, R. M. (1972) Periodontal involvement in eosinophilic granuloma. *J. Periodont.* 43, 427–432.

CASSAZZA, A. R., DUVALL, C. P. & CARBONE, P. P. (1966) Infection in lymphoma. Histology, treatment and duration in relation to incidence and survival. *J. Amer. Med. Assoc.* 197, 710–716.

CASSINGHAM, R. J. (1971) Infectious mononucleosis. A review of the literature, including recent findings on etiology. *Oral Surg.* **31**, 610–623.

CATALDO, E. & MEYER, I. (1966) Solitary and multiple plasma cell tumours of the jaws and oral cavity. *Oral Surg.* **22**, 628–639.

CATENA, D. L. (1975) Oral manifestations of the haemoglobinopathies. *Dent. Clin. N. Amer.* **19**, 1, 77–85.

CAWSON, R. A. (1965) Gingival changes in Wegener's granulomatosis. *Br. dent. J.* **118**, 30–32.

CHAUDHRY, A. P. & VICKERS, R. A. (1962) Primary reticulum cell sarcoma of the mouth. Report of a case. *J. oral Surg.* **20**, 159–162.

CHEDIAK, M. M. (1952) Nouvelle anomalie leucocytaire de caractère constitutionel et familial. *Revue Hématol.* **7**, 362–367.

CHENITZ, J. E. (1976) Herpes zoster in Hodgkin's disease: unusual oral sequelae. *J. Dent. Child.* **43**, 184–186.

CHRISTIAN, H. A. (1919) Defects in membranous bones, exophthalmos and diabetes insipidus, an unusual syndrome of dyspituitarism. *Med. Clin. N. Amer.* **3**, 849–871.

CHRISTOPHERSON, W. M. & MILLER, A. J. (1950) A re-evaluation of solitary plasma-cell myeloma of bone. *Cancer* **3**, 240–252.

CLARK, R. A. & KIMBALL, H. R. (1971) Defective granulocyte chemotaxis in the Chediak–Higashi syndrome. *J. Clin. Invest.* **50**, 2645–2652.

COHEN, D. W. & MORRIS, A. L. (1961) Periodontal manifestations of cyclic neutropenia. *J. Periodont.* **32**, 159–168.

COHEN, L. (1965) Recurrent oral ulceration and cutaneous infections associated with cyclical neutropenia. *Dent. Pract.* **16**, 97–98.

COHEN, M. M. (1977) Stomatologic alterations in childhood, Part III. *J. Dent. Child.* **44**, 396–400.

CONTRATTO, A. W. (1944) Infectious mononucleosis. A study of one hundred and ninety-six cases. *Archs. Intern. Med.* **73**, 449–459.

COOK, H. P. (1961) Oral lymphomas. *Oral Surg.* **14**, 690–704.

COOKE, B. E. D. (1958) Biopsy procedures. *Oral Surg.* **11**, 750–761.

COURANT, P. & SOBKOV, T. (1969) Oral manifestations of infectious mononucleosis. *J. Periodont.* **40**, 279–283.

CURTIS, A. B. (1971) Childhood leukaemias: osseous changes in jaws on panoramic dental radiographs. *J. Amer. dent. Assoc.* **83**, 844–847.

CUTTING, H. D. & LANG, J. E. (1964) Familial benign chronic neutropenia. *Ann. Intern. Med.* **61**, 876–887.

DAVEY, K. W. & KONCHAK, P. A. (1969) Agranulocytosis. Dental case report. *Oral Surg.* **28**, 166–171.

DAVIES, J. N. P. (1964) Lymphomas and leukemias in Uganda Africans. In: *Symposium on Lymphomatous Tumours in Africa,* Paris, 1963, F. C. ROULET (ed.), p. 67. Basel, Karger.

DAY, P. L., LANGSTON, W. C. & DARBY, W. J. (1938) Failure of nicotinic acid to prevent nutritional cytopenia in the monkey. *Proc. Soc. Exp. Biol. Med.* **38**, 860–863.

DEASY, M. J., VOGEL, R. I., ANNES, I. K. & SIMON, B. I. (1976) Periodontal disease associated with pre-leukaemic syndrome. *J. Periodont.* **47**, 41–45.

DELAIRE, J., GALLARD, A., BILLET, J. & RENAUD, Y. (1964) Le zona et ses manifestations faciales. *Acta Odontostomatol.* **65**, 7–22.

DENT, P. B., FISH, L. A., WHITE, J. G. & GOOD, R. A. (1966) Chediak–Higashi syndrome. Observations on the nature of the associated malignancy. *Lab. Invest.* **15**, 1634–1642.

DEUTSCH, C. M., DREIZEN, S. & STAHL, S. S. (1969) The effects of chronic iron deficiency anaemia on the periodontium of the adult rat. *J. Periodont.* **40**, 736–739.

DORFMAN, R. F. (1974) Classification of non-Hodgkin's lymphomas. *Lancet* **2**, 961–962.

DREIZEN, A. (1971) Oral indications of the deficiency states. *Postgrad. Med.* **49**, 97–102.

DREIZEN, S., BODEY, G. P. & BROWN, L. R. (1974) Opportunist Gram-negative bacillary infections in leukaemia. Oral manifestations during immunosuppression. *Postgrad. Med.* **55**, 133–139.

DREIZEN, S., LEVY, B. M. & BERNICK, S. (1969) Studies on the biology of the periodontium of marmosets. VII. The effect of vitamin C deficiency on the marmoset periodontium. *J. periodont. Res.* **4**, 274–280.

DREIZEN, S., LEVY, B. M. & BERNICK, S. (1970) Studies on the biology of the periodontium of marmosets. VIII. The effect of folic acid deficiency on the marmoset oral mucosa. *J. dent. Res.* **49**, 616–620.

DUFFY, J. H. & DRISCOLL, E. J. (1958) Oral manifestations of leukaemia. *Oral Surg.* **11**, 484–490.

DUNNET, W. N. (1963) Infectious mononucleosis. *Br. Med. J.* **1**, 1187–1191.

DUPUY, J. M., KOURILSKY, F. M., FRADELIZZI, D., FEINGOLD, N., JACQUILLAT, C., BERNARD, J. & DAUSSET, J. (1971) Depression of immunologic reactivity of patients with acute leukaemia. *Cancer* **27**, 323–331.

EDINGTON, G. M., MacLEAN, C. H. U. & OKUBADEJO, O. A. (1964) 101 necropsies on tumours of the reticulo-endothelial system in Ibadan, Nigeria, with special reference to childhood lymphoma. In: *Symposium on Lymphomatous Tumours in Africa,* Paris, 1963, F. C. ROULET (ed.), p. 236. Basel, Karger.

EDWARDS, M. B. & BUCKERFIELD, J. P. (1978) Wegener's granulomatosis: a case with primary mucocutaneous lesions. *Oral Surg.* **46**, 53–63.

EL-ASHIRY, G. M., RINGSDORF, W. M. J. & CHERASKIN, E. (1964) Local and systemic influences in periodontal disease. II. Effect of prophylaxis and natural versus synthetic vitamin C upon gingivitis. *J. Periodont.* **35**, 250–259.

EVANS, A. S. (1972) Infectious mononucleosis and other monolike syndromes. *New Engl. J. Med.* **286**, 836–838.

EVANS, A. S. (1974) The history of infectious mononucleosis. *Amer. J. Med. Sci.* **267**, 189–195.

EVANS, A. S., NIEDERMAN, J. C. & McCOLLUM, R. W. (1968) Seroepidemiologic studies of infectious mononucleosis with EB virus. *New Engl. J. Med.* **279**, 1121–1127.

EWING, M. R. & FOOTE, F. W. (1952) Plasma-cell tumours of the mouth and upper air passages. *Cancer* **5**, 499–513.

FASULO, C. P. & VANGAASBEEK, J. B. (1966) Hand–

Schüller–Christian disease. Medical and surgical problems involved. *Oral Surg.* 22, 555–563.

FERGUSON, M. M. (1975) Oral mucous membrane markers of internal disease: Part II, disorders of the endocrine system, haematopoietic system and nutrition. In: *Oral mucosa in health and disease*, A. E. DOLBY (ed.), pp. 232–299. Oxford, Blackwell.

FLANAGAN, V., BROWN, L. R., ROTH, G. D., HOOVER, D. R., NIELSEN, A. H. & WERDER, A. A. (1970) Histopathologic changes in the oral tissue of leukaemic and non-leukaemic mice. *J. Periodont.* 41, 526–531.

FORMAN, G. H. & WESSON, C. M. (1970) Hodgkin's disease of the mandible. *Br. J. oral Surg.* 7, 146–152.

FOX, P. C., GORDON, R. E. & WILLIAMS, A. C. (1977) Thrombotic thrombocytopenic purpura: report of a case. *J. oral Surg. Anaesth. Hosp. Dent. Serv.* 35, 921–923.

FRANKLIN, A. L., STOKSTAD, E. L. R., BELT, M. & JUKES, T. H. (1947) Biochemical experiments with a synthetic preparation having an action antagonistic to that of pteroylglutamic acid. *J. Biol. Chem.* 169, 427–435.

FRASER-MOODIE, W. (1959) Oral lesions in infectious mononucleosis. *Oral Surg.* 12, 685–691.

FRIEDMAN, I. (1964) Midline granuloma. *Proc. R. Soc. Med.* 57, 289–297.

FULLER, L. M., BANKER, F. L., BUTLER, J. J., GAMBLE, J. F. & SULLIVAN, M. P. (1975) The natural history of non-Hodgkin's lymphomata stages I and II. *Br. J. Cancer* 31, Suppl. II, 270–285.

FUSCILLA, I. S. & HANNAM, A. (1961) Hodgkin's disease in bone. *Radiology* 77, 53–60.

GARRETT, J. R. & LUDMAN, H. (1965) Delayed healing of an extraction socket caused by a malignant granulomatous condition. *Br. J. oral Surg.* 3, 92–96.

GATES, G. F. (1969) Chronic neutropenia presenting with oral lesions. *Oral Surg.* 27, 563–567.

GEORGIEWA, S., GEORGIEV, G., HADJIOLOV, A. I. & ZANRUSCHANOV, I. (1965) Histiochemie der Lipide in den Reticulohistiocyten bei einem Fall von Letterer–Siwescher Krankheit. *Arch. Klin. Exp. Derm.* 221, 348–357.

GERARD-MARCHANT, R., HAMLIN, I., LENNERT, K., RILKE, F., STANFELD, A. G. & VAN UNNIK, J. A. M. (1974) Classification of non-Hodgkin's lymphomas. *Lancet* 2, 406–408.

GERRY, R. G. & WILLIAMS, S. F. (1955) Primary reticulum cell sarcoma of the mandible. *Oral Surg.* 8, 568–581.

GILLIG, J. L. & CALDWELL, C. H. (1970) The Chediak–Higashi Syndrome: case report. *J. dent. Child.* 37, 527–529.

GINWALLA, T. M. S., BHOWEER, A. L. & D'SILVA, I. R. (1977) Plasmacytosis of the gingiva. *J. oral Med.* 32, 75–78.

GLICKMAN, I. (1948) Acute vitamin C deficiency and periodontal disease. II. The effect of acute vitamin C deficiency upon the response of the periodontal tissues of the guinea pig to artificially induced inflammation. *J. dent. Res.* 27, 201–210.

GLICKMAN, I. (1964) Nutrition in the prevention and treatment of gingival and periodontal diseases. *J. dent. Med.* 19, 179–183.

GODMAN, G. C. & CHURG, J. (1954) Wegener's granulomatosis. Pathology and review of the literature. *Archs. Path.* 58, 533–553.

GOFFINET, D. R., GLATSTEIN, E. J. & MERIGAN, T. C. (1972) Herpes zoster varicella infections and lymphoma. *Ann. Intern. Med.* 76, 235–240.

GOLD, B. G. (1961) Amyloidosis. *J. oral Surg.* 19, 136–139.

GOLDENFARB, P. B. & FINCH, S. C. (1973) Thrombotic thrombocytopenic purpura: A ten year survey. *J. Amer. Med. Assoc.* 226, 644–647.

GOOD, R. A. & FISHER, D. W. (1971) *Immunobiology*, pp. 55–61. Stamford, Sinaver.

GORLIN, R. J. & CHAUDHRY, A. P. (1960) The oral manifestations of cyclic (periodic) neutropenia. *Archs. Derm.* 82, 344–347.

GORLIN, R. J. & GOTTSEGEN, R. (1949) The role of the gingival biopsy in secondary amyloid disease. *Oral Surg.* 2, 864–866.

GOULD, J. F. & MAIN, J. H. P. (1969) Primary lymphosarcoma of the maxillary alveolar process. *Oral Surg.* 28, 106–108.

GREEN, D. (1974) Haemophilia. *Postgrad. Med.* 55, 129–133.

GROSSMAN, R. C. (1975) Orthodontics and dentistry for the haemophilic patients. *Amer. J. Orthodont.* 68, 391–403.

GUSTAFFSON, G. T. (1969) Increased susceptibility to periodontitis in mink affected by a lysosomal disease. *J. periodont. Res.* 4, 259–267.

HALSTEAD, C. L. (1970) Oral manifestations of haemoglobinopathies. A case of homozygous haemoglobin C disease diagnosed as a result of dental radiographic changes. *Oral Surg.* 30, 615–623.

HAMILTON, M. K., SHERRER, E. L. & SCHWARTZ, D. S. (1965) Lethal midline granuloma: report of a case. *J. oral Surg.* 23, 514–520.

HAMILTON, R. E. & GIANSANTI, J. S. (1974) The Chediak–Higashi Syndrome. *Oral Surg.* 37, 754–761.

HAND, A. Jr. (1893) Polyuria and tuberculosis. *Archs. Pediat.* 10, 673.

HARRINGTON, W. J., MINNICH, V. & ARIMURA, G. (1956) The autoimmune thrombocytopenias. *Prog. Hemat.* 1, 166–192.

HARVEY, W. & THOMSON, A. D. (1966) A case of reticulum cell sarcoma of gums and skin. *Br. J. oral Surg.* 3, 152–157.

HELLEM, A. J. (1960) The adhesiveness of human blood platelets *in vitro*. *Scand. J. Clin. Lab. Invest.* 12, Suppl. 51.

HENLE, G., HENLE, W. & DIEHL, V. (1968) Relation of Burkitt's tumour-associated herpes type virus to infectious mononucleosis. *Proc. Natl Acad. Sci., USA* 59, 74–101.

HERSH, E. M., BODEY, G. P., NIES, B. A. & FREIREICH, E. J. (1965) The causes of death in acute leukaemia. A study of 414 patients from 1954–1963. *J. Amer. Med. Assoc.* 193, 105–109.

HIGASHI, O. (1954) Congenital giantism of peroxidase granules. *Tohuku J. Exp. Med.* 59, 315–332.

HILL, J. B. & COOPER, W. M. (1968) Thrombotic thrombocytopenic purpura. Treatment with corticosteroids and splenectomy. *Archs. Intern. Med.* 122, 353–358.

HINDS, E. C., PLEASANTS, J. E. & BELL, W. E. (1956)

Solitary plasma cell myeloma of the mandible. *Oral Surg.* **9**, 193–202.

HOAGLAND, R. J. (1960) The clinical manifestations of infectious mononucleosis. *Amer. J. Med. Sci.* **240**, 55–63.

HOAGLAND, R. J. (1964) The incubation period of infectious mononucleosis. *Amer. J. Publ. Hlth* **54**, 1699–1705.

HODGES, R. E., HOOD, J., CANHAM, J. E., SAUBERLICH, H. E. & BAKER, E. M. (1971) Clinical manifestations of ascorbic acid deficiency in man. *Amer. J. Clin. Nutr.* **24**, 432–443.

HOLST, G., HUSTED, E. & PINDBORG, J. J. (1953) On the eosinophilic bone granuloma with regard to localisation in the jaws and relation to general histiocytosis. *Acta odont. Scand.* **10**, 148–179.

HORNOVA, J. & DLUHOSOVA, A. (1968) Primary amyloidosis of gingiva and conjunctiva and mental disorder in a brother and sister. *Oral Surg.* **25**, 457–464.

HUBLER, W. R. & NETHERTON, E. W. (1947) Cutaneous manifestations of monocytic leukaemia. *Archs. Derm. Syph.* **56**, 70–89.

JACKSON, H. & PARKER, F. (1945) Hodgkin's disease. IV. Involvement of certain organs. *New Engl. J. Med.* **232**, 547–559.

JOHNSON, R. E., CHRETIEN, P. B., O'CONOR, G. T., DEVITA, V. T. & THOMAS, L. B. (1974) Radiotherapeutic implications of prospective staging in non-Hodgkin's lymphoma. *Radiology* **110**, 655–657.

JOHNSON, R. P. & MOHNAC, A. H. (1967) Histiocytosis X: report of 7 cases. *J. oral Surg.* **25**, 7–21.

JOHNSTON, R. B. Jr. & BAEHNER, R. L. (1971) Chronic granulomatous disease: correlation between pathogenesis and clinical findings. *Pediatrics* **48**, 730–739.

JONES, J. H. (1973) The oral mucous membrane marker of internal disease. *Br. dent. J.* **134**, 81–87.

JONES, J. H. (1975) Healthy and diseased gingiva. *Practitioner* **214**, 356–364.

JORDAN, M. C. (1975) Nomenclature for mononucleosis syndromes. *J. Amer. Med. Assoc.* **234**, 45–46.

JORDAN, M. C., ROUSSEAU, W. E., STEWART, J. A., NOBLE, G. R. & CHIN, T. D. Y. (1973) Spontaneous cytomegalovirus mononucleosis. Clinical and laboratory observations in nine cases. *Ann. Intern. Med.* **79**, 153–160.

JOYNSON, D. M. H., JACOBS, A., WALKER, M. & DOLBY, A. E. (1972) Defect of cell mediated immunity in patients with iron-deficiency anaemia. *Lancet* **II**, 1058–1059.

JUDSON, S. C., HENLE, W. & HENLE, G. (1977) A cluster of Epstein–Barr virus associated American Burkitt's lymphoma. *New Engl. J. Med.* **297**, 464–468.

KAKEHASHI, S., HAMNER, J. E., BAER, P. N. & McINTIRE, J. A. (1965) Wegener's granulomatosis. Report of a case involving the gingiva. *Oral Surg.* **19**, 120–127.

KAUFMAN, J. & LOWENSTEIN, L. (1940) A study of the acute leukoses. *Ann. Intern. Med.* **14**, 903–915.

KAUFMAN, M. (1951) Eosinophilic granuloma of bone. *J. oral Surg.* **9**, 273–281.

KAY, A. B., WHITE, A. G., BARCLAY, G. R., DARG, C., RAEBURN, J. A., UTTLEY, W. S., McCRAE, W. M. & INNES, E. M. (1976) Leukocyte function in a case of chronic benign neutropenia of infancy

associated with circulating leucoagglutinins. *Br. J. Haemat.* **32**, 451–457.

KEENE, J. J., HUSSMAN, L., & BRUNER, G. (1972) Terminal oral manifestations of acute lymphoblastic leukaemia. *J. oral Med.* **27**, 117–119.

KENNEDY, D. J. (1957) Reticulum cell sarcoma of the maxilla. *Oral Surg.* **10**, 819–823.

KEUSCH, K. D., POOLE, C. A. & KING, D. R. (1966) The significance of 'floating teeth' in children. *Radiology* **86**, 215–219.

KLEMOLA, E. & KAARIAINEN, L. (1965) Cytomegalovirus as a possible cause of a disease resembling infectious mononucleosis. *Br. Med. J.* **2**, 1099–1102.

KLEMOLA, E., VON ESSEN, R., HENLE, G. & HENLE, W. (1970) Infectious mononucleosis-like disease with negative heterophil agglutination test: clinical features in relation to Epstein–Barr virus and cytomegalovirus antibodies. *J. Infect. Dis.* **121**, 608–614.

KOSTMAN, R. (1956) Infantile genetic agranulocytosis (agranulocytosis infantilis hereditaria), new recessive lethal disease in man. *Acta Paediat. Stockh.* Suppl. 105, **45**, 1–78.

KRAMER, I. R. H. (1965) Malignant lymphoma of children in Africa. *Int. dent. J.* **15**, 200–208.

KRITZLER, R. A., TERNER, J. Y., LINDENBAUM, J., MAGIDSON, J., WILLIAMS, R., PREISIG, R. & PHILLIPS, G. B. (1964) Chediak–Higashi syndrome. Cytologic and serum lipid observations in a case and family. *Amer. J. Med.* **36**, 583–594.

KYLE, R. A. & LINMAN, J. W. (1970) Gingivitis and chronic idiopathic neutropenia: report of two cases. *Proc. Staff Meet. Mayo Clin.* **45**, 494–504.

LAINSON, P. A., BRADY, P. P. & FRALEIGH, C. M. (1968) Anaemia, a systemic cause of periodontal disease. *J. Periodont.* **39**, 35–38.

LAMPERT, F. & FESSELER, A. (1975) Periodontal changes during chronic benign granulocytopenia in childhood. *J. Clin. Periodont.* **2**, 105–110.

LANE, S. L. (1952) Plasmacytoma of the mandible. *Oral Surg.* **5**, 434–442.

LASKIN, J. L. (1974) Oral haemorrhage after the use of quinidine. *J. Amer. Dent. Assoc.* **88**, 137–139.

LAVINE, W. S., PAGE, R. C. & PADGETT, G. A. (1976) Host response in chronic periodontal disease. V. The dental and periodontal status of mink and mice affected by Chediak–Higashi syndrome. *J. Periodont.* **47**, 621–635.

LEADER, R. W., PADGETT, G. A. & GORHAM, J. R. (1963) Studies of abnormal leucocyte bodies in the mink. *Blood* **22**, 477–484.

LEHRER, R. I., GOLDBERG, L. S., APPLE, M. A. & ROSENTHAL, N. P. (1972) Refractory megaloblastic anaemia with myeloperoxidase-deficient neutrophils. *Ann. Intern. Med.* **76**, 447–453.

LENNERT, K., STEIN, H. & KAISERLING, E. (1975) Cytological and functional criteria for the classification of malignant lymphomata. *Br. J. Cancer* **31**, Suppl. II, 29–43.

LERMAN, R. L. & GRODIN, M. A. (1977) Necrotising stomatitis in a pediatric burn victim. *J. Dent. Child.* **44**, 36–38.

LETTERER, E. (1924) Aleukämische Retikulose. *Frankf. Z. Path.* **30**, 377–394.

LEVINE, S. (1959) Chronic familial neutropenia with marked

periodontal lesions. *Oral Surg.* **12**, 310–314.

LEWIN, R. W. & CATALDO, E. (1967) Multiple myeloma discovered from oral manifestations: report of a case. *J. oral Surg.* **25**, 68–72.

LICHTENSTEIN, L. (1953) Histiocytosis X: Integration of eosinophilic granuloma of bone 'Letterer–Siwe disease', and 'Schüller–Christian disease' as related manifestations of a single nosologic entity. *Archs. Path.* **56**, 84–102.

LICHTENSTEIN, L. (1964) Histiocytosis X (eosinophilic granuloma of bone, Letterer–Siwe disease, Hand–Schüller–Christian disease): further observations of pathological and clinical importance. *J. Bone Jt. Surg.* **46**, 76–90.

LICHTENSTEIN, L. & JAFFE, H. L. (1940) Eosinophilic granuloma of bone, with report of a case. *Amer. J. Path.* **16**, 595–604.

LINARZI, L. R. (1951) Diagnostic and therapeutic aspects of multiple myeloma. *Med. Clin. N. Amer.* **35**, 189–226.

LOVETT, D. W., CROSS, K. R. & VAN ALLEN, M. (1965) The prevalence of amyloids in gingival tissues. *Oral Surg.* **20**, 444–448.

LUCAS, R. B. (1976a) *Pathology of tumours of the oral tissues* (3rd ed.), p. 250. Edinburgh, Churchill Livingstone.

LUCAS, R. B. (1976b) *Pathology of tumours of the oral tissues* (3rd ed.), p. 254. Edinburgh, Churchill Livingstone.

LUCAYA, J. (1971) Histiocytosis X. *Amer. J. Dis. Child.* **121**, 289–295.

LUKES, R. & BUTLER, J. J. (1966) The pathology and nomenclature of Hodgkin's disease. *Cancer Res.* **26**, 1063–1081.

LUKES, R. J. & COLLINS, R. D. (1974) Immunologic characterisation of human malignant lymphomas. *Cancer* **34**, 1488–1503.

LUKES, R. J. & COLLINS, R. D. (1975) New approaches to the classification of the lymphomata. *Br. J. Cancer* **31**, Suppl. II, 1–28.

LUKES, R. J. & COLLINS, R. D. (1977) Lukes–Collins classification and its significance. *Cancer Treat. Rep.* **61**, 971–979.

LYNCH, M. A. & SHIP, I. I. (1967a) Initial oral manifestations of leukaemia. *J. Amer. dent. Assoc.* **75**, 932–940.

LYNCH, M. A. & SHIP, I. I. (1967b) Oral manifestations of leukaemia: a postdiagnostic study. *J. Amer. dent. Assoc.* **75**, 1139–1144.

McCARTHY, F. P. & KARCHER, D. H. (1946) The oral lesions of monocytic leukaemia. *New England J. Med.* **234**, 787–790.

MacGILLWRAY, J. B., PACIE, J. V., HENRY, J. R. K., SACKER, L. S. & TIGARD, J. P. M. (1964) Congenital neutropenia: a report of five cases. *Acta Paediat., Stockh.* **53**, 188–203.

McGOWAN, D. A., GORMAN, J. M. & OTRIDGE, D. W. (1970) Intensive dental care in adult acute leukaemia. *Dent. Pract.* **20**, 239–243.

McKEE, L. C. & COLLINS, R. D. (1974) Intravascular leukocyte thrombi and aggregates as a cause of morbidity and mortality in leukaemia. *Medicine* **53**, 463–478.

McKELVY, B., SATINOVER, F. & SANDERS, B. (1976)

Idiopathic thrombocytopenic purpura manifesting as gingival hypertrophy: case report. *J. Periodont.* **47**, 661–663.

McNELIS, F. L. & PAI, V. T. (1969) Malignant lymphoma of head and neck. *Laryngoscope, St. Louis* **79**, 1076–1087.

MALLETT, S. P., GOLAN, H. P., ENGLAND, L. C. & KUTCH, J. H. (1947) Acute myelogenous leukemia with primary oral manifestations. *J. oral Surg.* **5**, 209–214.

MARKERT, J. (1967) Zur Ultrastruktur des eosinophilen Granulom des Knochens. *Frankf. Z. Path.* **76**, 157–163.

MASSUCCO, R. L. (1966) Sickle cell anaemia. A case of dental interest. *Oral Surg.* **31**, 397–402.

MATHE, G., RAPPAPORT, H., O'CONNOR, G. T. & TORLONI, H. (1976) Histological and cytological typing of neoplastic diseases of haematopoietic and lymphoid tissues. In: *WHO International histological classification of tumours*, No. 14, Geneva, WHO.

MATSANIOTIS, N., KOSSOGLAU, K., KARPOUZAS, J. & ANASTASEA-VLACHOU, K. (1966) Chromosomes in Kostmann's disease. *Lancet* **2**, 104.

MATTHEWS, J. B. & BASU, M. K. (in press) Primary extranodal lymphoma of the oral cavity: an immunohistochemical study. *Br. J. oral Surg.*

MELOY, T. M., GUNTER, J. H. & SAMPSON, D. A. (1945) Mandibular lesion as first evidence of multiple myeloma. *Amer. J. Orthod.* **31**, 685–689.

MERANUS, H., CARLIN, R., SURPRENANT, P. & SELDIN, R. (1968) Histiocytosis X: problems in diagnosis. *Oral Surg.* **26**, 759–768.

MERRIL, A. & PETERSON, L. J. (1970) Gingival haemorrhage secondary to uraemia. Review and report of a case. *Oral Surg.* **29**, 530–535.

MESROBIAN, A. Z. & SHKLAR, G. (1971) Experimental oral malignant lymphoma using alveolar socket carcinogen implantation. *J. Periodont.* **42**, 105–108.

MEYER, G., ROSWIT, B. & UNGER, S. M. (1959) Hodgkin's disease of the oral cavity. *Amer. J. Roentg.* **81**, 430–432.

MICHAUD, M., BAEHMER, R. L., BIXLER, D. & KAFRANY, A. H. (1977) Oral manifestations of acute leukaemia in children. *J. Amer. dent. Assoc.* **95**, 1145–1150.

MILLER, A. S. & CLARK, P. G. (1968) Experimental amyloidosis: deposition in the general and oral tissues of mice. *J. oral Surg.* **26**, 175–179.

MILLER, M. E., OSKI, F. A. & HARRIS, M. B. (1971) Lazy-leucocyte syndrome. A new disorder of leucocyte formation. *Lancet* **1**, 665–668.

MISHKIN, D. J., AKERS, J. O. & DARBY, C. P. (1976) Congenital neutropenia. Report of a case and a biorationale for dental management. *Oral Surg.* **42**, 738–745.

MITTELMAN, D. & KABAN, L. B. (1976) Recurrent 'non-Hodgkin's' lymphoma presenting with gingival enlargement. *Oral Surg.* **42**, 792–800.

MORGAN, A. D. & O'NEIL, R. (1956) The oral complications of polyarteritis and giant cell granulomatosis (Wegener's granulomatosis). *Oral Surg.* **9**, 845–857.

MORRIS, A. L. & STAHL, S. S. (1954) Intra-oral roentgenographic changes in sickle cell anaemia. A case report. *Oral Surg.* **7**, 787–791.

MOSCHCOWITZ, E. (1925) An acute febrile pleiochromic

anemia with hyaline thrombosis of the terminal arterioles and capillaries. An undescribed disease. *Archs. Intern. Med.* **36**, 89–93.

NALLY, F. E. (1968) Myeloma-like plasma cell lesion of the maxilla. *Ir. J. Med. Sci.* **7**, 227–236.

NIEDERMAN, J. C., McCOLLUM, R. W., HENLE, G. & HENLE, W. (1968) Infectious mononucleosis: clinical manifestations in relation to EB virus antibodies. *J. Amer. Med. Assoc.* **203**, 205–209.

NILSSON, I. M., BLOMBACK, M., JORRES, E., BLOMBACK, B. & JOHANSSON, S. A. (1957) On an inherited autosomal haemorrhagic diathesis with anti-hemophilic globulin (AHG) deficiency and prolonged bleeding time. *Acta Med. Scand.* **159**, 179–188.

NIXON, K. C., KEYS, D. W. & BROWN, G. (1975) Oral management of Glanzmann's thrombasthenia. A case report. *J. Periodont.* **46**, 364–367.

O'LEARY, T. J., RUDD, K. D., CRUMP, P. P. & KRAUSE, R. E. (1969) The effect of ascorbic acid supplementation on tooth mobility. *J. Periodont.* **40**, 284–286.

ORLEAN, S. L. & BLEWITT, G. (1965) Multiple myeloma with manifestation of a bony lesion in the maxilla. *Oral Surg.* **19**, 817–824.

ORSOS, S. (1958) Primary lymphosarcoma of the gingivae. *Oral Surg.* **11**, 426–430.

PADGETT, G. A., LEADER, R. W., GORHAM, J. R. & O'MARY, C. C. (1964) The familial occurrence of the Chediak–Higashi syndrome in mink and cattle. *Genetics, Princeton* **49**, 505–512.

PADGETT, G. A., REIQUAM, C. W., GORHAM, J. R., HENSON, J. B. & O'MARY, C. C. (1967) Comparative studies of the Chediak–Higashi syndrome. *Amer. J. Path.* **51**, 553–571.

PAGANO, J. S., HUANG, C. H. & LEVINE, P. (1973) Absence of Epstein–Barr viral DNA in American Burkitt's lymphoma. *New Engl. J. Med.* **289**, 1395–1399.

PAGE, A. R. & GOOD, R. A. (1957) Studies on cyclic neutropenia: a clinical and experimental investigation. *Amer. J. Dis. Child.* **94**, 623–661.

PARKER, F. Jr. & JACKSON, H. Jr. (1949) Primary reticulum cell sarcoma of bone. *Surgery, St. Louis* **68**, 45–53.

PAUL, J. R. & BUNNELL, W. W. (1932) The presence of heterophile antibodies in infectious mononucleosis. *Amer. J. Med. Sci.* **183**, 90–104.

PETERS, M. V., HASSELBACK, R. & BROWN, T. C. (1968) The natural history of the lymphomas related to the clinical classification. In: *Proceedings of the International Conference on Leukaemia-lymphoma,* C. J. D. ZARAFONETIS (ed.), pp. 357–371. Philadelphia, Lea & Febiger.

PETTERSSON, T. & WEGELIUS, D. (1972) Biopsy diagnosis of amyloidosis in rheumatoid arthritis. Malabsorption caused by intestinal amyloid deposits. *Gastroenterology,* **62**, 22–27.

PINDBORG, J. J. (1949) The effect of methyl folic acid on the periodontal tissues in rat molars (experimental granulocytopenia). *Oral Surg.* **2**, 1485–1496.

POGREL, M. A. (1978) Acute leukaemia. An atypical case presenting with gingival manifestations. *Int. J. oral Surg.* **7**, 119–122.

POSWILLO, D. (1967) Plasmacytosis of the gingiva. *Br. J. oral Surg.* **5**, 194–202.

PRESANT, C. A., SAFDAR, S. H. & CHERRICK, H. (1973) Gingival leukaemic infiltration in chronic lymphocytic leukaemia. *Oral Surg.* **36**, 672–674.

PRETTY, H. M., GOSSELIN, G., COLPRON, G. & LONG, L. A. (1965) Agranulocytosis: a report of 30 cases. *Canad. Med. Assoc. J.* **93**, 1058–1064.

PRIEST, R. E. (1970) Formation of epithelial basement membrane is restricted by scurvy *in vitro* and is stimulated by vitamin C. *Nature* **225**, 744–745.

PROWLER, J. R. & SMITH, E. W. (1965) Dental bone changes occurring in sickle cell diseases and abnormal haemoglobin traits. *Radiology* **65**, 762–769.

RAMON, Y., MARBERG, K., SAMRA, H. & KAUFMAN, A. (1965) Severe post-extraction bleeding as a presenting feature in a case of multiple myeloma. *Oral Surg.* **19**, 720–722.

RAPPAPORT, H. (1966) Tumours of haematopoietic system. In: *Armed Forces Institute of Pathology, Atlas of Tumor Pathology,* Section II, Fascicle 8, Washington D.C.

RAPPAPORT, H. (1977) In: BERARD, C. W., Discussion II: round table discussion of histopathologic classification. *Cancer Treat. Rep.* **61**, 1037–1048.

RAPPAPORT, H., WINTER, W. J. & HICKS, E. B. (1956) Follicular lymphoma: a re-evaluation of its position in the scheme of malignant lymphoma based on a survey of 253 cases. *Cancer* **9**, 792–821.

REED, W. B., JENSEN, A. K., KONWALER, B. E. & HUNTER, D. (1963) The cutaneous manifestations in Wegener's granulomatosis. *Acta Derm. Venereol. Stockh.* **43**, 250–264.

REICHART, P. A. & DORNOW, H. (1978) Gingivoperiodontal manifestations in chronic benign neutropenia. *J. Clin. Periodont.* **5**, 74–80.

REIMANN, H. A. & DE BARADINIS, C. T. (1949) Periodic (cyclic) neutropenia, an entity: collection of sixteen cases. *Blood* **4**, 1109–1116.

RITTER, R. A. (1966) Histiocytosis X: a case report with electron microscopic observations. *Cancer* **19**, 1155–1169.

ROATH, S., ISRAELS, M. S. & WILKINSON, J. F. (1964) The acute leukaemias: a study of 580 patients. *Q. Jl Med.* **33**, 257–283.

ROBINSON, I. B. & SARNAT, B. G. (1952) Roentgen studies of the maxillae and mandible in sickle cell anaemia. *Radiology* **58**, 517–523.

ROSENBERG, S. A., DIAMOND, H. D., JASLOWITZ, B. & CRAVER, L. F. (1961) Lymphosarcoma: a review of 1,269 cases. *Medicine* **49**, 31–84.

RYLANDER, H., ATTSTRÖM, R. & LINDHE, J. (1975) Influence of experimental neutropenia in dogs with chronic gingivitis. *J. periodont. Res.* **10**, 315–323.

SCHILIRO, G., PIZZARELLI, G., RUSSO, A. & SCIACCA, A. (1977) Dental care in leukaemia. *New Engl. J. Med.* **296**, 109.

SCHLUGER, S., YUODELIS, R. A. & PAGE, R. C. (1977) *Periodontal disease,* p. 98. Philadelphia, Lea & Febiger.

SCHNITZER, B., LOESEL, L. S. & REED, R. E. (1970) Lymphosarcoma cell leukaemia. A clinico-pathologic study. *Cancer* **26**, 1082–1096.

SCHNITZER, B. & WEAVER, D. K. (1979) Lymphoreticular

disorders. In: *Tumours of the head and neck* (2nd ed.), J. G. BATSAKIS, pp. 448–491. Baltimore, Williams & Wilkins.

SCHOFIELD, I. D. F. & GARDNER, D. G. (1971) Histiocytosis X: A case diagnosed from the oral findings. *J. Canad. dent. Assoc.* 37, 343–346.

SCHÜLLER, A. (1915) Über eigenartige Schädeldefekte im Jugendalter. *Fortschr. Geb. Röntgstrahl.* 23, 12–18.

SCHWARTZ, J., ROSENBERG, A. & COOPERBERG, A. A. (1972) Thrombotic thrombocytopenic purpura: a successful treatment of two cases. *Canad. med. Assoc. J.* 106, 1200–1205.

SCOTT, J. & FINCH, L. D. (1972a) Wegener's granulomatosis presenting as gingivitis. *Oral Surg.* 34, 920–933.

SCOTT, J. & FINCH, L. D. (1972b) Histiocytosis X with oral lesions. *J. oral Surg.* 30, 748–753.

SEDANO, H. O., CERNEA, P., HOSKE, G. & GORLIN, R. J. (1969) Histiocytosis X: Clinical, radiologic and histologic findings with special attention to oral manifestations. *Oral Surg.* 27, 760–771.

SEGELMAN, A. E. & DOKU, H. C. (1977) Treatment of the oral complications of leukaemia. *J. oral Surg.* 35, 469–477.

SELDIN, H. M., SELDIN, S. D. & RAKOWER, W. (1954) Oral lymphosarcoma. *J. oral Surg.* 12, 3–15.

SELIKOFF, I. J. & ROBIZEK, E. H. (1947) Gingival biopsy for the diagnosis of generalised amyloidosis. *Amer. J. Path.* 23, 1099–1111.

SHAFER, W. G., HINE, M. K. & LEVY, B. M. (1974) *A textbook of oral pathology* (3rd ed.), pp. 687–688. Philadelphia, Saunders.

SHAW, M. T. (1978) The distinctive features of acute monocytic leukaemia. *Amer. J. Haematol.* 4, 97–103.

SHERMAN, R. A. (1951) Résumé of the roentgen diagnosis of tumours of the jaw bones. *Oral Surg.* 4, 1427–1443.

SHILLITOE, E. J., LEHNER, T., LESSOF, M. H. & HARRISON, D. F. N. (1974) Immunological features of Wegener's granulomatosis. *Lancet* I, 281–284.

SHIVER, C. B., BERG, P. & FRENKEL, E. P. (1956) Palatine petechiae, an early sign in infectious mononucleosis. *J. Amer. med. Assoc.* 161, 592–594.

SIDDONS, R. C. (1974) Experimental nutritional folate deficiency in the baboon (*Papio cynocephalus*). *Br. J. Nutr.* 32, 579–587.

SIGALA, J. L., SILVERMAN, S., BRODY, H. A. & KUSHNER, J. H. (1972) Dental involvement in histiocytosis. *Oral Surg.* 33, 42–48.

SILVERMAN, L. M. (1955) Lymphosarcoma of gingivae. *Oral Surg.* 8, 1108–1114.

SILVERMAN, L. M. & SHKLAR, G. (1962) Multiple myeloma: report of a case. *Oral Surg.* 15, 301–309.

SINN, C. M. & DICK, F. W. (1956) Monocytic leukaemia. *Amer. J. Med.* 20, 588–602.

SINROD, H. S. (1957) Leukaemia as a dental problem. *J. Amer. dent. Assoc.* 55, 809–818.

SIWE, S. (1933) Die Reticuloendotheliose – ein neues Krankheitsbild unter den Hepatosplenomegalien. *Z. Kinderheilk.* 52, 212–217.

SLEEPER, E. L. (1951) Eosinophilic granuloma of bone. Its relationship to Hand–Schüller–Christian and Letterer–Siwe diseases, with emphasis upon oral symptoms and findings. *Oral Surg.* 4, 896–918.

SMILLIE, A. C. & COWMAN, S. C. (1969) Pulp and peri-

apical involvement in leukaemia. *N. Z. dent. J.* 65, 32–34.

SMITH, D. B. (1957) Multiple myeloma involving the jaws. *Oral Surg.* 10, 910–919.

SMITH, E. W. & CONLEY, C. L. (1953) Filter paper electrophoresis of human hemoglobins with special reference to the incidence and clinical significance of Hemoglobin C. *Bull. Johns Hopkins Hosp.* 93, 94–106.

SONI, N. N. (1966) Microradiographic study of dental tissues in sickle cell anaemia. *Archs. oral Biol.* 11, 561–564.

SOUTHAM, C. M., CRAVER, L. F., DARGEON, H. W. & BURCHENAL, J. H. (1951) Study of the natural history of acute leukaemia with special reference to duration of disease and occurrence of remissions. *Cancer* 4, 39–59.

SPITZER, R. & PRICE, L. W. (1948) Solitary myeloma of the mandible. *Br. Med. J.* I, 1027–1028.

STAMPS, J. T. (1974) The role of oral hygiene in a patient with idiopathic aplastic anaemia. *J. Amer. dent. Assoc.* 88, 1025–1027.

STEG, R. F., DAHLIN, D. C. & GORES, R. J. (1959) Malignant lymphoma of the mandible and maxillary region. *Oral Surg.* 12, 128–141.

STEINER, P. E. (1943) Hodgkin's disease. The incidence, distribution, nature and possible significance of lymphogranulomatous lesions in the bone marrow. A review with original data. *Archs. Path.* 36, 627–637.

STERN, M. H. & COLE, W. L. (1973) Radiographic changes in the mandible associated with leukaemic cell infiltration in a case of acute myelogenous leukaemia. *Oral Surg.* 36, 343–348.

STOUT, A. P. & KENNEY, F. R. (1949) Primary plasmacell tumours of the upper air passages and oral cavity. *Cancer* 2, 261–277.

SWENSON, H. M., REDISH, C. H. & MANNE, M. (1965) Agranulocytosis: two case reports. *J. Periodont.* 36, 466–470.

SYMMERS, W. ST. C. (1956) Primary amyloidosis: a review *J. Clin. Pathol.* 9, 187–211.

TALIANO, A. D. & WAKEFIELD, B. G. (1966) Atypical oral symptoms in acute myeloblastic leukaemia: report of a case. *J. oral Surg.* 24, 440–444.

TAUBMAN, S. B., COGEN, R. B. & LEPOW, A. H. (1974) Granule enzymes from human leukocytes. Their effects on HeLa cells. *Proc. Soc. Exp. Biol. Med.* 145, 952–957.

TELSEY, B., BEUBE, F. E., ZEGARELLI, E. V. & KUTSCHER, A. H. (1962) Oral manifestations of cyclical neutropenia associated with hypergammaglobulinaemia. *Oral Surg.* 15, 540–543.

TEMPEL, T. R., KIMBALL, H. R., KAKEHASHI, S. & AMEN, C. R. (1972) Host factors in periodontal disease: periodontal manifestations of Chediak–Higashi syndrome. *J. periodont. Res.* Suppl. 10, 26–27.

TILLMAN, H. M. (1957) Oral manifestations of generalised systemic amyloid disease. *Oral Surg.* 10, 743–748.

TILLMAN, H. M. (1965) Malignant lymphomas involving the oral cavity and surrounding structures. *Oral Surg.* 19, 60–72.

TIWARI, R. M. (1973) Hodgkin's disease of maxilla. *J. Lar. Otol.* 87, 85–88.

TRIEGER, N., COHEN, A. S. & CALKINS, E. (1960)

Gingival biopsy as a diagnostic aid in amyloid disease. *Archs. oral Biol.* **1**, 187–192.

UTHMAN, A. A. (1974) Hand–Schüller–Christian disease. *J. oral Med.* **29**, 22–24.

VALENTINE, W. N. (1971) Infectious mononucleosis. In: P. B. BEESON & W. McDERMOTT (eds.), *Cecil–Loeb textbook of medicine,* pp. 1565–1566. Philadelphia, Saunders.

VAN DER WAAL, I., FEHMERS, M. C. O. & KRAAL, E. R. (1973) Amyloidosis: its significance in oral surgery. *Oral Surg.* **36**, 469–481.

VANN, W. F. & OLDENBURG, T. R. (1976) Atypical hereditary neutropenia: case reports of two siblings. *J. Dent. Child.* **43**, 265–269.

VICKERY, I. M. & MIDDA, M. (1976) Dental complications of cytotoxic therapy in Hodgkin's disease – a case report. *Br. J. oral Surg.* **13**, 282–288.

WADE, A. B. & STAFFORD, J. L. (1963) Cyclical neutropenia. *Oral Surg.* **16**, 1443–1448.

WALTON, E. W. (1958) Giant cell granuloma of the respiratory tract (Wegener's granulomatosis). *Br. Med. J.* **2**, 265–270.

WARSON, R., & PREIS, F. (1969) A nonexophytic plasma-cell granuloma of the mandible. *Oral Surg.* **28**, 791–796.

WEARY, P. E. & BENDER, A. S. (1967) Chediak–Higashi syndrome with severe cutaneous involvement. Occurrence in two brothers 14 and 15 years of age. *Archs. Intern. Med.* **119**, 381–386.

WEGENER, F. (1936) Uber generalisierte, septische Gafässerkrankungen. *Verh. Dt. Path. Ges.* **29**, 202–209.

WHITE, G. E. (1970) Oral manifestations of leukaemia in children. *Oral Surg.* **29**, 420–427.

WHITE, J. G. (1966) The Chediak–Higashi syndrome: a possible lysosomal disease. *Blood* **28**, 143–156.

WHITEHEAD, F. I. H. (1972) Histiocytosis X. *Br. J. oral Surg.* **10**, 199–204.

WHITLOCK, R. I. H. & HUGHES, N. C. (1960) Solitary myeloma of mandible. *Oral Surg.* **13**, 23–32.

WHO BULLETIN (1969) Histiopathological definition of Burkitt's tumor. Memorandum Review. *Bull. WHO* **40**, 601.

WILLIS, R. A. (1967) *Pathology of tumours* (4th ed.), pp. 795–802. London, Butterworths.

WILSON, J. F., MARSA, G. W. & JOHNSON, R. E. (1972) Herpes zoster in Hodgkin's disease. Clinical, histologic and immunologic correlations. *Cancer* **29**, 461–465.

WINTHER, J. E., FEJERSKOV, O. & PHILIPSEN, H. P. (1972) Oral manifestations of histiocytosis X. *Archs. Derm. Stockh.* **52**, 75–79.

WOLBACH, S. B. & BESSY, O. A. (1942) Tissue changes in vitamin deficiencies. *Physiol. Rev.* **22**, 233–289.

WOLF, J. E. & EBEL, L. K. (1978) Chronic granulomatous disease: report of a case and review of the literature. *J. Amer. dent. Assoc.* **96**, 292–295.

WOLFF, E. & NOLAN, L. E. (1944) Multiple myeloma first discovered in the mandible. *Radiology* **42**, 76–78.

WONG, D. S., FULLMER, L. M., BUTLER, J. J. & SHULLENBERGER, C. C. (1975) Extranodal non-Hodgkin's lymphomas of the head and neck. *Amer. J. Roentg.* **123**, 471–481.

WOOD, G. D. (1975) Myelomatosis: a case report. *Br. dent. J.* **139**, 472–474.

WRIGHT, D. H. (1971) Burkitt's lymphoma: a review of the pathology, immunology, and possible etiologic factors. *Path. Ann.* **6**, 337–363.

YEAGER, D. A. (1975) Idiopathic thrombocytopenic purpura: report of a case. *J. Amer. dent. Assoc.* **30**, 640–643.

ZIEGLER, J. L. (1977) Treatment results of 54 American patients with Burkitt's lymphoma are similar to the African experience. *New Engl. J. Med.* **297**, 75–80.

Chapter 18

PERIODONTAL CYSTS
K. W. Lee

The periodontal ligament is occasionally involved by non-neoplastic cysts. These lesions are pathological cavities having fluid, semi-fluid or gaseous contents and which are not created by the accumulation of pus (Kramer, 1974). They have soft tissue sacs, which are frequently, but not always, lined by epithelium. The epithelium lining these cysts originates in the majority of cases from the odontogenic apparatus; in a few areas of the jaws, it is possible that the epithelium may be non-odontogenic in origin.

(Oral cysts which do not involve the periodontal ligament have not been included in the present chapter. Readers are referred to Shear (1976) for a recent account of these entities.)

ODONTOGENIC CYSTS

Inflammatory periodontal

RADICULAR (DENTAL, PERIAPICAL) CYST

The radicular cyst is the commonest non-neoplastic cyst involving the periodontal ligament. It arises usually as a result of chronic inflammatory changes at the periapical region of a non-vital tooth, commonly the end result of caries. Less commonly they may arise as a result of trauma, or the presence of a developmental defect, i.e. an invagination or evagination allowing direct bacterial ingress. Chronic inflammatory changes consequent to the spread of infection to the periapical tissues lead to the formation of a periapical granuloma. This is a mass of granulation tissue with fibroblasts, capillaries and a diffuse infiltrate of lymphocytes, plasma cells, macrophages and polymorphonuclear leucocytes (see Chapter 15). Within this mass, proliferated epithelium is seen. This is presumed to originate from epithelial cell rests of Malassez in the periodontal ligament (Fig. 1).

Further proliferation of epithelium leads to tissue breakdown and the formation of a cavity lined with stratified squamous epithelium. If the causative tooth is removed, leaving behind the cyst, this is referred to as a residual cyst.

The exact mechanism of cystic change is still unknown, but there are three main hypotheses (Stones, 1951):

1. As the mass of epithelium proliferates, stimulated by the inflammation, the cells in the central part of the mass become removed from their blood supply and undergo degeneration. This breakdown leads to cavity formation, and the rest of

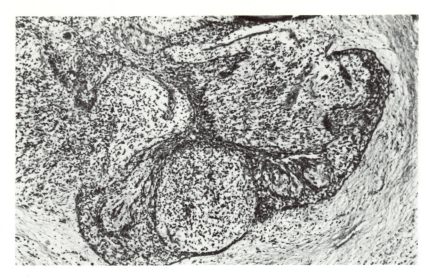

FIG. 1. Strands of proliferating epithelium within a periapical granuloma. Haematoxylin and eosin. ×75.

the epithelium forms a lining around this cavity.

2. The mass of proliferating epithelium encircles connective tissue islands forming loops around them. As a result of enzymatic action this core of connective tissue may break down and liquefy, undergoing cavity formation.

3. The periapical granuloma frequently undergoes abscess formation. When an abscess cavity is formed, the epithelium within the granuloma proliferates to line the abscess cavity and converts it into a cyst. A modification to this hypothesis suggests the oral epithelium as a possible alternative source of epithelium for the lining. The oral epithelium is deemed to have proliferated through the opening of a sinus through which the pus has tracked (Warwick James and Counsell, 1932).

Summers (1974) examined frozen sections of human periapical granulomas histochemically for aminopeptidase activity and proteolytic activity. He found that aminopeptidase activity was located in the mesodermal polymorphonuclear leucocytes and macrophages, and that maximal activity appeared within connective tissue not as yet surrounded by epithelium, although there was some activity in the epithelium from migrated polymorphonuclear leucocytes. The finding of aminopeptidase activity in the mesoderm within the proliferating loops of epithelium

suggested to him that cavitation in granulomas was due to enzymic proteolytic activity occurring in the mesoderm. Shear (1976) believed that both intra-epithelial and connective tissue breakdown were feasible and that they might operate independently of one another. There was morphological evidence in support of the intra-epithelial breakdown hypothesis as the proliferating epithelial masses showed considerable intercellular oedema. The intercellular accumulations of fluid coalesced to form microcysts containing epithelial and inflammatory cells. As Summers (1974) also found weak proteolytic activity within the proliferating epithelium, this suggested that the cells were undergoing autolysis. The microcysts might increase in size by coalescing with adjacent microcysts.

Enlargement of the cyst

Regardless of the mode of pathogenesis of the cyst, once a cavity is formed, the cyst gradually expands within the marrow spaces and the surrounding bone is resorbed. The mechanism of cyst expansion is also imperfectly understood. The classical explanation is that the cyst fluid exerts a higher osmotic pressure than the surrounding tissues and results in attraction of fluid into the cyst cavity, which in turn exerts a pressure effect on the surrounding bone, leading to osteoclastic resorption. Toller (1970) has shown that the mean osmolality of the fluid from twenty-one radicular cysts was 290 ± 14.93 milliosmoles compared to a mean serum osmolality of 279 ± 4.68 milliosmoles. The increased osmotic pressure of the cyst fluid probably arises as a result of lytic products of the epithelial and inflammatory cells in the cyst cavity. Skaug (1976a) has measured the intracystic fluid pressure of apical cysts by means of a pressure transducer following cannulation of the cyst cavity and found that the average radicular cyst exerted a pressure of $+47$ mm Hg. Using a tissue culture technique, Harris (1978) has shown that odontogenic cyst linings may liberate significant quantities of bone-resorbing prostaglandins. Chromatography on silica gel-impregnated paper further revealed that the prostaglandins were principally PGE 2, PGE 3 and PGF 3a.

On the outer aspect of the bone, osteoblastic activity attempts to compensate by laying down new bone. However, resorption outstrips repair, and the covering bone is gradually thinned, and eventually produces the 'ping-pong' ball feel on pressure. When the bone is thinned sufficiently a translucent bluish fluctuant swelling is seen clinically (Fig. 2). In the maxilla the enlargement may be buccal or palatal while in the mandible expansion usually takes place on the buccal aspect (Shear, 1976). On aspiration, a straw-coloured fluid rich in cholesterol crystals is obtained. These appear in a smear preparation as rhomboid plates with one corner cut off.

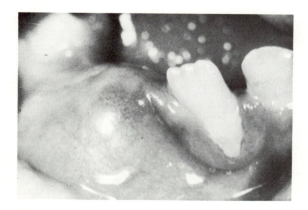

FIG. 2. Radicular cyst presenting as a translucent bluish fluctuant swelling.

Radiological features

Radiographically, a typical radicular cyst appears as a well-circumscribed radiolucent area with a radiopaque margin (Fig. 3). When the cyst is secondarily infected the radiopaque margin is replaced by an irregular radiolucent zone. It is generally accepted that in the early stages it is not possible to tell if a periapical radiolucency is a granuloma, cyst, or abscess.

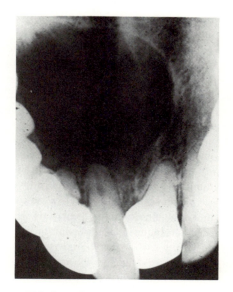

FIG. 3. Radiograph of a radicular cyst. Note the well-circumscribed radiolucent area with a radiopaque margin.

Histology

The soft tissue sac that comprises the cyst is lined with a non-keratinized stratified squamous epithelium of varying thickness. Near the causative tooth the epithelium may proliferate in the form of arcades or rings around islands of connective tissue (Fig. 4). Sometimes the lining is incomplete or discontinuous, due to secondary infection with consequent destruction of the epithelium or to an inherent incompleteness *de novo*. Goblet and ciliated cell metaplasia of the superficial cells may be seen (Fig. 5). Nodules of cholesterol are often seen attached to the cyst sac in areas of epithelial discontinuity. The source of the cholesterol in the cyst is a subject of considerable debate. Browne (1971a) found a statistically significant correlation ($p < 0.01$) between the presence of cholesterol and haemosiderin. He postulated that disintegrating red blood cells provided the main source of cholesterol in a form which crystallized readily in the tissues. Shear (1976) thought that the beta-lipoproteins in the plasma might also serve as a source. As the beta-lipoproteins passed through the fragile thin-walled blood vessels in the inflamed portions of the cyst wall, they split into cholesterol and its esters which were retained, and other lipid components such as phospholipids which were absorbed by the lymphatics. Once the cholesterol crystals were deposited in the fibrous wall of the cyst they were extruded by a foreign-body giant-cell reaction through the epithelial lining into the cyst lumen. Skaug (1976b) examined the lipoprotein content of cyst fluids by cellulose acetate membrane (CAM) electrophoresis and immuno-electrophoresis. By CAM electrophoresis cyst fluids showed alpha-1-lipoprotein and beta-lipoprotein bands but no pre-beta-lipoprotein band. The relative amount of alpha-1-lipoprotein was higher in cyst fluid than in serum. Single radial immunodiffusion showed that the content of beta-lipoprotein was low. Skaug hypothesized that the cholesterol in cysts was derived in part, at least, from the beta-lipoprotein originating from the plasma.

Hyaline bodies of Rushton are occasionally seen within the epithelium lining the cyst (Fig. 6). They are straight, curved, or of hair-pin shape, and sometimes laminated. There is considerable uncertainty

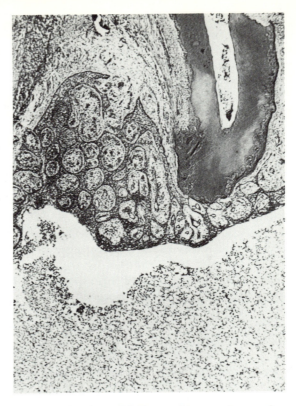

FIG. 4. Proliferating epithelium making arcades or rings around islands of connective tissue. Haematoxylin and eosin. ×30.

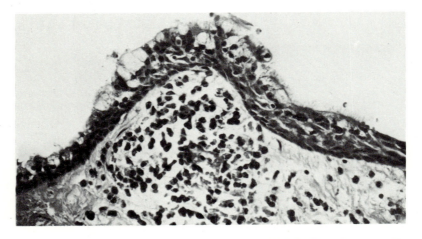

FIG. 5. Goblet and ciliated cell metaplasia in the epithelial lining. Haematoxylin and eosin. ×300.

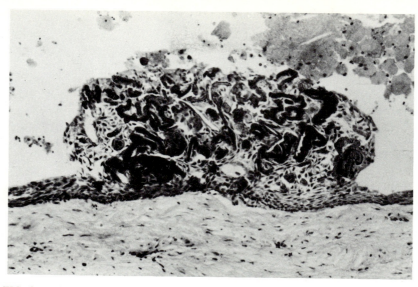

FIG. 6. Hyaline bodies of Rushton within the epithelial lining. Haematoxylin and eosin. ×120.

about the nature and origin of these hyaline bodies. Early investigations (Rushton, 1955; Shear, 1961) suggested that they may be keratinous in nature. Bouyssou and Guilhem (1965), Hodson (1966, 1967) and Sedano and Gorlin (1968) suggested a haematogenous origin. Morgan and Johnson (1974) concluded from histochemical and ultrastructural studies that they were a secretory product of odontogenic epithelium deposited on the surface of particulate matter such as cell debris or cholesterol crystals in a manner analogous to the formation of dental cuticle on the unerupted portions of enamel surfaces. Allison (1977) studied these bodies by electron microprobe analysis and revealed that they contained sulphur, chlorine, calcium and in some instances iron. His microradiographic studies showed that the density increased progressively towards the core and he concluded that his observations conformed with the hypothesis that hyaline bodies originated as epithelial secretions. In an electron-microscopic investigation El-Labban (1979) observed that the lamellar type of hyaline body was composed of alternating electron dense and electron lucent layers, the outermost layer always being electron dense. The granular type of hyaline body was composed of amorphous material in which fragments of red blood cells were seen. She concluded that the granular type formed from degenerating red

blood cells and that the lamellar type might have resulted from segregation of components within the mass.

The connective tissue wall of the cyst is usually divisible into two zones: a subepithelial, vascular, granulation tissue zone that is diffusely infiltrated with chronic inflammatory cells, including lymphocytes, plasma cells and macrophages which may be laden with lipids (foam cells) or haemosiderin, and a more collagenous zone of fibrous tissue which lies outside the granulation tissue zone forming a capsule.

The main non-inflammatory cell present in the fibrous wall is a spindle-shaped cell, which has been assumed to be a fibroblast. A recent study of these cells (Lee and El-Labban, 1980), however, revealed that some possessed the morphological characteristics of smooth muscle cells with parallel intracytoplasmic myofibrils demonstrable on phosphotungstic acid haematoxylin staining, and dense patches and fine myofilaments ultrastructurally. Some of these cells may be myofibroblasts, a recently recognized cell type possessing features of smooth muscle and fibroblast (Gabbiani, Ryan and Majno, 1971). Harris (1978) suggests that they may contribute to the elasticity of the cyst wall.

Buchner and David (1978) demonstrated that some of the pigmented cells manifested sudanophilia, acid-fastness, PAS-positivity, possessed a silver reduction capacity and exhibited yellow autofluorescence in ultraviolet light. They concluded that these cells may be macrophages containing lipopigments in the form of ceroids. They suggested that the latter were formed from locally liberated lipids with haemosiderin acting as an oxidation catalyst.

Developmental cysts

DENTIGEROUS (FOLLICULAR) CYST

The dentigerous cyst is one which encloses the crown of an unerupted tooth and is less common than the radicular cyst. The pathogenesis of this cyst is uncertain, but it is not thought to be of inflammatory origin. Following completion of crown development, the dental organ shrinks to a few layers of cells to become the reduced enamel epithelium. Accumulation of fluid between either the enamel surface and the reduced enamel epithelium, or more commonly between the layers of the reduced enamel epithelium itself, results in the formation of a cyst which envelops the crown of the unerupted tooth. Main (1970) suggests that the accumulation of fluid is the result of obstruction of venous outflow due to pressure exerted by the tooth on an impacted follicle. This is thought to induce a transudation of fluid across the capillary walls (Main, 1970).

Clinical features

Dentigerous cysts present as painless fluctuant swellings in the maxilla or mandible, associated with a missing tooth. The mandibular third molar, maxillary canine, a supernumerary mesiodens and mandibular premolar are the teeth most frequently involved. Pain is usually not a feature unless the cyst is secondarily infected.

Radiological features

Radiographs show a well-circumscribed radiolucent area related to the crown of the associated tooth (Fig. 7). In the central variety the radiolucency

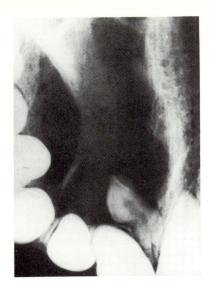

FIG. 7. Radiograph of a dentigerous cyst. The radiolucent area is associated with the conical supernumerary tooth.

envelops the crown while in the lateral variety the radiolucent area lies on one side of the crown. It is important to remember that not all radiographs showing these features will turn out to be dentigerous cysts at operation, as a number of these will be superimposed images, and the cyst and tooth may not be in dentigerous relationship with each other.

Histology

The epithelium lining the cyst is usually a non-keratinized stratified squamous epithelium (Fig. 8) attached to the tooth at the level of the amelocemental junction (Fig. 9). Goblet and ciliated cell metaplasia are common and hyaline bodies are seen occasionally. The connective tissue capsule is uniform unless the cyst becomes inflamed or infected, and islands of odontogenic epithelium are seen in the fibrous wall (Pindborg, Kramer and Torloni, 1971). The enamel of the associated tooth is usually normal although Crabb (1963) examined ground sections of these teeth by polarized light and observed that there were areas of lower mineralization in the sub-surface enamel corresponding to zones of natural enamel caries. He thought that these areas might be related to

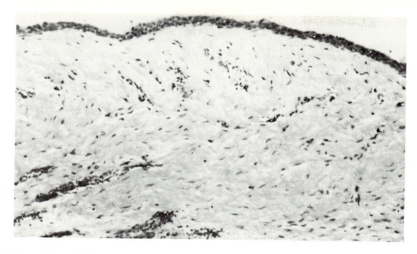

FIG. 8. Typical lining of a dentigerous cyst, comprising a thin, non-keratinized, stratified squamous epithelium. Haematoxylin and eosin. ×120.

faults in mineralization or to an attack on the enamel surface by cyst fluid.

THE PARADENTAL CYST

Craig (1976) described a cyst related to partly erupted mandibular third molars which had been involved by pericoronitis. The available teeth always possessed an enamel projection extending from the amelo-cemental junction into the buccal bifurcation. Craig concluded that these enamel projections might have a role in the pathogenesis of these cysts which appeared to originate from the reduced enamel epithelium. It is possible, however, that these cysts may have originated as dentigerous cysts with the tooth erupting through the cyst.

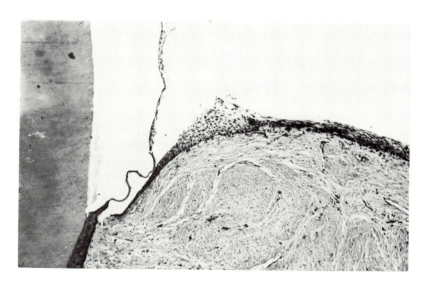

FIG. 9. Attachment of the cyst to the tooth at the level of the amelo-cemental junction. Note relationship of cyst lining to reduced enamel epithelium. Haematoxylin and eosin. ×75.

ODONTOGENIC KERATOCYST (PRIMORDIAL CYST)

Much confusion surrounds the use of the terms odontogenic keratocyst and primordial cyst. The terms are used here as synonyms as recommended by the World Health Organisation (WHO, 1978). The term primordial cyst was originally used by Robinson to designate a cyst which developed in place of a tooth (Robinson, 1975). Hence patients had to show an incomplete dentition with no history of tooth loss. Where a full dentition existed, supernumerary tooth germs were postulated. Philipsen (1956) coined the term 'odontogenic keratocyst' to describe cysts of odontogenic origin which possessed linings of keratinized stratified squamous epithelium. These were thought to be radicular or dentigerous cysts where inflammation had subsided. Shear (1960) detailed several criteria whereby primordial cysts could be diagnosed histologically and Pindborg and Hansen (1963) correlated these criteria with many of their odontogenic keratocysts. They further focused attention on the clinical behaviour of this cyst and showed that they had a high recurrence rate (62% in their series), a finding endorsed by Toller (1967), who found a recurrence rate of 51%. The detailed clinical and histological features of the condition have been reviewed by Browne (1970, 1971b) and Brannon (1976, 1977).

It is current thought (Kramer, 1974) that it is no longer necessary to postulate tooth germs that failed to develop into teeth as the source of epithelium for the development of a keratocyst, and there is general acceptance that it is an odontogenic cyst of developmental origin that has formed from the dental lamina. Stoelinga and Peters (1973) suggest, however, that these cysts originate from the oral mucosa as they were able to observe epithelial islands only within the oral mucosa superficial to the operated keratocysts and the developing dental lamina in human foetuses.

The lesion commonly develops in the region of the angle of the mandible and presents as a multilocular cyst radiographically (Fig. 10). Clinical swelling is often not marked, even when radiographic examination reveals extensive involvement of the mandible. In addition the cyst may develop in the tooth-bearing part of the jaws, presenting clinically and radiographically as lateral periodontal cysts, globulomaxillary cysts, median mandibular and median alveolar cysts,

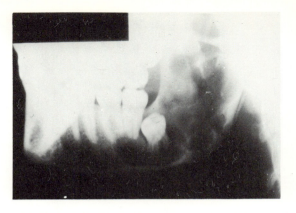

FIG. 10. Typical radiographic appearance of an odontogenic keratocyst. Note the multilocular appearance of the radiolucent area affecting the angle and ascending ramus of the mandible.

contributing to the confusion that surrounds several of the so-called 'fissural' cysts. Less commonly the cyst exists in true dentigerous relationship with a tooth, but it is assumed that this is a secondary dentigerous cyst. In edentulous mouths they may also be misdiagnosed as residual radicular cysts.

On aspiration, a material resembling inspissated pus without the characteristic smell is often obtained. Smears prepared from the aspirate reveal the presence of squames, and the soluble protein content of the aspirate has been shown to be frequently less than 4 g/100 ml. These two findings have been used by Kramer and Toller (1973) to complement the accuracy of pre-operative diagnoses.

Histology

The criteria listed for the diagnosis of primordial cysts by Shear (1960) were as follows:
1. The epithelium is keratinized or parakeratinized and is about five to eight cells thick.
2. The basal layer is cuboidal or columnar and the nuclei are intensely basophilic.
3. The epithelium is devoid of rete processes and the underlying connective tissue is free from inflammatory cell infiltration (Fig. 11).

These histological criteria remain the most important for the identification of the odontogenic keratocyst. Subsequently additional features have been observed. These include the increased mitotic

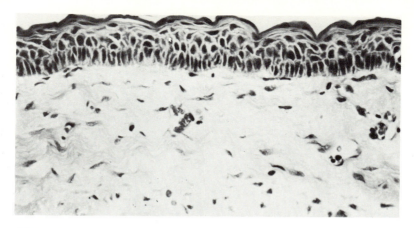

FIG. 11. Histological appearance of the lining of an odontogenic keratocyst. Note the thin parakeratinized stratified squamous epithelium devoid of rete processes and the columnar basal layer. Haematoxylin and eosin. ×300.

activity of the linings when compared with those of cysts with non-keratinized epithelial linings; the frequent separation of epithelium from connective tissue; the presence of islands of odontogenic epithelium and daughter cysts in the fibrous wall (Fig. 12) and the change from a keratinized to a non-keratinized lining when inflammation supervenes, with features becoming indistinguishable from those of radicular and dentigerous cysts.

Enlargement of the cyst

Kramer (1974) has suggested that keratocysts enlarge by accumulation of keratin within the cyst cavity. If one part of the epithelial lining is producing keratin at a greater rate, this locally increased production of a rather firm material might account for the uneven pushing out of the cyst wall. Harris and Toller (1975) suggest as an alternative explanation the fact that keratocysts are poor bone resorbers and extend preferentially along the cancellous bone with little resorption and expansion of the dense cortex.

Clinical behaviour

The high recurrence rate of the odontogenic keratocyst is probably attributable to several factors:

(i) the cyst lining is friable, and thus small frag-

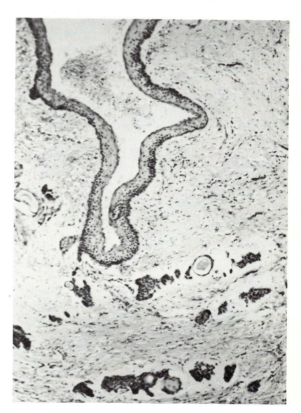

FIG. 12. Islands of odontogenic epithelium in the fibrous wall of an odontogenic keratocyst. Haematoxylin and eosin. ×75.

ments of cyst may be left behind during removal, resulting in recurrence;

(ii) the higher mitotic activity is an indicator of a more active epithelium;

(iii) the presence of islands of odontogenic epithelium and daughter cysts in the fibrous wall.

However, more recent studies (McIvor, 1972; Eversole *et al.*, 1975; Brannon, 1976, 1977) indicate that the rate of recurrence has been reduced in recent years to less than 20%. This may be due to more thorough removal of the cyst consequent to the recognition of its true nature.

Enzyme histochemistry

Donoff *et al.* (1972) demonstrated that explants of keratocysts exhibit collagenase activity which might be related to the expansile growth of keratocysts within bone. Magnusson (1978) studied the activity of NADH2- and NADPH2-diaphorase, glucose-6-phosphate dehydrogenase, glutamate dehydrogenase, acid phosphatase, leucine aminopeptidase and ATPase in keratocysts. He found that the oxidative enzymes showed strong activity in keratocyst epithelium, which contrasted with weak activity in other cysts. Acid phosphatase activity was similarly strong in keratocysts, while the fibrous walls of keratocysts showed a high activity of leucine aminopeptidase. The significance of these findings remains to be established.

Multiple keratocysts (Multiple naevoid basal cell carcinoma syndrome)

Odontogenic keratocysts occur as part of the multiple naevoid basal cell carcinoma syndrome (Gorlin, Pindborg and Cohen, 1976). In this syndrome, which involves autosomal dominant inheritance, the patients exhibit frontal and temporoparietal bossing, giving the skull a somewhat pagetoid appearance. Multiple cysts occur in the jaws and lesions microscopically indistinguishable from basal cell carcinomas occur on the skin of the face and neck, back and thorax, abdomen and upper extremities. In addition there are skeletal anomalies and intracranial calcifications. The skin lesions appear usually between puberty and the 35th year as papules varying from flesh-coloured to pale brown. The jaw cysts are typical keratocysts

with epithelial islands and microcysts in the connective tissue of the fibrous wall, which may account for the high recurrence rate of cysts seen in naevoid basal cell carcinoma syndrome patients. Donatsky *et al.* (1976) showed that 85% of the patients experienced recurrence within 2 years of cyst removal. Skeletal anomalies are present in 60–75% of patients, most commonly a splayed or bifid rib. Other costal anomalies include synostosis, partial agenesis, pseudoarthrosis, and cervical rudimentary ribs. Intracranial calcifications occur chiefly in the form of lamellar calcifications of the falx cerebri. Congenital communicating hydrocephaly and medulloblastomas have also been described in these patients.

LATERAL PERIODONTAL CYST

The term lateral periodontal cyst has been applied to at least three different entities, none of which truly represent the entity under discussion. Radicular cysts which form on the lateral aspect of the root as a result of inflammatory changes related to lateral canals have been called lateral periodontal cysts. Odontogenic keratocysts which anatomically fulfil the definition have likewise been referred to as lateral periodontal cysts. Still other cysts in this location have been shown to take origin from the reduced enamel epithelium and probably represent 'residual' dentigerous cysts. This is one of the modes of origin of the lateral periodontal cyst suggested by Shear and Pindborg (1975). Lateral periodontal cysts should, however, only be diagnosed when these entities have been excluded. Defined in this way, the lateral periodontal cyst is a developmental cyst of the periodontal ligament, with cystic change taking place within epithelial cell rests in this location.

Clinically they are found chiefly distal to the mandibular third molar or in the canine–premolar region. They are usually discovered on incidental radiographic examination and seldom grow to large size.

Histology

The lining is composed of a thin non-keratinized stratified squamous epithelium backed by fibrous tissue. Shear and Pindborg (1975) state that plaque formation is an important characteristic of the epithelium. These plaques are localized thickenings of the epithelial lining (Fig. 13). Some of these are small whereas others are larger and extend into the cyst cavity. Some cysts contain a number of plaques. The cells of the plaque are sometimes fusiform with their long axes parallel to the basement membrane. Frequently, they are large and clear, showing the features of intracellular oedema, and contain small pyknotic nuclei.

CALCIFYING ODONTOGENIC CYST

The calcifying odontogenic cyst was delineated as an entity by Gorlin *et al.* in 1962. Before then, it was probably regarded as an atypical ameloblastoma. The clinical and radiographical presentation are as for any cyst involving the periodontal ligament. However, radiopaque foci may be associated with the lesion

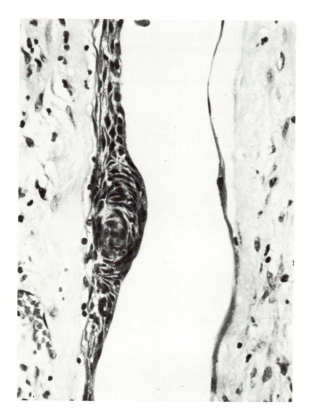

FIG. 13. Epithelial plaque formation in the lining of a lateral periodontal cyst. Haematoxylin and eosin. ×300.

for it may occur in association with a complex odontome and its calcifications may become large enough to be visible radiographically.

Histologically the lesion has a spectrum of appearances (Pindborg, Kramer and Torloni, 1971). In its simplest form, the cyst is lined with an epithelium of tall columnar basal cells, the nuclei being polarized away from the basal end of the cell. Faintly eosinophilic cells called ghost cells are prominent within the remainder of the epithelium (Fig. 14). These may undergo calcification and become visible on the radiograph. In addition to these features, the cyst may show areas of dysplastic dentine adjacent to the epithelium. As islands of odontogenic epithelium mimicking that of ameloblastoma are often seen within the fibrous wall, these foci of dysplastic dentine may distinguish the cyst from an ameloblastoma.

Areas of complex odontome sometimes form within the cyst wall, and the calcified masses of ghost cells may extrude into the fibrous wall producing a foreign-body giant-cell reaction. These features resemble those seen in odonto-ameloblastoma and ameloblastic fibro-odontoma. The clinical behaviour of lesions of this type which may grow to large size suggests that they may be neoplasms rather than malformations (Binnie *et al.*, 1975).

The ultrastructure of the cyst has been studied by Chen and Miller (1975). They identified four types of cells. These were the basal cell, the stellate reticulum type cell, the ghost cell and the hornified cell. The first two contained various amounts of tonofilaments and organelles. The ghost cell contained coarse bundles of tonofilaments intermingled with dilated membranous organelles. The hornified cell contained densely packed tonofilaments. The authors considered that the hornified cells may have derived from either the stellate reticulum type of cell or the ghost cells. Both the hornified cells and the ghost cells were considered as non-vital cell residues, and the mineralization of these cells was regarded as dystrophic calcification.

The fluid contents of odontogenic cysts

Browne (1976) determined the proportion of soluble protein and total protein content of fluids from various odontogenic cysts. He found that radicular cysts

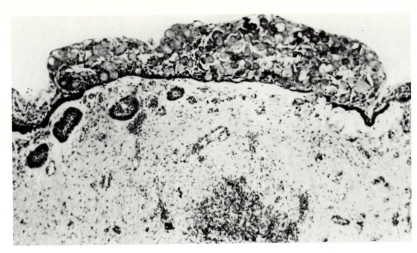

FIG. 14. Typical appearance of the lining of a calcifying odontogenic cyst. Note the presence of ghost cells in the epithelial lining and islands of odontogenic epithelium mimicking an ameloblastoma in the fibrous wall. Haematoxylin and eosin. ×75.

contained an average of 51.19% albumin, 17.25% β-globulin, 22.04% γ-globulin, and 6.30 g/100 ml protein. Dentigerous cysts contained an average of 61.35% albumin, 12.60% globulin and 4.86 g/100 ml protein. He also determined the immunoglobulin content by single radial immunodiffusion and found that radicular cysts contained an average of 488.9 mg/100 ml IgA, 2535.4 mg/100 ml IgG, and 135.6 mg/100 ml IgM. Dentigerous cysts contained an average of 308.4 mg/100 ml IgA, 1618.2 mg/100 ml IgG, and 155.6 mg/100 ml IgM. Odontogenic keratocysts contained mean levels of 135.6 mg/100 ml IgA, 491.9 mg/100 ml IgG, and 54.1 mg/100 ml IgM. Compared with serum the fluid of radicular cysts contains higher quantities of soluble protein, comprising proportionally less albumin and more β- and γ-globulins. The protein is likely to be derived from an inflammatory exudate modified by some activity of the cyst wall. Dentigerous cysts contained similar quantities of soluble protein, but it was thought that the fluid was less modified by cellular activity of the cyst wall. Skaug (1977) also determined the soluble proteins in fluids from non-keratinizing jaw cysts. He too found that the fluids from non-keratinizing cysts contained the main proteins found in plasma and exhibited the characteristics of an inflammatory exudate. He found that the non-immunoglobulin proteins occurred in concentrations lower than those of auto-

logous serum, and that there was an inverse relationship between the concentrations in cyst fluids of non-immunoglobulin proteins and their molecular weights. These low relative concentrations of macromolecular non-immunoglobulin proteins show that there is no free passage of plasma proteins into the cyst fluid. Presumably selective protein passage is due to restricted vascular permeability and a molecular-sieve effect exerted by the cyst capsule. With respect to immunoglobulins he found that cyst fluid contained on average IgG, IgA and IgM concentrations respectively 1.2, 1.7 and 0.9 times those of autologous serum. He considered that the immunoglobulins of cyst fluid were partly produced locally and partly derived from plasma.

NON-ODONTOGENIC CYSTS

Nasopalatine cyst

The nasopalatine cyst occurs in the maxillary incisor region characteristically as a heart-shaped area of radiolucency between the two maxillary central incisors (Fig. 15). Clinically it appears as a fluctuant swelling palatal to the maxillary incisors. Occasionally, it may present as a swelling on the labial aspect of the

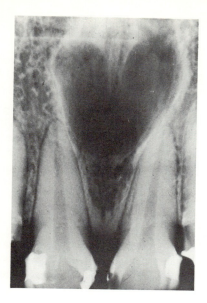

FIG. 15. Nasopalatine cyst presenting as a heart-shaped area of radiolucency between the two maxillary central incisor teeth.

alveolus or both. Very large cysts extend posteriorly and these probably account for most of the median palatal cysts that have been reported.

Histology

Nasopalatine cysts are thought to originate from epithelial remnants of the nasopalatine duct. The cyst is lined with either pseudostratified ciliated columnar epithelium or non-keratinized stratified squamous epithelium or both. Those lined with squamous epithelium are thought to have arisen from the oral end of the duct while those originating from the nasal end are lined with respiratory epithelium. Those originating in an intermediate position are lined by both. Shear (1976) feels that this should not be regarded as a rule, but that variability of the linings is suggestive of their origin from pluripotential epithelium or the result of metaplasia. In the fibrous wall are found thick-walled blood vessels, nerves (Fig. 16) and occasionally mucous glands and adipose tissue. This is thought to be due to the inclusion of the long sphenopalatine nerves and vessels which traverse the incisive canal.

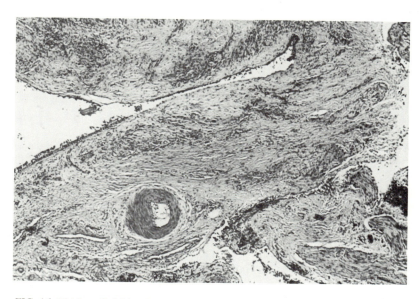

FIG. 16. Thick-walled blood vessels and nerve bundles in the fibrous wall of a naso-palatine cyst. Haematoxylin and eosin. × 30.

Globulomaxillary cyst

Situated between the maxillary lateral incisor and the maxillary canine the globulomaxillary cyst was at one time thought to have arisen as a result of enclavement of epithelium between the globular and maxillary processes (Fig. 17). However, the modern embryo-

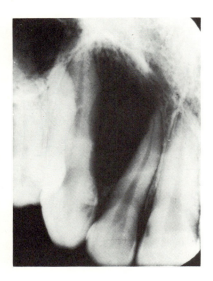

FIG. 17. Globulomaxillary cyst presenting as a well-circumscribed radiolucent area between the maxillary lateral incisor and canine.

logical view is that there is no meeting of facial processes in this region, and that there is continuity of the ectoderm in the earliest stages, with the 'facial processes' being due to growth of the underlying mesenchyme (Arey, 1965). It is therefore unlikely that the cyst develops from enclaved epithelium in early embryological development of the anterior maxilla.

Most cysts in this region are either radicular cysts related to the maxillary lateral incisor or canine, or odontogenic keratocysts. It is also necessary to exclude a cyst arising from a palatal invagination in the maxillary lateral incisor. Shear (1976) points out that a number of them fulfil the criteria for the diagnosis of a lateral periodontal cyst, being lined with a thin non-keratinized stratified squamous epithelium with areas of localized plaque formation.

Median cysts

There are two rare cyst entities which may involve the periodontal ligament in the median region of the jaws.

The median mandibular cyst is in the symphyseal region, and all teeth must be vital and an odontogenic keratocyst excluded before the diagnosis of median mandibular cyst can be accepted. It will then have to be lined with non-keratinized stratified squamous epithelium or pseudostratified ciliated columnar epithelium. Soskolne and Shteyer (1977) have reviewed the literature and have reported one further case which would appear to have fulfilled all the criteria for such a diagnosis.

The median alveolar cyst lies between the maxillary central incisor teeth in front of the incisive foramen. Sicher (1962) doubts the possibility that it develops from epithelium enclaved at the site of fusion between the right and left globular processes. The median alveolar cyst lies between the maxillary central incisor teeth in front of the incisive foramen. The solitary example seen by the author at this site turned out to be an odontogenic keratocyst.

Solitary bone cyst

The solitary bone cyst is alternatively known as a traumatic, or haemorrhagic bone cyst. Although it chiefly involves the basal bone the periodontal ligament may become involved as a result of extension to the alveolar bone. Radiographically this may be seen as a scalloping outline around the roots of the teeth (Fig. 18).

The cyst occurs in young individuals and is usually detected by routine radiographic examination, as it causes little or no expansion of bone. The cyst cavity is either empty or contains a small amount of sero-sanguinous fluid. Seward (1963) stated that, upon careful aspiration, these lesions yield a golden-yellow fluid which contains a high concentration of bilirubin. The tenuous fibrous lining lacks an epithelium and the surrounding bone exhibits osteoclastic resorption (Fig. 19).

The pathogenesis of the cyst is obscure. Howe reviewed the literature in 1965 and proposed the

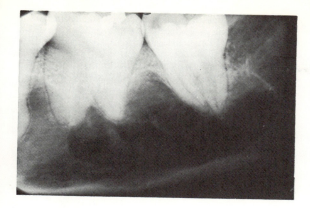

FIG. 18. Radiograph of a solitary bone cyst with scalloping outline around the roots of the teeth.

NEOPLASTIC CHANGE IN PERIODONTAL CYSTS

Rarely, neoplastic change may take place in periodontal cysts. Examples of radicular, dentigerous and odontogenic keratocysts undergoing carcinomatous change have been reported in the literature. Gardner (1975) has reviewed the published cases and accepted twenty-five of them. There is a clinical suspicion that odontogenic keratocysts are more likely to undergo a neoplastic change than other cysts but there are no statistical data to support such a contention.

There is also a long-standing view that the dentigerous cyst is a potential ameloblastoma (Cahn, 1933). This view arose from a study of lesions that appeared clinically and radiologically to be dentigerous cysts but which proved in fact to be ameloblastomas, and Cahn advanced the view that all dentigerous cysts should be considered as potential ameloblastomas. Shear (1976) feels that the confusion may have arisen for three reasons. Firstly, an unerupted tooth may be involved by an ameloblastoma, and this may be interpreted incorrectly as a dentigerous cyst on radiographs. Secondly, biopsies of ameloblastomas may be taken of an expanded locule lined apparently by a thin layer of epithelium similar to a non-neoplastic cyst. Thirdly, non-neoplastic islands of odontogenic epithelium in the wall of non-neoplastic cysts may be interpreted as ameloblastoma. Shear (1976) and Lucas (1976) concluded that while such a change is theoretically possible, it must be an extremely rare occurrence.

following hypothesis. Disruption of a thin-walled sinusoid in the red bone marrow leads to the formation of an intra-medullary haematoma. This haemorrhage may result from trauma. Resorption of the affected bone marrow and trabeculae occurs, the process being triggered partly by a rise in intramedullary pressure and partly by the action of breakdown products of haemolysis and a resultant rise in hydrogen ion concentration. The bone cavity so formed enlarges by means of osteoclastic action aided by transudation into the lesion from the breakdown of the blood proteins. Finally the pressure falls, bone resorption ceases and the resultant serous fluid is absorbed by cellular action, leaving an empty cavity within the bone.

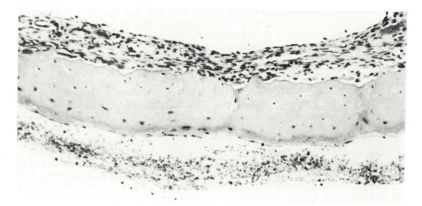

FIG. 19. Lining of a solitary bone cyst, comprising a tenuous fibrous tissue without epithelium and outer bony wall.

REFERENCES

ALLISON, R. T. (1977) Microprobe and microradiographic studies of hyaline bodies in odontogenic cysts. *J. oral Path.* **6**, 44–50.

AREY, L. B. (1965) *Developmental anatomy* (7th ed.), p. 205. Philadelphia and London, Saunders.

BINNIE, W. H., DE LATHOUWER, Cl., BROCHERIOU, Cl., PANDERS, A. K. & PRAETORIUS, F. (1975) Symposium on maxillofacial bone pathology. *Int. J. oral Surg.* **4**, 80–92.

BOUYSSOU, M. & GUILHEM, A. (1965) Recherches morphologiques et histochimiques sur les corps hyalins intrakystiques de Rushton. *Bull. Grpmt. Int. Rech. scient. Stomat.* **8**, 81–104.

BRANNON, R. B. (1976, 1977) The odontogenic keratocyst. A clinico-pathological study of 312 cases. Part I. *Oral Surg.* **42**, 54–72. Part II. *Ibid.* **43**, 233–255.

BROWNE, R. M. (1970) The odontogenic keratocyst – clinical aspects. *Br. dent. J.* **128**, 225–231.

BROWNE, R. M. (1971a) The origin of cholesterol in odontogenic cysts in man. *Archs. oral Biol.* **16**, 107–113.

BROWNE, R. M. (1971b) The odontogenic keratocyst – histological features and their correlation with clinical behaviour. *Br. dent. J.* **131**, 249–259.

BROWNE, R. M. (1976) Some observations on the fluids of odontogenic cysts. *J. oral Path.* **5**, 74–87.

BUCHNER, A. & DAVID, R. (1978) Lipopigment in odontogenic cysts. *J. oral Path.* **7**, 311–317.

CAHN, L. R. (1933) The dentigerous cyst is a potential ameloblastoma. *Dent. Cosmos* **75**, 889–893.

CHEN, S. Y. & MILLER, A. S. (1975) Ultrastructure of the keratinizing and calcifying odontogenic cyst. *Oral Surg.* **39**, 769–780.

CRABB, H. S. M. (1963) Areas simulating carious lesions in the enamel of teeth from dentigerous cysts. *Br. dent. J.* **114**, 499–511.

CRAIG, G. T. (1976) The paradental cyst. A specific inflammatory odontogenic cyst. *Br. dent. J.* **141**, 9–14.

DONATSKY, O., HJORTING-HANSEN, E., PHILIPSEN, H. P. & FEJERSKOV, O. (1976) Clinical, radiologic, and histopathological aspects of 13 cases of naevoid basal cell carcinoma syndrome. *Int. J. oral Surg.* **5**, 19–28.

DONOFF, R. B., HARPER, E. & GURALNICK, W. C. (1972) Collagenolytic activity in keratocysts. *J. oral Surg.* **30**, 879–884.

EL-LABBAN, N. G. (1979) Electron microscopic investigation of hyaline bodies in odontogenic cysts. *J. oral Path.* **8**, 81–93.

EVERSOLE, L. R., SABES, W. R. & ROVIN, S. (1975) Aggressive growth and neoplastic potential of odontogenic cysts. *Cancer* **35**, 270–282.

GABBIANI, G., RYAN, G. B. & MAJNO, G. (1971) Presence of modified fibroblasts in granulation tissue and their possible role in wound contraction. *Experientia* **27**, 549–550.

GARDNER, A. F. (1975) A survey of odontogenic cysts and their relationship to squamous cell carcinoma. *J. Canad. dent. Assoc.* **41**, 161–167.

GORLIN, R. J. PINDBORG, J. J., CLAUSEN, F. P. & VICKERS, R. A. (1962) The calcifying odontogenic cyst – a possible analogue of the cutaneous calcifying epithelioma of Malherbe. *Oral Surg.* **15**, 1235–1245.

GORLIN, R. J., PINDBORG, J. J. & COHEN, M. M. (1976) *Syndromes of the head and neck* (2nd ed.), pp. 520–526. New York, McGraw-Hill.

HARRIS, M. (1978) Odontogenic cyst growth and prostaglandin-induced bone resorption. *Ann. R. Coll. Surg. Engl.* **60**, 86–91.

HARRIS, M. & TOLLER, P. A. (1975) Pathogenesis of dental cysts. *Br. med. Bull.* **31**, 159–163.

HODSON, J. J. (1966) Origin and nature of the cuticula dentis. *Nature* **209**, 990–993.

HODSON, J. J. (1967) The distribution, structure, origin and nature of the dental cuticle of Gottlieb. *Periodontics* **5**, 237–256, 295–302.

HOWE, G. L. (1965) 'Haemorrhagic cysts' of the mandible *Br. J. oral Surg.* **3**, Part I, 55–76; Part II, 77–91.

KRAMER, I. R. H. (1974) Changing views on oral disease. *Proc. R. Soc. Med.* **67**, 271–276.

KRAMER, I. R. H. & TOLLER, P. A. (1973) The use of exfoliative cytology and protein estimations in preoperative diagnosis of odontogenic keratocysts. *Int. J. oral Surg.* **2**, 143–151.

LEE, K. W. & EL-LABBAN, N. G. (1980) A light and electron-microscopic study of smooth muscle-like cells in the walls of radicular (dental) cysts in man. *Archs. oral Biol.* **25**, 403–408.

LUCAS, R. B. (1976) *Pathology of tumours of the oral tissues* (3rd ed.), pp. 46–50. Edinburgh, Churchill, Livingstone.

MAGNUSSON, B. C. (1978) Odontogenic keratocyst. A clinical and histological study with special reference to enzyme histochemistry. *J. oral Path.* **7**, 8–18.

MAIN, D. M. G. (1970) The enlargement of epithelial jaw cysts. *Odont. Revy* **21**, 29–49.

McIVOR, J. (1972) The radiological features of odontogenic keratocysts. *Br. J. oral Surg.* **10**, 116–125.

MORGAN, P. R. & JOHNSON, N. W. (1974) Histological, histochemical and ultrastructural studies on the nature of hyaline bodies in odontogenic cysts. *J. oral Path.* **3**, 127–147.

PHILIPSEN, H. P. (1956) Om keratocyster (kolesteatom) i kaeberne. *Tandlaegebladet* **60**, 963–981.

PINDBORG, J. J. & HANSEN, J. (1963) Studies of odontogenic cyst epithelium. 2. Clinical and roentgenologic aspects of odontogenic keratocysts. *Acta path. microbiol. Scand.* (A) **58**, 283–294.

PINDBORG, J. J., KRAMER, I. R. H. & TORLONI, H. (1971) *Histological typing of odontogenic tumours, jaw cysts, and allied lesions*, pp. 28, 40–41. Geneva, World Health Organisation.

ROBINSON, H. B. G. (1975) Primordial cyst vs. keratocyst. *Oral Surg.* **40**, 362–364.

RUSHTON, M. A. (1955) Hyaline bodies in the epithelium of dental cysts. *Proc. R. Soc. Med.* **48**, 407–409.

SEDANO, J. O. & GORLIN, R. J. (1968) Hyaline bodies of Rushton. Some histochemical considerations concerning their aetiology. *Oral Surg.* **26**, 198–201.

SEWARD, G. R. (1963) Radiology in general dental practice. *Br. dent. J.* **115**, 231.

SHEAR, M. (1960) Primordial cysts. *J. dent. Assoc. S. Afr.* **15**, 211–217.

SHEAR, M. (1961) The hyaline and granular bodies in dental cysts. *Br. dent. J.* **110**, 301–307.

SHEAR, M. (1976) *Cysts of the oral regions.* Bristol, John Wright & Sons.

SHEAR, M. & PINDBORG, J. J. (1975) Microscopic features of the lateral periodontal cyst. *Scand. J. dent. Res.* **83**, 103–110.

SICHER, H. (1962) Anatomy and oral pathology. *Oral Surg.* **15**, 1264–1269.

SKAUG, N. (1976a) Intracystic fluid pressure in non-keratinizing jaw cysts. *Int. J. oral Surg.* **5**, 59–65.

SKAUG, N. (1976b) Lipoproteins in fluids from non-keratinizing jaw cysts. *Scand. J. dent. Res.* **84**, 98–105.

SKAUG, N. (1977) Soluble proteins in fluids from non-keratinizing jaw cysts in man. *Int. J. oral Surg.* **6**, 107–121.

SOSKOLNE, W. A. & SHTEYER, H. (1977) Median mandibular cyst. *Oral Surg.* **44**, 84–88.

STOELINGA, P. J. W. & PETERS, J. H. (1973) A note on the origin of keratocysts of the jaws. *Int. J. oral Surg.* **2**, 37–44.

STONES, H. H. (1951) *Oral and dental diseases* (2nd ed.), pp. 805–809. Edinburgh, Livingstone.

SUMMERS, L. (1974) The incidence of epithelium in peri-apical granulomas and the mechanism of cavitation in apical dental cysts in man. *Archs. oral Biol.* **19**, 1177–1180.

TOLLER, P. A. (1967) Origin and growth of cysts of the jaws. *Ann. R. Coll. Surg., Engl.* **40**, 306–336.

TOLLER, P. A. (1970) The osmolality of fluids from cysts of the jaws. *Br. dent. J.* **129**, 275–278.

WARWICK JAMES, W. & COUNSELL, A. (1932) A histological study of the epithelium associated with chronic apical infection of the teeth. *Br. dent. J.* **53**, 463–483.

WORLD HEALTH ORGANISATION (1978) *Application of the International Classification of Diseases to Dentistry and Stomatology.* Geneva.

Chapter 19

SOFT CONNECTIVE-TISSUE DISORDERS AND THE PERIODONTAL LIGAMENT

D. M. Chisholm

INTRODUCTION

The connective-tissue disorders comprise a group of diseases affecting connective tissues which at present can only be classified together on the basis of the similarity of the tissue changes. Indeed, it is not unusual for a number of these disorders to occur together in one individual. Whilst the aetiology of these disorders is unknown, recent evidence suggests that they have an autoimmune basis. Despite unresolved problems concerning aetiology and pathogenesis, however, in all probability the diseases are multi-factorial, with genetic, infective, immunological and environmental components playing varying parts.

By their multi-organ involvement, the connective-tissue disorders may alter the oral environment by impeding oral hygiene such that periodontal disease occurs as a secondary consequence of the primary disease state. However, involvement of the periodontal ligament as a direct result of a connective-tissue disorder appears to obtain for progressive systemic sclerosis (scleroderma) only and for none of the other 'collagen diseases' of man. For this reason, this short chapter will be concerned mainly with scleroderma, only brief mention being made of other disorders. In addition, although not classically belonging to the connective-tissue-disorders group, information will also be given about the effects of

lathyrogens on the periodontal ligament and about atrophy of this tissue due to reduced function. Mention will also be made of the effects of mucopolysaccharidoses.

PROGRESSIVE SYSTEMIC SCLEROSIS

Progressive systemic sclerosis or scleroderma is a chronic disease characterized by diffuse sclerosis of the skin, gastrointestinal tract, cardiac muscle, lungs and kidney (Winkelmann, 1971).

The disease most commonly affects females between the ages of 20 and 50 years. The onset is usually insidious. Among the changes in skin are induration, hyperpigmentation and telangiectasia. Raynaud's phenomenon (digital arterial insufficiency provoked by cold) is a common feature, while calcification of subcutaneous tissue (calcinosis universalis) tends to be a late manifestation. The clinical symptoms vary according to the extent and organ involvement. Thus, cardiac, pulmonary, renal and gastrointestinal symptoms may be present. Morphoea or localized scleroderma is a localized benign, self-limiting form of the disease affecting the skin.

The clinical association of progressive systemic sclerosis with other connective-tissue diseases (including systemic lupus erythematosus, rheumatoid arthritis, Sjögren's syndrome and mixed connective tissue disease) suggests an immunological cause or causes. Although some evidence of cell-mediated cytotoxicity against embryonic fibroblasts is available, inflammatory cell infiltration is slight and humoral changes are not directly suggestive of a pathogenic mechanism. Hypergammaglobulinaemia and circulating serum autoantibodies are often present. The hypergammaglobulinaemia is usually polyclonal and rheumatoid factors are often found. The fluorescent anti-nuclear antibody test shows a speckled or nucleolar pattern in 70% of cases. Those patients with mixed connective-tissue disease have high levels of anti-ribonuclease-sensitive extractable nuclear antigen (Rothfield and Rodman, 1968; Sharp, Irwin and Tan, 1972).

Weisman and Calcaterra (1978) found that 80% of scleroderma patients show head and neck manifestations, while 30% have head and neck features as the presenting symptoms. These features included dysphagia, tight facial skin and telangiectasia, decreased mouth opening (Fig. 1), microstomia and

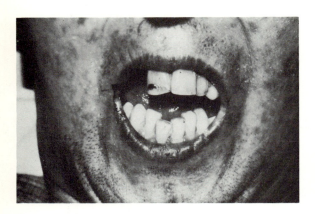

FIG. 1. Progressive systemic sclerosis. Reduced mouth opening, gross dental and periodontal disease, angular cheilitis and mottled skin.

dryness of the mouth. Progressive systemic sclerosis may also present as the connective tissue manifestation of Sjögren's syndrome. Involvement of the lips and cheeks restricts mastication and temporomandibular joint movement. Indeed, the joint may become fixed. Induration and immobility of the tongue interfere with mastication, swallowing and speech. Exposure of the teeth following lip retraction

(Fig. 2) may result in increased caries and periodontal disease, while immobile mucous membranes are particularly susceptible to trauma from mastication or dentures.

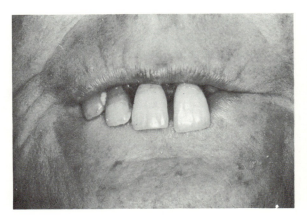

FIG. 2. Female patient with advanced progressive systemic sclerosis. Lip retraction together with acquired microstomia results in exaggerated prominence of upper anterior dentition.

Radiographically, there is often widening of the periodontal space (Fig. 3). This feature is found in 30–100% of cases (Stafne and Austin, 1944; Rowell and Hopper, 1977; White et al., 1977). Rowell and Hopper (1977) found no direct relationship between widening of the ligament and other systemic changes. Thickening of the periodontal ligament is associated with an insidious gingival recession. A meticulous

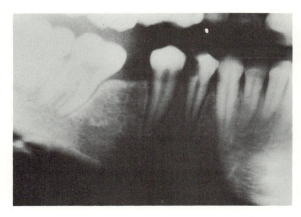

FIG. 3. Radiograph indicating the periodontal ligament thickening in a case of progressive systemic sclerosis.

approach to periodontal therapy is required. Should tooth extraction become necessary a surgical technique is advisable. In spite of the wider ligament, however, the teeth in scleroderma are not hypermobile (Fullmer and Witte, 1962; Jayson, 1976). Posterior teeth seem to be affected more than anterior teeth.

Investigation of periodontal ligament affected by scleroderma revealed a ligament up to 3 mm thick with collagen fibres in apical and middle thirds of the ligament running almost parallel to the root (Fig. 4) and an absence of cellular cementum (Stafne and Austin, 1944; Gores, 1957). Continuity of the fibres seemed to be lost a short distance from the cementum. Scattered through the fibrous tissue were many spicules of bone. The walls of blood vessels were thickened and their lumina narrowed (Stafne and Austin, 1944; Gores, 1957) as in other tissues affected by the disease (Krogh, 1950). Bailey (1976) observed that sites of scleroderma contain many thin, apparently newly formed fibres reminiscent of embryonic collagen.

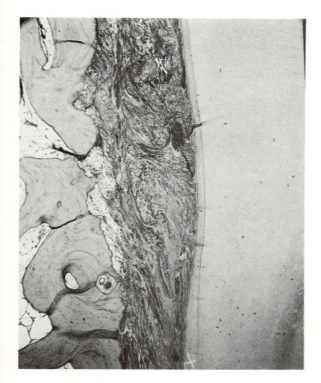

FIG. 4. Scleroderma. Note widened ligament and fibres **almost parallel** to root. ×21.

In a detailed histological and histochemical study, Fullmer and Witte (1962) showed that the scleroderma-affected ligament contained collagen, oxytalan and elastin fibres. The collagen was more dense, mature and hyalinized than normal, especially adjacent to the teeth. The number of oxytalan fibres increased proportionately with the collagen. The fibres were aligned normally in the transseptal region. Elsewhere they were aligned almost parallel to the root with occasional sites of indiscriminate orientation. Some sites contained many mast cells. These workers found no alteration in cementum in amount or type. They concluded that the thickening of the periodontal ligament was due to bone resorption and a proportionate increase in collagen and oxytalan fibre content, including areas of degenerating fibres. Sclerosis and hyalinization of collagen and development of elastic fibres were most marked adjacent to the cementum.

Regarding possible chemical factors underlying the ligament changes in scleroderma, it has been shown that there is a considerable increase in the proportion of reducible aldimine bond cross-links in scleroderma-affected connective tissue. These intermolecular cross-links (which are responsible for the high tensile strength of collagen fibres) are replaced by more stable non-reducible cross-links during maturation (Herbert *et al.*, 1974; Jayson, 1976). The older tissue from the centre of lesions in morphoea (the localized form of scleroderma) also contains lower levels of detectable cross-links than younger tissue from the edge of the lesion, where collagen is being synthesized (Herbert *et al.*, 1974). Jayson (1976) was unable to find a serum factor to which might be attributed the increased production of collagen (as shown by ^{3}H-proline uptake in skin cultures) occurring in sites of active scleroderma (Herbert *et al.*, 1974).

Concerning the treatment of scleroderma, the drug D-penicillamine is used because it binds to the aldehyde cross-link precursor, thus inhibiting cross-linking, and producing a more fragile fibre. The drug has no effect on mature sclerodermatous collagen (Herbert *et al.*, 1974).

As mentioned previously, with the exception of scleroderma there is little evidence of direct periodontal ligament involvement in these disorders although indirectly periodontitis may result from difficulties in maintaining satisfactory oral hygiene. However, a fortuitous case of periodontosis has been diagnosed in a patient with disseminated dermato-myositis (Newman and Dunn, unpublished finding).

Bailey (1976) has reviewed the sparse information available concerning possible periodontal ligament effects in some other connective-tissue disorders. (Developmental disorders are considered in more detail in Chapter 11.)

LATHYRISM

Lathyrism is the name given to denote the condition caused by administering drugs which specifically inhibit cross-linking in collagen, acting on the enzyme lysyl oxidase (e.g. Siegel and Martin, 1970). This results in fragile collagen fibres in the connective tissues (at least in those in which collagen is turning over, such as the periodontal ligament). The drugs include aminoacetonitrile, B-aminopropionitrile and cysteamine. They have been of particular use in studying eruptive mechanisms (see Chapter 10). Since collagen contraction has been implicated in generating the eruptive force, the effects on eruption rates following the administration of lathyrogens have been studied. By inhibiting cross-linking, these drugs should significantly reduce any contraction occurring during collagen maturation and thus retard eruption. However, though lathyritic drugs retard impeded eruption in continuously growing rodent incisors (e.g. Sarnat and Sciaky, 1965; Thomas, 1965; Berkovitz, Migdalski and Solomon, 1972; Michaeli et al., 1975), there is little effect on unimpeded eruption rates (e.g. Berkovitz et al., 1972; Tsuruta, Eto and Chiba, 1974).

Following administration of lathyritic agents to rodents, loss of tooth support due to damage of periodontal ligament fibres is indicated by looseness of the teeth and the subsequent ease with which they can be extracted (Dasler, 1954; Sciaky and Ungar, 1961; Berkovitz et al., 1972). Interference with the tooth-support mechanisms is also indicated by the occurrence of dilaceration of the root, particularly the continuously growing maxillary incisors.

The most significant change occurring in the periodontal ligament of the rat dentition is a gradual hyalinization of its structure (Fig. 5) (Gardner, Dasler and Weinmann, 1958; Sciaky and Ungar, 1961; Krikos, Beltran and Cohen, 1965; Sarnat and Sciaky, 1965; Thomas, 1965). The collagen fibres lose their coarse, fibrous appearance and characteristic orientation. Instead, they appear as fine fibrils embedded in increased amounts of an amorphous, eosinophilic material which is surrounded by palisading fibroblasts (Fig. 5). The fibrils lack any preferential orientation. The cells bordering the hyalinized zone were more cuboidal than normal fibroblasts. The general histological appearance seems to be related to the mechanical stresses placed on the tooth since, if the opposing teeth are extracted, the ligament appears normal (Krikos et al., 1965).

Studies of periodontal changes in lathyrism to date have been at the light microscope level. More detailed ultrastructural studies are awaited.

MUCOPOLYSACCHARIDOSES AND MUCOLIPIDOSES

The mucopolysaccharidoses (MPS) are conditions in which there are inherited defects of ground substance metabolism. They have received little attention regarding possible periodontal effects. The only histological finding seems to be the presence around some teeth affected by delayed eruption of hyperplastic dental follicles containing excess dermatan sulphate in some cases (Gorlin et al., 1976). Gorlin et al. (1976) also note that gingival and alveolar enlargement can occur. Teeth may be widely spaced. Tooth abscesses have been noted in the final stages of MPS III. Eruption of permanent molars is retarded in MPS VI, and some of the affected teeth may be deeply buried and angulated in the mandible. The teeth may also be surmounted by radiolucent bony defects that represent the accumulation of dermatan sulphate in hyperplastic follicles (Gorlin et al., 1976). Dorst (1972 – in Gorlin et al., 1976) has reported on the accumulation of storage material about unerupted first permanent molars in some cases of gangliosidosis. Tooth spacing has been found in mucolipidoses. In mucolipidoses II the teeth may be buried in hypertrophied alveolus and gingiva and may not erupt at all. There is accumula-

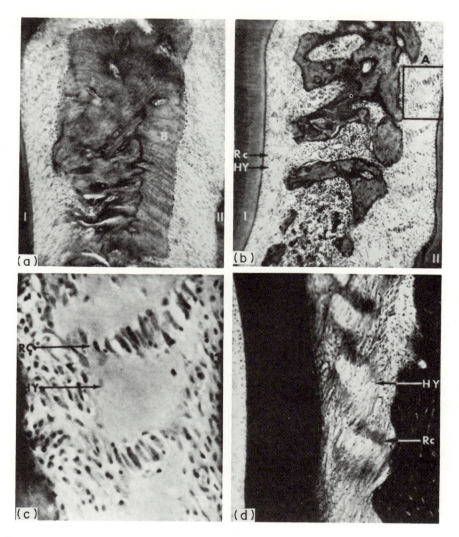

FIG. 5. Lathyrism. (a) Mesiodistal section of interdental alveolar septum and periodontal membrane between the upper first (I) and second (II) molars of control animals, 43 days of age, fed a 50% edible pea diet for 3 weeks. Principal fibres run from the surface of the alveolar process to a more apical area at the surface of the cementum, the marrow spaces are small, and bundle bone is wide at B. (Haematoxylin and eosin stain; orig. mag. ×115.) (b) Mesiodistal section of the interdental alveolar septum and periodontal membrane between the upper first (I) and second (II) molars of experimental animals, 43 days of age, fed a 50% sweet pea diet for 3 weeks. Note hyaline layers separated by palisade-arranged cells in the periodontal membrane, enlarged marrow spaces in the alveolar septum, and the lack of bundle bone formation. Rc – rows of palisade cells, HY – hyalinization. (Haematoxylin and eosin stain; orig. mag. ×115.) (c) Photomicrograph of area A in (b). Note hyaline layers separated by palisade-arranged cells in the periodontal membrane. RC – rows of palisade cells, HY – hyalinization. (Haematoxylin and eosin stain; orig. mag. ×560.) (d) Photomicrograph of a mesiodistal section of the periodontal membrane of an experimental animal, 43 days of age, fed a 50% sweet pea diet for 3 weeks. Note the large numbers of fibres in areas of cells (Rc) and the few fibres in areas of hyalinization (HY). (Mallory stain; orig. mag. ×270.)

tion of storage material about the crowns of unerupted first molars (as in gangliosidosis). Widely spaced teeth occur also in mannosidosis and aspartylglucosaminuria (Gorlin *et al.,* 1976).

DISUSE ATROPHY

The subject of connective-tissue disorders affecting the periodontal ligament, on a practical basis, may include atrophy due to reduced function. The main features are narrowing of the ligament and reduction in the number of principal fibres (Henry and Weinmann, 1951). The remaining collagen fibres are orientated more or less parallel to the long axis of the root, and the ligament shows reduced rate of collagen turnover (Henry and Weinmann, 1951; Ruben *et al.,* 1970). In spite of the term atrophy, some ligament function appears to persist even if only from contact of tooth with surrounding oral soft tissues. The atrophic ligament is thought to adapt poorly to sudden stress (Ruben *et al.,* 1970). In mouse molars, loss of function without any apparent infection caused progressive ligament atrophy. This led to almost total disappearance of the periodontal ligament within 900 days (the approximate life span of the animal). At this time, only traces of ligament remained (Cohn, 1965). Periodontal ligament around rat molars 3 days after extraction of the opponent teeth showed increased remodelling of collagen, as measured by ^{3}H-proline uptake (Kanoza *et al.,* 1980). This the authors suggested was related to reactivated eruption, although it seems unrelated to the long-term atrophic changes described previously.

REFERENCES

BAILEY, A. J. (1976) In: *The eruption and occlusion of teeth,* D. F. G. POOLE and M. V. STACK (eds.), pp. 277–278. London, Butterworths.

BERKOVITZ, B. K. B., MIGDALSKI, A. & SOLOMON, M. (1972) The effect of the lathyritic agent amino-acetonitrile on the unimpeded eruption rate in normal and root-resected rat lower incisors. *Archs. oral Biol.* 17, 1755–1763.

COHN, S. A. (1965) Disuse atrophy of the periodontium in mice. *Archs. oral Biol.* 10, 909–919.

DASLER, W. (1954) Incisor ash versus femur ash in sweet pea lathyrism (Odoratism). *J. Nutr.* 54, 397–402.

FULLMER, H. M. & WITTE, W. E. (1962) Periodontal membrane affected by scleroderma. *Arch. Path.* 73, 184–189.

GARDNER, A. F., DASLER, W. & WEINMANN, J. P. (1958) Masticatory apparatus of albino rats in experimental lathyrism. *J. dent. Res.* 37, 492–515.

GORES, R. J. (1957) Dental characteristics associated with acrosclerosis and diffuse scleroderma. *J. Amer. dent. Assoc.* 54, 755–759.

GORLIN, R. J., PINDBORG, J. J. & COHEN, M. M. (1976) *Syndromes of the head and neck* (2nd ed.), pp. 476–509. New York, McGraw-Hill.

HENRY, J. L. & WEINMANN, J. P. (1951) The pattern of resorption and repair of human cementum. *J. Amer. dent. Assoc.* 42, 270–290.

HERBERT, C. M., LINDBERG, K. A., JAYSON, M. I. V. & BAILEY, A. J. (1974) Biosynthesis and maturation of skin collagen in scleroderma, and effect of D-penicillamine. *Lancet* 1, 187–192.

JAYSON, M. I. V. (1976) Collagen studies in connective tissue diseases. In: *The eruption and occlusion of teeth,* D. F. G. POOLE & M. V. STACK (eds.), pp. 267–270 and 277. London, Butterworths.

KANOZA, R. J. J., KELLEHER, L., SODEK, J. & MELCHER, A. H. (1980) A biochemical analysis of the effect of hypofunction on collagen metabolism in the rat molar periodontal ligament. *Archs. oral Biol.* 25, 663–668.

KRIKOS, G. A., BELTRAN, R. & COHEN, A. (1965) Significance of mechanical stress on the development of periodontal lesions in lathyritic rats. *J. dent. Res.* 44, 600–607.

KROGH, H. W. (1950) Dental manifestations of scleroderma. Report of case. *J. oral Surg.* 8, 242–244.

MICHAELI, Y., PITURA, S., ZAJICEK, G. & WEINREB, M. M. (1975) Role of attrition and occlusal contact in the physiology of the rat incisor. IX. Impeded and unimpeded eruption in lathyritic rats. *J. dent. Res.* 54, 891–896.

ROTHFIELD, N. F. & RODMAN, G. P. (1968) Serum antinuclear antibodies in progressive systemic sclerosis. *Arthritis and rheumatism* 11, 607–616.

ROWELL, N. R. & HOPPER, F. E. (1977) The periodontal membrane in systemic sclerosis. *Br. J. Dermatol.* 96, 15–20.

RUBEN, M. P., GOLDMAN, H. M. & SCHULMAN, S. M. (1970) Diseases of the periodontium. In: *Thoma's oral pathology,* Vol. I, R. J. GORLIN & H. M. GOLDMAN (eds.), pp. 394–444. St. Louis, Mosby.

SARNAT, H. & SCIAKY, I. (1965) Experimental lathyrism in rats; effects of removing incisal stress. *Periodontics* 3, 128–134.

SCIAKY, I. & UNGAR, H. (1961) Effects of experimental lathyrism on the suspensory apparatus of incisors and molars in rats. *Ann. Dent.* 20, 90–99.

SHARP, G. C., IRWIN, W. S. & TAN, E. M. (1972) Mixed connective tissue disease. *Amer. J. Med.* 52, 148–159.

SIEGEL, R. C. & MARTIN, G. R. (1970) Collagen cross-linking. Enzymatic synthesis of lysine-derived aldehydes and the production of cross-linked components. *J. biol. Chem.* 245, 1653–1658.

STAFNE, E. C. & AUSTIN, L. T. (1944) A characteristic

dental finding in acrosclerosis and diffuse scleroderma. *J. oral Surg.* **30**, 25–29.

THOMAS, N. R. (1965) The process and mechanisms of tooth eruption. Ph.D. Thesis. University of Bristol.

TSURUTA, M., ETO, K. & CHIBA, M. (1974) Effect of daily or 4-hourly administrations of lathyrogens on the eruption rates of impeded and unimpeded mandibular incisors of rats. *Archs. oral Biol.* **19**, 1221–1226.

WEISMAN, R. A. & CALCATERRA, T. C. (1978) Head and neck manifestations of scleroderma. *Ann. Otol. Rhinol. Laryngol.* **87**, 332–339.

WHITE, S. C., FREY, N. W., BLASCHKNE, D. D., ROSS, M. D., CLEMENTS, P. J., FURST, D. E. & PAULUS, H. E. (1977) Oral radiographic changes in patients with progressive systemic sclerosis (scleroderma). *J. Amer. dent. Assoc.* **94**, 1178–1182.

WINKELMANN, R. K. (1971) Classification and pathogenesis of scleroderma. *Mayo Clin. Proc.* **46**, 83–91.

Chapter 20

THE EFFECTS OF HORMONES AND NUTRITIONAL FACTORS ON THE PERIODONTAL LIGAMENT
M. M. Ferguson

INTRODUCTION

Little is known about the influence of the nutritional and hormonal status of an individual on the condition of the periodontal ligament. However, knowledge about this is not only essential for appreciating how changes outside the normal range of metabolism induce a pathological disturbance but also for understanding the normal structure and function of the tissue.

Clearly, the condition of a connective tissue is governed by its anabolism and catabolism which in turn are influenced by local biochemical factors, availability of essential dietary substances and controlling factors, both neurogenic and hormonal. It is not unreasonable, therefore, to propose that a first step towards improving our understanding of the mechanisms which control the metabolism of the periodontal ligament involves a full appreciation of the manner of synthesis and degradation of its various components. Information concerning this for periodontal ligament fibres, ground substance and cells are described in Chapters 4, 6 and 2 respectively. As these reviews indicate, however, much still needs to be discovered and consequently the study of hormonal and nutritional influences is handicapped. A further complication concerns the compartmentalization of periodontal ligament research. It is apparent that many of the problems related to this tissue can be solved only by an approach more integrated than has been attempted hitherto. An additional difficulty arises because some of the changes seen in connective tissues are common to several kinds of nutritional or hormonal imbalances and are therefore non-specific. Further problems (often seen in man) occur as a result of multiple deficiencies or excesses.

The functional state of the periodontal ligament also has a bearing on these matters. For example, it seems likely that the age of the tissue plays a role in its sensitivity to a given substrate deficiency. Also, it has been suggested that the higher the rate of turnover of a connective tissue, the more easily its metabolism is influenced (e.g. Neuberger, Perrone and Slack, 1951; Neuberger and Slack, 1953; Neuberger, 1955). On this basis, the rapid turnover of the periodontal ligament (Carneiro and Fava de Moraes, 1965) (see Chapter 4) suggests that it may be readily influenced by hormonal and nutritional disturbances.

It is well to remember that nutritional factors and hormones interrelate so that a dietary deficiency can affect the functional state of endocrine glands. In spite of this integration, for ease of description, the effects of hormones and diet will here be discussed separately. Finally, two general points concerning this topic must be borne in mind. Firstly, what little is known is based on studies of relatively gross deficiencies or excesses of dietary factors or hormones. Secondly, much of the information is based upon animal experimentation. The difficulties of extrapolating the results of such experiments to man cannot be too strongly emphasised.

HORMONES AND THE PERIODONTAL LIGAMENT

Metabolic control leading to body homeostasis is regulated by the secretions of the endocrine system. The actions of most hormones are widespread, involving many tissues, and where fibroblasts and osteoblasts in particular are influenced at any site in the body, it may be anticipated that the same effects will be manifest within the periodontal ligament. In addition, the immune system is also influenced by endocrine (and nutritional) factors and this is of particular relevance in the periodontium.

The variation in the molecular configuration of hormones is considerable and target cell receptor mechanisms differ. Whereas steroids attach to cytoplasmic receptors and subsequently nuclear receptors, the remainder of hormones are considered to bind to surface receptor mechanisms on the plasma membrane and exert their effect by altering intra-cellular cyclic-AMP synthesis.

The production rates of different hormones are frequently interrelated and in any experimental procedure designed to alter a particular hormonal status cognizance should be taken of other compensatory fluctuations. Furthermore, the nervous system has a major influence upon the endocrine system. For example, the anterior pituitary gland (a producer of many of the trophic hormones controlling other endocrine glands) is regulated by the activity of the hypothalamus. Consequently, experimental procedures affecting one system can lead to compensatory changes in the other. Indeed, should the effects be extreme enough, pathological changes may result.

Since it is the reviewer's remit to emphasize what little is known about the specific hormonal effects on the periodontal ligament, the reader is referred elsewhere to the considerable number of comprehensive texts on endocrinology for more general information. Nevertheless, a few general statements to introduce each hormone are necessary to provide some basis for understanding its action.

Pituitary gland

The pituitary gland secretes a series of peptide hormones from both the anterior and posterior lobes.

Hypophysectomy in rats has been seen to result in reduced vascularity of the periodontal ligaments of incisors and molars (Schour and Van Dyke, 1932 a and b; Schour, 1934; Shapiro and Shklar, 1962) (Fig. 1). Degeneration of the ligament with cystic degeneration and calcification of many of the epithelial rests has also been reported. Further, the junctional epithelium is often atrophic or absent. Whether such changes are the direct result of the hypophysectomy or are attributable to the reduction in blood supply or to changes in other endocrine glands has not been assessed.

Since the periodontal ligament appears to be the site of the eruptive mechanism (see Chapter 10), a hormonal effect on eruption may be regarded as evidence in favour of the view that the hormone has produced periodontal changes. Following hypophysectomy, decreased eruption has been reported in the rat incisor (Schour and Van Dyke, 1931, 1932 a, b, 1934; Baume et al., 1954a; Bryer, 1957; Garren and Greep, 1960; Kusner, Michaeli and Weinreb, 1973). Hypopituitarism was associated with delayed and hyperpituitarism with accelerated eruption

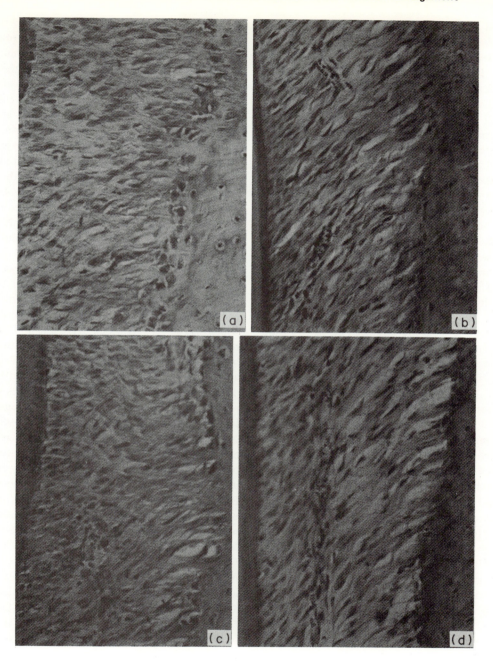

FIG. 1. The effect of hypophysectomy on (rat) periodontal ligament. (a) Control. Note large number of osteoblasts lining bone surface. The ligament is regular in appearance and highly cellular. ×350. (b) Hypophysectomized animal. The ligament fibres present some separation and the fibroblasts are smaller, more deeply staining, and fewer in number. The osteoblasts are reduced in number and have smaller nuclei. ×350. (c) Hypophysectomized animal. The ligament fibres show separation and degeneration. ×350. (d) Hypophysectomized animal. Osteoblasts are absent, ligament fibroblasts are reduced in number and the fibres show degenerative changes. ×350.

(Schour and Massler, 1943). Studies confirm that the pituitary effects on eruption are not due to changes in blood levels of growth hormone (e.g. Baume, Becks and Evans, 1954b; Bryer, 1957) but most probably act through the thyroid gland (Baume, Becks and Evans, 1954c; Domm and Wellband, 1961) and adrenal cortex (Domm and Wellband, 1961). Growth hormone and thyroxine produce the same eruption rate as thyroxine alone (Baume, Becks and Evans, 1954c).

With respect to the anterior pituitary, only growth hormone is known to influence the oral tissues: this may be either from the direct action or secondarily by the stimulation of somatedin, a sulphation factor from the liver and kidneys. In children an excessive secretion of growth hormone leads to gigantism and, depending upon the age of onset, the rate of tooth eruption may be increased. Conversely, in hypopituitarism there is a decrease in the secretion of growth hormone and dental eruption is retarded. These effects are also seen in the eruption of the rat incisor (e.g. Schour and Van Dyke, 1932 a, b). In the acromegalic adult there is enlargement of the entire facial skeleton and this is particularly striking in the mandible. The expansion of the dental arches results in the teeth being spaced apart. Stahl and Joly (1958) observed that injection of growth hormone resulted in increased cellularity of the (rat) periodontal ligament. Administration of cortisone to young adult (male) rats was associated with reduced cellularity of the ligament. The effect was reversed by somatotropic hormone (Stahl and Gerstner, 1960).

Little information is available concerning the effects of the hormones of the posterior pituitary. However, Litvin and De Marco (1973) claim that twice-daily injections of antidiuretic vasopressin to rabbits increased the unimpeded rate of eruption of their incisors.

Thyroid gland

The action of thyroxine and triiodothyronine (which are secreted from the follicles of the thyroid gland) is to generally increase the basic metabolic rate. Calcitonin, a peptide from the C-cells, appears to suppress osteoblastic activity and also causes a reduction in the plasma calcium and phosphorus concentrations. The effect of calcitonin on the periodontium is considered along with other aspects of calcium metabolism.

When the thyroid is excised from rats the enamel organ undergoes partial atrophy (Baume and Becks, 1952). Thyroidectomy in the new-born rat has been reported to produce a reduction in cellularity of the incisor periodontal ligament (Baume *et al.*, 1954c). This effect was reversed with the administration of thyroxine or growth hormone. In rabbits, surgically induced hypothyroidism causes degeneration and fragmentation of periodontal ligament collagen fibres (Rosenberg, Goldman and Garber, 1961).

The experimental excision of the thyroid gland must include the C-cells of the thyroid itself and possibly the parathyroid glands. An alternative procedure has been to dose animals with propylthiouracil which will selectively block thyroxine and triiodothyronine synthesis. In rats treated in this manner there is both a delay in the organization of the collagen fibres and a decrease in the amount of fibres in the periodontal ligament: myxoid tissue becomes apparent relatively early and is particularly prominent adjacent to the alveolar bone surface (Paynter, 1954; Pinto, 1974) (Fig. 2). Likewise in rabbits there is a decreased cellularity, hydropic degeneration and interstitial oedema (Rosenberg *et al.*, 1961). In thiouracil-induced hypothyroidism in the rat, Glickman and Pruzansky (1947) have seen retardation of alveolar bone apposition. Hypothyroidism is also associated with delayed eruption of human teeth (Schour and Massler, 1943).

Thyroidectomy has resulted in decreased eruption in the rat (Baume *et al.*, 1954a; Bryer, 1957; Domm and Wellband, 1961), while a similar effect occurs after administration of propylthiouracil (Garren and Greep, 1955; Bryer, 1957). Baume *et al.* (1954c) found that growth hormone did not restore the eruption rate following thyroidectomy. Delays in tooth eruption have been recorded also in hypothyroid humans (Garn, Lewis and Blizzard, 1965).

Early eruption is said to occur in hyperthyroidism. In man an increase in the eruption rate of normal rats has followed the administration of thyroxine (Herzberg and Schour, 1941; Bryer, 1957; Schumer

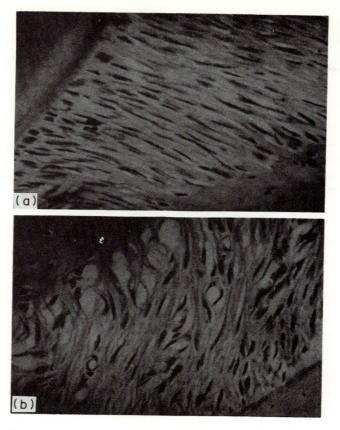

FIG. 2. The effect of hypothyroidism on the (rat) periodontal ligament. (a) Control specimen showing normal ligament. ×300. (b) Myxoid structure of the ligament in a hypothyroid animal (condition induced 85 days previously by 6-propylthiouracil administration). ×300.

and Wells, 1958; Moxham and Berkovitz, 1980), thyroid gland powder (Garren and Greep, 1955; Bryer, 1957) and triiodothyroacetic acid (Schumer and Wells, 1958). Thyroid powder (Garren and Greep, 1955) or thyroxine (Baume, Becks and Evans, 1954c) have been found to substitute for lost thyroid tissue.

Goldman (1943) has reported that hyperthyroidism in guinea pigs produced by the administration of very large doses of thyroxine results in an increased periodontal vascularity. Also, a widened periodontal space was seen. In rats fed thyroid extract for up to 16 weeks, an increase in the periodontal ligament

width and vascularity was also reported (Baume and Becks, 1952).

Hypothyroidism in rabbits has been observed to lead to the degeneration, fragmentation and moderate disorganization of the ligament fibres. There was also diminished cellularity and areas of hydropic degeneration. Hyperthyroidism produced a highly cellular, well-organized, slightly thickened ligament (Baume, Becks and Evans, 1954c; Rosenberg, Goldman and Garber, 1961). The combination of growth hormone with thyroxine produces a more vascular and cellular ligament than normal (Baume, Becks and Evans, 1954c).

Parathyroid glands

Parathormone is a polypeptide secreted by the para-thyroid glands in response to low concentrations of plasma calcium and magnesium. The action of para-thormone is to increase intestinal absorption of calcium, increase bone resorption and inhibit phos-phorus reabsorption in the renal tubules. In bone, parathormone appears to cause calcium resorption by affecting both the osteocytes and the osteoclasts. Collagen formation may also be inhibited.

The influence of parathormone on the periodontal ligament is discussed in the section on calcium metabolism.

The adrenals

The adrenal cortex is a source of glucocorticos-teroids, mineralocorticosteroids and some sex hor-mones. The adrenal medulla secretes adrenaline. Shklar (1965) has studied the effects of adrenalec-tomy on the periodontal tissues. He reported that although there was a marked reduction in osteo-blastic activity in the interdental septum in rats, no changes in periodontal ligament collagen fibres were seen. Glickman, Stone and Chawla (1953) observed a loss of tooth-supporting bone in adrenalectomized mice. Shklar (1965) reported that osteogenesis in alveolar bone, which was reduced in adrenalectomized rats, was restored by cortisone replacement. With respect to the hormones of the adrenal cortex, no changes in the gingivae or periodontal ligament are described in hypoadrenocorticism (Addison's disease). A reduced rate of eruption of rat incisors was reported by Garren and Greep (1960) and Domm and Wellband (1960, 1961) following adrenal-ectomy. This rate was restored to normal levels by cortisone.

Administration of high doses of cortisone to mice leads to a reduction in cellularity and loss of definition of fibre bundles of the periodontal ligament and to osteoporosis of the alveolar bone (Glickman et al., 1953; Applebaum and Seeling, 1955; Glickman and Shklar, 1955; Stahl and Gerstner, 1960; Labelle and Schaffer, 1966) (Fig. 3). Glickman, Stone and Chawla (1953) reported that cortisone injections in mice result in vascular disturbances within the perio-dontal ligament and degenerative changes within the collagen fibres (associated with inflammation caused by local irritation). In addition, osteoporosis occurred in the alveolar bone. The simultaneous administration of oestrogen caused an increase in the number of fibroblasts which had larger nuclei than normal. It also increased the number of fibres although these lacked the normal arrangement (Glickman and Shklar, 1954) (Fig. 3). Hydrocortisone also caused a loss of ligament fibres in rats. The effect was almost completely prevented by fluoride (Zipkin, Bernick and Menczel, 1965; Lipari, Blake and Zipkin, 1974). Mucopolysaccharide synthesis is also affected with diminished production of hyaluronic acid, chondroitin-6-sulphate and heparin (Kofoed and Bozzini, 1970). The changes in alveolar bone can be inhibited by the administration of relatively high doses of fluoride (Zipkin, Bernick and Menczel, 1965; Lipari, Blake and Zipkin, 1974).

In marmosets to which cortisone was given there was a very substantial reduction in the number of acute and chronic inflammatory cells within the gingivae: this seemed to facilitate invasion of the papillae by numerous micro-organisms (Dreizen, Levy and Bernick, 1971) (Fig. 4). In addition, there was reduced fibroblast activity with a decrease in the size and number of fibroblasts and impaired collagen synthesis; collagen bundles became thinned and fibrillar degeneration occurred with oedema of the ligament. These findings have also been noted with dexamethasone administration where the alveolar bone of the marmosets became osteoporotic and the periodontal fibres reduced in quantity due to a reduction in collagen synthesis (Sallum et al., 1976) (Fig. 5).

Regarding tooth eruption, Domm and Wellband (1960) and Garren and Greep (1960) found that daily doses of cortisone resulted in a significant increase in the eruption of rat incisors. Ball (1977) noted that maintaining mature rates in a hyper-glucocorticoid state (using weekly subcutaneous injections of methylprednisolone acetate) produced a significant increase in the eruption rates of the mandibular incisors. In all these studies the erup-tion rates were impeded. It has been shown, how-ever, that hydrocortisone also increases unimpeded rates in normal (Moxham and Berkovitz, 1980)

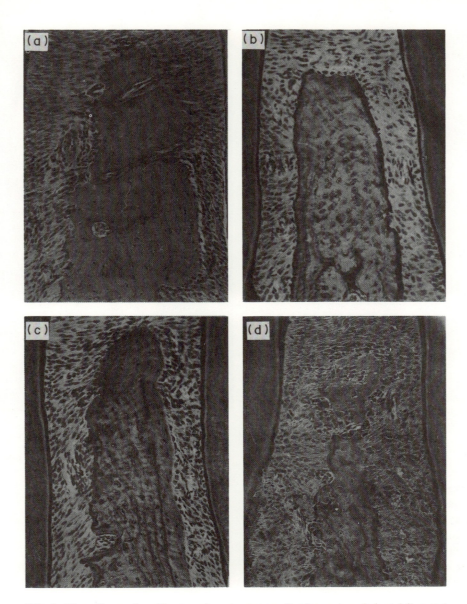

FIG. 3. The effects of cortisone and oestrogen on the (mouse) periodontal ligament.
(a) Control. ×145. (b) Cortisone-treated animal. With the exception of isolated areas, the
periodontal ligament fibres are replaced by a homogeneous, minutely fibrillar stroma. The
fibroblasts are fewer in number and less regular in appearance than in the control animal.
×145. (c) Oestrogen-treated animal. There appears to be an increase in numbers of fibroblasts and cementoblasts. ×145. (d) Cortisone- and oestrogen-treated animal. Note area
of new bone formation at crest with a bordering zone of fibroblasts. ×145.

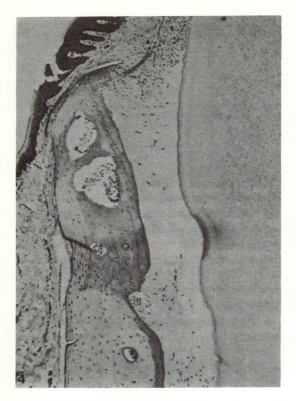

FIG. 4. Cortisone-induced changes in primate (marmoset) periodontal ligament. Reduction in fibroblast content of periodontal ligament in marmoset treated with cortisone for 4 months. ×20.

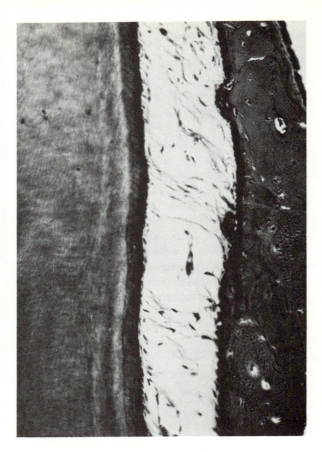

FIG. 5. Effects on the (marmoset) periodontal ligament of occlusal traumatism and dexamethasone. The ligament shows reduced cellularity and loss of fibres compared with control specimens subjected to trauma alone. ×60.

and root-resected teeth (Berkovitz, 1971). Parmer, Katonah and Argrist (1951) and Domm and Marzano (1954) noted that cortisone hastened tooth eruption in new-born rats.

No information is available concerning periodontal effects of adrenaline. However, there have been studies on the effects of nor-adrenaline on tooth support and the eruptive mechanism. Slatter and Picton (1972) and Wills, Picton and Davies (1976) have recorded changes in mobility of macaque monkey teeth with intrusive loading following the submucosal injection of nor-adrenaline. Similar influences were reported by Körber (1961) for horizontal tooth mobility. Moxham (1979) and Myhre, Preus and Aars (1979) have observed intrusive movements of previously erupting rabbit incisors after nor-adrenaline administration.

Pancreatic islets

Insulin is secreted from the B-cells in the islets of Langerhans and has widespread effects on carbohydrate, protein and lipid metabolism. In diabetes mellitus there is a lack of available insulin which may be due to a number of causes including a lack of insulin secretion, altered plasma membrane surface receptors for insulin and antibodies directed towards insulin. The severity of diabetes mellitus is variable but is in general more marked in the juvenile onset form which requires the regular injection of insulin.

In uncontrolled diabetes mellitus there is hyperglycaemia and ketosis. Vascular changes develop with thickening of blood vessel walls and basement membrane due to deposition of mucoprotein and collagen. Anoxia of the arterial intima is thought to lead to the development of atherosclerosis.

Chronic inflammatory periodontal disease is more severe in diabetics whether adequately or inadequately controlled (Williams, 1928; Rutledge, 1940; Lovestedt and Austin, 1943; Mackenzie and Millard, 1963; Belting, Hiniker and Dummett, 1964; Cheraskin and Ringsdorf, 1965; Chinn et al., 1966; Glavind, Lund and Löe, 1968; Cohen et al., 1969, 1970, 1971; Hove and Stallard, 1970; Bernick et al., 1975; Ringelberg et al., 1977). Not all studies show a correlation in controlled diabetes (Benveniste, Bixler and Conneally, 1967; El Geneidy et al., 1974). However, opinions still differ regarding the exact relationship between diabetes and the oral disease. Indeed, some claim that when the two conditions exist together, it is coincidental, there being no cause and effect relationship (e.g. Badanes, 1933; Bonheim, 1943; O'Leary, Shannon and Prigmore, 1962; Reeve and Winkelmann, 1962; Ulrich, 1962; Mackenzie and Millard, 1963). It is often presumed that diabetes alters the response of the periodontal tissue to local irritants. Shklar, Cohen and Yerganian (1962), Cohen, Shklar and Yerganian (1963) and Cohen et al. (1969) have shown an increase in chronic inflammatory periodontal disease in laboratory animals.

The histopathological changes in the periodontal ligament in diabetics have had limited attention. Vascular changes comparable to those found elsewhere in the body with thickening of the walls have been noted in some small blood vessels of the ligament (Russell, 1966, 1967; Keene, 1969 a, b, 1972). Necrotic foci in the periodontal collagen have also been reported (Benveniste et al., 1967). There is more basement membrane material (Keene, 1969 a, b; Listgarten et al., 1974). The vessel thickening is due to increased collagen production and that of the capillary basement lamina to periendothelial deposition of basement membrane-like material. These changes may impede oxygen diffusion and waste-product elimination and this may explain the poor tissue response to plaque in diabetes (Frantzis, Reeve and Brown, 1971). Following the induction of diabetes in rats by the drug alloxan, Bissada,

Schaffer and Lazarow (1966) observed infrequent fragmentation of the bundles of periodontal collagen fibres and widening of the ligament due to alveolar bone resorption. The fibres became disorganized and the collagen appeared more granular than fibrillar. The ligament was more vascular than normal and the blood capillaries were engorged, many being thrombosed. If local irritants were present, there was degeneration and oedema of the ligament especially in the furcation regions. Unlike human diabetes there were no histological changes in the vessels themselves. In other animal studies, osteoporosis and reduction in height of alveolar bone have been reported without much change in the periodontal ligament. Sheehan and Cohen (1970) could not see ligament changes in animals with autosomal recessive diabetes. The combination of excessive occlusal forces with alloxan-induced diabetes results in greater periodontal tissue destruction, possibly since repair mechanisms are inhibited (Glickman, Smulow and Moreau, 1966). Post-surgical periodontal healing is also delayed in these animals, although local irritants were a more significant delaying factor than the diabetes (Glickman, Smulow and Moreau, 1967).

Another animal model for studying the effects of diabetes on the periodontium has been a strain of hamster with hereditary diabetes. In these the periodontal ligament shows a reduction in the numbers of fibroblasts and collagen fibres. The remaining fibroblasts are smaller than normal with small deeply staining pyknotic nuclei. The osteoblast layer on bone is absent. Chronic periodontitis is more severe than in control animals (Shklar, Cohen and Yerganian, 1962) (Fig. 6).

Thymus gland

Though no histological studies are available linking the thymus gland and periodontal tissues, Rowntree, Clark and Hanson (1934) and Barrett (1935) observed precocious eruption of teeth in rats following administration of thymus extract.

Sex hormones

The principal sources of steroid sex hormones are the

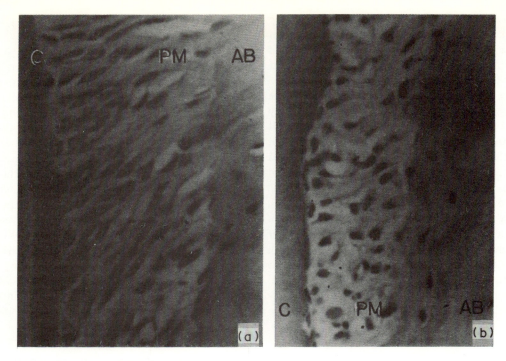

FIG. 6. The effect of diabetes mellitus on the periodontal ligament (in a strain of Chinese hamster with a hereditary form of the disease). (a) Control specimen. ×350. (b) Note diminution and granularity of the collagen fibres, and pyknotic changes in the ligament fibroblasts. Their cytoplasm is shrivelled and the nuclei small and deeply staining. The osteoblasts are also reduced in number along the bone margin (AB). C = cementum, PM = periodontal ligament. ×350.

testes and ovaries which secrete androgens or oestrogens and progestogens respectively.

The action of female sex hormones upon the periodontium has attracted substantial attention due to the increased severity of chronic inflammatory periodontal disease. However, as will be clear from what follows, most information available concerns the gingivae and not the periodontal ligament.

An increased incidence of gingivitis in females has been reported at both puberty (Massler, Schour and Chopra, 1950; Parfitt, 1957; Sutcliffe, 1972) and during pregnancy (Ziskin and Nesse, 1946; Maier and Orban, 1949; Hilming, 1952; Löe and Silness, 1963; Löe, 1965; Cohen et al., 1969; Hugoson, 1971; Adams, Carney and Dicks, 1974). Löe and Silness (1963) concluded from their study that there was no permanent periodontal damage from pregnancy gingivitis. Oral contraceptives most frequently include a synthetic oestrogen and progestogen. Several workers have considered that inges-

tion of oral contraceptives increases the prevalence of gingivitis although this finding is not unanimous (Lindhe and Bjorn, 1967; Lynn, 1967; Lindhe, Birch and Branemark, 1968; Lindhe, Branemark and Birch, 1968; Kaufman, 1969; Sperber, 1969; El Ashiry et al., 1970; Klinger and Klinger, 1970; Knight and Wade, 1974; Pearlman, 1974). Knight and Wade (1974) report no effect of hormonal contraceptives on plaque accumulation or gingivitis, but more severe periodontitis which they attribute to an altered host response. Current opinion indicates that it is progesterone which is most probably responsible for the major gingival inflammatory changes (Lindhe and Branemark, 1967 a, b, c). The reason for this requires elucidation: one possibility is that progesterone has a direct action upon capillary permeability (Mohammed, Waterhouse and Friederici, 1974). More recently it has been shown that progesterone in physiological concentrations stimulates the cell-mediated immune response to a standard antigenic challenge *in vitro*. In addition, a specific receptor for progesterone has been demonstrated in the neutrophil (Ferguson, 1981).

In terms of histopathology, most attention has focused on the gingival inflammatory response which is attributed to fluctuations in sex steroid levels. Again, there is negligible information on possible changes in the periodontal ligament.

At present, there is no clear consensus as to whether the gingivitis potentiated by these hormones is beneficial or detrimental in the long term.

Oestrogen receptors were not detected in the rabbit gingiva (Rubright, Termon and Yannone, 1973) and histological studies failed to show any response to systemic oestradiol administration (Rubright, Higa and Yannone, 1971). In mice, injections of oestradiol have been reported to produce sclerosis of the alveolar bone (Stahl *et al.*, 1950).

That sex hormones have an effect on the periodontal ligament is indicated by the observation that there is a progressive increase in horizontal tooth mobility during pregnancy (Mühlemann, 1951; Mühlemann, Savdis and Rateitschak, 1965; Rateitschak, 1967). It was reported that these changes were reduced to previous levels at full term. Friedman (1972) claims that horizontal tooth mobility is not changed during the menstrual cycle. Sex hormones may also have effects on tooth eruption. It is well documented that the development and eruption of teeth is earlier in girls than boys (e.g. Cattell, 1928; Garn *et al.*, 1958). Van Wagenen and Hurme (1950) accelerated canine eruption by injecting male monkeys with testosterone. Gonadectomy in squirrels resulted in a slight retardation in eruption (Schour, 1936). Increased secretion of gonadotrophin resulted in early eruption and formation of the teeth in man (Rushton, 1941). Hypergonadism is associated with more advanced deciduous eruption; hypogonadism has no marked effect on eruption but cases have occurred in which it has been slightly accelerated (Schour and Massler, 1943). Methyltestosterone has anacalciphylactic effects and has been found to reduce the periodontal damage caused by dihydrotachysterol intoxication (Ratcliff and Krajewski, 1966).

Histologically, when oestrogen was administered to 6-week-old mice for a period of 5 weeks, an increase in the cellularity of the periodontal ligament was observed (Shklar and Glickman, 1956). However, when the drug was given for a 10-week period, a reduction in both cellularity and collagen bundles was reported. These findings could be interpreted as the result of a possible decrease in the amount of FSH. Subsequently, Piroshaw and Glickman (1957) assessed the effects of ovariectomy in young adult mice. They observed a reduction in fibre density and cellularity in the periodontal ligament which reduced over 1 year, indicating a reduced susceptibility to the hormone with increasing age. Differentiation of mesenchyme cells to form osteoblasts and cementoblasts was impaired. There was no evidence of adrenal compensation (Glickman and Quintarelli, 1960) (Fig. 7). Schneider (1967) has noted fibrosis of the periodontal vasculature in ovariectomized rats. Shklar, Chauncey and Shapiro (1967) reported an increased cellularity of the periodontal ligament (Fig. 8) in hypophysectomized rats receiving testosterone.

Urogastrone — epidermal growth factor

A substance (Epidermal Growth Factor — EGF) has been isolated from mouse submandibular salivary glands which accelerates incisor tooth eruption and eyelid opening (Cohen, 1962; Carpenter, 1978). An almost identical 53-residue polypeptide termed urogastrone has been found in human urine and is thought to originate both in the submandibular glands and Brunner's glands of the duodenum (Gregory, Holmes and Willshire, 1979; Gregory, Walsh and Hopkins, 1979). It is secreted in the submandibular and parotid saliva where it is at a similar concentration to plasma.

NUTRITION AND THE PERIODONTAL LIGAMENT

There can be no doubt that one of the major contributions to the marked prolongation of the mean length of life in 'civilized' areas has been a sufficient availability of food of good quality. However, it is

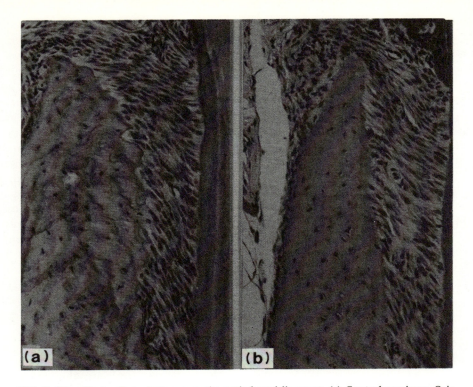

FIG. 7. The effects of ovariectomy on the periodontal ligament. (a) Control specimen. Orig. mag. ×400. (b) Ovariectomized animal, 6 months after operation. The ligament fibres are thinner, reduced in number and disorganized. The cellularity is diminished. Note the thin cementum layer compared with that in the control specimen. Orig. mag. ×400.

only in this century that the concept of nutritional deficiency diseases has evolved. A balanced diet is one containing proportional amounts of protein, minerals, fatty acids and vitamins. Carbohydrate is basically utilized for the production of energy. It is unusual for a single constituent to be deficient in the diet, and the clinical descriptions of nutritional deficiency may be due to a group of essential nutrients. However, it is possible to regulate the dietary intake in experimental animals, although it must still be appreciated that metabolism of the many nutrients are interrelated (e.g. folic acid and vitamin B12), and a change in one will inevitably involve others.

As will be evident from the review which follows, surprisingly few studies have been undertaken on the influence of nutritional factors on the connective tissues of the periodontal ligament. Two general points are worth emphasizing at this stage. Firstly, although animal experiments have shown that defi-

ciency or excess of nutrients in the diet can markedly affect the health of the periodontal tissues, the evidence for similar periodontal changes in humans is less convincing. Secondly, it is possible that some nutritional disturbances by themselves do not initiate lesions, but perhaps modify the response to local irritants.

Food texture

The texture of the diet is often not considered when assessing nutritional influences on health. Recently attention has been directed to the importance of dietary fibre (Robertson, 1972; Burkitt, 1973; Cleave, Campbell and Painter, 1973; Eastwood, 1973; Heaton, 1973; Southgate, 1973; Trowell, 1973). There has been little correlation between the advent of soft, fibre-deficient diet and dental health. This

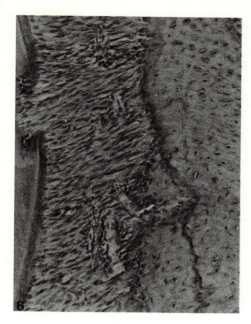

FIG. 8. The effect of testosterone on the (rat) periodontal ligament. Hypophysectomized animal receiving testosterone. The ligament is highly cellular and there is a dense fibre structure. There is some resorption of cementum and dentine. ×250.

is remarkable when one considers that probably the most significant factor in chronic inflammatory periodontal disease is the loss of natural masticatory function leading to the accumulation of dental plaque at sites prone to this condition (Newman, 1974). Indeed, one of the means of inducing chronic periodontitis in experimental animals is to feed them soft diets (Egelberg, 1965; Carlsson and Egelberg, 1965 a, b).

Diet consistency can affect the periodontal ligament not only indirectly in relation to the formation of local irritants (Ainamo, 1972; Newman, 1974), but also have a direct effect by influencing the pattern of mastication (and hence the mode of support offered by the ligament). The previous loading history has a bearing upon the reactions of a tooth to the application of a force (see Chapter 11). In mammalian dentitions where food having a 'natural' texture is masticated, there is some evidence that the extraction of teeth is usually more difficult, the muscles of mastication are stronger, and biting pressures are heavier than where the diet has a soft

consistency (Baaregaard, 1949; Davies and Pedersen, 1955). The effects of soft diet regarding more severe periodontitis apply both to domesticated animals (Keyes and Litkins, 1946; Klingsberg and Butcher, 1959; Hatt, Lyle-Stewart and Cresswell, 1968; Ferguson, 1969) and man (Sim Wallace, 1904; Colyer, 1931; Waugh, 1937; Waugh, 1940; Begg, 1954; Beyron, 1964; Klatsky and Klatell, 1943; Taylor, 1962, 1963; Rugg-Gunn, 1968; Lavelle, 1973). There is evidence, for the continuously growing incisors of rodents, that eruption (a property of the periodontal ligament, see Chapter 10) is influenced by biting behaviour and the degree of attrition (e.g. Ness, 1964). Further, Moxham and Berkovitz (in press) have shown that the periodontal tissues of these teeth show changes in resistance to loading when removed from the bite. Even in teeth of limited growth, attrition may be accompanied by compensatory 'eruption' (Philippas, 1952; Begg, 1954; Picton, 1957; Sarnäs, 1957; Brothwell and Carr, 1962; Murphy, 1959, 1964; Tait, 1965; Newman and Levers, 1979). Thompson and Kendrick (1964) and Ainamo and Talari (1976) claim that eruption in man is independent of attrition, since it has been shown to occur in the absence of the latter. Vigorous masticatory function is associated with a widening of the periodontal ligament (Coolidge, 1937).

For information concerning the effects on the periodontal ligament of disuse of a tooth, the reader is referred to Chapter 19.

Carbohydrates

Some findings exist suggesting that refined carbohydrates in the diet influence the severity of chronic inflammatory periodontal disease in man (Holloway, James and Slack, 1963) and in laboratory animals (Frandsen et al., 1953; Auskaps, Gupta and Shaw, 1957; Stahl, 1962, 1963 a, b). However, others report no correlation (Shannon and Gibson, 1964). Further, there is no evidence showing a direct effect of carbohydrates per se on the periodontal ligament, though in some circumstances there could be an influence as a result of modifying the diet consistency.

Proteins

Since the periodontal ligament shows a high turnover rate for many of its constituents, particularly collagen (e.g. Sodek, 1978), a deficiency of dietary protein might be expected to produce changes within it.

In rats fed protein-deficient diets, there is a reduction in periodontal ligament collagen fibres, particularly the transseptal component (Stein and Ziskin, 1949; Chawla and Glickman, 1951; Frandsen *et al.*, 1953; Stahl, Miller and Goldsmith, 1958; Ten Cate, Deporter and Freeman, 1976). Similar changes have been reported in monkeys (Goldman, 1954) and pigs (Platt and Stewart, 1962). The ligament is less cellular, with oedema and disorganization of fibre bundles. There is a reduction in the number of cementoblasts as well as fibroblasts. Occlusal trauma exacerbates these effects (Chawla and Glickman, 1951; Stahl, Sandler and Cahn, 1955; Stahl, Miller and Goldsmith, 1957; Miller, Stahl and Goldsmith,

1957) (Fig. 9). Periodontal healing is delayed in rats fed a protein-deficient diet (Stahl, 1962, 1963 a, b).

The only report of the effects of an amino acid deficiency on the periodontal ligament is that of Bavetta and Bernick (1956). They described severe alveolar destruction with loss of attachment of the periodontal ligament in tryptophan-deficient rats.

Bryer (1957) assessed the effect of a deficiency of proteins on eruption of the rat incisor. He reported that acute protein deficiency (accompanied by weight loss of between 25—45%) had little effect.

Fatty acids

Only two fatty acids (the unsaturated fatty acids linoleic acid and linolenic acid) are essential dietary components for humans, as the body can synthesize the remainder.

It is probable that essential fatty acid deficiency is

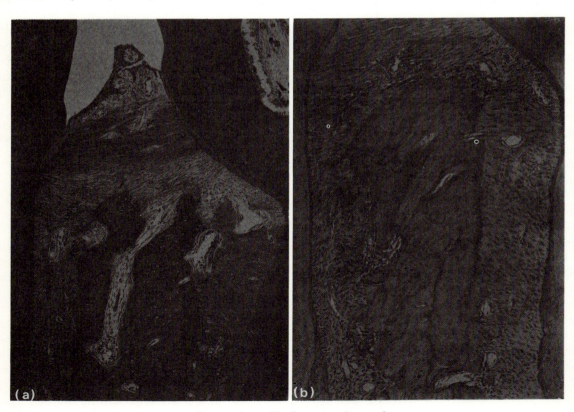

(For caption to Fig. 9 see opposite page.)

manifested by an inability to synthesize prostaglandins (El-Attar, 1978), although this is by no means certain. If essential fatty acid deficiency leads to a reduction in prostaglandin production, it is possible that periodontal changes may result which would be due, in part, to an altered inflammatory reaction (El-Attar, 1978). The mechanisms by which fatty acids affect collagen and bone metabolism remain to be established. Changes have been observed within the periodontal tissues of rats fed on fatty-acid-deficient diets. Rao, Shourie and Sharkwaller (1965) reported an increase in cellularity of the periodontal ligament with resorption of adjacent cementum and alveolar bone. Prout and Tring (1971, 1973) fed young rats a fat-free diet and noted that the collagen fibre bundles of the molar periodontal ligaments became more vascular, irregular and disorientated.

Vitamins

Vitamins are essential organic factors which cannot be synthesized within the body and are required in only small amounts. They are classified into fat-soluble vitamins (vitamins A, D, E and K) and water-soluble vitamins (vitamins B complex, C).

VITAMIN A

Vitamin A is concerned with the control of epithelial differentiation and bone formation. In dogs, vitamin A deficiency has been reported to be associated with periodontal inflammation (Mellanby, 1929; Mellanby, 1941; Frandsen, 1963). Vitamin A-deficient rats have been observed to have widened (molar) periodontal

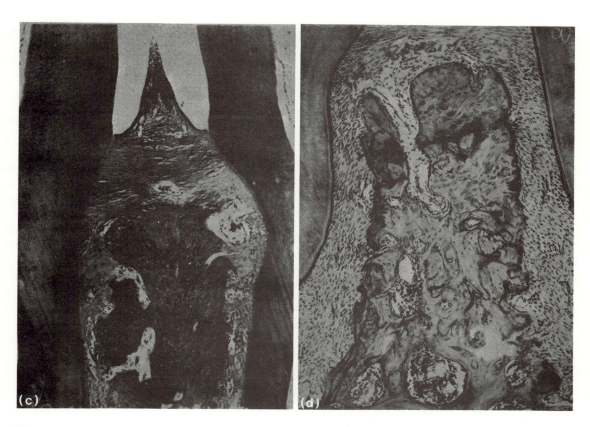

FIG. 9. Protein deprivation and the (rat) periodontal ligament. (a) and (b) Control specimens: (a) ×116, (b) ×150. (c) Note wavy outline of periodontal ligament collagen fibres, which are reduced in number. ×116. (d) Showing reduction in cellularity of ligament. The fibroblasts have small, flattened nuclei. ×150.

ligaments (Boyle and Bessey, 1941) and areas of hyaline necrosis where the roots impacted against bone (Boyle, 1947). The experiments of Wolbach and Howe (1933), Schour, Hoffman and Smith (1941) and Bryer (1957) suggest that eruption is retarded in vitamin A-deficient rats. Bryer (1957) reported that there was a marked decrease in vascularity of the periodontal ligament. He claimed that new osteoid tissue also resulted in a decrease in width of the ligament. Whereas Glickman and Stoller (1948) found deeper periodontal pockets in vitamin A-deficient rats, Miglani (1959) found no direct ligament effects. It is possible that any such changes are secondary to the main oral effect of the deficiency, i.e. xerostomia (Salley, Bryson and Eshleman, 1959; Hayes, McCombs and Faherty, 1970).

Excessive intake of vitamin A may be associated (in rats) with alveolar bone resorption (Wolbach and Bessey, 1942; Ferguson, 1969).

VITAMIN D

The principal action of vitamin D is to elevate plasma calcium and phosphate concentrations by stimulating their intestinal absorption and by resorption of bone. Dietary cholecalciferol is absorbed from the alimentary tract and converted into 25-hydroxy-cholecalciferol in the liver. This passes into the circulation and is subsequently transformed into 1:25-dihydroxycholecalciferol in the kidney and represents the active form of vitamin D. Synthesis of 1:25-dihydroxycholecalciferol is regulated by plasma levels of calcium, phosphate, parathyroid hormone and possibly calcitonin. A deficiency of vitamin D results in rickets in children and osteomalacia in adults. Both conditions are characterized by defective mineralization of the organic matrix. The effects of vitamin D on the periodontal ligament are considered under the section concerned with mineralization factors (pages 441–443).

VITAMIN E

This group of tocopherols acts as antioxidants protecting unsaturated fatty acids, vitamin A and vitamin C. There is some doubt as to vitamin E being essential in humans, particularly adults. In the continuously

growing incisors of rats, deficiency of this vitamin is associated with atrophic changes in the enamel organ (Irving, 1942; Pindborg, 1952) and in the periodontal ligament (Schneider and Pose, 1969).

VITAMIN K

Vitamins K_1 and K_2 are necessary for the hepatic synthesis of clotting factors. Deficiency does not lead to any direct periodontal changes. However, there may be increased gingival bleeding due to failure of the clotting mechanism.

VITAMIN B COMPLEX

This group of water-soluble vitamins are essential co-enzymes for the metabolism of carbohydrates, proteins and fats. The vitamin B complex includes the following substances: thiamine (vitamin B_1), riboflavin (vitamin B_2), nicotinic acid (niacin) or nicotinic acid amide (niacinamide), pantothenic acid, pyridoxine (vitamin B_6), biotin, para-aminobenzoic acid, inositol, choline, folic acid (folacin), and vitamin B_{12} (cyanocobalamin).

Severe periodontal destruction has been reported in riboflavin (Tomlinson, 1939; Topping and Fraser, 1939; Chapman and Harris, 1941), nicotinic acid and pantothenic acid-deficient rodents and primates (Tomlinson, 1939; Becks, Wainwright and Morgan, 1943; Ziskin *et al.*, 1947). Mice fed a pantothenic acid-deficient diet for 2 weeks were reported to have wider periodontal ligaments in which epithelial rest proliferation had occurred, together with an increase in the size of blood vessels on the bone side of the ligament (Levy, 1949). In a study of deficiencies of niacin, riboflavin, pyridoxine, pantothenic acid and folic acid in adult dogs (Afonsky, 1955), periodontal ligament involvement with alveolar crest fibre destruction was seen only with folic acid deficiency. There is also some evidence of a relationship between folic acid deficiency and partial necrosis of the ligament (Pindborg, 1949; Shaw, 1962).

VITAMIN C

Vitamin C is involved in oxidation—reduction reactions

and is concerned particularly with proline hydroxylation in the synthesis of collagen. Its other actions are less well understood, but it is involved also in the formation of epithelial basement membranes (Priest, 1970). Deficiency of vitamin C leads to scurvy with widespread disorders in bones and connective tissue as a result of defective collagen synthesis (e.g. Wolbach, 1953).

In the guinea pig, vitamin C deficiency leads to a failure in collagen formation and destruction of existing fibres in the periodontal ligament (Wolbach and Howe, 1926; Boyle, Bessey and Wolbach, 1937; Glickman and Stoller, 1948; Hunt and Paynter, 1959). Healing of gingival wounds is delayed and collagen formation is disordered (Turesky and Glickman, 1954).

Waerhaug (1960) reported that a vitamin C-deficient diet in monkeys results in breakdown of collagen fibres, although those in the epithelial cuff appeared to be more resistant. Widening of the periodontal ligament can occur which may be attributed to resorption of the adjoining alveolar bone (Dreizen, Levy and Bernick, 1969) (Fig. 10). Østergaard (1975) claims that the hydroxyproline content of the ligament is decreased by 66% in ascorbic acid-deficient monkeys, thus explaining the reduction in ligament collagen in these animals. However, several investigations into the status of vitamin C in relation to human chronic inflammatory periodontal disease have shown no convincing association (Blockley and Baenzigen, 1942; Stuhl, 1943; Restarski and Pijoun, 1944; Perlitsch, Nielsen and Stanmeyer, 1961; Glickman and Dines, 1963; El-Ashiry, Ringsdorf and Cheraskin, 1964).

With respect to the effects of vitamin C on tooth eruption, deficiency of the vitamin is associated with a decreased rate of eruption of impeded and unimpeded guinea pig incisors (Dalldorf and Zall, 1930; Berkovitz, 1974a).

Mineralization factors

This section is concerned with both hormonal and nutritional factors which are involved in calcification and which seem to affect periodontal ligament development and function.

Decreased availability of calcium may result from a dietary deficiency of the mineral or from a deficiency of vitamin D. A similar effect may be induced by renal disease or by excision of the parathyroid glands. Calcium metabolism is regulated by a series of interactions and an alteration of any one must inevitably result in a sequence of compensatory changes. It can be difficult, therefore, to separate primary from secondary actions. Hence, for any *in vivo* experimental procedure, cognizance should be taken of these potential effects even if they have not beeen recorded.

One way of overcoming this difficulty is to examine the effect of individual factors in organ or tissue culture. In one such investigation (Rao, Moe and Heersche, 1978), the influence on periodontal fibroblasts of calcitonin, parathormone and the prostaglandin PGE was examined. This showed that whilst calcitonin or parathormone had no effect on cyclic-AMP production, PGE_1 caused a very significant elevation. A study using hamster periodontal tissue also showed no effect of calcitonin (El Kafrawy and Mitchell, 1976).

Another approach involves giving diets to animals where only one factor is changed, the other factors being maintained at 'normal' levels. Consider the situation where there is a deficiency in the diet of vitamin D (with normal dietary calcium and phosphorus). Weinmann and Schour (1945 a and b) reported that such a diet in young dogs resulted in narrowing of the periodontal ligament, probably as a result of failure of the normal resorptive processes associated with the adjacent alveolar bone. There was also evidence of hyaline degeneration and partial obliteration of the ligament. Similar changes have been described by Bryer (1957) for the rat incisor and partial ligament necrosis has also been observed in vitamin D-deficient monkeys (Tomlinson, 1939). In contrast, however, Oliver (1969) found the periodontal ligament of young rats to be unaltered by such a diet. Where there was a deficiency of both vitamin D and calcium (with phosphorus levels remaining normal), Becks and Weber (1931) reported the presence of destructive changes within the periodontal ligament. They observed a widened periodontal ligament, with blood-containing, cyst-like structures in some sites.

Rats placed on a calcium-deficient diet show

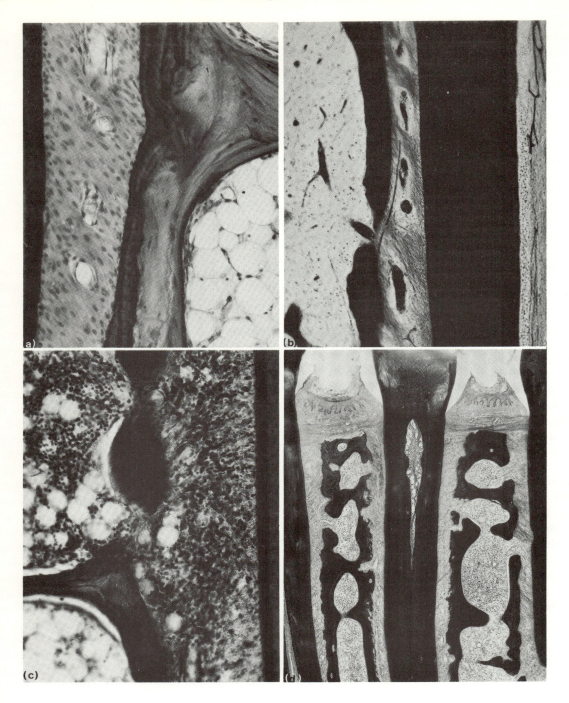

FIG. 10. Scurvy and the primate (marmoset) periodontal ligament. (a) Control specimen. ×160. (b) Scorbutic marmoset. Lack of fibre bundles around vascular spaces and congestion of periodontal blood vessels. ×160. (c) Scorbutic marmoset. Proliferating bone marrow encroaching into the ligament. ×160. (d) Scorbutic marmoset. Showing loss of attachment fibres, and reduction in ligament density. ×20.

osteoporotic changes in alveolar bone (Ferguson and Hartles, 1963, 1966) and a reduction in the number and diameter of periodontal ligament fibres (Oliver, 1969) (Figs. 11 and 12). Parathormone administration, which is probably analogous to calcium deficiency, has been shown to stimulate osteoclastic activity in the rat periodontium (Roberts, 1975). In studying cell kinetics in the rat maxillary first molar following the injection of parathyroid extract, Roberts (1975) found an increased cellularity of the periodontal ligament which could be accounted for only partly by local cell proliferation. He concluded that there must have been an influx of migrating cells into the periodontal ligament.

There seem to be no reports of changes in the periodontal ligament associated with a deficiency of phosphorus, though osteoporotic changes in alveolar bone have been described (Ferguson and Hartles, 1966). That there might be changes in the periodontium is indicated by reports that tooth eruption may be retarded in experimental animals fed a phosphorus-deficient diet (Burrill, 1943), though Bryer (1957) reported no change in eruption rates for rat incisors.

When high doses of vitamin D (in the form of dihydrotachysterol) are given to rats to induce local calcification, there is widespread degeneration, loss in fibre orientation and oedema of the periodontal ligament. Capillaries become enlarged, some haemorrhage is present, calcification of the transseptal fibres may occur, and multiple foci of calcification appear throughout the ligament (Ratcliff and Itokazu, 1964; Moskow, Baden and Zengo, 1966; Bernick, Ershoff and Lal, 1971) (Fig. 13). The effects are reduced by ferric dextran (Ratcliff and Itokazu, 1964) and methyltestosterone (Ratcliff and Krajewski, 1966). Hypervitaminosis D in the hamster is said to result in narrowing of the periodontal ligament, with calcification of the principal fibres (particularly for the molars) (Fahmy *et al.*, 1961) (Fig. 14).

As regards the effects of mineralization factors on tooth eruption, the eruption rate in rats was found to fall with vitamin D deficiency and excess (Bryer, 1957). There seems to be no effect on eruption of phosphorus deficiency (Bryer, 1957). Removal of the parathyroids does not appear to affect tooth eruption, at least for the rat incisor (Schour, Chandler and Tweedy, 1937; Bryer, 1957). Ziskin, Salmon and Applebaum (1940) reported that replacement

therapy of parathormone extract was without effect on eruption. The eruption of human teeth in subjects suffering from hypo- and hyperparathyroidism is not affected (Schour and Massler, 1943).

Inorganic elements

The effects of calcium and phosphorus are considered in the preceding section.

Widening of the periodontal ligament has been observed with magnesium deficiency (Klein, Orent and McCallum, 1935; Becks and Furuta, 1943). Furthermore, the eruption rate of rat incisors has been reported to decrease in animals fed magnesium-deficient diets (Klein, Orent and McCallum, 1935; Becks and Furuta, 1939, 1941; Gagnon, Schour and Patras, 1942; Bernick and Hungerford, 1965; Kusner, Michaeli and Weinreb, 1973). These effects may be related to the role of Mg^{++} ions in several enzyme systems. Only one study suggested a relationship between magnesium deficiency and the severity of periodontitis (Klein *et al.*, 1935).

Fluoride seems to reduce the destructive effects of excessive orthodontic tooth movement, at least in rats (Singer, Furstman and Bernick, 1967). In this study, female rats were given 100 ppm fluoride in distilled water and orthodontic elastics were inserted between molar teeth. It was observed that there were fewer areas of ligament hyalinization in fluoride-treated animals than in controls. Although it has been suggested that fluoride reduces the rate of eruption of the rat molar (Smith, 1934; Ness, 1964), Berkovitz (1974b) has reported that rats given 25–100 ppm fluoride exhibited no changes in incisor eruption rates.

Severe iron deficiency has been related to periodontal destruction in dogs (Hall and Robinson, 1937). In humans, however, there does not seem to be a clear correlation between iron-deficiency anaemia and chronic inflammatory periodontal disease. From clinical observations, Lainson, Brady and Fraleigh (1968) had the impression that patients with moderate to severe periodontitis sometimes had subnormal levels of iron. Animal experiments have not yet revealed any effects of iron deficiency on the periodontal ligament (Deutsch, Dreizen and Stahl, 1969).

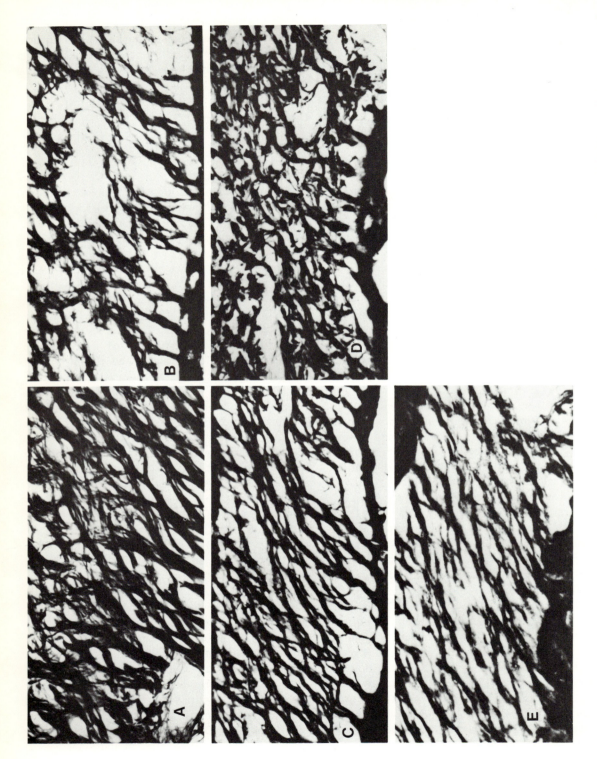

FIG. 11. Vitamin D deficiency and the (rat) periodontal ligament. (A) Adequate diet. (B), (D) Diet deficient in calcium. (C), (E) Diet deficient in calcium and vitamin D. ×80. There is reduction in number and diameter of these fibres in rats deficient in calcium or calcium and vitamin D.

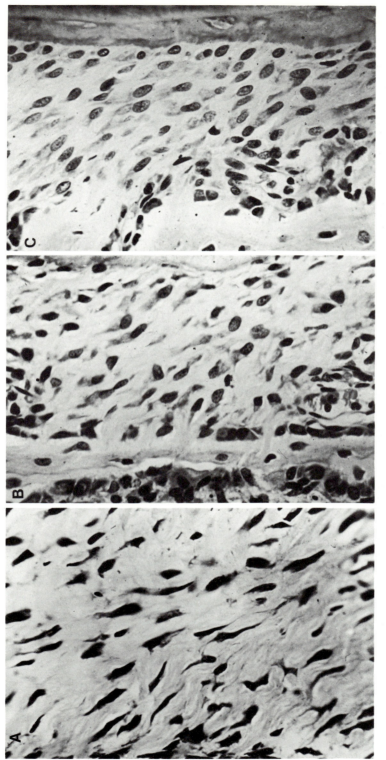

FIG. 12. Cells of (rat) periodontal ligament. (A) Adequate diet. (B) Deficient in calcium. (C) Deficient in calcium and vitamin D. ×80. Note reduction in cellularity and rounding of fibroblasts in (B) and (C). Figs. 11 and 12 indicate that vitamin D deficiency alone has no obvious effect on the rat periodontal ligament.

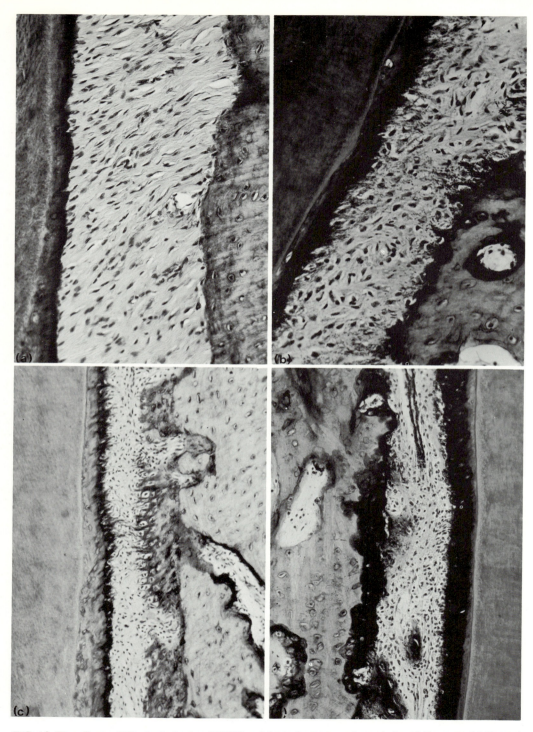

FIG. 13. The effects of dihydrotachysterol (DHT) and ferric dextran on the periodontal ligament. (a) Control. ×144. (b) Basophilic staining oral granules in ligament of 7-day DHT-treated animal. ×200. (c) Active osteoid formation obliterating periodontal ligament of 18-day DHT-treated animal. Note calcification of Sharpey's fibres. ×100. (d) Small islands of new bone in ligament of 37-day DHT-treated animal. ×128.

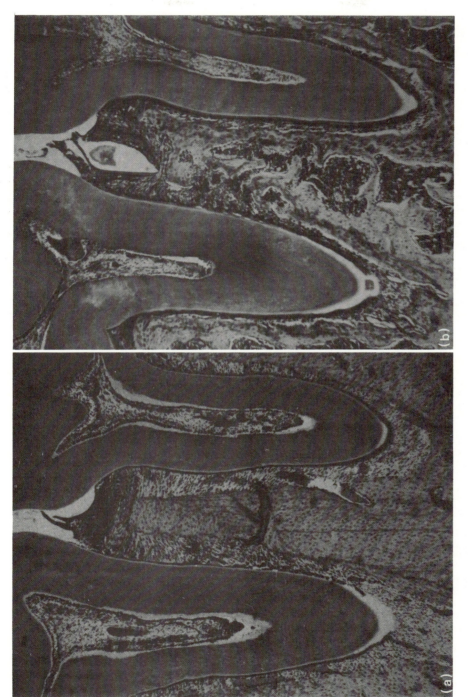

FIG. 14. Hypervitaminosis D and the (hamster) periodontal ligament. (a) Control animal. ×35. (b) Hamster given excess vitamin D. Note calcification of principal fibres and resorption of bone and osteoid. ×35.

Although cobalt is said to retard the eruption of the rat incisor (Bryer, 1957), no reports concerning the influence of this inorganic element on the structure of the periodontal ligament have been published. Even with Bryer's work, doubts may be expressed about his conclusions since the eruption rates were only marginally reduced (from 1.83 to 1.70 mm/ 48 h).

REFERENCES

ADAMS, D., CARNEY, J. S. & DICKS, D. A. (1974) Pregnancy gingivitis: a survey of 100 antenatal patients. *J. Dent.* **2**, 106–111.

AFONSKY, D. (1955) Oral lesions in niacin, riboflavin, pyridoxine, folic acid and pantothenic acid deficiencies in adult dogs. *Oral Surg.* **8**, 867–876.

AINAMO, J. (1972) Relationship between occlusal wear of the teeth and periodontal health. *Scand. J. dent. Res.* **80**, 505–509.

AINAMO, J. & TALARI, A. (1976) Eruptive movements of teeth in human adults. In: *The eruption and occlusion of teeth*, D. F. G. POOLE and M. V. STACK (eds.), pp. 97–107. London, Butterworths.

APPLEBAUM, E. & SEELING, A. (1955) Histologic changes in jaws and teeth of rats following nephritis, adrenalectomy and cortisone treatment. *Oral Surg.* **8**, 881–891.

AUSKAPS, A. M., GUPTA, O. P. & SHAW, J. H. (1957) Periodontal disease in the rice rat. III. Survey of dietary influences. *J. Nutr.* **63**, 325–343.

BAAREGAARD, A. (1949) Dental conditions and nutrition among natives in Greenland. *Oral Surg.* **2**, 995–1007.

BADANES, B. B. (1933) Diabetes, acidosis and the significance of acid mouth. *Dent. Cosmos* **75**, 476–484.

BALL, P. C. (1977) The effect of adrenal glucocorticoid administration on eruption rates and tissue dimensions in rat mandibular incisors. *J. Anat.* **124**, 157–163.

BARRETT, M. T. (1935) The effects of thymus extract (Hanson) on the early eruption and growth of the teeth of white rats. *Dent. Cosmos* **77**, 1088–1093.

BAUME, L. J. & BECKS, H. (1952) The effect of thyroid hormone in dental and paradental structures. *Paradentologie* **6**, 89–109.

BAUME, L. J., BECKS, H., RAY, J. C. & EVANS, H. M. (1954a) Hormonal control of tooth eruption. II. The effects of hypophysectomy on the upper rat incisor following progressively longer intervals. *J. dent. Res.* **33**, 91–103.

BAUME, L. J., BECKS, H. & EVANS, H. M. (1954b) Hormonal control of tooth eruption. III. The response of the incisors of hypophysectomized rats to growth hormone, thyroxin or the combination of both. *J. dent. Res.* **33**, 104–114.

BAUME, L. J., BECKS, H. & EVANS, H. M. (1954c) Hormonal control of tooth eruption, I. The effect of

thyroidectomy on the upper rat incisor and the response to growth hormone, thyroxin or the combination of both. *J. dent. Res.* **33**, 80–90.

BAVETTA, L. A. & BERNICK, S. (1956) Effect of tryptophan deficiency on bones and teeth of rats. II. Effect of prolongation. *Oral Surg.* **9**, 308–315.

BECKS, H. & FURUTA, W. J. (1939) Effect of magnesium deficient diets on oral and dental tissues. I. Changes in the enamel epithelium. *J. Amer. dent. Assoc.* **26**, 883–891.

BECKS, H. & FURUTA, W. J. (1941) Effect of magnesium deficient diets on oral and dental tissues. II. Changes in the dental structures. *J. Amer. dent. Assoc.* **28**, 1083–1088.

BECKS, H. & FURUTA, W. J. (1943) Effects of magnesium deficient diets on oral and dental structures. IV. Changes in paradental bone structure. *J. dent. Res.* **22**, 215–217.

BECKS, H., WAINWRIGHT, W. W. & MORGAN, A. F. (1943) Comparative study of oral changes in dogs due to deficiencies of pantothenic acid, nicotinic acid and unknowns of the B-vitamin complex. *Amer. J. Orthodont.* **29**, 183–207.

BECKS, H. & WEBER, M. (1931) The influence of diet on the bone system with special reference to the alveolar process and the labyrinthine capsule. *J. Amer. dent. Assoc.* **18**, 197–264.

BEGG, P. R. (1954) Stone Age Man's dentition – with reference to anatomically correct occlusion, the etiology of malocclusion, and a technique for its treatment. *Amer. J. Orthodont.* **40**, 292–312 and 373–383.

BELTING, C. M., HINIKER, J. J. & DUMMETT, C. O. (1964) Influence of diabetes mellitus on the severity of periodontal disease. *J. Periodont.* **35**, 476–480.

BENVENISTE, R., BIXLER, D. & CONNEALLY, P. M. (1967) Periodontal disease in diabetics. *J. Periodont.* **38**, 271–279.

BERKOVITZ, B. K. B. (1971) Effects of surgical interference and drug administration on eruption in the rat mandibular incisor. *J. dent. Res.* **50**, 654 (abs.).

BERKOVITZ, B. K. B. (1974a) Effect of fluoride on eruption rates of rat incisors. *J. dent. Res.* **53**, 334–337.

BERKOVITZ, B. K. B. (1974b) The effect of vitamin C deficient diet on eruption rates for the guinea pig lower incisor. *Archs. oral Biol.* **19**, 807–811.

BERNICK, S., COHEN, D. W., BAKER, L. & LASTER, L. (1975) Dental disease in children with diabetes mellitus. *J. Periodont.* **46**, 241–245.

BERNICK, S., ERSHOFF, B. H. & LAL, J. B. (1971) Effects of hypervitaminosis D on bones and teeth of rats. *Int. J. Vitam. Nutr. Res.* **41**, 480–489.

BERNICK, S. & HUNGERFORD, G. F. (1965) Effect of dietary magnesium deficiency on the bones and teeth of rats. *J. dent. Res.* **44**, 1317–1324.

BEYRON, H. (1964) Occlusal relations and mastication in Australian aborigines. *Acta odont. Scand.* **22**, 597–678.

BISSADA, N. F., SCHAFFER, E. M. & LAZAROW, A. (1966) Effect of alloxan diabetes and local irritating factors on the periodontal structures of the rat. *Periodontics* **4**, 233–240.

BLOCKLEY, C. H. & BAENZIGER, P. E. (1942) An investigation into the connection between the vitamin C content of the blood and periodontal disturbances. *Brit. dent. J.* **73**, 57–61.

BONHEIM, F. (1943) The endocrine system in periodontal disease. In: *Textbook of periodontia* (2nd ed.), S. C. MILLER (ed.), pp. 520–553. Philadelphia, Blakiston.

BOYLE, P. E. (1947) Effects of vitamin A deficiency on the periodontal tissues. *Amer. J. Orthodont.* **33**, 744–748.

BOYLE, P. E. & BESSEY, O. A. (1941) The effect of acute vitamin A deficiency on the molar teeth and paradontal tissues with a comment on deformed incisor teeth in this deficiency. *J. dent. Res.* **20**, 236–237 (abs.).

BOYLE, P. E., BESSEY, D. A. & WOLBACH, S. D. (1937) Experimental alveolar bone atrophy produced by ascorbic acid deficiency and its relation to pyorrhoea alveolaris. *Proc. Soc. exp. Biol. Med.* **36**, 733–735.

BROTHWELL, D. R. & CARR, H. G. (1962) The dental health of the Etruscans. *Br. dent. J.* **113**, 207–210.

BRYER, L. W. (1957) An experimental evaluation of the physiology of tooth eruption. *Int. dent. J.* **7**, 432–478.

BURKITT, D. P. (1973) Some diseases characteristic of modern Western civilisation. *Br. Med. J.* **1**, 274–278.

BURRILL, D. Y. (1943) The effect of low phosphorus intake on the growth of the jaws in dogs. *J. Amer. dent. Assoc.* **30**, 513–523.

CARLSSON, J. & EGELBERG, J. (1965a) Effect of diet on early plaque formation in man. *Odont. Revy* **16**, 112–125.

CARLSSON, J. & EGELBERG, J. (1965b) Local effect of diet on plaque formation and development of gingivitis in dogs. II. Effect of high carbohydrate versus high protein-fat diets. *Odont. Revy* **16**, 42–49.

CARNEIRO, J. & FAVA DE MORAES, F. (1965) Radioautographic visualisation of collagen metabolism in the periodontal tissue of the mouse. *Archs. oral Biol.* **10**, 833–848.

CARPENTER, G. (1978) The regulation of cell proliferation: advances in the biology and mechanisms of action of epidermal growth factor. *J. Invest. Dermatol.* **71**, 283–287.

CATTELL, P. (1928) The eruption and growth of the permanent teeth. *J. dent. Res.* **8**, 279–287.

CHAPMAN, O. D. & HARRIS, A. E. (1941) Oral lesions associated with dietary deficiencies in monkeys. *J. Infect. Dis.* **69**, 7–17.

CHAWLA, T. N. & GLICKMAN, I. (1951) Protein deprivation and the periodontal structures of the albino rat. *Oral Surg.* **4**, 578–602.

CHERASKIN, E. & RINGSDORF, W. M. (1965) Gingival state and carbohydrate metabolism. *J. dent. Res.* **44**, 480–486.

CHINN, H., BRODY, H., SILVERMAN, S. & DI RAIMONDO, V. (1966) Glucose tolerance in patients with oral symptoms. *J. oral Therap. Pharmacol.* **2**, 261–269.

CLEAVE, T. L., CAMPBELL, G. D. & PAINTER, N. S. (1973) *Diabetes coronary thrombosis and the saccharine disease* (2nd ed.). Bristol, Wright.

COHEN, D. W., FRIEDMAN, L., SHAPIRO, J. & KYLE, G. C. (1969) Studies on periodontal patterns in diabetes mellitus. *J. periodont. Res.* suppl. 4, 35–36.

COHEN, D. W., FRIEDMAN, L. A., SHAPIRO, J., KYLE,

G. C. & FRANKLIN, S. (1970) Diabetes mellitus and periodontal disease: two year longitudinal observations. *J. Periodont.* **41**, 709–712.

COHEN, D. W., SHAPIRO, J., FRIEDMAN, L., KYLE, G. C. & FRANKLIN, S. (1971) Diabetes mellitus and periodontal disease. II. 3 year longitudinal study. *J. dent. Res.* **50**, 206 (abs.).

COHEN, M. M., SHKLAR, G. & YERGANIAN, G. (1963) Pulpal and periodontal disease in Chinese hamsters with hereditary diabetes mellitus. *Oral Surg.* **16**, 104–112.

COHEN, S. (1962) Isolation of a mouse submaxillary gland protein accelerating incisor eruption and eyelid opening in the newborn animal. *J. Biol. Chem.* **237**, 1555–1562.

COLYER, F. (1931) *Abnormal conditions of the teeth of animals in their relationship to similar conditions in man,* pp. 39–63 and 81–108. London, The Dental Board of the United Kingdom.

COOLIDGE, E. D. (1937) The thickness of the human periodontal membrane. *J. Amer. dent. Assoc. and Dent. Cosmos* **24**, 1260–1270.

DALLDORF, G. & ZALL, C. (1930) Tooth growth in experimental scurvy. *J. exp. Med.* **52**, 57–63.

DAVIES, T. G. H. & PEDERSEN, P. O. (1955) The degree of attrition of the deciduous teeth and first permanent molars of primitive and urbanised Greenland natives. *Br. dent. J.* **99**, 35–43.

DEUTSCH, C. M., DREIZEN, S. & STAHL, S. S. (1969) The effects of chronic iron deficiency anaemia on the periodontium of the adult rat. *J. Periodont.* **40**, 736–739.

DOMM, L. V. & MARZANO, R. (1954) Observations on the effect of certain hormones on the growth rate of the incisors of the albino rat. *Anat. Rec.* **118**, 383–384.

DOMM, L. V. & WELLBAND, W. A. (1960) Effect of adrenalectomy and cortisone on eruption rate of incisors of young female albino rats. *Proc. Soc. exp. Biol.* **104**, 582–584.

DOMM, L. V. & WELLBAND, W. A. (1961) Effect of adrenalectomy, thyroidectomy, thyro-adrenalectomy and cortisone on eruption rate of incisors in adult female rats. *Proc. Soc. exp. Biol.* **107**, 268–272.

DREIZEN, S., LEVY, B. M. & BERNICK, S. (1969) Studies on the biology of the periodontium of marmosets. VII. The effect of vitamin C deficiency on the marmoset periodontium. *J. periodont. Res.* **4**, 274–280.

DREIZEN, S., LEVY, B. M. & BERNICK, S. (1971) Studies on the biology of the periodontium of marmosets. Cortisone induced periodontal and skeletal changes in adult cotton top marmosets. *J. Periodont.* **42**, 217–224.

EASTWOOD, M. (1973) Vegetable dietary fibre food-fad or farrago. In: *Getting the most out of food,* 8, pp. 39–59. London, van der Bergh's and Jurgens.

EGELBERG, J. (1965) Local effect of diet on plaque formation and development of gingivitis in dogs. I. Effect of hard and soft diets. *Odont. Revy* **16**, 31–41.

EL-ASHIRY, G. M., RINGSDORF, W. M. & CHERASKIN, E. (1964) Local and systemic influences in periodontal disease. II. Effect of prophylaxis and natural versus synthetic vitamin C upon gingivitis. *J. Periodont.* **35**, 250–259.

EL-ASHIRY, G. M., EL KAFRAWY, A. H., NASR, M. F. & YOUNIS, H. (1970) Comparative study of the influence of pregnancy and oral contraceptives on the gingiva. *Oral Surg.* 30, 472–475.

EL-ATTAR, T. M. A. (1978) Prostaglandins: Physiology, biochemistry, pharmacology and clinical applications. *J. oral Pathol.* 7, 175–208 and 239–282.

EL GENEIDY, A. K., STALLARD, R. E., FILLIOS, L. C. & GOLDMAN, H. M. (1974) Periodontal and vascular alteration: their relationship to the changes in tissue glucose and glycogen in diabetic mice. *J. Periodont.* 45, 394–401.

EL KAFRAWY, A. H. & MITCHELL, D. F. (1976) Dental and periodontal effects of calcitonin in hamsters. *J. dent. Res.* 55, 554.

FAHMY, H., ROGERS, W. E., MITCHELL, D. F. & BREMER, H. E. (1961) Effects of hypervitaminosis D on the periodontium of the hamster. *J. dent. Res.* 40, 870–877.

FERGUSON, H. W. (1969) Effect of nutrition on the periodontium. In: *Biology of the periodontium,* A. H. MELCHER & W. H. BOWEN (eds.), pp. 421–451. London, Academic Press.

FERGUSON, H. W. & HARTLES, R. L. (1963) Effect of vitamin D on the bones of young rats receiving diets low in calcium or phosphorus. *Archs. oral Biol.* 8, 407–418.

FERGUSON, H. W. & HARTLES, R. L. (1966) The effect of diets deficient in calcium or phosphorus in the presence and absence of supplement of vitamin D on the incisor teeth and bone of adult rats. *Archs. oral Biol.* 11, 1345–1364.

FERGUSON, M. M. (1981) Unpublished data.

FRANDSEN, A. M. (1963) Periodontal tissue changes in vitamin A deficient young rats. *Acta odont. Scand.* 21, 19–34.

FRANDSEN, A. M., BECKS, H., NELSON, M. M. & EVANS, H. M. (1953) Effects of various levels of dietary protein on the periodontal tissues of young rats. *J. Periodont.* 24, 135–142.

FRANTZIS, T. G., REEVE, C. M. & BROWN, A. L. (1971) The ultrastructure of capillary basement membranes in the attached gingiva of diabetic and non-diabetic patients with periodontal disease. *J. Periodont.* 42, 406–411.

FRIEDMAN, L. A. (1972) Horizontal tooth mobility and the menstrual cycle. *J. periodont. Res.* 7, 125–130.

GAGNON, T., SCHOUR, I. & PATRAS, M. C. (1942) Effect of magnesium deficiency on dentine apposition and eruption in the incisor of rat. *Proc. Soc. exp. Biol.* 49, 662–666.

GARN, S. M., LEWIS, A. B. & BLIZZARD, R. M. (1965) Endocrine factors in dental development. *J. dent. Res.* 44 (suppl.), 243–258.

GARN, S. M., LEWIS, A. B., KOSKI, K. & POLACHEK, D. L. (1958) The sex difference in tooth calcification *J. dent. Res.* 37, 561–567.

GARREN, L. & GREEP, R. O. (1955) Effects of thyroid hormone and propylthiouracil on eruption rate of upper incisor teeth in rats. *Proc. Soc. exp. Biol.* 90, 652–655.

GARREN, L. & GREEP, R. O. (1960) Effect of adrenal cortical hormones on eruption rate of incisor teeth in the rat. *Endocrinology* 66, 625–628.

GLAVIND, L., LUND, B. & LÖE, H. (1968) The relationship between periodontal state and diabetes duration, insulin dosage and retinal changes. *J. Periodont.* 39, 341–343.

GLICKMAN, I. & DINES, M. M. (1963) Effect of increased ascorbic acid blood levels on the ascorbic acid level in treated and non-treated gingiva. *J. dent. Res.* 42, 1152–1158.

GLICKMAN, I. & PRUZANSKY, S. (1947) Propyl-thiouracil-hypothyroidism in the albino rat – its effect on the jaws. *J. dent. Res.* 26, 471 (abs.).

GLICKMAN, I., & QUINTARELLI, J. (1960) Low oestrogen levels due to oöphorectomy in rats. *J. Periodont.* 31, 31–37.

GLICKMAN, I. & SHKLAR, G. (1954) Modification of the effect of cortisone upon alveolar bone by the systemic administration of estrogen. *J. Periodont.* 25, 231–239.

GLICKMAN, I. & SHKLAR, G. (1955) The steroid hormones and tissues of the periodontium. A series of related experiments in white mice. *Oral Surg.* 8, 1179–1191.

GLICKMAN, I., SMULOW, J. B. & MOREAU, J. (1966) Effect of alloxan diabetes upon the periodontal response to excessive occlusal forces. *J. Periodont.* 37, 146–155.

GLICKMAN, I., SMULOW, J. B. & MOREAU, J. (1967) Postsurgical periodontal healing in alloxan diabetes. *J. Periodont.* 38, 93–99.

GLICKMAN, I. & STOLLER, M. (1948) The periodontal tissues of the albino rat in vitamin A deficiency. *J. dent. Res.* 27, 758 (abs.).

GLICKMAN, I., STONE, I. C. & CHAWLA, T. N. (1953) The effect of the systemic administration of cortisone upon the periodontium of white mice. *J. Periodont.* 24, 161–166.

GOLDMAN, H. M. (1943) Experimental hyperthyroidism in guinea pigs. *Amer. J. Orthodont. oral Surg.* 29, 665–681.

GOLDMAN, H. M. (1954) The effects of dietary protein deprivation and of age on the periodontal tissues of the rat and spider monkey. *J. Periodont.* 25, 87–96.

GREGORY, H., HOLMES, J. E. & WILLSHIRE, I. R. (1979) Urogastrone-epidermal growth factor. In: *Methods in hormone radioimmunoassay,* B. M. JAFFE & H. R. BEHRMAN (eds.), pp. 927–941. London, Academic Press.

GREGORY, H., WALSH, S. & HOPKINS, C. R. (1979) The identification of urogastrone in serum, saliva and gastric juice. *Gastroenterology* 77, 313–318.

HALL, J. F. & ROBINSON, H. B. G. (1937) Alveolar atrophy in anemic dogs. *J. dent. Res.* 16, 345–346 (abs.).

HATT, S. D., LYLE-STEWART, W. & CRESSWELL, E. (1968) Periodontal disease in sheep. *Dent. Practit.* 19, 123–127.

HAYES, K. C., McCOMBS, H. C. & FAHERTY, T. P. (1970) The fine structure of vitamin A deficiency. I. Parotid duct metaplasia. *Lab. Invest.* 22, 81–89.

HEATON, K. W. (1973) Are we getting too much out of food? *Nutrition* 27, 170–183.

HERZBERG, F. & SCHOUR, I. (1941) Effects of thyroxine on rate of eruption and dentine apposition. *J. dent. Res.* 20, 276 (abs.).

HILMING, F. (1952) Gingivitis gravidarum. *Oral Surg.* 5, 734–751.

HOLLOWAY, P. J., JAMES, P. M. C. & SLACK, G. L. (1963)

Dental disease in Tristan da Cunha. *Br. dent. J.* 115, 19–25.

HOVE, K. A. & STALLARD, R. E. (1970) Diabetes and the periodontal patient. *J. Periodont.* 41, 713–758.

HUGOSON, A. (1971) Gingivitis in pregnant women. A longitudinal clinical study. *Odont. Revy* 22, 65–84.

HUNT, A. M. & PAYNTER, K. J. (1959) The effects of ascorbic acid deficiency on the teeth and periodontal tissues of guinea pigs. *J. dent. Res.* 38, 232–243.

IRVING, J. T. (1942) Enamel organ of the rat's incisor tooth in vitamin E deficiency. *Nature* 150, 122–123.

KAUFMAN, A. Y. (1969) An oral contraceptive as an etiologic factor in producing hyperplastic gingivitis and a neoplasm of the pregnancy tumour type. *Oral Surg.* 28, 666–670.

KEENE, J. J. (1969a) Observations of small blood vessels in human nondiabetic and diabetic gingiva. *J. dent. Res.* 48, 967.

KEENE, J. J. (1969b) A histochemical evaluation for small vessel calcification in human nondiabetic and diabetic gingival biopsy specimens. *J. dent. Res.* 48, 968.

KEENE, J. J. (1972) An alternation in human diabetic arterioles. *J. dent. Res.* 51, 569–572.

KEYES, P. H. & LITKINS, R. C. (1946) Plaque formation, periodontal disease, and dental caries in Syrian hamsters. *J. dent. Res.* 25, 166 (abs.).

KLATSKY, M. & KLATELL, J. S. (1943) Anthropological studies in dental caries. *J. dent. Res.* 22, 267–274.

KLEIN, H., ORENT, E. R. & McCALLUM, E. V. (1935) The effect of magnesium deficiency on the teeth and their supporting structures in rats. *Amer. J. Physiol.* 112, 256–262.

KLINGER, G. & KLINGER, G. (1970) Untersuchungen über den Einfluss oraler Kontrazeptiva auf die Mund- und Vaginalschleimhaut. *Dtsch. Stomat.* 20, 664–669.

KLINGSBERG, J. & BUTCHER, E. O. (1959) Aging, diet, and periodontal lesions in the hamster. *J. dent. Res.* 38, 421.

KNIGHT, G. M. & WADE, A. B. (1974) The effects of hormonal contraceptives on the human periodontium. *J. periodont. Res.* 9, 18–22.

KÖRBER, K. H. (1961) Elektronisches Messen der Zahnbeweglichkeit. *Dtsch. Zahnärztebl.* 16, 605–613.

KOFOED, J. A. & BOZZINI, C. E. (1970) The effect of hydrocortisone on the concentration and synthesis of acid mucopolysaccharides in the rat gingiva. *J. periodont. Res.* 5, 259–262.

KUSNER, W., MICHAELI, Y., & WEINREB, M. M. (1973) Role of attrition and occlusal contact in the physiology of the rat incisor. VI. Impeded and unimpeded eruption in hypophysectomized and magnesium-deficient rats. *J. dent. Res.* 52, 65–73.

LABELLE, R. E. & SCHAFFER, E. M. (1966) The effects of cortisone and induced local factors on the periodontium of the albino rat. *J. Periodont.* 37, 483–490.

LAINSON, P. A., BRADY, P. P. & FRALEIGH, C. M. (1968) Anaemia, a systemic cause of periodontal disease? *J. Periodont.* 39, 35–38.

LAVELLE, C. L. B. (1973) Alveolar bone loss and tooth attrition in skulls from different population samples. *J. periodont. Res.* 8, 395–399.

LEVY, B. M. (1949) Effects of pantothenic acid deficiency on the mandibular joints and periodontal structures of mice. *J. Amer. dent. Assoc.* 38, 215–223.

LINDHE, J., BIRCH, J. & BRANEMARK, P. I. (1968) Vascular proliferation in pseudopregnant rabbits. *J. periodont. Res.* 3, 12–20.

LINDHE, J. & BJORN, A. L. (1967) Influence of hormonal contraceptives on the gingiva of women. *J. periodont. Res.* 2, 1–6.

LINDHE, J. & BRANEMARK, P. I. (1967a) The effect of sex hormones on vascularisation of a granulation tissue. *J. periodont. Res.* 3, 6–11.

LINDHE, J. & BRANEMARK, P. I. (1967b) Changes in microcirculation after local application of sex hormones. *J. periodont. Res.* 2, 185–193.

LINDHE, J. & BRANEMARK, P. I. (1967c) Changes in vascular permeability after local application of sex hormones. *J. periodont. Res.* 2, 259–265.

LINDHE, J., BRANEMARK, P. I., & BIRCH, J. (1968) Microvascular events in cheek pouch wounds of oöphorectomised hamsters following intramuscular injections of female sex hormones. *J. periodont. Res.* 3, 21–23.

LIPARI, W. A., BLAKE, L. C. & ZIPKIN, I. (1974) Preferential response of the periodontal apparatus and the epiphyseal plate to hydrocortisone and fluoride in the rat. *J. Periodont.* 45, 879–890.

LISTGARTEN, M. A., RICKER, F. H., LASTER, L., SHAPIRO, J. & COHEN, D. W. (1974) Vascular basement lamina thickness in the normal and inflamed gingiva of diabetics and non-diabetics. *J. Periodont.* 45, 676–684.

LITVIN, P. E. & DE MARCO, T. J. (1973) The effect of a diuretic and antidiuretic on tooth eruption. *Oral Surg.* 35, 294–298.

LÖE, H. (1965) Periodontal changes in pregnancy. *J. Periodont.* 36, 209–217.

LÖE, H. & SILNESS, J. (1963) Periodontal disease in pregnancy. *Acta odont. Scand.* 21, 533–551.

LOVESTEDT, S. A. & AUSTIN, L. T. (1943) Periodontoclasia in diabetes mellitus. *J. Amer. dent. Assoc.* 30, 273–275.

LYNN, B. P. (1967) 'The Pill' as an etiological agent in hypertrophic gingivitis. *Oral Surg.* 24, 333–334.

MACKENZIE, R. S. & MILLARD, H. D. (1963) Interrelated effects of diabetes, arteriosclerosis and calculus on alveolar bone loss. *J. Amer. dent. Assoc.* 66, 191–198.

MAIER, A. W. & ORBAN, B. (1949) Gingivitis in pregnancy. *Oral Surg.* 2, 334–373.

MASSLER, M., SCHOUR, I. & CHOPRA, B. (1950) Occurrence of gingivitis in suburban Chicago school children. *J. Periodont.* 21, 146–164.

MELLANBY, H. (1941) The effect of maternal dietary deficiency of vitamin A on dental tissues in rats. *J. dent. Res.* 20, 489–509.

MELLANBY, M. (1929) Diet and the teeth. Part I. Dental structure in dogs. *Spec. Rep. Ser. Med. Res. Coun. Lond.* No. 140.

MIGLANI, D. C. (1959) The effect of vitamin A deficiency on the periodontal structures of rat molars with emphasis on cementum resorption. *Oral Surg.* 12, 1372–1386.

MILLER, S. C., STAHL, S. S. & GOLDSMITH, E. D. (1957) The effects of vertical occlusal trauma on the periodontium of protein-deprived young adult rats. *J. Periodont.* 28, 87–97.

MOHAMMED, A. H., WATERHOUSE, J. P. & FRIEDERICI,

H. H. R. (1974) The microvasculature of the rabbit gingiva as affected by progesterone: an ultrastructural study. *J. Periodont.* **45**, 50–60.

MOSKOW, B. S., BADEN, E. & ZENGO, A. (1966) The effects of dihydrotachysterol and ferric dextran upon the periodontium in the rat. *Archs. oral Biol.* **11**, 1017–1026.

MOXHAM, B. J. (1979) The effects of some vaso-active drugs on the eruption of the rabbit mandibular incisor. *Archs. oral Biol.* **24**, 759–763.

MOXHAM, B. J. & BERKOVITZ, B. K. B. (1980) An approach to the investigation of a multifactorial basis for the mechanism of tooth eruption. *J. dent. Res.* **59**, 1840 (abs.).

MOXHAM, B. J. & BERKOVITZ, B. K. B. (in press) A quantitative assessment of the effects of axially directed extrusive loads on displacement of the impeded and unimpeded rabbit mandibular incisor. *Archs. oral Biol.*

MUHLEMANN, H. R. (1951) Periodontometry. A method for measuring tooth mobility. *Oral Surg.* **4**, 1220–1233.

MÜHLEMANN, H. R., SAVDIS, S. & RATEITSCHAK, K. H. (1965) Tooth mobility – its causes and significance. *J. Periodont.* **36**, 148–153.

MURPHY, T. R. (1959) Compensatory mechanisms in facial height adjustment to functional tooth attrition. *Aust. dent. J.* **4**, 312–323.

MURPHY, T. R. (1964) Reduction of the dental arch by approximal attrition, *Br. dent. J.* **116**, 483–488.

MYHRE, L., PREUS, H. R. & AARS, H. (1979) Influences of axial load and blood pressure on the position of the rabbit's incisor tooth. *Acta odont. Scand.* **37**, 153–159.

NESS, A. R. (1964) Movement and forces in tooth eruption. In: *Advances in oral biology*, P. H. STAPLE (ed.), pp. 33–75. London, Academic Press.

NEUBERGER, A. (1955) Stoffwechsel von Kollagen unter normal Bedingungen. *Symp. Soc. exp. Biol.* **9**, 72–84.

NEUBERGER, A., PERRONE, J. C. & SLACK, H. G. (1951) The relative metabolic inertia of tendon collagen in the rat. *Biochem. J.* **49**, 199–204.

NEUBERGER, A. & SLACK, H. G. B. (1953) The metabolism of collagen from liver, bone, skin and tendon in the normal rat. *Biochem. J.* **53**, 47–52.

NEWMAN, H. N. (1974) Diet, attrition, plaque and dental disease. *Br. dent. J.* **136**, 491–497.

NEWMAN, H. N. & LEVERS, B. G. H. (1979) Tooth eruption and function in an early Anglo-Saxon population. *J. R. Soc. Med.* **72**, 341–350.

O'LEARY, T. M., SHANNON, I. L. & PRIGMORE, J. R. (1962) Clinical and systemic findings in periodontal disease. *J. Periodont.* **33**, 243–251.

OLIVER, W. M. (1969) The effect of deficiencies of calcium, vitamin D or calcium and vitamin D and or variations in the source of dietary protein on the supporting tissues of the rat molar. *J. periodont. Res.* **4**, 56–60.

ØSTERGAARD, E. (1975) The collagen content of skin and gingival tissues in ascorbic acid-deficient monkeys. *J. periodont. Res.* **10**, 103–114.

PARFITT, G. J. (1957) A five year longitudinal study of the gingival condition of a group of children in England. *J. Periodont.* **28**, 26–32.

PARMER, L. G., KATONAH, E. & ARGRIST, A. A. (1951) Comparative effects of ACTH, cortisone, corticosterone, deoxycorticosterone, pregnenolone, on growth and development in infant rats. *Proc. Soc. exp. Biol.* **77**, 215–218.

PAYNTER, K. J. (1954) The effect of propylthiouracil on the development of molar teeth in rats. *J. dent. Res.* **33**, 364–376.

PEARLMAN, B. A. (1974) An oral contraceptive drug and gingival enlargement; the relationship between local and systemic factors. *J. clin. Periodont.* **1**, 47–51.

PERLITSCH, M., NIELSEN, A. G. & STANMEYER, W. R. (1961) Ascorbic acid levels and gingival health in personnel wintering over in Antarctica. *J. dent. Res.* **40**, 789–799.

PHILIPPAS, G. G. (1952) Evidence of function on healthy teeth: the evidence of ancient Athenian remains. *J. Amer. dent. Assoc.* **45**, 443–453.

PICTON, D. C. A. (1957) Calculus, wear and alveolar bone loss in the jaws of sixth-century Jutes. *Dent. Practit.* **7**, 301–303.

PINDBORG, J. J. (1949) The effect of methyl folic acid on the periodontal tissues in rat molars (experimental granulocytopenia). *Oral Surg.* **2**, 1485–1496.

PINDBORG, J. J. (1952) Effect of vitamin E deficiency on the rat incisor. *J. dent. Res.* **31**, 805–811.

PINTO, A. C. G. (1974) Effect of hypothyroidism obtained experimentally in the periodontium of rat. *J. Periodont.* **45**, 217–221.

PIROSHAW, N. A. & GLICKMAN, I. (1957) The effect of ovariectomy upon the tissues of the periodontium and skeletal bones. *Oral Surg.* **10**, 133–147.

PLATT, B. S. & STEWART, R. J. C. (1962) Transverse trabecula and osteoporosis in bones in experimental protein-calorie deficiency. *Br. J. Nutr.* **16**, 483–495.

PRIEST, R. E. (1970) Formation of epithelial basement membrane is restricted by scurvy *in vitro* and is stimulated by vitamin C. *Nature* **225**, 744–745.

PROUT, R. E. S. & TRING, F. C. (1971) Effect of fat-free diet on ameloblast and enamel formation in incisors of rats. *J. dent. Res.* **50**, 1559–1561.

PROUT, R. E. S. & TRING, F. C. (1973) Dentinogenesis in incisors of rats deficient in essential fatty acids. *J. dent. Res.* **52**, 462–467.

RAO, L. G., MOE, H. K. & HEERSCHE, J. N. M. (1978) *In vitro* culture of porcine periodontal ligament cells: response of fibroblast-like and epithelial-like cells to prostaglandin E_1, parathyroid hormone and calcitonin and separation of a pure population of fibroblast-like cells. *Archs. oral Biol.* **23**, 957–964.

RAO, S. S., SHOURIE, K. L. & SHARKWALLER, G. B. (1965) Effect of dietary fat variations on the periodontium. *Periodontics* **3**, 66–76.

RATCLIFF, P. A. & ITÔKAZU, H. (1964) The effect of dihydrotachysterol and ferric dextran on the teeth and periodontium of the rat. *J. oral Therap. Pharmacol.* **1**, 7–22.

RATCLIFF, P. A. & KRAJEWSKI, J. (1966) The influence of methyl testosterone on dihydrotachysterol intoxication as it affects the periodontium. *J. oral Therap. Pharmacol.* **2**, 353–361.

RATEITSCHAK, K. H. (1967) Tooth mobility changes in pregnancy. *J. periodont. Res.* **2**, 199–206.

REEVE, C. M. & WINKELMANN, R. K. (1962) Glycogen

storage in gingival epithelium of diabetic and non-diabetic patients. *J. dent. Res.* **40**, 31 (abs.).

RESTARSKI, J. S. & PIJOUN, M. (1944) Gingivitis and vitamin C. *J. Amer. dent. Assoc.* **31**, 13–23.

RINGELBERG, M. L., DIXON, D. O., FRANCIS, A. D. & PLUMMER, R. W. (1977) Comparison of gingival health and gingival crevicular fluid flow in children with and without diabetes. *J. dent. Res.* **56**, 108–111.

ROBERTS, W. E. (1975) Cell kinetic nature and diurnal periodicity of the rat periodontal ligament. *Archs. oral Biol.* **20**, 465–471.

ROBERTSON, J. (1972) Changes in the fibre of the British diet. *Nature* **238**, 290–292.

ROSENBERG, M. M., GOLDMAN, H. M. & GARBER, E. (1961) Effects of experimental thyrotoxicosis and myxoedema on the periodontium of rabbits. *J. dent. Res.* **40**, 708–709 (abs.).

ROWNTREE, L. G., CLARK, J. H. & HANSON, A. M. (1934) The biologic effects of thymus extract (Hanson). *J. Amer. Med. Assoc.* **103**, 1425–1430.

RUBRIGHT, W. C., HIGA, L. H. & YANNONE, M. E. (1971) Histological quantification of the biological effects of estradiol benzoate on the gingiva and genital mucosa of castrated rabbits. *J. periodont. Res.* **6**, 55–64.

RUBRIGHT, W. C., TERMON, S. A. & YANNONE, M. E. (1973) A comparative study of an *in vitro* ^{3}H-17β-estradiol binding in gingiva skeletal muscle and uterus of ovariectomised rabbits. *J. periodont. Res.* **8**, 304–313.

RUGG-GUNN, A. J. (1968) Caries resistance in the Kuria Muria Islands. Report of a dental health survey. *Br. dent. J.* **124**, 75–77.

RUSHTON, M. A. (1941) Cases of accelerated and retarded dentition. *Br. dent. J.* **71**, 277–279.

RUSSELL, B. G. (1966) Gingival changes in diabetes mellitus. *Acta Pathol. Microbiol. Scand.* **68**, 161–168.

RUSSELL, B. G. (1967) The dental pulp in diabetes mellitus. *Acta Pathol. Microbiol. Scand.* **70**, 319–320.

RUTLEDGE, C. E. (1940) Oral and roentgenographic aspects of teeth and jaws of juvenile diabetics. *J. Amer. dent. Assoc.* **27**, 1740–1750.

SALLEY, J. J., BRYSON, W. F. & ESHLEMAN, J. R. (1959) The effect of chronic vitamin A deficiency on dental caries in the Syrian hamster. *J. dent. Res.* **38**, 1038–1043.

SALLUM, A. W., DO NASCIMENTO, A., BOZZO, L. & DE TOLEDO, S. (1976) The effect of dexamethasone in traumatic changes of the periodontium of marmosets (*Callithrix jacchus*). *J. Periodont.* **47**, 63–66.

SARNÅS, K. V. (1957) Growth changes in skulls of ancient man in North America. An X-ray cephalometric investigation of some cranial and facial changes during growth in the Indian knoll skeletons. *Acta odont. Scand.* **15**, 213–271.

SCHNEIDER, H. G. (1967) Veränderungen am Parodont der Ratte nach Ovarektomie. Der Einfluss der Kastration auf das Epithel der Gingiva propria. *Parodontologie Acad. Rev.* **1**, 106–114.

SCHNEIDER, H. G. & POSE, G. (1969) Influence of tocopherol on the periodontium of molars in rats fed a diet lacking in vitamin E. *Archs. oral Biol.* **14**, 431–433.

SCHOUR, I. (1934) The effects of hypophysectomy on the periodontal tissues. *J. Periodont.* **5**, 15–24.

SCHOUR, I. (1936) Changes in the incisor of the 13-lined ground squirrel (*Citellus tridecemlineatus*) following bilateral gonadectomy. *Anat. Rec.* **65**, 177–199.

SCHOUR, I., CHANDLER, S. B. & TWEEDY, W. R. (1937) Changes in teeth following parathyroidectomy. *Amer. J. Pathol.* **13**, 945–970.

SCHOUR, I., HOFFMAN, M. M. & SMITH, M. C. (1941) Changes in incisor teeth of albino rats with vitamin A deficiency and effects of replacement therapy. *Amer. J. Pathol.* **17**, 529–533.

SCHOUR, I. & MASSLER, M. (1943) Endocrines and dentistry. *J. Amer. dent. Assoc.* **30**, 595–603, 763–773 and 943–950.

SCHOUR, I. & VAN DYKE, H. B. (1931) Histologic changes in the rat incisor following hypophysectomy. *J. dent. Res.* **11**, 873–875.

SCHOUR, I. & VAN DYKE, H. B. (1932a) Changes in the teeth following hypophysectomy. I. Changes in the incisor of the white rat. *Amer. J. Anat.* **50**, 397–433.

SCHOUR, I. & VAN DYKE, H. B. (1932b) Effect of replacement therapy on eruption of the incisor of the hypophysectomized rat. *Proc. Soc. exp. Biol. Med.* **29**, 378–382.

SCHOUR, I. & VAN DYKE, H. B. (1934) Changes in teeth following hypophysectomy. II. Changes in the molar of the white rat. *J. dent. Res.* **14**, 69–91.

SCHUMER, S. & WELLS, H. (1958) Effect of thyroxine and triiodothyroacetic acid on incisor eruption rate. *J. dent. Res.* **37**, 980 (abs.).

SHANNON, I. L. & GIBSON, W. A. (1964) Oral glucose tolerance responses in healthy young adult males classified as to caries experience and periodontal status. *Periodontics* **2**, 292–297.

SHAPIRO, S. & SHKLAR, G. (1962) The effect of hypophysectomy on the periodontium of the albino rat. *J. Periodont.* **33**, 364–371.

SHAW, J. H. (1962) The relation of nutrition to periodontal disease. *J. dent. Res.* **41**, 264–274.

SHEEHAN, R. & COHEN, M. (1970) The periodontium of diabetic mice. *J. dent. Res.* **49**, 111 (abs.).

SHKLAR, G. (1965) The effect of adrenalectomy and cortisone replacement on the periodontium of the rat. *Periodontics* **3**, 239–242.

SHKLAR, G., CHAUNCEY, H. H. & SHAPIRO, S. (1967) The effect of testosterone on the periodontium of normal and hypophysectomized rats. *J. Periodont.* **38**, 203–210.

SHKLAR, G., COHEN, M. M. & YERGANIAN, G. (1962) A histopathologic study of periodontal disease in the Chinese hamster with hereditary diabetes. *J. Periodont.* **33**, 14–21.

SHKLAR, G. & GLICKMAN, I. (1956) The effect of oestrogenic hormone on the periodontium of white mice. *J. Periodont.* **27**, 16–23.

SIM WALLACE, J. (1904) Physical deterioration in relation to the teeth. *Br. dent. J.* **25**, 861–867.

SINGER, J., FURSTMAN, L. & BERNICK, S. (1967) A histologic study of the effect of fluoride on tooth movement in the rat. *Amer. J. Orthodont.* **53**, 296–308.

SLATTER, J. M. & PICTON, D. C. A. (1972) The effect on intrusive tooth mobility of noradrenaline injected locally in monkeys (*Macaca irus*). *J. periodont. Res.* **7**, 144–150.

SMITH, M. C. (1934) Effects of fluorine upon rate of eruption of rat incisors and its correlation with bone development and body growth. *J. dent. Res.* **14,** 139–144.

SODEK, J. (1978) A comparison of collagen and non-collagenous protein metabolism in rat molar and incisor periodontal ligament. *Archs. oral Biol.* **23,** 977–982.

SOUTHGATE, D. A. T. (1973) Dietary fibre. *Plant foods for man,* **1,** 45–47.

SPERBER, G. H. (1969) Oral contraceptive hypertrophic gingivitis. *J. dent. Assoc. S. Afr.* **24,** 37–40.

STAHL, S. S. (1962) The effect of a protein free diet on the healing of gingival wounds in rats. *Archs. oral Biol.* **7,** 551–556.

STAHL, S. S. (1963a) Healing of gingival wounds in female rats fed a low-protein diet. *J. dent. Res.* **42,** 1511–1516.

STAHL, S. S. (1963b) Soft tissue healing following experimental gingival wounding in female rats of various ages. *Periodontics* **1,** 142–146.

STAHL, S. S. & GERSTNER, R. (1960) The response of the oral mucosa and periodontium to simultaneous administration of cortisone and somatotropic hormone in young adult male rats. *Archs. oral Biol.* **1,** 321–324.

STAHL, S. S. & JOLY, O. (1958) Response of periodontal tissues to intraoral injections of somatotropic hormone in young adult male rats. *Oral Surg.* **11,** 475–483.

STAHL, S. S., MILLER, S. C. & GOLDSMITH, E. D. (1957) The effects of vertical occlusal trauma on the periodontium of protein-deprived young adult rats. *J. Periodont.* **28,** 87–97.

STAHL, S. S., MILLER, S. C. & GOLDSMITH, E. D. (1958) Effects of protein deprivation on the periodontium of young adult male hamsters. *J. dent. Res.* **37,** 984 (abs.).

STAHL, S. S., SANDLER, H. C. & CAHN, L. (1955) The effects of protein deprivation upon the oral tissues of the rat and particularly upon periodontal structures under irritation. *Oral Surg.* **8,** 760–768.

STAHL, S. S., WEINMANN, J. P., SCHOUR, I. & BRADY, A. M. (1950) The effect of estrogen on the alveolar bone and teeth of mice and rats. *Anat. Rec.* **107,** 21–41.

STEIN, G. & ZISKIN, D. E. (1949) The effect of a protein free diet on the teeth and periodontium of the albino rat. *J. dent. Res.* **28,** 529 (abs.).

STUHL, F. (1943) Vitamin C subnutrition in gingivo-stomatitis. *Lancet* **1,** 640–642.

SUTCLIFFE, P. (1972) A longitudinal study of gingivitis and puberty. *J. periodont. Res.* **7,** 52–58.

TAIT, R. V. (1965) Tooth grinding in preventive dentistry. *Dental magazine and oral topics* **82,** 119–121.

TAYLOR, R. M. S. (1962) Non-metrical studies of the human palate and dentition in Morori and Maori skulls. *J. Polynes. Soc.* **71,** 167–187.

TAYLOR, R. M. S. (1963) Cause and effect of wear of teeth. Further non-metrical studies of the teeth and palate in Moriori and Maori skulls. *Acta Anat.* **53,** 97–157.

TEN CATE, A. R., DEPORTER, D. A. & FREEMAN, E. (1976) The role of fibroblasts in the remodeling of periodontal ligament during physiologic tooth move-ment. *Amer. J. Orthod.* **69,** 155–168.

THOMPSON, J. L. & KENDRICK, G. S. (1964) Changes in the vertical dimensions of the human male skull during the third and fourth decades of life. *Anat. Rec.* **150,** 209–213.

TOMLINSON, T. H. (1939) Oral pathology in monkeys in various experimental dietary deficiencies. *U.S. Publ. Hlth Rep.* **54,** 1, 431–439.

TOPPING, N. H. & FRASER, H. F. (1939) Mouth lesions associated with dietary deficiencies in monkeys. *U.S. Publ. Hlth Rep.* **54,** 416–431.

TROWELL, H. (1973) Dietary fibre, coronary heart disease and diabetes mellitus. I. Historical aspects of fibre in the food of western man. *Plant foods for man* **1,** 11–16.

TURESKY, S. & GLICKMAN, I. (1954) Histochemical evaluation of gingival healing in experimental animals on adequate and vitamin C deficient rats. *J. dent. Res.* **33,** 273–280.

ULRICH, K. (1962) Über Vorkommen und Ursachen von Parodontopathien bei jugendlichen Diabetes mellitus. *Dtsch. zahnärztl. Zeit.* **17,** 221–225.

VAN WAGENEN, G. & HURME, V. C. (1950) Effects of testosterone propionate on permanent canine tooth eruption in the monkey (*Macaca mulatta*). *Proc. Soc. exp. Biol.* **73,** 296–301.

WAERHAUG, J. (1960) The role of ascorbic acid in periodontal tissue. *J. dent. Res.* **39,** 1089 (abs.).

WAUGH, D. B. (1940) On the biting strength of Alaskan Eskimos. *J. dent. Res.* **19,** 324–325 (abs.).

WAUGH, L. M. (1937) Dental observations among Eskimo. VII: Survey of mouth conditions, nutritional study, and gnathodynamometer data in most primitive and populous native village in Alaska. *J. dent. Res.* **16,** 355–356 (abs.).

WEINMANN, J. P. & SCHOUR, I. (1945a) Experimental studies in calcification. I. The effect of a rachitogenic diet on the dental tissues of the white rat. *Amer. J. Pathol.* **21,** 821–831.

WEINMANN, J. P. & SCHOUR, I. (1945b) Experimental studies in calcification. II. The effect of a rachitogenic diet on the alveolar bone of the white rat. *Amer. J. Pathol.* **21,** 833–855.

WILLIAMS, J. B. (1928) Diabetic periodontoclasia. *J. Amer. dent. Assoc.* **15,** 523–529.

WILLS, D. J., PICTON, D. C. A. & DAVIES, W. I. R. (1976) A study of the fluid systems of the periodontium in macaque monkeys. *Archs. oral Biol.* **21,** 175–185.

WOLBACH, S. B. (1953) Experimental scurvy: its employment for the study of intercellular substances. *Proc. Nutr. Soc.* **12,** 247–255.

WOLBACH, S. B. & BESSEY, O. A. (1942) Tissue changes in vitamin deficiencies. *Physiol. Rev.* **22,** 233–289.

WOLBACH, S. B. & HOWE, P. R. (1933) The incisor teeth of albino rats and guinea pigs in vitamin A deficiency and repair. *Amer. J. Path.* **9,** 275–279.

WOLBACH, S. B. & HOWE, P. R. (1926) Intracellular substance in experimental scorbutus. *Arch. Path.* **1,** 1–24.

ZIPKIN, I., BERNICK, S. & MENCZEL, J. (1965) A morphological study of the effect of fluoride on the periodontium of the hydrocortisone-treated rat. *Periodontics* **3,** 111–114.

ZISKIN, D. E. & NESSE, G. J. (1946) Pregnancy gingivitis.

Amer. J. Orthodont. oral Surg. **32**, 390–432.

ZISKIN, D. E., SALMON, T. N. & APPLEBAUM, R. (1940) The effect of thyro-parathyroidectomy at birth and at 7 days on dental and skeletal development of rats. *J. dent. Res.* **19**, 93–102.

ZISKIN, D. E., STEIN, G., GROSS, P. & RUNNE, E. (1947) Oral, gingival and periodontal pathology induced in rats on a low pantothenic acid diet by toxic doses of zinc carbonate. *Amer. J. Orthodont. oral Surg.* **33**, 407–446.

INDEX

Numbers *in italics* refer to information in figures